Infectious Diseases

A Clinical Short Course

Notice

Medicine is an ever-changing science. As new research and clinical experience broaden our Despite dire warnings that we are approaching the end of the antibiotic era, the incidence of antibiotic-resistant bacteria continues to rise. The proportions of penicillin-resistant Streptococcus pneumoniae, hospital-acquired methicillin-resistant Staphylococcus aureus (MRSA), and vancomycin-resistant Enterococcus (VRE) strains continue to increase. Community-acquired MRSA (cMRSA) is now common throughout the world. Multiresistant Acinetobacter and Pseudomonas are everyday realities in many of our hospitals. The press is now warning the lay public of the existence of "dirty hospitals." As never before, it is critical that health care providers understand the principles of proper anti-infective therapy and use anti-infective agents judiciously. These agents need to be reserved for treatable infections-not used to calm the patient or the patient's family. Too often, patients with viral infections that do not warrant anti-infective therapy arrive at the physician's office expecting to be treated with an antibiotic. And health care workers too often prescribe antibiotics to fulfill those expectations. Physicians unschooled in the principles of microbiology utilize anti-infective agents just as they would more conventional medications, such as anti-inflammatory agents, anti-hypertensive medications, and cardiac drugs. They use one or two broad-spectrum antibiotics to treat all patients with. They use one or two broad-spectrum antibiotics to treat all patients with.

Infectious Diseases

A Clinical Short Course

Second Edition

FREDERICK S. SOUTHWICK, M.D.

Professor of Medicine
Chief of Infectious Diseases
Vice Chairman of Medicine
University of Florida College of Medicine
Gainesville, Florida

McGraw-Hill

Medical Publishing Divison

New York   ncago   San Fracisco   Lisbon   London   Madrid   Mexico City   Milan
New Delhi   San Juan   Seoul   Singapore   Sydney   Toronto

Infectious Diseases: A Clinical Short Course, Second Edition

Copyright © 2008 by The McGraw-Hill Companies, Inc. All rights reserved. Printed in the United States of America. Except as permitted under the United States Copyright Act of 1976, no part of this publication may be reproduced or distributed in any form or by any means, or stored in a data base or retrieval system, without the prior written permission of the publisher.

Previous edition copyright © 2004 by The McGraw-Hill Companies, Inc.

1 2 3 4 5 6 7 8 9 0   FGR/FGR   0 9 8 7

ISBN: 978-0-07-1477222
MHID: 0-07-1477225

**WC
100
S728i
2008**

This book was set in AGaramond by Aptara, Inc.
The editors were James Shanahan and Regina Y. Brown
The production supervisor was Sherri Souffarance
Project Management was provided by Aptara Inc.

Quebecor Fairfield was printer and binder

This book is printed on acid-free paper.

Library of Congress Cataloging-in-Publication Data

Catalog-in-Publication data is on file for this title
at the Library of Congress.

International Edition ISBN-13: 978-0-07-128725-8; ISBN-10: 0-07-128725-6
Copyright © 2007. Exclusive rights by the McGraw-Hill Companies, Inc., for manufacture and export. This book cannot be re-exported from the country to which it is consigned by McGraw-Hill. The International Edition is not available in North America.

Dedication

To my mother and father, Ann and Wayne Southwick, and to my beautiful wife, Kathie Southwick for all their loving encouragement

Contents

Color insert appears between pages 418 and 419.

Contributors   ix
Preface   xi
Acknowledgments   xiii

1   ANTI-INFECTIVE THERAPY   1

2   THE SEPSIS SYNDROME   57

3   THE FEBRILE PATIENT   66

4   PULMONARY INFECTIONS   79

5   EYE, EAR, NOSE, AND THROAT INFECTIONS   120

6   CENTRAL NERVOUS SYSTEM INFECTIONS   139

7   CARDIOVASCULAR INFECTIONS   167

8   GASTROINTESTINAL AND HEPATOBILIARY INFECTIONS   190

9   GENITOURINARY TRACT INFECTIONS AND SEXUALLY TRANSMITTED DISEASES (STDs)   231

10   SKIN AND SOFT TISSUE INFECTIONS   256

11   OSTEOMYELITIS, PROSTHETIC JOINT INFECTIONS, DIABETIC FOOT INFECTIONS, AND SEPTIC ARTHRITIS   273

12   PARASITIC INFECTIONS   288

13   ZOONOTIC INFECTIONS   322

14   BIOTERRORISM   349

15   SERIOUS VIRAL ILLNESSES IN THE ADULT PATIENT   365

16   INFECTIONS IN THE IMMUNOCOMPROMISED HOST   384

17   HIV INFECTION   396

Index   434

Contributors

Bernard Hirschel, M.D.
Professor of Medicine
Division of Infectious Diseases
University of Geneva
Geneva, Switzerland

P. Daniel Lew, M.D.
Professor of Medicine and Chief
  of Infectious Diseases
University of Geneva
Geneva, Switzerland

Reuben Ramphal, M.D.
Professor of Medicine
Division of Infectious Diseases
University of Florida College
  of Medicine
Gainesville, Florida

Frederick S. Southwick, M.D.
Professor of Medicine
Chief of Infectious Diseases
Vice Chairman of Medicine
University of Florida College
  of Medicine
Gainesville, Florida

Sankar Swaminathan, M.D.
Associate Professor of Medicine
Division of Infectious Diseases
University of Florida College
  of Medicine
Gainesville, Florida

Preface

THE END OF THE ANTIBIOTIC ERA?

Time and *Newsweek* magazines have heralded the "End of the Antibiotic Era". Echoing the concerns of many infectious disease and health policy experts, *The Chicago Tribune*'s feature on "Unhealthy Hospitals" warns that the "overuse of antibiotics are spawning drug-resistant germs that are spreading from hospitals into the community at unprecedented rates". Vancomycin resistant enterococcus (VRE), methicillin-resistant *Staphylococcus aureus* (MRSA) are now commonly found in our hospitalized patients and a new highly virulent community-acquired methicillin resistant *Staphylococcus aureus* (cMRSA) is infecting high school and college athletes. Extensively drug-resistant tuberculosis (XDR-TB) has resulted in near 100% mortality in an outbreak in South Africa. Newly discovered infectious diseases such as SARS, Avian Influenza, Ehrlichia, Lyme Disease, and West Nile Encephalitis are emerging as threats to our well-being. Malaria remains a leading cause of death in many parts of the world. The 2001 bioterrorist attack launched by mailing anthrax spores illustrates the critical need for all health providers to recognize the manifestations of this nearly forgotten pathogen and others that can be used as weapons of mass destruction. The AIDS epidemic continues to devastate sub-Saharan Africa, and is spreading at an alarming rate in Asia and the former Soviet Union. HIV strains resistant to antiretroviral therapy are increasing throughout the United States and Europe. Diseases long believed to have non-infectious etiologies are now confirmed as having microbial origins. Infectious diseases have re-emerged as one of the world's top healthcare priorities, and to meet the needs of the 21st Century, health care providers must possess a solid grounding in clinical infectious diseases.

FEATURES OF THE SECOND EDITION

This is the second edition of a textbook envisioned as a 30-day tutorial designed to provide a solid grounding in the principles of clinical infectious diseases. The title has been changed from *infectious Diseases in 30 Days* to *Infectious Diseases: A Clinical Short Course;* however the design and intention of our book has not changed. As our title emphasizes we have created a concise overview of this important field that will allow the busy physician, medical student, nurse practioner, and physician assistant to understand, diagnose and treat common infectious diseases.

Mastering the field of infectious diseases seems daunting, and many textbooks in the field are over a thousand pages in length. Our goal has been to make this task easier and more enjoyable. By indicating the number of days that should be allotted to the study of each chapter, we have a created a schedule for completion of each lesson. By taking one small step at a time, a seemingly difficult task can be more readily achieved. The book has been shortened to make completion within 30 days feasible. This has been made possible by creating a wide array of tables that summarize the methods of clinical assessment, anti-infective agent doses, and drug toxicities; facts that do not require memorization, but do need to be referred to when caring for patients.

Chapters are organized by organ system when possible, because this is how clinicians encounter infectious diseases. As in the last edition, guiding questions begin each chapter to encourage the reader to actively inquire as he or she reads the text. The potential severity of each disease is assessed to give the inexperienced clinician a sense of the speed with which care must be initiated. Key points are included in shaded areas to emphasize the most important facts the clinician should know when managing each infection. When possible simple diagrams summarize management approaches, as well as principles of pathogenesis. All chapters have been updated to reflect the current treatment and diagnostic guidelines of the Infectious Disease Society of America (IDSA) and up-to-date references have been included at the end of each chapter. Our goal is to improve healthcare providers understanding of infectious diseases and provide them with the latest approaches managing infections. It is our firm belief that only through a concerted educational campaign to teach the principles of infectious diseases and the judiciously use anti-infective agents we can help to prevent the "End of the Antibiotic Era".

Acknowledgments

I wish to thank Dr. Morton Swartz who first inspired my love for Infectious Diseases. I will always be grateful to Drs. James McGuigan, and Tom Stossel for serving as my mentors throughout my career. Thank you to my contributors, Drs. P. Daniel Lew, Reuben Ramphal, Sankar Swaminathan, and Bernard Hirschel for their prompt and well written submissions. Dr. Hirschel and I want to acknowledge the assistance of Drs. Markus Flepp, Véronique Schiffer, and Rainer Weber with sections of Chapter 17. I also want to thank the many medical students at the University of Florida who provided helpful feedback on the first edition. Their input has guided many of the improvements in the second edition.

A special thanks to James Shanahan of McGraw-Hill who has been my sounding board throughout the writing process, and was instrumental making the second edition a Lange series publication. Finally, I wish to acknowledge the excellent artwork of Roger Hoover.

Anti-Infective Therapy

Time Recommended to complete: 3 days

Frederick Southwick, M.D.

GUIDING QUESTIONS

1. Are we at the end of the antibiotic era?

2. Why are "superbugs" suddenly appearing in our hospitals?

3. How do bacteria become resistant to antibiotics?

4. How can the continued selection of highly resistant organisms be prevented?

5. Is antibiotic treatment always the wisest course of action?

6. Does one antibiotic cure all infections?

7. What are the strategies that underlie optimal antibiotic usage?

8. How is colonization distinguished from infection, and why is this distinction important?

Despite dire warnings that we are approaching the end of the antibiotic era, the incidence of antibiotic-resistant bacteria continues to rise. The proportions of penicillin-resistant *Streptococcus pneumoniae*, hospital-acquired methicillin-resistant *Staphylococcus aureus* (MRSA), and vancomycin-resistant *Enterococcus* (VRE) strains continue to increase. Community-acquired MRSA (cMRSA) is now common throughout the world. Multiresistant *Acinetobacter* and *Pseudomonas* are everyday realities in many of our hospitals. The press is now warning the lay public of the existence of "dirty hospitals." As never before, it is critical that health care providers understand the principles of proper anti-infective therapy and use anti-infective agents judiciously. These agents need to be reserved for treatable infections—not used to calm the patient or the patient's family. Too often, patients with viral infections that do not warrant anti-infective therapy arrive at the physician's office expecting to be treated with an antibiotic. And health care workers too often prescribe antibiotics to fulfill those expectations.

Physicians unschooled in the principles of microbiology utilize anti-infective agents just as they would more conventional medications, such as anti-inflammatory agents, anti-hypertensive medications, and cardiac drugs. They use one or two broad-spectrum antibiotics to treat all patients with suspected infections.

Many excellent broad-spectrum antibiotics can effectively treat most bacterial infections without requiring a specific causative diagnosis. However, overuse of empiric broad-spectrum antibiotics has resulted in the selection of highly resistant pathogens. A simplistic approach to anti-infective therapy and establishment of a fixed series of simple rules concerning the use of these agents is unwise and has proved harmful to patients. Such an approach ignores the remarkable adaptability of bacteria, fungi, and viruses. It is no coincidence that these more primitive life forms have survived for millions of years, far longer than the human race.

The rules for the use of anti-infective therapy are dynamic and must take into account the ability of these pathogens to adapt to the selective pressures exerted by the overuse of antibiotic, antifungal, and antiviral agents. The days of the "shotgun" approach to infectious diseases must end, or more and more patients will become infected with multiresistant organisms that cannot be treated. Only through the judicious use of anti-infective therapy can we hope to slow the arrival of the end of the antibiotic era.

<table>
<tr><td>

KEY POINTS

About Anti-Infective Therapy

1. Too often, antibiotics are prescribed to fulfill the patient's expectations, rather than to treat a true bacterial infection.
2. A single antibiotic cannot meet all infectious disease needs.
3. Physicians ignore the remarkable adaptability of bacteria, fungi, and viruses at their patient's peril.
4. Anti-infective therapy is dynamic and requires a basic understanding of microbiology.
5. The "shotgun" approach to infectious diseases must end, or we may truly experience the end of the antibiotic era.

</td></tr>
</table>

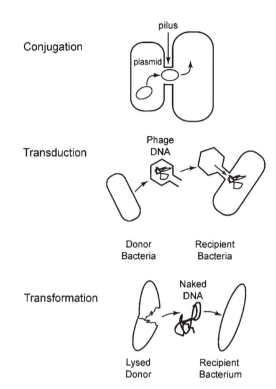

Figure 1–1. Mechanisms by which bacteria transfer antibiotic resistance genes.

■ ANTIBIOTIC RESISTANCE

GENETIC MODIFICATIONS LEADING TO ANTIMICROBIAL RESISTANCE

To understand why antibiotics must be used judiciously, the physician needs to understand how bacteria are able to adapt to their environment. Point mutations can develop in the DNA of bacteria as they replicate. These mutations occur in the natural environment, but are of no survival advantage unless the bacteria are placed under selective pressures. In the case of a mutation that renders a bacterium resistant to a specific antibiotic, exposure to the specific antibiotic allows the bacterial clone that possesses the antibiotic resistance mutation to grow, while bacteria without the mutation die and no longer compete for nutrients. Thus the resistant strain becomes the dominant bacterial flora. In addition to point mutations bacteria can also use three major mechanisms to transfer genetic material among themselves:

1. **Conjugation.** Bacteria often contain circular, double-stranded DNA structures called plasmids. These circular DNA structures lie outside the bacterial genome (Figure 1.1). Plasmids often carry resistance ("R") genes. Through a mechanism called "conjugation," plasmids can be transferred from one bacterium to another. The plasmid encodes for the formation of a pilus on the donor bacteria's outer surface. The pilus attaches to a second bacterium and serves as bridge for the transfer of the plasmid DNA from the donor to the recipient bacterium. Using this mechanism, a single resistant bacterium can transfer resistance to other bacteria.

2. **Transduction.** Bacteriophages are protein-coated DNA segments that attach to the bacterial wall and inject DNA in a process called "transduction." These infective particles can readily transfer resistance genes to multiple bacteria.

3. **Transformation.** Donor bacteria can also release linear segments of chromosomal DNA, which is then taken up by recipient bacteria and incorporated into the recipient's genome. This process is called "transformation," and the naked DNA capable of incorporating into the genome of recipient bacteria is called a transposon (Figure 1.1). Natural transformation most commonly occurs in *Streptococcus*, *Haemophilus*, and *Neisseria* species. Transposons can transfer multiple antibiotic resistance genes in a single event and have been shown to be responsible for high-level vancomycin resistance in enterococci.

KEY POINTS

About Antibiotic Resistance

1. Bacteria can quickly alter their genetic makeup by
   a) point mutation.
   b) transfer of DNA by plasmid conjugation.
   c) transfer of DNA by bacteriophage transduction.
   d) transfer of naked DNA by transposon transformation.
2. The ability of bacteria to share DNA provides a survival advantage, allowing them to quickly adapt to antibiotic exposure.
3. Biochemical alterations leading to antibiotic resistance include
   a) degradation or modification of the antibiotic.
   b) reduction of the bacterial antibiotic concentration by inhibiting entry or by efflux pumps.
   c) modification of the antibiotic target.
4. Under the selection pressure of antibiotics, the question is not *whether*, but *when* resistant bacteria will take over.

Thus bacteria possess multiple ways to transfer their DNA, and they promiscuously share genetic information. This promiscuity provides a survival advantage, allowing bacteria to quickly adapt to their environment.

BIOCHEMICAL MECHANISMS FOR ANTIMICROBIAL RESISTANCE

What are some of the proteins that these resistant genes encode for, and how do they work?

The mechanisms by which bacteria resist antibiotics can be classified into three major groups:

- Degradation or modification of the antibiotic
- Reduction of the bacterial antibiotic concentration
- Modification of the antibiotic target

Degradation or Modification of the Antibiotic

β-LACTAMASES

Many bacteria synthesize one or more enzymes called β-lactamases that inactivate antibiotics by breaking the amide bond on the β-lactam ring. Transfer of β-lactamase activity occurs primarily through plasmids and transposons.

Multiple classes of β-lactamases exist. Some preferentially break down penicillins; others preferentially destroy specific cephalosporins or carbenicillin. Extended-spectrum β-lactamases (ESBLs) readily destroy most cephalosporins. Another class of β-lactamase is resistant to clavulanate, an agent added to numerous antibiotics to inhibit β-lactamase activity. Some bacteria are able to produce β-lactamases called carbapenemases that are capable of inactivating imipenem and meropenem.

Gram-negative bacilli produce a broader spectrum of β-lactamases than do gram-positive organisms, and therefore infections with gram-negative organisms more commonly arise in patients treated for prolonged periods with broad-spectrum antibiotics. In some instances, β-lactamase activity is low before the bacterium is exposed to antibiotics; however, following exposure, β-lactamase activity is induced. *Enterobacter* is a prime example. This gram-negative bacterium may appear sensitive to cephalosporins on initial testing. Following cephalosporin treatment, β-lactamase activity increases, resistance develops, and the patient's infection relapses. For this reason, third-generation cephalosporins are not recommended for serious *Enterobacter* infections.

OTHER ENZYME MODIFICATIONS OF ANTIBIOTICS

Erythromycin is readily inactivated by an esterase that hydrolyzes the lactone ring of the antibiotic. This esterase has been identified in *Escherichia coli*. Other plasmid-mediated erythromycin inactivating enzymes have been discovered in *Streptococcus* species and *S. aureus*. Chloramphenicol is inactivated by chloramphenicol acetyltransferase, which has been isolated from both gram-positive and gram-negative bacteria. Similarly, aminoglycosides can be inactivated by acetyltransferases. Bacteria also inactivate this class of antibiotics by phosphorylation and adenylation.

These resistance enzymes are found in many gram-negative strains and are increasingly detected in enterococci, *S. aureus* and *S. epidermidis*.

Reduction of the Bacterial Antibiotic Concentration

INTERFERENCE WITH ANTIBIOTIC ENTRY

For an antibiotic to work, it must be able to penetrate the bacterium and reach its biochemical target. Gram-negative bacteria contain an outer lipid coat that impedes penetration by hydrophilic reagents (such as most antibiotics). The passage of hydrophilic antibiotics is facilitated by the presence of porins—small channels in the cell walls of gram-negative bacteria that allow the passage of charged molecules. Mutations leading to the loss of porins can reduce antibiotic penetration and lead to antibiotic resistance.

PRODUCTION OF EFFLUX PUMPS

Transposons have been found that encode for an energy-dependent pump that can actively pump tetracycline out of bacteria. Active efflux of antibiotics has been observed in many enteric gram-negative bacteria, and this mechanism is used to resist tetracycline, macrolide, and fluoroquinolone antibiotic treatment. *S. aureus*, *S. epidermidis*, *S. pyogenes*, group B streptococci, and *S. pneumoniae* also can utilize energy-dependent efflux pumps to resist antibiotics.

Modification of the Antibiotic Target

ALTERATIONS OF CELL WALL PRECURSORS

Alteration of cell wall precursors is the basis for VRE. Vancomycin and teicoplanin binding requires that D-alanine-D-alanine be at the end of the peptidoglycan cell wall precursors of gram-positive bacteria. Resistant strains of *Enterococcus faecium* and *Enterococcus faecalis* contain the vanA plasmid, which encodes a protein that synthesizes D-alanine-D-lactate instead of D-alanine-D-alanine at the end of the peptidoglycan precursor. Loss of the terminal D-alanine markedly reduces vancomycin and teicoplanin binding, allowing the mutant bacterium to survive and grow in the presence of these antibiotics.

CHANGES IN TARGET ENZYMES

Penicillins and cephalosporins bind to specific proteins called penicillin-binding proteins (PBPs) in the bacterial cell wall. Penicillin-resistant *S. pneumoniae* demonstrate decreased numbers of PBPs or PBPs that bind penicillin with lower affinity, or both. Decreased penicillin binding reduces the ability of the antibiotic to kill the targeted bacteria.

The basis for antibiotic resistance in MRSA is production of a low affinity PBP encoded by the *mecA* gene. Mutations in the target enzymes dihydropteroate synthetase and dihydrofolate reductase cause sulfonamide and trimethoprim resistance respectively. Single amino-acid mutations that alter DNA gyrase function can result in resistance to fluoroquinolones.

ALTERATIONS IN RIBOSOMAL BINDING SITE

Tetracyclines, macrolides, lincosamides, and aminoglycosides all act by binding to and disrupting the function of bacterial ribosomes (see the descriptions of individual antibiotics later in this chapter). A number of resistance genes encode for enzymes that demethylate adenine residues on bacterial ribosomal RNA, inhibiting antibiotic binding to the ribosome.

Ribosomal resistance to gentamicin, tobramycin, and amikacin is less common because these aminoglycosides have several binding sites on the bacterial ribosome and require multiple bacterial mutations before their binding is blocked.

CONCLUSIONS

Bacteria can readily transfer antibiotic resistance genes. Bacteria have multiple mechanisms to destroy antibiotics, lower the antibiotic concentration, and interfere with antibiotic binding. Under the selective pressures of prolonged antibiotic treatment, the question is not *whether*, but *when* resistant bacteria will take over.

■ ANTI-INFECTIVE AGENT DOSING

The characteristics that need to be considered when administering antibiotics include absorption (when dealing with oral antibiotics), volume of distribution, metabolism, and excretion. These factors determine the dose of each drug and the time interval of administration. To effectively clear a bacterial infection, serum levels of the antibiotic need to be maintained above the minimum inhibitory concentration (MIC) for a significant period. For each pathogen, the MIC is determined by serially diluting the antibiotic into liquid medium containing 10^4 bacteria per milliliter. Inoculated tubes are incubated overnight until broth without added antibiotic has become cloudy or turbid as a result of bacterial growth. The lowest concentration of antibiotic that prevents active bacterial growth—that is, the liquid media remains clear—constitutes the MIC (Figure 1.2). Automated analyzers can now quickly determine, for individual pathogens, the MICs for multiple antibiotics, and these data serve to guide the physician's choice of antibiotics.

The mean bactericidal concentration (MBC) is determined by taking each clear tube and inoculating a plate of solid medium with the solution. Plates are then incubated to allow colonies to form. The lowest concentration of antibiotic that blocks all growth of bacteria—that is, no colonies on solid medium—represents the MBC.

Successful cure of an infection depends on multiple host factors in addition to serum antibiotic concentration. However, investigators have attempted to predict successful treatment by plotting serum antibiotic levels against time. Three parameters can be assessed (Figure 1.3): time above the MIC (T>MIC), ratio of the peak antibiotic concentration to the MIC (Cmax/MIC), and the ratio of the area under the curve (AUC) to the MIC (AUC/MIC).

Cure rates for β-lactam antibiotics are maximized by maintaining serum levels above the MIC for >50% of the time. Peak antibiotic concentrations are of less

MIC & MBC

Inoculate all tubes with 10⁴ bacteria incubate 38°C X 12 hrs

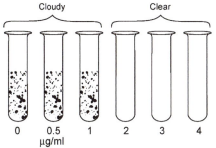

Minimal Inhibitory Concentration (MIC) = 2µg/ml

Then take a sample from each clear tube and inoculate a culture plate. Incubate 38° X 12 hrs.

Minimal Bactericidal concentration (MBC) = 3µg/ml

Figure 1–2. Understanding the minimum inhibitory concentration and the minimal bactericidal concentration.

importance for these antibiotics, and serum concentrations above 8 times the MIC are of no benefit other than to enhance penetration into less permeable body sites.

Unlike β-lactam antibiotics, aminoglycosides and fluoroquinolones demonstrate concentration-dependent killing. In vitro studies show that these antibiotics demonstrate greater killing the more their concentrations

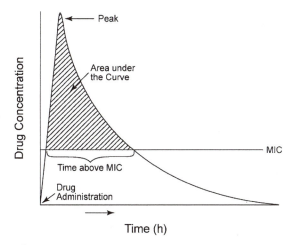

Figure 1–3. Pharmacokinetics of a typical antibiotic.

exceed the MIC. High peak levels of these antibiotics may be more effective than low peak levels at curing infections. Therefore, for treatment with aminoglycosides and fluoroquinolones Cmax/MIC and AUC/MIC are more helpful for maximizing effectiveness. In the treatment of gram-negative bacteria, aminoglycosides have been suggested to achieve maximal effectiveness when Cmax/MIC is 10 to 12. For fluoroquinolones, best outcomes in community-acquired pneumonia may be achieved when the AUC/MIC is >34. To prevent the development of fluoroquinolone resistance to *S. pneumoniae*, in vitro studies have suggested that AUC/MIC should be >50. For *P. aeruginosa*, an AUC/MIC of >200 is required.

In vitro studies also demonstrate that aminoglycosides and fluoroquinolones demonstrate a post-antibiotic effect: when the antibiotic is removed, a delay in the recovery of bacterial growth occurs. Gram-negative bacteria demonstrate a delay of 2 to 6 hours in the recovery of active growth after aminoglycosides and fluoroquinolones, but no delay after penicillins and cephalosporins. But penicillins and cephalosporins generally cause a 2-hour delay in the recovery of gram-positive organisms. Investigators suggest that antibiotics with a significant post-antibiotic effect can be dosed less frequently; those with no post-antibiotic effect should be administered by constant infusion. Although these in vitro effects suggest certain therapeutic approaches, it must be kept in mind that concentration-dependent killing and post-antibiotic effect are both in vitro phenomena, and treatment strategies based on these effects have not been substantiated by controlled human clinical trials.

KEY POINTS

About Antibiotic Dosing

1. Absorption, volume of distribution, metabolism, and excretion all affect serum antibiotic levels.
2. Mean inhibitory concentration (MIC) is helpful in guiding antibiotic choice.
3. To maximize success with β-lactam antibiotics, serum antibiotic levels should be above the MIC for at least 50% of the time (T>MIC > 50%).
4. To maximize success with aminoglycosides and fluoroquinolones, high peak concentration, Cmax/MIC, and high AUC/MIC ratio are recommended.
5. The clinical importance of concentration-dependent killing and post-antibiotic effect for aminoglycosides and fluoroquinolones remain to be proven by clinical trials.

BASIC STRATEGIES FOR ANTIBIOTIC THERAPY

The choice of antibiotics should be carefully considered. A step-by-step logical approach is helpful (Figure 1.4).

1. Decide Whether The Patient Has a Bacterial Infection

One test that has traditionally been used to differentiate an acute systemic bacterial infection from a viral illness is the peripheral white blood cell (WBC) count. In patients with serious systemic bacterial infections, the peripheral WBC count may be elevated and may demonstrate an increased percentage of neutrophils. On occasion, less mature neutrophils such as band forms and, less commonly, metamyelocytes are observed on peripheral blood smear. Most viral infections fail to induce a neutrophil response. Viral infections, particularly Epstein–Barr virus, induce an increase in lymphocytes or monocytes (or both) and may induce the formation of atypical monocytes. Unfortunately, the peripheral WBC count is only a rough guideline, lacking both sensitivity and specificity. Recently, serum procalcitonin concentration has been found to be a far more accurate test for differentiating bacterial from viral infection. In response to bacterial infection, this precursor of calcitonin is synthesized and released into the serum by many organs of the body; production of interferon in response to viral infection inhibits its synthesis. The serum procalcitonin test may also be of prognostic value, serum procalcitonin levels being particularly high in severe sepsis (see Chapter 2).

2. Make a Reasonable Statistical Guess as to the Possible Pathogens

Based on the patient's symptoms and signs, as well as on laboratory tests, the anatomic site of the possible infection can often be determined. For example, burning on urination, associated with pyuria on urinalysis, suggests a urinary tract infection. The organisms that cause uncomplicated urinary tract infection usually arise from the bowel flora. They include *E. coli*, *Klebsiella*, and *Proteus*. Antibiotic treatment needs to cover these potential pathogens. Later chapters review the pathogens commonly associated with infections at specific anatomic sites and the recommended antibiotic coverage for those pathogens.

3. Be aware of the Antibiotic Susceptibility Patterns in Your Hospital and Community

In patients that develop infection while in hospital ("nosocomial infection), empiric therapy needs to take into account the antibiotic susceptibility patterns of the

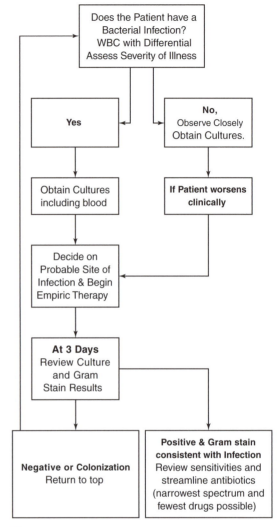

Figure 1-4. Algorithm for the initial use of anti-infective therapy.

flora associated with the hospital and the floor where the patient became ill. Many hospitals have a high incidence of MRSA and therefore empiric antibiotic treatment for a possible staphylococcal infection must include vancomycin, pending culture results. Other hospitals have a large percentage of *Pseudomonas* strains that are resistant to gentamicin, eliminating that antibiotic from consideration as empiric treatment of possible gram-negative sepsis. In many communities, individuals who have never been hospitalized are today presenting with soft-tissue infections caused by cMRSA, and physicians in these communities must adjust their empiric antibiotic selection (see Chapter 10).

4. Take into Account Previous Antibiotic Treatment

The remarkable adaptability of bacteria makes it highly likely that a new pathogen will be resistant to previously administered antibiotics. If the onset of the new infection was preceded by a significant interval when antibiotics were not given, the resident flora may have recolonized with less resistant flora. However, the re-establishment of normal flora can take weeks, and patients in hospital are likely to recolonize with highly resistant hospital flora.

5. Take into Consideration Important Host Factors

a. **Penetration into the site of infection.** For example, patients with bacterial meningitis should not be treated with antibiotics that fail to cross the blood–brain barrier (examples include 1st-generation cephalosporins, gentamicin, and clindamycin).

b. **Peripheral WBC count.** Patients with neutropenia have a high mortality rate from sepsis. Immediate broad-spectrum, high-dose intravenous antibiotic treatment is recommended as empiric therapy for these patients.

c. **Age and underlying diseases (hepatic and renal dysfunction).** Elderly patients tend to metabolize and excrete antibiotics more slowly; longer dosing intervals are therefore often required. Agents with significant toxicity (such as aminoglycosides) should generally be avoided in elderly patients because they exhibit greater toxicity. Antibiotics metabolized primarily by the liver should generally be avoided or reduced in patients with significant cirrhosis. In patients with significant renal dysfunction, antibiotic doses need to be modified.

d. **Duration of hospitalization.** Patients who have just arrived in the hospital tend to be colonized with community-acquired pathogens; patients who have been in the hospital for prolonged periods and have received several courses of antibiotics tend to be colonized with highly resistant bacteria and with fungi.

e. **Severity of the patient's illness.** The severely ill patient who is toxic and hypotensive requires broad-spectrum antibiotics; the patient who simply has a new fever without other serious systemic complaints can usually be observed off antibiotics.

6. Use the Fewest Drugs Possible

a. **Multiple drugs may lead to antagonism rather than synergy.** Some regimens, such as penicillin and an aminoglycoside for *Enterococcus*, have been shown to result in synergy—that is, the combined effects are greater than simple addition of the MBCs of the two agents would suggest. In other instances, certain combinations have proved to be antagonis-

tic. The use of rifampin combined with oxacillin is antagonistic in some strains of *S. aureus*, for example. Many combination regimens have not been completely studied, and the natural assumption that more antibiotics lead to more killing power often does not apply.

b. **Use of multiple antibiotics increases the risk of adverse reactions.** Drug allergies are common. When a patient on more than one antibiotic develops an allergic reaction, all antibiotics become potential offenders, and these agents can no longer be used. In some instances, combination therapy can increase the risk of toxicity. The combination of gentamicin and vancomycin increases the risk of nephrotoxicity, for example.

c. **Use of multiple antibiotics often increases costs and the risk of administration errors.** Administration of two or more intravenous antibiotics requires multiple intravenous reservoirs, lines, and pumps. Nurses and pharmacists must dispense each antibiotic dose, increasing labor costs. The more drugs a patient receives, the higher the probability of an administration error. Use of two or more drugs usually increases the acquisition costs.

d. **Use of multiple antibiotics increases the risk of infection with highly resistant organisms.** Prolonged use of broad-spectrum antibiotic coverage increases the risk of infection with MRSA, VRE, multiresistant gram-negative bacilli, and fungi. When multiple antibiotics are used, the spectrum of bacteria killed increases. Killing most of the normal flora in the pharynx and gastrointestinal tract is harmful to the host. The normal flora compete for nutrients, occupy binding sites that could otherwise be used by pathogenic bacteria, and produce agents that inhibit the growth of competitors. Loss of the normal flora allows resistant pathogens to overgrow.

7. Switch to Narrower-Spectrum Antibiotic Coverage Within 3 Days

(Table 1.1, Figure 1.5). Within 3 days following the administration of antibiotics, sequential cultures of mouth flora reveal that the numbers and types of bacteria begin to change significantly. The normal flora die, and resistant gram-negative rods, gram-positive cocci, and fungi begin to predominate. The more quickly the selective pressures of broad-spectrum antibiotic coverage can be discontinued, the lower the risk of selecting for highly resistant pathogens. Broad coverage is reasonable as initial empiric therapy until cultures are available. By the 3rd day, the microbiology laboratory can generally identify the pathogen or pathogens, and a narrower-spectrum, specific antibiotic

Table 1.1. Classification of Antibiotics by Spectrum of Activity

Narrow	Moderately Broad	Broad	Very Broad
Penicillin	Ampicillin	Ampicillin–sulbactam	Ticarcillin–clavulinate
Oxacillin/Nafcillin	Ticarcillin	Amoxicillin–clavulanate	Piperacillin–tazobactam
Cefazolin	Piperacillin	Ceftriaxone,	Cefepime
Cephalexin/Cephradine	Cefoxitin	Cefotaxime	Imipenem
Aztreonam	Cefotetan	Ceftizoxime	Meropenem
Aminoglycosides	Cefuroxime–axetil	Ceftazidime	Ertapenem
Vancomycin	Cefaclor	Cefixime	Gatifloxacin
Macrolides	Ciprofloxacin	Cefpodoxime proxetil	Moxifloxacin
Clindamycin	Azithromycin	Tetracycline	Tigecycline
Linezolid	Clarithromycin	Doxycycline	
Quinupristin/dalfopristin	Talithromycin	Chloramphenicol	
Daptomycin	Trimethoprim–sulfamethoxazole	Levofloxacin	
Metronidazole			

regimen can be initiated. Despite the availability of culture results, clinicians too often continue the same empiric broad-spectrum antibiotic regimen, and that behavior is a critical factor in explaining subsequent infections with highly resistant superbugs. Figure 1.5 graphically illustrates the spectrum of available antibiotics as a guide to the antibiotic choice.

Obey the 3-day rule. Continuing broad-spectrum antibiotics beyond 3 days drastically alters the host's resident flora and selects for resistant organisms. After 3 days, streamline antibiotic coverage. Use narrower-spectrum antibiotics to treat the specific pathogens identified by culture and Gram stain.

8. All Else Being Equal, Choose The Least Expensive Drug

As is discussed in later chapters, more than one antibiotic regimen can often be used to successfully treat a specific infection. Given the strong economic forces driving medicine today, the physician needs to consider the cost of therapy whenever possible. Too often, new, more expensive antibiotics are chosen over older generic antibiotics that are equally effective. In this book, the review of each specific antibiotic tries to classify that antibiotic's cost range to assist the clinician in making cost-effective decisions.

However, in assessing cost, factoring in toxicity is also important. For example, the acquisition cost of gentamicin is low, but when blood-level monitoring, the requirement to closely follow blood urea nitrogen

---

KEY POINTS

About the Steps Required to Design an Antibiotic Regimen

1. Assess the probability of bacterial infection. (Antibiotics should be avoided in viral infections.)
2. Be familiar with the pathogens primarily responsible for infection at each anatomic site.
3. Be familiar with the bacterial flora in the local hospital and community.
4. Take into account previous antibiotic treatment.
5. Take into account the specific host factors (age, immune status, hepatic and renal function, duration of hospitalization, severity of illness).
6. Use the minimum number and narrowest spectrum of antibiotics possible.
7. Switch to a narrower-spectrum antibiotic regimen based on culture results.
8. Take into account acquisition cost and the costs of toxicity.

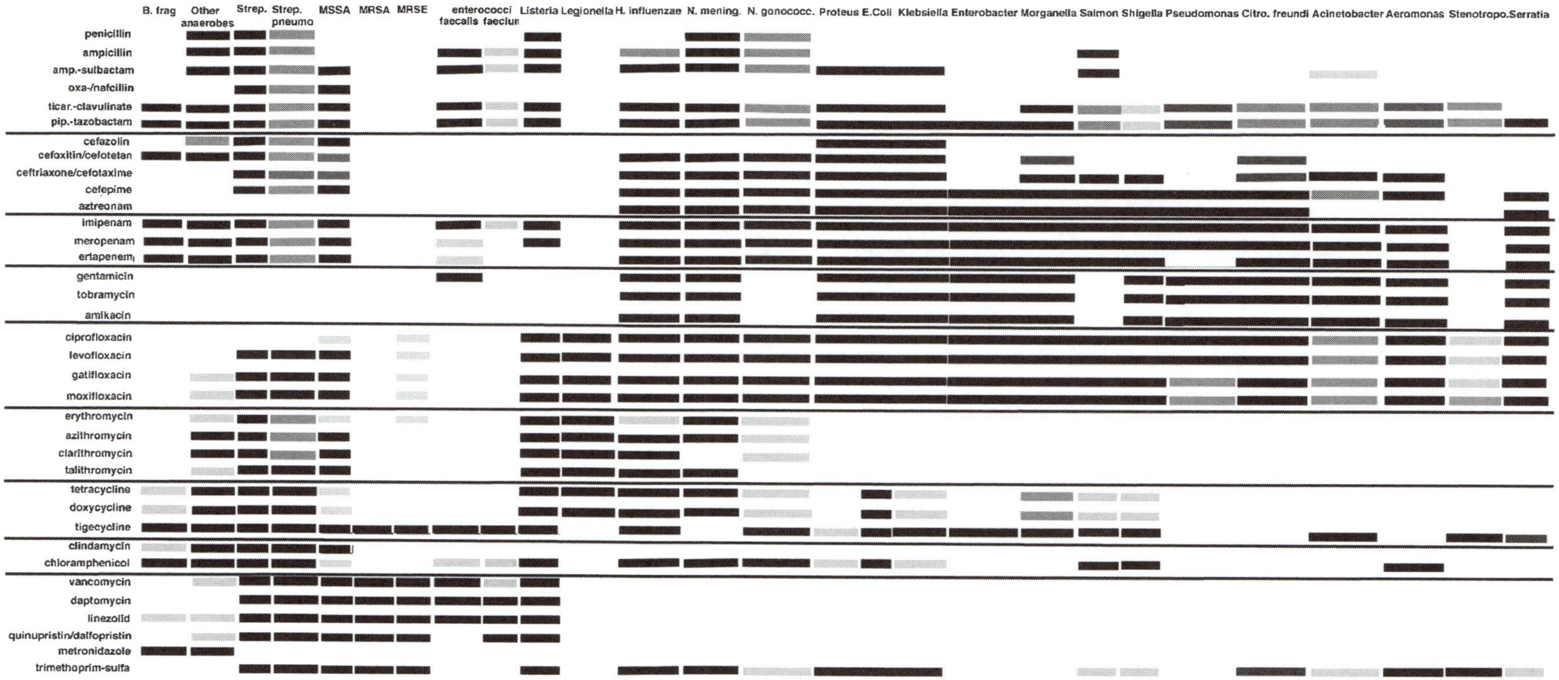

Blank = not recommended
Light gray = < 30% susceptibility
Darker gray = 30–60% susceptibility
Black = 61–95% susceptibility

Figure 1–5. Antibiogram of all major antibiotics.

9

and serum creatinine, and the potential for an extended hospital stay because of nephrotoxicity are factored into the cost equation, gentamicin is often not cost-effective.

Obey the 3-day rule. Continuing broad-spectrum antibiotics beyond 3 days drastically alters the host's normal flora and selects for resistant organisms. After 3 days streamline the antibiotics. Use narrower-spectrum antibiotics to treat the specific pathogens identified by culture and Gram stain.

COLONIZATION VERSUS INFECTION

CASE 1.1

Following a motor vehicle accident, a 40-year-old man was admitted to the intensive care unit with 4 fractured ribs and a severe lung contusion on the right side. Chest X-ray (CXR) demonstrated an infiltrate in the right lower lobe. Because of depressed mental status, this man required respiratory support.

Initially, Gram stain of the sputum demonstrated few polymorphonuclear leukocytes (PMNs) and no organisms. On the third hospital day, this patient developed a fever to 103°F (39.5°C), and his peripheral WBC increased to 17,500 from 8000 (80% PMNs, 15% band forms). A new CXR demonstrated extension of the right lower lobe infiltrate. Gram stain of sputum revealed abundant PMNs and 20 to 30 gram-positive cocci in clusters per high-power field. His sputum culture grew methicillin-sensitive S. aureus. Intravenous cefazolin (1.5 g every 8 hours) was initiated. He defervesced, and secretions from his endotracheal tube decreased over the next 3 days. On the fourth day, a repeat sputum sample was obtained. Gram stain revealed a moderate number of PMNs and no organisms; however, culture grew E. coli resistant to cefazolin. The physician changed the antibiotic to intravenous cefepime (1 g every 8 hours).

Case 1.1 represents a very typical example of how antibiotics are misused. The initial therapy for a probable early *S. aureus* pneumonia was appropriate, and the patient responded (fever resolved, sputum production decreased, gram-positive cocci disappeared from the Gram stain, and *S. aureus* no longer grew on

culture). However, because the sputum culture was positive for a resistant *E. coli*, the physician switched to a broader-spectrum antibiotic. The correct decision should have been to continue cefazolin.

One of the most difficult and confusing issues for many physicians is the interpretation of culture results. Wound cultures and sputum cultures are often misinterpreted. Once a patient has been started on an antibiotic, the bacterial flora on the skin and in the mouth and sputum will change. Often these new organisms do not invade the host, but simply represent new flora that have colonized these anatomic sites. Too often, physicians try to eradicate the new flora by adding new more-powerful antibiotics. The result of this strategy is to select for organisms that are multiresistant. The eventual outcome can be the selection of a bacterium that is resistant to all antibiotics.

No definitive method exists for differentiating between colonization and true infection. However, several clinical findings are helpful in guiding the physician. Evidence supporting the onset of a new infection include a new fever or a change in fever pattern, a rise in the peripheral WBC with a increase in the percentage of PMNs and band forms (left shift), Gram stain demonstrating an increased number of PMNs in association with predominance of bacteria that are morphologically consistent with the culture results. In the absence of these findings, colonization is more likely, and the current antibiotic regimen should be continued.

KEY POINTS

About Differentiating Colonization from Infection

1. Growth of resistant organisms is the rule in the patient on antibiotics.
2. Antibiotics should be switched only on evidence of a new infection.
3. Evidence for a new superinfection includes
   a) new fever or a worsening fever pattern,
   b) increased peripheral leukocyte count with left shift,
   c) increased inflammatory exudate at the original site of infection,
   d) increased polymorphonuclear leukocytes on Gram stain, and
   e) correlation between bacterial morphology and culture on Gram stain.

SPECIFIC ANTI-INFECTIVE AGENTS

ANTIBIOTICS

Before prescribing a specific antibiotic, clinicians should be able to answer these questions:

- How does the antibiotic kill or inhibit bacterial growth?
- What are the antibiotic's toxicities and how should they be monitored?
- How is the drug metabolized, and what are the dosing recommendations? Does the dosing schedule need to be modified in patients with renal dysfunction?
- What are the indications for using each specific antibiotic?
- How broad is the antibiotic's antimicrobial spectrum?
- How much does the antibiotic cost?

Clinicians should be familiar with the general classes of antibiotics, their mechanisms of action, and their major toxicities. The differences between the specific antibiotics in each class can be subtle, often requiring the expertise of an infectious disease specialist to design the optimal anti-infective regimen. The general internist or physician-in-training should not attempt to memorize all the facts outlined here, but rather should read the pages that follow as an overview of anti-infectives. The chemistry, mechanisms of action, major toxicities, spectrum of activity, treatment indications, pharmacokinetics, dosing regimens, and cost are reviewed. The specific indications for each anti-infective are briefly covered here. A more complete discussion of specific regimens is included in the later chapters that cover infections of specific anatomic sites.

Upon prescribing a specific antibiotic, physicians should reread the specific sections on toxicity, spectrum of activity, pharmacokinetics, dosing, and cost. Because new anti-infectives are frequently being introduced, prescribing physicians should also take advantage of hand-held devices, online pharmacology databases, and antibiotic manuals so as to provide up-to-date treatment (see Further Reading at the end of the current chapter). When the proper therapeutic choice is unclear, on-the-job training can be obtained by requesting a consultation with an infectious disease specialist. Anti-infective agents are often considered to be safe; however, the multiple potential toxicities outlined below, combined with the likelihood of selecting for resistant organisms, emphasize the dangers of over-prescribing antibiotics.

β-Lactam Antibiotics

CHEMISTRY AND MECHANISMS OF ACTION

The β-Lactam antibiotics have a common central structure (Figure 1.6) consisting of a β-lactam ring and a thiazolidine ring [in the penicillins and carbapenems, Figure 1.6(A)] or a β-lactam ring and a dihydrothiazine ring [in the cephalosporins, Figure 1.6(B)]. The side chain attached to the β-lactam ring (R_1) determines many of the antibacterial characteristics of the specific antibiotic, and the structure of the side chain attached to the dihydrothiazine ring (R_2) determines the pharmacokinetics and metabolism.

The β-lactam antibiotics bind to various PBPs. The PBPs represent a family of enzymes important for bacterial cell wall synthesis, including the carboxypeptidases, endopeptidases, transglycolases, and transpeptidases. Strong binding to PBP-1, a cell wall transpeptidase and transglycolase causes rapid bacterial death. Inhibition of this transpeptidase prevents the cross-linking of the cell wall peptidoglycans, resulting in a loss of integrity of the bacterial cell wall. Without its protective outer coat, the hyperosmolar intracellular contents swell, and the bacterial cell membrane lyses. Inhibition of PBP-3, a

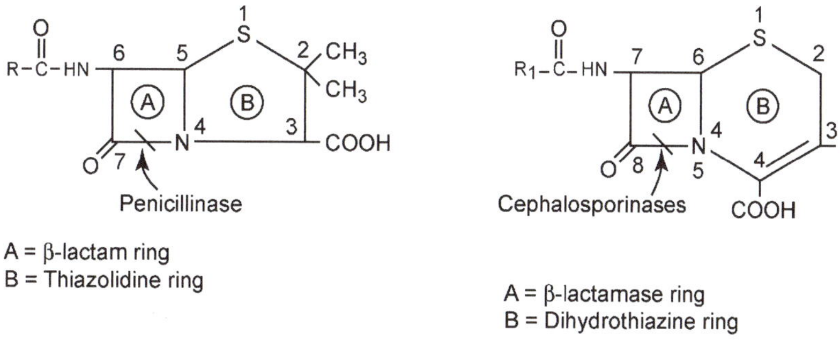

A = β-lactam ring
B = Thiazolidine ring

A = β-lactamase ring
B = Dihydrothiazine ring

Figure1-6. Basic structure of the **A** penicillins and **B** the cephalosporins.

> **KEY POINTS**
>
> **About β-Lactam Antibiotics**
>
> 1. Penicillins, cephalosporins, and carbapenems are all b-lactam antibiotics:
>   a) All contain a β-lactam ring.
>   b) All bind to and inhibit penicillin-binding proteins, enzymes important for cross-linking bacterial cell wall peptidoglycans.
>   c) All require active bacterial growth for bacteriocidal action.
>   d) All are antagonized by bacteriostatic antibiotics.

and bacterial death. Inhibition of other PBPs blocks cell wall synthesis in other ways, and activates bacterial lysis.

The activity of all β-lactam antibiotics requires active bacterial growth and active cell wall synthesis. Therefore, bacteria in a dormant or static phase will not be killed, but those in an active log phase of growth are quickly lysed. Bacteriostatic agents slow bacterial growth and antagonize β-lactam antibiotics, and therefore, in most cases, bacteriostatic antibiotics should not be combined with β-lactam antibiotics.

TOXICITY

Table 1.2 summarizes the toxicities of the β-lactam antibiotics.

Hypersensitivity reactions are the most common side effects associated with the β-lactam antibiotics. Penicillins are the agents that most commonly cause allergic reactions, at rates ranging from 0.7% to 10%. Allergic reactions to cephalosporins have been reported in 1% to 3% of patients, and similar percentages have been reported with carbapenems. However,

transpeptidase and transglycolase that acts at the septum of the dividing bacterium, causes the formation of long filamentous chains of non-dividing bacteria

Table 1.2. Toxicities of β-Lactam Antibiotics

Clinical symptom	Penicillins	Cefazolin	Cefotetan	Ceftriaxone	Cefepime	Aztreonam	Imipenem	Meropenem
Allergic skin rash	■	░	░	░	░	░	■	■
Anaphylaxis	░							
Steven–Johnson	░							
Seizures	░				░	░	■	░
Encephalopathy				░ (a)	░			
Diarrhea (*Clostridium difficile*)	░	░	░	■	░		░	■
Cholelithiasis				■				
Phlebitis	■	■	■	■	░	░	■	■
Laboratory tests:								
Coagulation			░					
Creatinine↑		░	░				░	
Cytopenias	░	░	░			░	░	
Eosinophilia						░	■	░
AST/ALT↑				░	░	░	░	░

[a] Encephalopathy associated with myoclonus has been reported in elderly patients.

Black = principal side effect; dark gray = less common side effect; light gray = rare side effect; white = not reported or very rare; ↑ = rise; AST/ALT = aspartate aminotransferase/ alanine transaminase.

the incidence of serious, immediate immunoglobulin E (IgE)–mediated hypersensitivity reactions is much lower with cephalosporins than with penicillins. Approximately 1% to 7% of patients with penicillin allergies also prove to be allergic to cephalosporins and carbapenems.

Penicillins are the most allergenic of the β-lactam antibiotics because their breakdown products, particularly penicilloyl and penicillanic acid, are able to form amide bonds with serum proteins. The resulting antigens increase the probability of a host immune response. Patients who have been sensitized by previous exposure to penicillin may develop an immediate IgE-mediated hypersensitivity reaction that can result in anaphylaxis and urticaria. In the United States, penicillin-induced allergic reactions result in 400 to 800 fatalities annually. Because of the potential danger, patients with a history of an immediate hypersensitivity reaction to penicillin should never be given any β-lactam antibiotic, including a cephalosporin or carbapenem. High levels of immunoglobulin G anti-penicillin antibodies can cause serum sickness, a syndrome resulting in fever, arthritis, and arthralgias, urticaria, and diffuse edema.

Other less common toxicities are associated with individual β-lactam antibiotics. Natural penicillins and imipenem lower the seizure threshold and can result in grand mal seizures. Ceftriaxone is excreted in high concentrations in the bile and can crystallize, causing biliary sludging and cholecystitis. Antibiotics containing a specific methylthiotetrazole ring (cefamandole, cefoperazone, cefotetan) can induce hypoprothrombinemia and, in combination with poor nutrition, may increase postoperative bleeding. Cefepime has been associated with encephalopathy and myoclonus in elderly individuals. All broad-spectrum antibiotics increase the risk of pseudomembranous colitis (see Chapter 8). In combination with aminoglycosides, cephalosporins demonstrate increased nephrotoxicity.

Penicillins

Tables 1.3 and 1.4, together with Figure 1.5, summarize the characteristics of the various penicillins.

Penicillins vary in their spectrum of activity. Natural penicillins have a narrow spectrum. The aminopenicillins have an intermediate spectrum, and combined with β-lactamase inhibitors, the carboxy/ureidopenicillins have a very broad spectrum of activity.

NATURAL PENICILLINS

Pharmacokinetics—All natural penicillins are rapidly excreted by the kidneys, resulting in short half-lives (Table 1.3). As a consequence, the penicillins must be dosed frequently, and dosing must be adjusted in patients with renal dysfunction. Probenecid slows renal excretion, and this agent can be used to sustain higher serum levels.

KEY POINTS

About β-Lactam Antibiotic Toxicity

1. Allergic reactions are most common toxicity, and they include both delayed and immediate hypersensitivity reactions.
2. Allergy to penicillins (PCNs) seen in 1% to 10% of patients; 1% to 3% are allergic to cephalosporins and carbapenems. 1% to 7% of patients with a PCN allergy are also allergic to cephalosporins and carbapenems.
3. Seizures are associated with PCNs and imipenem, primarily in patients with renal dysfunction.
4. Ceftriaxone is excreted in the bile and can crystallize to form biliary sludge.
5. Cephalosporins with methylthiotetrazole rings (cefamandole, cefoperazone, moxalactam, cefotetan) can interfere with vitamin K and increase prothrombin time.
6. Pseudomembranous colitis can develop as a result of overgrowth of *Clostridium difficile*.
7. Nephrotoxicity sometimes occurs when cephalosporins are given in combination with aminoglycosides.

KEY POINTS

About the Natural Penicillins

1. Very short half-life (15–30 minutes).
2. Excreted renally; adjust for renal dysfunction; probenecid delays excretion.
3. Penetrates most inflamed body cavities.
4. Narrow spectrum. Indicated for *Streptococcus pyogenes, S. viridans* Gp., mouth flora, *Clostridia perfringens, Neisseria meningitidis, Pasteurella*, and spirochetes.
5. Recommended for penicillin-sensitive *S. pneumoniae* [however, penicillin resistant strains are now frequent (>30%)]; infections caused by mouth flora; *Clostridium perfringens* or spirochetes.

Table 1.3. Penicillins: Half-Life, Dosing, Renal Dosing, Cost, and Spectrum

Antibiotic (trade name)	Half-life (h)	Dose	Dose for reduced creatinine clearance (mL/min)	Cost[a]	Spectrum
Natural penicillins (PCNs)					
PCN G	0.5	$2-4 \times 10^6$ U IV q4h	<10: Half dose	$	Narrow
Procaine PCN G		$0.6-1.2 \times 10^6$ U IM q24h		$	Narrow
Benzathine PCN G		2.4×10^6 U IM weekly		$	Narrow
PCN V–K	0.5	250–500 mg PO q6–8h		$	Narrow
Aminopenicillins					
Ampicillin (Omnipen)	1	Up to 14 g IV daily, given q4–6h	30–50: q8h <10: q12h	$	Moderate
Amoxicillin (Amoxil)	1	500 mg PO q8h or 875 mg q12h	<10: q24h	$	Moderate
Amoxicillin–clavulanate (Augmentin)		Same as amoxicillin PO	Same as amoxicillin	$$$$	Broad
Ampicillin–sulbactam (Unasyn)	1	1.5–2 g q6h IV	30–50: q8h <10: q12h	$$$$	Broad
Penicillinase–resistant PCNs					
Oxacillin (Prostaphlin)	0.5	1–2 g q4h IV	None	$	Narrow
Nafcillin (Unipen)	0.5	0.5–2 g q4h IV	None	$$$$	Narrow
Cloxacillin/dicloxacillin (Dynapen)	0.5	0.25–1 g q6h	None	$	Narrow
Carboxy/ureido–PCNs					
Ticarcillin–clavulanate (Timentin)	1	3.1 g q4–6h IV	10–50: 3.1 g q6–8h <10: 2 g q12h	$	Very broad
Piperacillin–tazobactam (Zosyn)	1	3.375 g q6h or 4.5 g q8h	10–50: 2.25 g q6h <10: 2.5 g q8h	$$	Very broad

[a] Intravenous preparations (daily cost dollars): $ = 20 to 60; $$ = 61 to 100; $$$ = 101 to 140; $$$$ = 140 to 180; $$$$$ = more than 180; oral preparations (10-day course cost dollars): $ = 10 to 40; $$ = 41 to 80; $$$ = 81 to 120; $$$$ = 121 to 160; $$$$$ ≥ 160.

Depending on the specific drug, penicillins can be given intravenously or intramuscularly. Some penicillins have been formulated to withstand the acidity of the stomach and are absorbed orally. Penicillins are well distributed in the body and are able to penetrate most inflamed body cavities. However, their ability to cross the blood–brain barrier in the absence of inflammation is poor. In the presence of inflammation, therapeutic levels are generally achievable in the cerebrospinal fluid.

Spectrum of Activity and Treatment Recommendations—Penicillin G (Table 1.4) remains the treatment of choice for *S. pyogenes* ("group A strep") and the *S. viridans* group. It also remains the most effective agent for the treatment of infections caused by mouth flora. Penicillin G is also primarily recommended for *Clostridium perfringens, C. tetani, Erysipelothrix rhusiopathiae, Pasteurella multocida,* and spirochetes including syphilis and *Leptospira.* This antibiotic also remains the primary recommended therapy for *S. pneumoniae* sensitive to penicillin (MIC < 0.1 μg/mL). However, in many areas of the United States, more than 30% of strains are moderately resistant to penicillin (MIC = 0.1–1 μg/mL). In these cases, ceftriaxone, cefotaxime, or high-dose penicillin (>12 million units daily) can be used. Moderately resistant strains of *S. pneumoniae* possess a lower-affinity PBP, and this defect in binding can be overcome

Table 1.4. Organisms That May Be Susceptible to Penicillins

Natural penicillins (PCNs)	Aminopenicillins (with or without clavulanate)	Anti-staphylococcal penicillin (nafcillin/oxacillin)	Carboxy/ureidopenicillins plus clavulanate or tazobactam
Streptococcus pyogenes S. pneumoniae (increasing numbers of PCN-resistant strains) S. viridans PCN-sensitive enterococci Mouth flora including: Actinomyces israeli, Capnocytophaga canimorsus, Fusobacterium nucleatum, Eikenella corrodens Clostridium perfringens Clost. tetani Pasteurella multocida Erysipelothrix rhusiopathiae Spirochetes: Treponema pallidum, Borrelia burgdorferi, Leptospira interrogans Neisseria gonorrhoeae Neiss. meningitidis Listeria monocytogenes	Covers same organisms as natural penicillins plus: Escherichia coli Proteus PCN-sensitive enterococci Salmonella spp. Shigella spp. Addition of clavulanate adds susceptibility to: H. influenzae (β-lactamase strains) Moraxella catarrhalis Methicillin-sensitive Staph. aureus (MSSA)	Narrower spectrum than natural penicillins, No activity against anaerobes, Enterococcus, or gram-negative organisms. Drug of choice for MSSA.	Covers same organisms as natural penicillins plus: MSSA E. coli Proteus mirabilis Klebsiella pneumoniae Enterobacter spp. Citrobacter freundii Serratia spp. Morganella spp. Pseudomonas aeruginosa Bacteroides fragilis

by high serum levels of penicillin in the treatment of pneumonia, but not of meningitis. Infections with high-level penicillin-resistant *S. pneumoniae* (MIC > 2 µg/mL) require treatment with vancomycin or another alternative antibiotic.

AMINOPENICILLINS

Pharmacokinetics—In aminopenicillins, a chemical modification of penicillin increases resistance to stomach acid, allowing these products to be given orally (Table 1.3). They can also be given intramuscularly or intravenously. Amoxicillin has excellent oral absorption: 75% as compared with 40% for ampicillin. Absorption is not impaired by food. The higher peak levels achievable with aminopenicillins allow for a longer dosing interval, making them a more convenient oral antibiotic than ampicillin. As observed with the natural penicillins, the half-life is short (1 hour) and these drugs are primarily excreted unmodified in the urine.

Spectrum of Activity and Treatment Recommendations—The spectrum of activity in the aminopenicillins is slightly broader than in the natural penicillins (Table 1.4). Intravenous ampicillin is recommended for treatment of *Listeri monocytogenes*, sensitive enterococci, *Proteus mirabilis*, and non–β-lactamase-producing

Haemophilus influenzae. Aminopenicillins are also effective against *Shigella flexneri* and sensitive strains of nontyphoidal *Salmonella*. Amoxicillin can be used to treat otitis media and air sinus infections. When combined with a β-lactamase inhibitor (clavulanate or sulbactam), aminopenicillins are also effective against methicillin-sensitive *S. aureus* (MSSA), β-lactamase-producing strains of *H. influenzae*, and *Moraxella catarrhalis*. The latter two organisms are commonly cultured from middle ear and air sinus infections (see Chapter 5). However, the superiority of amoxicillin–clavulanate over amoxicillin for middle ear and air sinus infections has not been proven.

PENICILLINASE-RESISTANT PENICILLINS

Pharmacokinetics—The penicillinase-resistant penicillins have the same half-life as penicillin (30 minutes) and require dosing at 4-hour intervals or constant intravenous infusion (Table 1.3). Unlike the natural penicillins, these agents are cleared hepatically, and doses of nafcillin and oxacillin usually do not need to be adjusted for renal dysfunction. But the efficient hepatic excretion of nafcillin means that the dose needs to be adjusted in patients with significant hepatic dysfunction. The liver excretes oxacillin less

---

KEY POINTS

About the Aminopenicillins

1. Short half-life (1 hour), and clearance similar to natural penicillins.
2. Slightly broader spectrum of activity.
3. Parenteral ampicillin indicated for *Listeria monocytogenes*, sensitive enterococci, *Proteus mirabilis*, and non–b-lactamase-producing *Haemophilus influenzae*.
4. Ampicillin plus an aminoglycoside is the treatment of choice for enterococci. Whenever possible, vancomycin should be avoided.
5. Amoxicillin has excellent oral absorption; it is the initial drug of choice for otitis media and bacterial sinusitis.
6. Amoxicillin–clavulanate has improved coverage of *Staphylococcus*, *H. influenzae*, and *Moraxella catarrhalis*, but it is expensive and has a high incidence of diarrhea. Increased efficacy compared with amoxicillin is not proven in otitis media. However, covers amoxicillin-resistant *H. influenzae*, a common pathogen in that disease.

---

efficiently, and so dose adjustment is usually not required in liver disease.

Spectrum of Activity and Treatment Recommendations—The synthetic modification of penicillin to render it resistant to the β-lactamases produced by *S. aureus* reduces the ability of these agents to kill anaerobic mouth flora and *Neisseria* species (Table 1.4). These antibiotics are strictly recommended for the treatment of MSSA. They are also used to treat cellulitis when the most probable pathogens are *S. aureus* and *S. pyogenes*. Because oral preparations result in considerably lower serum concentration levels, cloxacillin or

---

KEY POINTS

About Penicillinase-Resistant Penicillins

1. Short half-life, hepatically metabolized.
2. Very narrow spectrum, poor anaerobic activity.
3. Primarily indicated for methicillin-sensitive *Staphylococcus aureus* and cellulitis.

---

dicloxacillin should not be used to treat *S. aureus* bacteremia. These oral agents are used primarily for mild soft-tissue infections or to complete therapy of a resolving cellulitis.

CARBOXYPENICILLINS AND UREIDOPENICILLINS

Pharmacokinetics—The half-lives of ticarcillin and piperacillin are short, and they require frequent dosing (Table 1.3). Sale of ticarcillin and piperacillin alone has been discontinued in favor of ticarcillin–clavulanate and piperacillin–tazobactam.

Dosing every 6 hours is recommended for piperacillin–tazobactam to prevent accumulation of tazobactam. In *P. aeruginosa* pneumonia, the dose of piperacillin–tazobactam should be increased from 3.375 g Q6h to 4.5 g Q8h to achieve cidal levels of piperacillin in the sputum. In combination with an aminoglycoside, piperacillin–tazobactam often demonstrates synergy against *P. aeruginosa*. However, the administration of the piperacillin–tazobactam needs to be separated from the administration of the aminoglycoside by 30 to 60 minutes.

Spectrum of Activity and Treatment Recommendations—Ticarcillin and piperacillin are able to resist β-lactamases produced by *Pseudomonas*, *Enterobacter*, *Morganella*, and *Proteus–Providencia* species. At high doses, ticarcillin and piperacillin can also kill many strains of *Bacteroides fragilis* and provide effective anaerobic coverage. These antibiotics can be used for empiric coverage of moderate to severe intra-abdominal infections. They have been combined with a β-lactamase inhibitor (clavulanate or tazobactam) to provide effective killing of MSSA.

These agents are reasonable alternatives to nafcillin or oxacillin when gram-negative coverage is also

---

KEY POINTS

About Carboxypenicillins and Ureidopenicillins

1. More effective resistance to gram-negative β-lactamases.
2. Carboxypenicillin or ureidopenicillin combined with aminoglycosides demonstrate synergistic killing of *Pseudomonas aeruginosa*.
3. Ticarcillin–clavulanate and piperacillin–tazobactam have excellent broad-spectrum coverage, including methicillin-sensitive *Staphylococcus aureus* and anaerobes. They are also useful for intra-abdominal infections, acute prostatitis, in-hospital aspiration pneumonia, and mixed soft-tissue and bone infections.

Table 1.5. Cephalosporins: Half-Life, Dosing, Renal Dosing, Cost, and Spectrum

Antibiotic (trade name)	Half-life (h)	Dose	Dose for reduced creatinine clearance (mL/min)	Cost[a]	Spectrum
1st generation					
Cefazolin (Ancef)	1.8	1–1.5 g IV or IM q6–8h	10–50: 0.5–1 g q8–12h <10: 0.25–0.75 g q18–24h	$	Narrow
Cephalexin (Keflex)	0.9	0.25–1 g PO q6–8h		$	Narrow
Cephradine (Velocef)	0.7	0.25–1 g PO q6h		$–$$	
Cefadroxil (Duricef)	1.2	0.5–1 g PO q12h		$$–$$$$	Narrow
2nd generation					
Cefoxitin (Mefoxin)	0.8	1–2 g IV or IM q4–6h, not to exceed 12 g daily	50–80: q8–12h 10–50: q12–24h <10: 0.5–1 g q12–24h	$$	Moderately broad
Cefotetan (Cefotan)	3.5	1–2 g IV or IM q12h	10–50: q24h <10: q48h	$	Moderately broad
Cefuroxime (Zinacef)	1.3	0.75–1.5 g IV q8h	10–50: q12h <10: 0.75 g q24h	$	Moderately broad
Cefuroxime–axetil (Ceftin)	1.5	0.25–0.5 g PO q12h	<10: 0.25 g q12h	$$$$	Moderately broad
Cefaclor (Ceclor)	0.8	0.25–0.5 g PO q8h	No change required	$$$$	Moderately broad
3rd generation					
Ceftriaxone (Rocephin)	8	1–2 g IV q12–24h	No change required	$$	Broad
Cefotaxime (Claforin)	1.5	2 g IV q4–8h (maximum 12 g daily)	10–30: q8–12h <10: q12–24h	$$	Broad
Ceftizoxime (Cefizox)	1.7	1–4 g IV q8–12h (maximum 12 g daily)	10–30: q12h <10: q24h	$$	Broad
Ceftazidime (Fortaz)	1.9	1–3 g IV or IM q8h, up to 8 g daily	10–50: 1 g q12–24h <10: 0.5 q24–48h	$$	Broad
Cefixime (Suprax)	3.7	400 mg PO q12h or q24h	10–30: 300 mg q24h <10: 200 mg q24h	$$$$	Broad
Cefpodoxime proxetil (Vantin)	2.2	200–400 g PO q12h	10–30: ×3 weekly <10: ×1 weekly	$$$	Broad
4th generation					
Cefepime (Maxipime)	2.1	0.5–2 g IV q12h	10–30: 0.5–1 g q24h <10: 250–500 mg q24h q12h	$–$$	Very broad
Cefpirome (IV–Cef)	2	1–2 g IV q12h	Same as cefepime	$$	Very broad
Monobactams					
Aztreonam (Azactam)	2	1–2 g IV q6h	10–30: q12–18h <10: q24h	$$–$$$$	Narrow

Intravenous preparations (daily cost dollars): $ = 20–70; $$ = 71–110; $$$ = 111–150; $$$$ = 150–200; $$$$$ ≥ 200; oral preparations (10-day course cost dollars): $ = 10–50; $$ = 51–100; $$$ = 101–140; $$$$ = 141–180; $$$$$ ≥ 180.

Table 1.6. Organisms That May Be Susceptible to Cephalosporins

1st generation (cefazolin)	2nd generation (cefoxitin, cefotetan)	3rd generation (ceftriaxone, cefotaxime)	4th generation (cefepime)
Methicillin-sensitive	Covers same organisms	Covers same organisms	Covers same organisms
Staphylococcus aureus (best activity)	as cefazolin, but weaker gram-positive activity.	as cefazolin, but often weaker gram-	as cefazolin and ceftriaxone. Excellent gram-positive and gram-negative activity.
Streptococcus pyogenes	Also covers:	positive and stronger gram-negative	Also covers:
Penicillin (PCN)–sensitive	*Haemophilus influenzae*	activity.	Intermediate
S. pneumoniae	*Moraxella catarrhalis*	Also covers:	PCN-resistant
Escherichia coli (some species)	*Neisseria gonorrhoeae*	*H. influenzae*	*S. pneumoniae*
Klebsiella pneumoniae (some species)	*N. meningitidis*	*M. catarrhalis*	*Enterobacter* spp.
Proteus mirabilis (some species)	*Bacteroides fragilis* (some strains)	*N. gonorrhoeae*	*Pseudomonas aeruginosa*
		N. meningitidis *Citrobacter freundii*	*Serratia* spp.
		Morganella spp. *Salmonella* spp.	
		Shigella spp.	

required. Both agents can be used for in-hospital aspiration pneumonia to cover for mouth flora and gram-negative rods alike, and they can also be used for serious intra-abdominal, gynecologic, and acute prostate infections. They have been used for skin and bone infections thought to be caused by a combination of gram-negative and gram-positive organisms.

Cephalosporins

Tables 1.5 and 1.6, together with Figure 1.5, summarize the characteristics of the various cephalosporins.

In an attempt to create some semblance of order, the cephalosporins have been classified into generations based on spectrum of activity (Table 1.5). First-generation cephalosporins are predominantly effective against gram-positive cocci. Second-generation cephalosporins demonstrate increased activity against aerobic and anaerobic gram-negative bacilli, but have variable activity against gram-positive cocci. The third-generation cephalosporins demonstrate even greater activity against gram-negative bacilli, but only limited activity against gram-positive cocci. Finally, the fourth-generation cephalosporins demonstrate the broadest spectrum of activity, being effective against both gram-positive cocci and gram-negative bacilli.

Classification of the cephalosporins by generation naturally leads to the assumption that newer, later-generation cephalosporins are better than the older cephalosporins. However, it is important to keep in mind that, for many infections, earlier-generation, narrower-spectrum cephalosporins are preferred to the more recently developed broader-spectrum cephalosporins.

FIRST-GENERATION CEPHALOSPORINS

Pharmacokinetics—Cefazolin, the preferred parenteral first-generation cephalosporin, has a longer half-life than penicillin, and it is primarily excreted by the kidneys (Table 1.5). The first-generation cephalosporins penetrate most body cavities, **but they fail to cross the blood–brain barrier.** Oral preparations (cephalexin, cephradine, cefadroxil) are very well absorbed, achieving excellent peak serum concentrations (0.5 g cephalexin results in a 18 μg/mL peak). Absorption is not affected

---

KEY POINTS

About First-Generation Cephalosporins

1. Excellent gram-positive coverage, some gram-negative coverage.
2. Do not cross the blood–brain barrier.
3. Inexpensive.
4. Useful for treating soft-tissue infections and for surgical prophylaxis. Can often be used as an alternative to oxacillin or nafcillin.

by food. The half-lives of cephalexin and cephradine are short, requiring frequent administration. These agents need to be corrected for renal dysfunction.

Spectrum of Activity and Treatment Recommendations—The first-generation cephalosporins are very active against gram-positive cocci, including MSSA, and they also have moderate activity against some community-acquired gram-negative bacilli (Table 1.6). They are active against oral cavity anaerobes, but are ineffective for treating *B. fragilis*, *H. influenzae*, *L. monocytogenes*, MRSA, penicillin-resistant *S. pneumoniae*, and *Enterococcus*.

First-generation cephalosporins are an effective alternative to nafcillin or oxacillin for soft-tissue infections thought to be caused by MSSA or *S. pyogenes*. Cefazolin is also the antibiotic of choice for surgical prophylaxis. Because of its inability to cross the blood–brain barrier, cefazolin should never be used to treat bacterial meningitis. Oral preparations are commonly used to treat less severe soft-tissue infections, including impetigo, early cellulitis, and mild diabetic foot ulcers.

SECOND-GENERATION CEPHALOSPORINS

Pharmacokinetics—The second-generation cephalosporins are cleared primarily by the kidney (Table 1.5). They have half-lives that range from 0.8 to 3.5 hours, and they penetrate all body cavities.

Spectrum of Activity and Treatment Recommendations—The second-generation cephalosporins possess increased activity against some gram-negative strains, and they effectively treat MSSA and non-enterococcal streptococci (Table 1.6). Given the availability of the first-, third-, and fourth-generation cephalosporins and the newer penicillins, second-generation cephalosporins are rarely recommended as primary therapy.

Because cefoxitin and cefotetan demonstrate increased anaerobic coverage, including many strains of *B. fragilis*, and also cover gonococcus, these two agents are used as part of first-line therapy in pelvic inflammatory disease. They are also used for the treatment of moderately severe intra-abdominal infections and mixed aerobic–anaerobic soft-tissue infections, including diabetic foot infections. The oral preparation cefuroxime achieves serum levels that are approximately one tenth that of intravenous preparations, and this agent is recommended for the outpatient treatment of uncomplicated urinary tract infections and otitis media. Other less costly oral antibiotics effectively cover the same pathogens.

Cefaclor, the other second-generation oral preparation, is inactivated by β-lactamases produced by *H. influenzae* and *M. catarrhalis*. Although cefaclor has been recommended for otitis media, other oral antibiotics are generally preferred.

THIRD-GENERATION CEPHALOSPORINS

Pharmacokinetics—With the exception of ceftriaxone, the third-generation cephalosporins are excreted by the kidneys (Table 1.5). Ceftriaxone is cleared primarily by the liver, but high concentrations of the drug are also excreted in the biliary system. The half-lives of these agents vary, being as short as 1.5 hours (cefotaxime) and as long as 8 hours (ceftriaxone). They penetrate most body sites effectively.

Spectrum of Activity and Treatment Recommendations—As compared with the first- and second-generation, third-generation cephalosporins have enhanced activity against many aerobic gram-negative bacilli, but they do not cover *Serratia marcescens*, *Acinetobacter*, and *Enterobacter cloacae*. With the exceptions of ceftazidime and cefoperazone, third-generation cephalosporins are ineffective against *P. aeruginosa*.

These agents have excellent cidal activity against *S. pneumoniae* (including moderately penicillin-resistant strains), *S. pyogenes*, and other streptococci. All members of this generation are ineffective for treating *Enterococcus*, MRSA, highly penicillin-resistant pneumococcus, and *L. monocytogenes*.

The ESBLs are increasing in frequency, and they promise to reduce the effectiveness of the third- and fourth-generation cephalosporins. A large number of third-generation cephalosporins are available, all with similar indications. Small deficiencies in coverage and less-desirable pharmacokinetics have affected the popularity of a number of these drugs.

Ceftriaxone and cefotaxime are recommended for empiric treatment of community-acquired pneumonia and community-acquired bacterial meningitis (see Chapters 4 and 6). Third-generation cephalosporins can be used

KEY POINTS

About Second-Generation Cephalosporins

1. Improved activity against Haemophilus influenzae, Neisseria species, and Moraxella catarrhalis.
2. Cefoxitin and cefotetan have anaerobic activity and are used in mixed soft-tissue infections and pelvic inflammatory disease.
3. Cefotetan and cefamandole have a methylthiotetrazole ring that decreases prothrombin production. Vitamin K prophylaxis is recommended in malnourished patients.
4. Cefuroxime–axetil is a popular oral cephalosporin; less expensive alternative oral antibiotics are available, however.
5. Overall, this generation is of limited usefulness.

in combination with other antibiotics to empirically treat the septic patient. Ceftriaxone is recommended for treatment of *N. gonorrhoeae*. Cefotaxime is cleared renally and does not form sludge in the gallbladder. For this reason, this agent is preferred over ceftriaxone by some pediatricians, particularly for the treatment of bacterial meningitis in children—where high-dose therapy has been associated with symptomatic biliary sludging. Ceftazidime is the only third-generation cephalosporin that has excellent activity against *P. aeruginosa*; however, the fourth-generation cephalosporin cefepime (and the monobactam aztreonam) are now more commonly utilized for anti-*Pseudomonas* therapy in many institutions.

The oral third-generation cephalosporin cefixime has a long half-life, allowing for once-daily dosing. Cefixime provides effective coverage for *S. pneumoniae* (penicillin-sensitive), *S. pyogenes*, *H. influenzae*, *M. catarrhalis*, *Neisseria* species, and many gram-negative bacilli, but it is ineffective against *S. aureus*. Its absorption is not affected by food. This agent is a potential second-line therapy for community-acquired pneumonia, and it is an alternative to penicillin for the treatment of bacterial pharyngitis. The other oral preparation, cefpodoxime proxetil, has an antimicrobial spectrum similar to that of cefixime. In addition, it has moderate activity against *S. aureus*. The indications for use are similar to those for cefixime, and cefpodoxime proxetil has also been recommended as an alternative treatment for acute sinusitis.

KEY POINTS

About the Third-Generation Cephalosporins

1. Improved gram-negative coverage.
2. Excellent activity against Neisseria gonorrhoeae, N. meningitidis, Haemophilus influenzae, and Moraxella catarrhalis.
3. Ceftriaxone has a long half-life that allows for once-daily dosing. In children, acalculous cholecystitis can occur with large doses.
4. Cefotaxime has a shorter half-life but activity identical to that of ceftriaxone; does not cause biliary sludging.
5. Ceftazidime has excellent activity against most *Pseudomonas aeruginosa* strains, but reduced activity against *Staphylococcus aureus*.
6. Extended spectrum β-lactamases are increasing in frequency and endangering the effectiveness of third-generation cephalosporins.
7. Recommended for community-acquired pneumonia and bacterial meningitis

FOURTH-GENERATION CEPHALOSPORINS

Pharmacokinetics—Clearance of the fourth-generation cephalosporins is renal, and the half-lives of these agents are similar to the renally cleared third-generation cephalosporins (Table 1.5). The R_2 substitution of the fourth-generation cephalosporins contains both a positively and negatively charged group that, together, have zwitterionic properties that permit these antibiotics to penetrate the outer wall of gram-negative bacteria and concentrate in the periplasmic space. This characteristic also allows for excellent penetration of all body compartments, including the cerebrospinal fluid.

Spectrum of Activity and Treatment Recommendations—The fourth-generation cephalosporins are resistant to most β-lactamases, and they only weakly induce β-lactamase activity (Table 1.6, Figure 1.5). These agents also bind gram-positive PBPs with high affinity.

The only agent currently available in the United States is cefepime. In addition to having broad antimicrobial activity against gram-negative bacilli, including *P. aeruginosa*, cefepime provides excellent coverage for *S. pneumoniae* (including strains moderately resistant to penicillin), *S. pyogenes*, and MSSA. Cefepime and ceftazidime provide comparable coverage for *P. aeruginosa*. To maximize the likelihood of cure of serious *P. aeruginosa* infection, more frequent dosing (q8h) has been recommended.

Cefepime is not effective against *L. monocytogenes*, MRSA, or *B. fragilis*. As compared with third-generation cephalosporins, cefepime is more resistant to β-lactamases, including the ESBLs. It has been effectively used to treat gram-negative meningitis. Cefepime is effective as a single agent in the febrile neutropenic

KEY POINTS

About Fourth-Generation Cephalosporins

1. Zwitterionic properties allow for excellent penetration of the bacterial cell wall and of human tissues and fluids.
2. Weakly induce β-lactamases.
3. More resistant to extended-spectrum β-lactamases and chromosomal β-lactamases.
4. Excellent gram-positive (including methicillin-sensitive *Staphylococcus aureus*) and gram-negative coverage (including *Pseudomonas aeruginosa*).
5. Excellent broad-spectrum empiric therapy. Useful in nosocomial infections.

patient, and it is an excellent agent for initial empiric coverage of nosocomial infections.

Cefpirome is available in Europe. It has an antimicrobial spectrum similar to that of cefepime, although it is somewhat less active against *P. aeruginosa*.

Monobactams

AZTREONAM

Chemistry and Pharmacokinetics—Aztreonam was originally isolated from *Chromobacterium violaceum* and subsequently modified. This antibiotic has a distinctly different structure from the cephalosporins, and it is the only available antibiotic in its class. Rather than a central double ring, aztreonam has a single ring ("monocyclic β-lactam structure"), and has been classified as a monobactam.

Because of its unique structure, aztreonam exhibits no cross-reactivity with other β-lactam antibiotics. It can be used safely in the penicillin-allergic patient. The drug penetrates body tissue well and crosses the blood–brain barrier of inflamed meninges. Aztreonam is renally cleared and has a half-life similar to to that of the renally cleared third- and fourth-generation cephalosporins.

Spectrum of Activity and Treatment Recommendations—Aztreonam does not bind to the PBPs of gram-positive organisms or anaerobes; rather, it binds with high affinity to PBPs, particularly PBP-3 (responsible for septum formation during bacterial division), of gram-negative bacilli including *P. aeruginosa*. Gram-negative organisms exposed to aztreonam form long filamentous structures and are killed.

Aztreonam is effective against most gram-negative bacilli, and this agent has been marketed as a non-nephrotoxic replacement for aminoglycosides. However, unlike aminoglycosides, aztreonam does not provide synergy with penicillins for *Enterococcus*. A major advantage of

> ## KEY POINTS
>
> ### About Aztreonam
>
> 1. A distinctly different structure than that of the cephalosporins.
> 2. No cross-reactivity with penicillin,
> 3. Binds the penicillin-binding proteins of gram-negative, but not of gram-positive bacteria.
> 4. Narrow spectrum, with excellent activity against aerobic gram-negative rods.
> 5. Marketed as a non-nephrotoxic replacement for aminoglycosides. However, as compared with aminoglycosides, it
>   a) has no synergy with penicillins in enterococcal infections.
>   b) is not helpful for treating *Streptococcus viridans* endocarditis.
> 6. Excellent empiric antibiotic when combined with an antibiotic with good gram-positive activity. Useful for the treatment of pyelonephritis.

aztreonam is its restricted antimicrobial spectrum, which allows for survival of the normal gram-positive and anaerobic flora that can compete with more resistant pathogens.

Aztreonam can be used for the treatment of most infections attributable to gram-negative bacilli. It has been used effectively in pyelonephritis, nosocomial gram-negative pneumonia, gram-negative bacteremia, and gram-negative intra-abdominal infections. Importantly, though, aztreonam provides no gram-positive or anaerobic coverage. Therefore, when it is used for empiric treatment of potential gram-positive pathogens in the seriously ill patient,

Table 1.7. Carbapenems: Half-Life, Dosing, Renal Dosing, Cost, and Spectrum

Antibiotic (trade name)	Half-life (h)	Dose	Dose for reduced creatinine clearance (mL/min)	Cost[a]	Spectrum
Imipenem–cilastin (Primaxin)	1	0.5–1 g IV q6h	50–80: 0.5 g q6–8h 10–50: 0.5 g q8–12h <10: 0.25–0.5 g q12h	$$$–$$$$$	Very broad
Meropenem (Merrem)	1	1 g IV q8h	10–50: 0.5 g q8h <10: 0.5 g q24h	$$$$	Very broad
Ertapenem (Invanz)	4	1 g IV or IM q24h	<30: 500 mg q24h	$	Very broad

Intravenous preparations (daily cost dollars): $ = 20–70; $$ 71–110; $$$ = 111–150; $$$$ = 150–200; $$$$$ ≥ 200.

aztreonam should be combined with vancomycin, clindamycin, erythromycin, or a penicillin.

Carbapenems

Table 1.7, together with Figure 1.5, summarizes the characteristics of the various carbapenems.

CHEMISTRY AND PHARMACOKINETICS

The carbapenems have both a modified thiazolidine ring and a change in the configuration of the side chain that renders the β-lactam ring highly resistant to cleavage. Their hydroxyethyl side chain is in a *trans* rather than *cis* conformation, and this configuration is thought to be responsible for the group's remarkable resistance to β-lactamase breakdown. At physiologic pH, these agents have zwitterionic characteristics that allow them to readily penetrate tissues. The carbapenems bind with high affinity to the high molecular weight PBPs of both gram-positive and gram-negative bacteria.

Imipenem is combined in a 1:1 ratio with cilastatin to block rapid breakdown by renal dehydropeptidase I. Meropenem and ertapenem are not significantly degraded by this enzyme and do not require co-administration with cilastatin. These drugs are all primarily cleared by the kidneys.

SPECTRUM OF ACTIVITY AND TREATMENT RECOMMENDATIONS

The carbapenems have a very broad spectrum of activity, effectively killing most strains of gram-positive and gram-negative bacteria, including anaerobes. Overall, imipenem has slightly better activity against gram-positive organisms. Meropenem and ertapenem have somewhat better activity against gram-negative pathogens (except *Pseudomonas*, as described later in this subsection).

These agents are cidal not only against *S. pneumoniae*, *S. pyogenes*, and MSSA, but also against organisms that are not covered by the cephalosporins, including *Listeria*, *Nocardia*, *Legionella*, and *Mycobacterium avium intracellulare* (MAI). They have static activity against penicillin-sensitive enterococci; however, many penicillin-resistant strains are also resistant to carbapenems. MRSA, some penicillin-resistant strains of *S. pneumoniae*, *C. difficile*, *Stenotrophomonas maltophilia*, and *Burkholderia cepacia* are also resistant. Resistance in gram-negative bacilli is most often secondary to loss of an outer membrane protein called D2 that is required for intracellular penetration of the carbapenems. Increasing numbers of gram-negative strains can also produce β-lactamases called carbapenemases that can hydrolyze these drugs.

Imipenem and meropenem can be used as empiric therapy for sepsis, and they are particularly useful if polymicrobial bacteremia is a strong possibility. They can also be used to treat severe intra-abdominal infections and complicated pyelonephritis. Infections attributable to gram-negative bacilli resistant to cephalosporins and aminoglycosides may be sensitive to imipenem or meropenem. Imipenem or meropenem are recommended as primary therapy for *Serratia*. Meropenem can be used for meningitis, achieving therapeutic levels in the cerebrospinal fluid. Imipenem is not recommended for this purpose because of its propensity to cause seizures. In general, imipenem and meropenem should be reserved for the seriously ill patient or the patient infected with a highly resistant bacterium that is sensitive only to this antibiotic.

Ertapenem has a longer half-life and can be given just once daily, making it a useful agent for home intravenous therapy. This agent is not effective against *P. aeruginosa*, but otherwise it has a spectrum similar to that of meropenem. It is recommended for complicated intra-abdominal infections, postpartum and postoperative acute pelvic infections, and complicated soft-tissue infections.

Because the carbapenems are extremely broad-spectrum agents, they kill nearly all normal flora. The loss of normal flora increases the risk of nosocomial infections with resistant pathogens including MRSA, *Pseudomonas*, and *Candida*.

KEY POINTS

About the Carbapenems

1. β-Lactam ring is highly resistant to cleavage.
2. Have zwitterionic characteristics, and penetrate all tissues.
3. Frequent cross-reactivity in penicillin-allergic patients (7%).
4. Imipenem causes seizures at high doses; be cautious in renal failure patients. Meropenem is less epileptogenic.
5. Bind penicillin binding proteins of all bacteria with high affinity.
6. Very broad cidal activity for aerobic and anaerobic gram-positive and gram-negative bacteria. Also covers *Listeria monocytogenes* and *Nocardia*.
7. Imipenem and meropenem are useful for empiric therapy of suspected mixed aerobic and anaerobic infection or a severe nosocomial infection, pending culture results. Reserve for the severely ill patient.
8. Ertapenem can be given once daily. Lacks *Pseudomonas aeruginosa* coverage.
9. Treatment markedly alters the normal bacterial flora.

Aminoglycosides

Tables 1.8 and 1.9, together with Figure 1.5, summarize the characteristics of the various aminoglycosides.

CHEMISTRY AND MECHANISM OF ACTION

Aminoglycosides were originally derived from *Streptomyces* species. These agents have a characteristic 6-member ring with amino-group substitutions, and they are highly soluble in water. At neutral pH, they are positively charged, and this positive charge contributes to their antibacterial activity. At a low pH, the charge is reduced, impairing antimicrobial activity. Their positive charge also causes aminoglycosides to bind to and become inactivated by β-lactam antibiotics. Therefore aminoglycosides should never be in the same solution with β-lactam antibiotics.

Upon entering the bacterium, the antibiotic molecules interact with and precipitate DNA and other anionic components. Aminoglycosides also bind to the 30S subunit of bacterial 16S ribosomal RNA and interfere with translation. These combined effects are bactericidal.

TOXICITY

The aminoglycosides have a narrow ratio of therapeutic effect to toxic side effect, and monitoring serum levels is generally required to prevent toxicity. These agents are among the most toxic drugs prescribed today, and they should be avoided whenever safer alternative antibiotics are available (Table 1.10).

Two major toxicities are observed:

1. **Nephrotoxicity.** Injury to the proximal convoluted tubules of the kidney leads to a reduction in creatinine clearance. The brush border cells of the proximal tubule take up aminoglycosides by endocytosis, and intracellular entry is associated with cell necrosis. Aminoglycosides cause significant reductions of glomerular filtration in 5% to 25% of patients. Patient characteristics associated with an increased risk of nephrotoxicity include older age, pre-existing renal disease, hepatic dysfunction, volume depletion, and hypotension. Re-exposure to aminoglycosides increases risk, as do the use of larger doses, more frequent dosing intervals, and treatment for more than 3 days. The risk of renal failure is also associated with co-administration of vancomycin, amphotericin B, clindamycin, piperacillin, cephalosporins, foscarnet, or furosemide. Because renal tubular cells have regenerative power, renal dysfunction usually reverses on discontinuation of the aminoglycoside. Because aminoglycosides are primarily renally cleared, aminoglycoside serum levels are useful for detecting worsening renal function. Trough aminoglycoside serum levels often rise before a significant rise in serum creatinine can be detected.

2. **Ototoxicity.** Aminoglycosides enter the inner ear fluid and damage outer hair cells important to the detection of high-frequency sound. Loss of high-frequency hearing occurs in 3% to 14% of patients treated with aminoglycosides. The risk of hearing loss is greater after prolonged treatment, with most cases developing after 9 or more days of therapy. Hearing loss is irreversible and can occur weeks after therapy has been discontinued. A genetic predisposition has been observed, with certain families having a high incidence of deafness after receiving aminoglycosides. The risk of hearing loss depends on the specific aminoglycoside. Neomycin has the highest risk of toxicity, followed in order of decreasing frequency by gentamicin, tobramycin, amikacin, and netilmicin. Concomitant use of furosemide or vancomycin, and exposure to loud noises increase the risk. As compared with dosing at 8-hour intervals, once-daily dosing reduces the toxic risk.

Less commonly, aminoglycosides can cause neuromuscular blockade; they should be avoided in myasthenia gravis. Given the high risk of toxicity, aminoglycosides should be used only when alternative antibiotics are unavailable. When aminoglycosides are required, the duration of therapy should be as brief as possible. Pretreatment and periodic testing of high-frequency hearing should be performed, and serum creatinine and aminoglycoside serum levels should be monitored.

PHARMACOKINETICS

Following intravenous infusion, aminoglycosides take 15 to 30 minutes to distribute throughout the body. Therefore, to determine peak serum level, blood samples should be drawn 30 minutes after completion of the intravenous infusion. The half-life of aminoglycosides is 2 to 5 hours, and these agents are cleared by the kidneys.

Proper dosing of aminoglycosides is more complicated than for most other antibiotics, and these agents require close monitoring. In many hospitals, a pharmacist is consulted to assist in dose management. For daily multiple-dose therapy, a loading dose is first given to rapidly achieve a therapeutic serum level; maintenance doses are then administered. Doses are calculated based on ideal body weight. In the setting of renal dysfunction, dosing must be carefully adjusted, and peak and trough serum levels monitored. As renal impairment worsens, the dosage interval should be extended.

Once-daily aminoglycoside dosing is now the preferred therapy in nearly all instances. As compared with multidose therapy, once-daily administration reduces

Table 1.8. Aminoglycosides: Half-Life, Dosing, Renal Dosing, Cost, and Spectrum

Antibiotic (trade name)	Half-life (h)	Dose	Dose for reduced creatinine clearance (mL/min)	Cost[a]	Spectrum
Gentamicin and tobramycin (Garamycin and Nebcin)	2	2 mg/kg load, then 1.7–2 mg/kg q8h; or 5 mg/kg q24h	0.03 mg/kg × CrCl q8h, adjusting peak to 5–10 µg/mL and trough 1–2 µg/mL; or 60–79: 4 mg/kg q24h 50: 3.5 mg/kg q24h 40: 2.5 mg/kg q24h <30: Conventional dosing, adjusting trough to <0.5 µg/mL	$$$$–$$$$$	Narrow
Amikacin (Amikin)	2	8 mg/kg load, then 7.5–8 mg/kg q8h, or 15 mg/kg daily	0.12 mg/kg × CrCl q8h, adjusting peak to 20–40 µg/mL, and trough 5–10 µg/mL, or 60–79: 12 mg/kg q24h 50: 7.5 mg/kg q24h 40: 4.0 mg/kg q24h <30: Conventional dosing, adjusting trough to <5 µg/mL	$$$$–$$$$$	Narrow
Netilmicin	2.5	2 mg/kg load, then 2 mg/kg q8h	Same as gentamicin and tobramycin	$$$$–$$$$$	Narrow
Streptomycin	2–5	7.5 mg/kg load, then 7.5 mg/kg q12h	50–80: 15 mg/kg q24–72h 10–40: 15 mg/kg q72–96h <10: 7.5 mg/kg q72–96h, adjusting peak to 15–25 µg/mL and trough to 5–10 µg/mL	$$$$–$$$$$	Narrow

Intravenous preparations (daily cost dollars): $ = 20–70; $$ = 71–110; $$$ = 111–150; $$$$ = 150–200; $$$$$ ≥ 200. Includes costs of monitoring and toxicity.

Table 1.9. Organisms That May Be Susceptible to Aminoglycosides

Gentamicin	Tobramycin	Amikacin	Streptomycin
Most Enterobacteriaceae (see Figure 1.5)	Most Enterobacteriaceae (see Figure 1.5)	Most Enterobacteriaceae (see Figure 1.5)	*Yersinia pestis* *Francisella tularensis*
Francisella tularensis *Brucella* spp. (combined with doxycycline)	*Pseudomonas aeruginosa* (synergy with anti-*Pseudomonas* penicillin or cephalosporins)	*Mycobacterium avium* complex	*Brucella* spp. (combined with doxycycline)
Synergy with penicillins, vancomycin, and ceftriaxone for *S. viridans*			*M. tuberculosis*
Synergy with penicillins and vancomycin for *Enterococcus*			

Table 1.10. Toxicities of Miscellaneous Antibiotics

Clinical symptom	Aminoglycosides	Vancomycin	Macrolides	Clindamycin	Tetracyclines	Chloramphenicol	Quinolons	Linezolid	Quinu/dalfopristin	Daptomycin	Meronidazole	Sulfas
Allergic skin rash	░	▓ [a]	░	░	░ [b]	░	░ [c]	░	░		░	■
Steven–Johnson												■
Diarrhea (*Clost. difficile*)			▓	■	░	░	▓		░		░	
Gastrointestinal intolerance			■	▓	▓	░	░				■	
Hearing loss	▓	░	░									
Dizziness	▓				░		▓					░
Neurotoxicity	░	░	░	░	░	░	░		░	░	░	
Seizure											░	
Musculoskeletal							░		■			
Phlebitis		▓	░	░								
Laboratory tests:												
Coagulation						░	░					
Creatinine↑	■	░		░								
Cytopenias		░	░	░		▓		■			░	
Eosinophilia			░	░			░					
AST/ALT↑			░ [d]				░	▓	░		▓	
Bilirubin↑									■			
QT prolonged			░				▓					
Glucose↑ or ↓							░					
Amylase↑											░	

[a] "Red man syndrome" common, but not a true allergic reaction (see text).
[b] Also photosensitivity.
[c] Gemifloxacin is associated with frequent skin rash in women under 40 years of age.
[d] Severe and occasionally fatal hepatitis associated with talithromycin.

Black = principle side effect; dark gray = less common side effect; light gray = rare side effect; white = not reported or very rare; ↑ = rise; AST/ALT = aspartate aminotransferase/alanine transaminase.

the concentration of the aminoglycoside that accumulates in the renal cortex and lowers the incidence of nephrotoxicity. Because aminoglycosides demonstrate concentration-dependent killing, the high peak levels achieved with this regimen increase the bactericidal rate and prolong the post-antibiotic effect. In addition, a once-daily regimen is simpler and less expensive to administer. This regimen has not been associated with a higher incidence of neuromuscular dysfunction. To adjust for renal impairment, the daily dose should be reduced.

Monitoring of serum levels is recommended for both multidose and once-daily regimens. With multidose therapy, blood for a peak level determination should be drawn 30 minutes after intravenous infusion is complete, and for a trough level, 30 minutes before the next dose. Blood for peak and trough determinations should be drawn after the third dose of

---

KEY POINTS

About Aminoglycoside Toxicity

1. Very low ratio of therapeutic benefit to toxic side effect.
2. Monitoring of serum levels usually required.
3. Nephrotoxicity commonly occurs (usually reversible). Incidence is higher in
   a) elderly individuals,
   b) patients with pre-existing renal disease,
   c) patients with volume depletion and hypotension, and
   d) patients with liver disease.
4. Higher incidence with co-administration of vancomycin, cephalosporins, clindamycin, piperacillin, foscarnet, or furosemide.
5. The loss of high-frequency hearing and vestibular dysfunction resulting from ototoxicity is often devastating for elderly individuals.
6. Neuromuscular blockade is rare.
7. Once-daily therapy may be less toxic.

---

advantage of this characteristic. Aminoglycosides also demonstrate persistent suppression of bacterial growth for 1 to 3 hours after the antibiotic is no longer present. The higher the concentration of the aminoglycoside, the longer the post-antibiotic effect. Aminoglycosides also demonstrate synergy with antibiotics that act on the cell wall (β-lactam antibiotics and glycopeptides). The effect of these combinations is greater than the sum of the anti-microbial effects of each individual agent. Synergy has been achieved in the treatment of enterococci, *S. viridans*, *S. aureus*, coagulase-negative staphylococci, *P. aeruginosa*, *L. monocytogenes*, and JK corynebacteria.

An aminoglycoside in combination with other antibiotics is generally recommended for treatment of the severely ill patients with sepsis syndrome to assure broad coverage for gram-negative bacilli. An aminoglycoside combined with penicillin is recommended for empiric coverage of bacterial endocarditis. Tobramycin combined with an anti-pseudomonal penicillin or an anti-pseudomonal cephalosporin is recommended as primary treatment of *P. aeruginosa*. Streptomycin or gentamicin is the treatment of choice for tularemia and *Yersinia pestis*, and either agent can

antibiotic to assure full equilibration within the distribution volume. In the critically ill patient, blood for a peak level determination should be drawn after the first dose to assure achievement of an adequate therapeutic level.

For once-daily dosing, trough levels need to be monitored to assure adequate clearance. Serum level at 18 hours should be <1 μg/mL. Alternatively, blood for a level determination can be drawn between 6 and 14 hours, and the value applied to a nomogram to help decide on subsequent doses. In the seriously ill patient, blood for a peak level determination should also be drawn 30 minutes after completion of the infusion to assure that a therapeutic level is being achieved (for gentamicin–tobramycin, a target concentration of 16 to 24 μg/mL should be achieved). Once-daily dosing is not recommended for the treatment of enterococcal endocarditis and has not been sufficiently studied in pregnancy or in patients with osteomyelitis or cystic fibrosis.

SPECTRUM OF ACTIVITY AND TREATMENT RECOMMENDATIONS

The aminoglycosides are cidal for most aerobic gram-negative bacilli, including *Pseudomonas* species. These agents kill rapidly, and the killing is concentration-dependent—that is, the rate increases as the concentration of the antibiotic increases. Once-daily dosing takes

---

KEY POINTS

About Dosing and Serum Monitoring of Aminoglycosides

1. Aminoglycosides take 15 to 30 minutes to equilibrate in the body.
2. For multidose therapy, blood for a peak serum level determination should be drawn 30 minutes after infusion.
3. Blood for trough serum level determinations should be drawn just before the next dose.
4. Conventionally, aminoglycosides are given 3 times daily. Dosing should be based on lean body weight.
5. Once-daily dosing takes advantage of concentration-dependent killing and the post-antibiotic effects of aminoglycosides.
6. Once-daily dosing reduces, but does not eliminate, nephrotoxicity.
7. In most cases, trough serum levels need to be monitored only during once-daily dosing. Toxicity correlates with high trough levels.
8. Once-daily dosing is not recommended for enterococcal endocarditis or pregnant women.

also be used to treat *Brucella*. Gentamicin combined with penicillin is the treatment of choice for both *S. viridans* and *Enterococcus faecalis*.

Glycopeptide Antibiotics

Table 1.11, together with Figure 1.5, summarizes the characteristics of the glycopeptide antibiotics.

CHEMISTRY AND MECHANISM OF ACTION

Vancomycin and teicoplanin are complex glycopeptides of approximately 1500 Da molecular weight. These agents act primarily at the cell wall of gram-positive organisms by binding to the D-alanine–D-alanine precursor and preventing it from being incorporated into the peptidoglycan. The binding of vancomycin to this cell wall precursor blocks the transpeptidase and transglycolase enzymes, interfering with cell wall formation and increasing permeability of the cell. These agents may also interfere with RNA synthesis. They bind rapidly and tightly to bacteria and rapidly kill actively growing organisms. They also have a 2-hour post-antibiotic effect.

TOXICITY

The most common side effect of the glycopeptide antibiotics is "red man syndrome," which occurs most often when vancomycin is infused rapidly (Table 1.10). The patient experiences flushing of the face, neck, and upper thorax. This reaction is thought to be caused by sudden histamine release secondary to local hyperosmolality and not to be a true hypersensitivity reaction. Infusing vancomycin over a 1-hour period

usually prevents this reaction. There is less experience with teicoplanin; however, this agent does not cause significant thrombophlebitis, and skin flushing after rapid infusion is uncommon. Ototoxicity has been reported.

PHARMACOKINETICS

The half-lives of vancomycin (4 to 6 hours) and teicoplanin (40 to 70 hours) are prolonged Table 1.11). Both drugs are excreted primarily by the kidneys, and in the anuric patient, the half-life of vancomycin increases to 7 to 9 days. For vancomycin, peak levels should reach 20 to 50 μg/mL, with trough levels being maintained at 10 to 12 μg/mL. Vancomycin penetrates most tissue spaces, but does not cross the blood–brain barrier in the absence of inflammation. Therapeutic cerebrospinal levels are achieved in patients with meningitis. Unlike vancomycin, which is minimally bound to protein, teicoplanin is 90% protein-bound, accounting for its slow renal clearance. Tissue penetration has not been extensively studied, and little data are available on penetration of bone, peritoneal, or cerebrospinal fluid.

Table 1.11. Glycopeptides, Macrolides, Clindamycin, Tetracyclines, and Chloramphenicol: Half-Life, Dosing, Renal Dosing, Cost, and Spectrum

Antibiotic (trade name)	Half-life (h)	Dose	Dose for reduced creatinine clearance (mL/min)	Cost[a]	Spectrum
Vancomycin (Vancocin)	4–6	15 mg/kg IV q12h (usual dose: 1 g q12h)	40–60: 1 g q12–24h 20–40: q24–48h 10–20: q48–72h <10: q3–7d Exact dose based on levels: peak: 25–50 μg/mL; trough: 10–12 μg/mL	$	Narrow
Teicoplanin (Targocid)	40–70	6 mg/kg IV or IM followed by 3 mg/kg q24h	10–50: Half the dose <10: One third the dose	Not sold in United States	Narrow
Erythromycin	1.2–1.6	250-500 mg PO q6h 1 g IV q6h	No change required	$	Narrow
Clarithromycin (Biaxin, Biaxin XL)	4	250–500 mg PO q12h XL: 1 g PO q24h	<10: 250–500 mg q24h	$–$$	Narrow
Azithromycin (Zithromax)	68	500 mg PO, followed by 250 mg PO q24h, or 500 mg IV q24h	Probably no change required <10: Not studied	$	Narrow
Talithromycin (Ketek)	10	800 mg PO q24h	<30: 600 mg q24h	$$	Narrow
Clindamycin (Cleocin)	2.5	150–300 mg PO q6h 300–900 mg IV q6–8h	No change required	PO: $$$$$ IV: $	Narrow
Tetracycline	8	250–500 mg PO twice daily	50–80: q12h 10–50: q12–24h <10: q24h	$	Broad
Doxycycline (Vibramycin, Doxy)	18	100 mg PO twice daily	No change required	$	Broad
Minocycline (Minocin, Dynacin)	16	200 mg PO twice daily	No change required	$	Broad
Tigecycline (Tygecil)	42	100 mg IV, followed by 50 mg IV q12h	No change required. For severe hepatic dysfunction, maintenance dose: 25 mg IV q12h	$$	Very broad
Chloramphenicol (Chloromycetin)	4	0.25–1 g IV q6h	No change required. Serum levels should be monitored in hepatic failure.	$	Broad

[a] Intravenous preparations (daily cost dollars): $ = 20–70; $$ 5 71–110; $$$ = 111–150; $$$$ = 150–200; $$$$$ ≥ 200; oral preparations (10-day course cost dollars): $ = 10–50; $$ = 51–100; $$$ = 101–140; $$$$ = 141–180; $$$$$ ≥ 180.

ANTIMICROBIAL SPECTRUM AND TREATMENT RECOMMENDATIONS

Vancomycin and teicoplanin both cover MRSA and MSSA, and they are the recommended treatment for MRSA. These agents also kill most strains of coagulase-negative staphylococci (*S. epidermidis*), which are usually methicillin-resistant. They are recommended for the treatment of coagulase-negative staphylococcal line sepsis and bacterial endocarditis. For the latter infection, the glycopeptide antibiotic should be combined with one or more additional antibiotics (see Chapter 7). Vancomycin-intermediately-resistant strains of *S. aureus* were first discovered in Japan and have also been identified in Europe and the United States. These strains have MICs of 8 to 16 μg/mL and are cross-resistant to teicoplanin. The increasing use of vancomycin has selected for these strains and warns us that the indiscriminant use of the glycopeptide antibiotics must be avoided.

Vancomycin and teicoplanin not only have excellent activity against *Staphylococcus*, but also against penicillin-resistant and susceptible strains of *S. pneumoniae*, and they are recommended for empiric treatment of the seriously ill patient with pneumococcal meningitis to cover for highly penicillin-resistant strains. The glycopeptide antibiotics also effectively treat *S. pyogenes*, GpB streptococci, *S. viridans*, and *S. bovis*, and they are recommended for treatment of these infections in the penicillin-allergic patient. *Corynebacterium jeikeium* (previously called JK diphtheroids) is sensitive to vancomycin, and that antibiotic is recommended for its treatment. Oral vancomycin clears *C. difficile* from the bowel, and in the past it was recommended for *C. difficile* toxin–associated diarrhea. However, because of the increased risk of developing VRE following oral vancomycin, this regimen is recommended only for cases that are refractory to metronidazole or for patients who are very seriously ill.

Vancomycin is frequently used to treat *Enterococcus faecalis* and *faecium*; however, an increasing number of strains have become resistant. Three gene complexes transfer resistance. The van A gene cluster directs peptidoglycan cell wall synthesis and coverts D-alanine–D-alanine (the site of vancomycin action) to D-alanine–D-lactate, markedly reducing vancomycin and teicoplanin binding. The other two resistance gene clusters, van B and van C, result in vancomycin resistance, but do not impair teicoplanin activity.

Macrolides and Ketolides

Tables 1.11 and 1.12, together with Figure 1.5, summarizes the chracteristics of the macrolides and ketolides.

KEY POINTS

About the Treatment Recommendations for Vancomycin

1. Treatment of choice for methicillin-resistant *Staphylococcus aureus*; vancomycin-tolerant strains have been reported.

2. Treatment of choice for coagulase-negative staphylococci.

3. Excellent activity against high-level penicillin-resistant *Streptococcus pneumoniae*.

4. In the penicillin-allergic patient, vancomycin is recommended for *Strep. pyogenes*, Gp B streptococci, Strep. viridans, and Strep. bovis.

5. Excellent activity against some strains of *Enterococcus*; however, van A gene–mediated vancomycin-resistant enterococci (VRE) are increasing in frequency.

6. Vancomycin use must be restricted to reduce the likelihood of selecting for VRE and vancomycin-tolerant *Staph. aureus*.

CHEMISTRY AND MECHANISM OF ACTION

The founding member of the macrolide family, erythromycin, was originally purified from a soil bacterium. It has a complex 14-member macrocyclic lactone ring (which gives rise to the class name "macrolides") attached to two sugars. Azithromycin has a 15-member lactone ring and a nitrogen substitution. Clarithromycin has a methoxy group modification at carbon 6 of the erythromycin molecule. These modifications enhance oral absorption and broaden the antimicrobial spectrum.

The newest class of macrolide-like agents are the semisynthetic derivatives of erythromycin called ketolides. The ketolides, represented by talithromycin, have a 14-member macrolactone ring with a keto group at position 3, with the hydroxyls at positions 11 and 12 replaced by a cyclic carbamate. These agents all inhibit protein biosynthesis by blocking the passage of nascent proteins through the ribosome exit tunnel. In the case of conventional macrolides, inhibition is accomplished by binding to a single domain of the 50S ribosomal subunit (domain V of the 23 rRNA molecule). As compared

Table 1.12. Organisms That May Be Susceptible to Macrolides and Ketolides

Erythromycin	Clarithromycin	Azithromycin	Talithromycin
Streptococcus pyogenes	More active against	Less active against *S. pyogenes*	Most active against *S. pyogenes*
Penicillin (PCN)–sensitive	*S. pyogenes*	Less active against PCN-sensitive	Active against some erythromycin-resistant strains
S. pneumoniae	More active against PCN-sensitive	*S. pneumoniae*	Active against multiresistant *S. pneumoniae*
Mouth flora including anaerobes, but not *Bacteroides fragilis*	*S. pneumoniae*	all pathogens covered by erythromycin, plus:	All pathogens covered by erythromycin, plus:
Neisseria gonorrhoeae	All pathogens covered by erythromycin, plus:	more active against *H. influenzae*	Most active against erythromycin-sensitive
Neisseria meningitides	*Haemophilus influenzae*	*Moraxella catarrhalis*	*S. aureus*
Campylobacter jejuni	*Moraxella catarrhalis*	Most active against *Legionella pneumophilia*	Good activity against *Enterococcus faecalis*, but not *Enterococcus faecium*
Bordetella pertussis	*Borrelia burgdorferi*	*M. avium* complex	
Legionella pneumophilia	*Mycoplasma leprae*	*Helicobacter pylori*	*H. influenzae*
Mycoplasma pneumoniae	*Mycobacterium avium* complex	*Plasmodium falciparum*	*Moraxella catarrhalis*
Ureaplasma urealyticum	*Toxoplasma gondii*		Poor activity against *M. avium* complex
Chlamydia trachomatis	*Helicobacter pylori*		
Chlamydophila pneumoniae			
Corynebacterium diphtheriae			
Bartonella quintana			

with the macro-lides, talithromycin binds to the 50S subunit with higher affinity, binding to two regions of the 23S rRNA molecule (domains II and V) rather than one region. This unique binding mode explains the enhanced antimicrobial activity of ketolides against macrolide-resistant pathogens.

TOXICITY

Macrolides and ketolides are among the safer classes of antibiotics (Table 1.10). The primary adverse reactions are related to these agents' ability to stimulate bowel motility. In fact, erythromycin can be used to treat gastric paresis. Particularly in younger patients, abdominal cramps, nausea, vomiting, diarrhea, and gas are common with erythromycin. These symptoms are dose-related and are more common with oral preparations, but can also occur with intravenous administration. Gastrointestinal toxicity can be debilitating, forcing the drug to be discontinued. Azithromycin and clarithromycin at the usual recommended doses are much less likely to cause these adverse reactions.

Talithromycin administration has been accompanied by difficulty with accommodation, resulting in blurred vision. Patients have also experienced diplopia following administration of this agent. Talithromycin treatment has also resulted in the sudden onset of severe and occasion-

ally fatal hepatitis. All patients receiving this agent should therefore be warned of this potential side effect, and the drug should be prescribed only for cases of pneumonia in which the incidence of penicillin-resistant *S. pneumoniae* is high. Under these circumstance a fluoroquinolone with gram-positive coverage may be preferred.

Macrolides and ketolides may exacerbate myasthenia gravis and should be avoided in patients with that illness. Macrolides prolong the QT interval, and erythromycin administration has, on rare occasions, been associated with ventricular tachycardia.

These agents are metabolized by the cytochrome P450 3A4 system, and they cause an increase in serum levels of other drugs metabolized by that system, including many of the statins, short-acting benzodiazepines, such as midazolam (Versed), cisapride (Propulsid), ritonavir (Norvir), and tacrolimus (Prograf).

PHARMACOKINETICS

The stearate, ethylsuccinate, and estolate forms of erythromycin are reasonably well absorbed on an empty stomach, reaching peak serum levels 3 hours after ingestion. Clarithromycin, azithromycin, and talithromycin are better absorbed orally than erythromycin is, resulting in peak concentrations within 1 hour. Erythromycin and azithromycin should be taken on an empty stomach. If cost is not a primary issue, the improved

<table>
</table>

KEY POINTS

KEY POINTS

About Macrolide Chemistry, Mechanism of Action, and Toxicity

1. Complex 14- to 15-member lactone ring structure.
2. Inhibit RNA-dependent protein synthesis, bind to 50S ribosomal subunit; talithromycin binds with higher affinity, binding to two sites rather than just one,
3. Can be bacteriostatic or cidal.
4. Gastrointestinal irritation, particularly with erythromycin, is the major toxicity.
5. Hypersensitivity reactions can occur.
6. Transient hearing loss with high doses, mainly in elderly individuals.
7. Talithromycin can cause blurred vision and diplopia. Also can result in fatal hepatitis.
8. Can exacerbate myasthenia gravis.
9. Prolonged QT interval; occasionally causes ventricular tachycardia.
10. Metabolized by the cytochrome P450 3A4 system; increase serum concentrations of other drugs metabolized by that system.

absorption and lower incidence of gastrointestinal toxicity make the three newer agents preferable to erythromycin in most instances (Table 1.11).

Most of the macrolides and ketolides are metabolized and cleared primarily by the liver. Azithromycin is not metabolized, being excreted unchanged in the bile. Small percentages of these drugs are also excreted in the urine. These agents are widely distributed in tissues, achieving concentrations that are several times the peak concentration achieved in serum in most areas the body, including the prostate and middle ear. Clarithromycin levels in middle ear fluid have been shown to be nearly 10 times serum levels. Azithromycin concentrations in tissue exceed serum levels by a factor of 10 to 100, and its average half-life in tissues is 2 to 4 days. Therapeutic levels of azithromycin have been estimated to persist for 5 days after the completion of a 5-day treatment course. With the exception of intravenous erythromycin, these agents fail to achieve significant levels in the cerebrospinal fluid.

SPECTRUM OF ACTIVITY AND TREATMENT RECOMMENDATIONS

Macrolides demonstrate excellent activity against most gram-positive organisms and some gram-negative

bacteria. Erythromycin can be bacteriostatic or bactericidal. Cidal activity increases when antibiotic concentrations are high and bacteria are growing rapidly.

These drugs are recommended for the treatment of community-acquired pneumonia (see Chapter 4). However S. pneumoniae resistance to macrolides has steadily increased and now ranges between 10% and 15%. Resistance is more likely in intermediately penicillin-resistant strains (40% macrolide resistant) and highly penicillin-resistant strains (60% macrolide resistance). Multiresistant S. pneumoniae can be treated with talithromycin as a consequence of that agent's different ribosomal binding sites.

In most countries, including the United States, 95% of S. pyogenes are sensitive to macrolides. However, in Japan, where macrolides are commonly used, 60% are resistant. Because S. aureus can develop resistance after a single mutation, macrolides are generally not recommended in their treatment. The macrolides and ketolides are effective against mouth flora, including anaerobes, but they do not cover the bowel anaerobe B. fragilis. The macrolides are also the treatment of choice for Legionella pneumophilia, with talithromycin, azithromycin, and clarithromycin being more potent than erythromycin.

Macrolides are the primary antibiotics used to treat the two major pathogens associated with atypical pneumonia: Mycoplasma pneumoniae and Chlamydophila pneumoniae (see Chapter 4). Talithromycin is also approved for acute bacterial sinusitis. In many instances the erythromycins can be used as an alternative to penicillin in the penicillin-allergic patient.

Clarithromycin is one of the primary antibiotics used for the treatment of atypical mycobacterial infections, particularly MAI complex. Azithromycin in combination with other antibiotics is also recommended for the treatment of MAI complex, and it can be used alone for MAI prophylaxis in HIV-infected patients with CD4 cell counts below 100 cells/mL.

In combination with antacid therapy, effective regimens for curing peptic ulcer disease caused by Helicobacter pylori include azithromycin or clarithromycin combined with bismuth salts and either amoxicillin, metronidazole, or tetracycline. Single high-dose azithromycin (1 g) effectively treats chancroid, as well as Chlamydia trachomatis urethritis and cervicitis. Single-dose therapy also cures male Ureaplasma urealyticum urethritis.

Clindamycin

CHEMISTRY AND MECHANISM OF ACTION

Although clindamycin is structurally different from erythromycin, many of its biologic characteristics are similar. Clindamycin consists of an amino acid linked to an amino sugar, and it was derived by modifying lincomycin. It binds to the same 50S ribosomal binding site used by the macrolides, blocking bacterial protein synthesis.

TOXICITY

Diarrhea is a major problem seen in 20% of patients taking clindamycin (Table 1.10). The incidence is highest with oral administration. In up to half of the affected patients, the cause of diarrhea is pseudomembranous colitis, a disease caused by overgrowth of the anaerobic bacteria *C. difficile* (see Chapter 8).

PHARMACOKINETICS

Clindamycin is well absorbed orally; however, the drug can also be administered intravenously and the intravenous route can achieve higher peak serum levels. Clindamycin penetrates most tissues, but it does not enter the cerebrospinal fluid. Clindamycin is metabolized primarily by the liver and is excreted in the bile. Therapeutic concentrations of clindamycin persist in the stool for 5 or more days after the antibiotic is discontinued, and the reduction of clindamycin-sensitive flora persists for up to 14 days. Small percentages of clindamycin metabolites are also excreted in the urine.

ANTIMICROBIAL SPECTRUM AND TREATMENT RECOMMENDATIONS

Clindamycin is similar to erythromycin in its activity against streptococci and staphylococci (Figure 1.5). Moderately penicillin-resistant *S. pneumoniae* are often sensitive to clindamycin. In the penicillin-allergic patient, clindamycin is a reasonable alternative for *S. pyogenes* pharyngitis. Because its activity against *H. influenzae* is limited, clindamycin is not recommended for the treatment of otitis media.

Clindamycin distinguishes itself from the macrolides by possessing excellent activity against most anaerobic bacteria. It is used effectively in combination with an aminoglycoside, aztreonam, or a third-generation cephalosporin to treat fecal soilage of the peritoneum. However, other less-toxic regimens have proved to be equally effective. Clindamycin in combination with a first-generation cephalosporin can be used to block toxin production in severe cellulitis and necrotizing fasciitis caused by MSSA or *S. pyogenes*. It is also effective for the treatment of anaerobic pulmonary and pleural infections. Clindamycin also has significant activity against *Toxoplasma gondii* and is recommended as alternative therapy in the sulfa-allergic patient.

Tetracyclines

CHEMISTRY AND MECHANISMS OF ACTION

The tetracyclines consist of four 6-member rings with substitutions at the 4, 5, 6, and 7 positions that alter the pharmacokinetics of the various preparations; however, with the exception of tigecycline, these changes have no effect on the antimicrobial spectrum. The tetracyclines enter gram-negative bacteria by passively diffusing through porins. They bind to the 30S ribosomal subunit and block tRNA binding to the mRNA ribosome complex. This blockade primarily inhibits protein synthesis in bacteria, but to a lesser extent, it also affects mammalian cell protein synthesis, particularly mitochondria. The inhibition of bacterial protein synthesis stops bacterial growth, but does not kill the bacterium. Therefore, tetracycline is termed a bacteriostatic agent.

TOXICITY

Photosensitivity reactions consisting of a red rash over sun-exposed areas can develop (Table 1.10). Hypersensitivity reactions are less common than with the penicillins, but they do occur. Tetracyclines interfere with enamel formation, and in children, teeth often become permanently discolored. Therefore these agents are not recommended for children 8 years of age or younger, or for pregnant women. Because the tetracyclines inhibit protein synthesis, they increase azotemia in renal failure patients. Minocycline can cause vertigo, and that side effect has limited its use. Benign intracranial hypertension (pseudotumor cerebri) is another rare neurologic side effect.

PHARMACOKINETICS

Tetracycline is reasonably well absorbed (70% to 80%) by the gastrointestinal tract (see Table 1.11). Food interferes with its absorption. Doxycycline is nearly completely absorbed in the gastrointestinal

tract. Calcium- or magnesium-containing antacids, milk, or multivitamins markedly impair absorption of all tetracycline preparations, and simultaneous ingestion of these products should be avoided. Tigecycline can be administered only intravenously. Tetracycline is cleared primarily by the kidneys; other agents, including doxycycline and tigecycline are cleared primarily by the liver.

ANTIMICROBIAL SPECTRUM AND TREATMENT RECOMMENDATIONS

The tetracyclines are able to inhibit the growth of a broad spectrum of bacteria (Table 1.13, Figure 1.5). However, for most conventional pathogens, other agents are more effective. High concentrations of tetracycline are achieved in the urine, and this agent can be used for uncomplicated urinary tract infections. Doxycycline combined with gentamicin is the treatment of choice for brucellosis. Tetracyclines are also recommended for the treatment of Lyme disease (*Borrelia burgdorferi*), and chlamydia infections (including *Chlamydia* pneumonia, psittacosis, epididymitis, urethritis, and endocervical infections). Tetracyclines are the treatment of choice for rickettsial infections (including Rocky Mountain spotted fever, ehrlichiosis, Q fever, and typhus fever). They are also often used in combination with other antibiotics for the treatment of pelvic inflammatory disease.

The most recently developed member of this family, tigecycline, was derived from minocycline. Tigecycline has a broader spectrum of activity. It effectively inhibits the growth of many resistant gram-positive bacteria (Table 1.13). This agent also

Table 1.13. Organisms That May Be Susceptible to the Tetracyclines

Tetra-, Doxy-, and Minocycline	Tigecycline
Vibrio spp.	Methicillin-resistant
Mycobacterium marinum	*Staphylococcus aureus (MRSA)*
Borrelia burgdorferi	Vancomycin intermediately resistant
Leptospira	*S. aureus (VISA)*
Chlamydia spp.	Vancomycin-resistant enterococci (VRE)
Rickettsia spp.	Penicillin-resistant *S. pneumoniae*
Brucella	*Acinetobacter baumannii* *Stenotrophomonas maltophilia*
	Enterobacteriaceae, including those with extended-spectrum β-lactamases *Bacteroides fragilis* *Clostridium perfringens* and *difficile*

demonstrates improved activity against many highly resistant nosocomial gram-negative bacteria, but it does not effectively cover *P. aeruginosa* or *Proteus* species. Tigecycline is approved for complicated intra-abdominal and soft-tissue infections.

Chloramphenicol

CHEMISTRY AND MECHANISMS OF ACTION

Chloramphenicol consists of a nitro group on a benzene ring and a side chain containing five carbons. Chloramphenicol uses an energy-dependent mechanism to enter bacteria, and once in the cell, binds to the larger 50S subunit of the 70S ribosome, blocking attachment of tRNA. It inhibits bacterial protein synthesis, making it bacteriostatic for most bacteria; however, chloramphenicol is cidal for *H. influenzae*, *S. pneumoniae*, and *N. meningitidis*.

TOXICITY

Probably as result of its binding to human mitochondrial ribosomes, this agent has significant bone marrow toxicity (see Table 1.10). Two forms are observed.

The first form is dose-related and is commonly observed in patients receiving chloramphenicol 4 g or more daily. The reticulocyte count decreases, and anemia develops in association with elevated serum iron. Leukopenia and thrombocytopenia are also commonly encountered. These changes reverse when the antibiotic is discontinued. The second form of marrow toxicity, irreversible aplastic anemia, is rare, but usually fatal. This complication can occur weeks or months after the antibiotic is discontinued. Any patient receiving chloramphenicol requires twice-weekly monitoring of peripheral blood counts. If the WBC drops below 2500/mm^3, the drug should be discontinued.

PHARMACOKINETICS

As a result of the much higher incidence of idiosyncratic aplastic anemia associated with oral administration as compared with intravenous administration, oral preparations of chloramphenicol are no longer available in the United States. The drug is well absorbed, and therapeutic serum levels can be achieved orally (Table 1.11). Chloramphenicol is metabolized by the liver. It diffuses well into tissues and crosses the blood–brain barrier in uninflamed as well as inflamed meninges. A serum assay is available, and serum levels should be monitored in patients with hepatic disease, maintaining the serum concentration between 10 and 25 µg/mL.

ANTIMICROBIAL SPECTRUM AND TREATMENT RECOMMENDATIONS

Chloramphenicol has excellent activity against most gram-positive organisms with the exception of enterococci and *S. aureus*, as well as many gram-negative pathogens (Figure 1.5). Chloramphenicol also is very active against spirochetes, as well as Rickettsiae, Chlamydiae, and mycoplasmas.

Because of its bone marrow toxicity, chloramphenicol is not considered the treatment of choice for any infection. Alternative, less-toxic agents are available for each indication. For the penicillin-allergic patient, chloramphenicol can be used for bacterial meningitis. Chloramphenicol can also be used as alternative therapy for brain abscess, *C. perfringens*, psittacosis, rickettsial infections including Rocky Mountain spotted fever, *Vibrio vulnificus*, and typhoid fever.

Quinolones

Tables 1.14 and 1.15, together with Figure 1.5, summarizes the characteristics of the quinolone antibiotics.

CHEMICAL STRUCTURE AND MECHANISMS OF ACTION

The quinolones all contain two 6-member rings (see Figure 1.7) with a nitrogen at position 1, a carbonyl group at position 4, and a carboxyl group attached to the carbon at position 3. Potency of the quinolones is greatly enhanced by adding fluorine at position 6, and gram-negative activity is enhanced by addition of a nitrogen-containing piperazine ring at position 7.

The quinolones inhibit two enzymes critical for DNA synthesis: DNA gyrase, which is important for regulating the superhelical twists of bacterial DNA, and topoisomerase IV, which is responsible for segregating newly

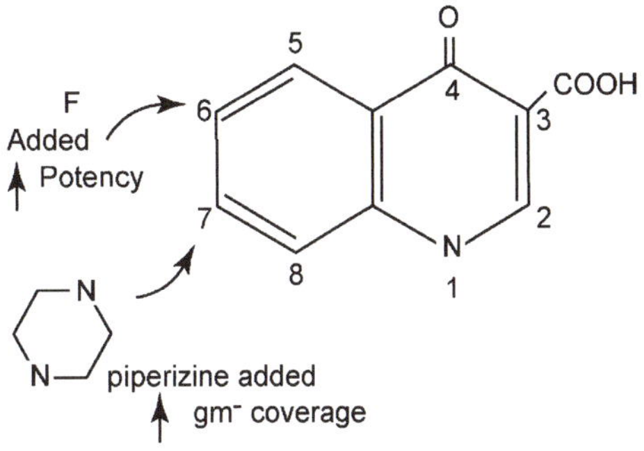

Figure 1–7. Basic structure of the quinolones.

formed DNA into daughter cells. The loss of these activities blocks DNA synthesis and results in rapid bacterial death. Killing is concentration-dependent.

TOXICITY

The most common side effects are mild anorexia, nausea, vomiting, and abdominal discomfort (Table 1.10). Quinolones can result in arthropathy because of cartilage damage and tendonitis. Although rare, this complication can be debilitating, but it usually reverses weeks to months after the quinolone is discontinued. Because of concerns about cartilage damage in children, quinolones are not recommended for routine administration in pediatric patients. Gatifloxacin administration can be associated with severe dysregulation of glucose homeostasis and can result in either severe hypo- or hyperglycemia. Fluoroquinolones are associated with a concentration-dependent delay in cardiac repolarization, causing a prolongation of the QT interval—a condition that can predispose to ventricular tachycardia. In combination with other agents that effect repolarization, moxifloxacin has occasionally been associated with life-threatening cardiac arrhythmias.

PHARMACOKINETICS

The quinolones are readily absorbed orally, but can also be given intravenously. Ciprofloxacin, levofloxacin, and gatifloxacin are cleared primarily by the kidneys. Moxifloxacin is also partially metabolized by the liver, and gemifloxacin is metabolized primarily by the liver. All quinolones demonstrate similar tissue penetration, being concentrated in prostate tissue, feces, bile, and lung tissue. These drugs tend to be very highly concentrated in macrophages and neutrophils.

SPECTRUM OF ACTIVITY AND TREATMENT RECOMMENDATIONS

Ciprofloxacin—Ciprofloxacin is the most potent quinolone for *P. aeruginosa* (Table 1.15, Figure 1.5). As a

---

KEY POINTS

About the Chemistry, Mechanisms of Action, and Toxicity of Quinolones

1. Inhibit bacterial DNA gyrase (important for coiling DNA) and topoisomerase (required to segregate DNA to daughter cells). Rapidly cidal, with concentration-dependent killing.

2. Main side effects are
   a) nausea and anorexia.
   b) allergic reactions (most common with gemifloxacin; less common with other quinolones).
   c) Arthropathy and tendonitis. May damage cartilage. Not routinely recommended in children.
   d) Gatifloxacin can cause hypo- or hyperglycemia.
   e) Moxifloxacin prolongs the QT interval.

Table 1.14. Quinolones, Linezolid, Quinupristin/Dalfopristin, Daptomycin, Metronidazole, and Sulfano-mides: Half-Life, Dosing, Renal Dosing, Cost, and Spectrum

Antibiotic (trade name)	Half-life (h)	Dose (loading/ maintenance)	Dose for reduced creatinine clearance (mL/min)	Cost[a]	Spectrum
Ciprofloxacin (Cipro)	4	250–750 mg PO q12h, or 200–400 mg IV q12h	10–50: q18h <10: q24h	PO: $$$ IV: $–$$	Moderately broad
Levofloxacin (Levoquin)	6–8	500 mg PO or IV q24h	10–50: 250 mg q24h <10: 250 mg q48h	PO: $$$ IV: $	Broad
Gatifloxacin (Tequin)	6–8	400 mg PO or IV q24h	10–50: 200 mg q24h <10: 200 mg q24h	PO: $$ IV: $	Very broad
Moxifloxacin (Avelox)	6–8	400 mg PO q24h	No change required	PO: $$ IV: $	Very broad
Gemifloxacin (Factive)	7	320 mg PO q24h	10–50: 160 mg q24h <10: 160 mg q24h	$$$$$	Broad
Linezolid (Zyvox)	5	600 mg PO or IV q12h	No change required	PO: $$$$$$ IV: $$$$	Narrow
Quinupristin/ dalfopristin (Synercid)	1.5	7.5 mg/kg IV q8–12h	No change required	$$$$$	Narrow
Daptomycin (Cubicin)	8–9	4 mg/kg IV q24h (soft-tissue infection) 6 mg/kg IV q24h (*Staphylococcus aureus* bacteremia)	<30: q48h	$$$$–$$$$$	Narrow
Metronidazole (Flagyl, Protostat, Metronid)	6–14	500 mg PO q8h, or 500 mg–1 g PO q12h 15 mg/kg followed by 7.5 mg/kg IV q6h or 15 mg/kg q12h (not to exceed 4 g)	No change required. In severe hepatic failure, half the dose.	$	Narrow
Sulfisoxazole		1–2 g PO q6h	10–50: 1 g q8–12h <10: 1 g q12–24h	$	Moderately Broad
Sulfadiazine		0.5–1.5 g PO q 4–6h	10–50: 0.5– 1.5 g q8–12h <10: 0.5–1.5 g q12–24h	$$	Moderately Broad
Trimethoprim– sulfamethoxazole		2–4 tablets q24h or 1–2 DS PO q24h Trimethoprim: 3–5 mg/kg IV q6–12h	Half the oral dose, and reduce the IV dose to 10–50: 3–5 mg/kg q12–24h <10: Don't give	$	Moderately Broad

[a] Intravenous preparations (daily cost dollars): $ = 20–70; $$ = 71–110; $$$ = 111–150; $$$$ = 150–200; $$$$$ ≥ 200; oral preparations (10-day course cost dollars): $ = 10–50; $$ = 51–100; $$$ = 101–140; $$$$ = 141–180; $$$$$ ≥ 180.

Table 1.15. Organisms That May Be Susceptible to the Quinolones

Ciprofloxacin	Levofloxacin, Gemifloxacin, Gatifloxacin, Moxifloxacin
Pseudomonas aeruginosa	Same as ciprofloxacin, plus:
Escherichia coli	Methicillin-sensitive
Enterobacter cloacae	Staphylococcus aureus
Proteus spp.	Streptococcus pneumoniae
Providencia	Vancomycin-sensitive Enterococcus
Salmonella, including Sal. typhi	Strep. pyogenes
Shigella spp.	Gatifloxacin and moxifloxacin: anaerobes
Yersinia spp.	
Campylobacter spp.	
Bacillus anthracis	
Mycoplasma pneumoniae	
Chlamydia spp.	
Ureaplasma urealyticum	
Bartonella henselae	
Neisseria gonorrhoeae	

result of an excellent gram-negative spectrum, ciprofloxacin is one of the primary antibiotics recommended for treatment of urinary tract infections. It concentrates in the prostate and is recommended for treatment of prostatitis. For gonococcal urethritis, it is a useful alternative to ceftriaxone. Ciprofloxacin has been used effectively for traveler's diarrhea most commonly caused by enterotoxigenic *E. coli* and *Shigella*. It is the drug of choice for *Salmonella typhi* (typhoid fever), and it also is recommended for treatment of *Salmonella* gastroenteritis when antibiotic treatment is necessary. Ciprofloxacin is the recommended treatment for cat scratch disease caused by *Bartonella henselae*.

Levofloxacin, Moxifloxacin, Gatifloxacin, and Gemifloxacin—These agents all demonstrate improved gram-positive coverage (Table 1.15, Figure 1.5) and have been recommended as one of the first-line treatments for community-acquired pneumonia in the otherwise healthy adult who does not require hospitalization. With the exception of gemifloxacin, these agents can also be used in soft-tissue infection in which a combination of gram-positive and gram-negative organisms is suspected. Given the worse toxicity profiles of the three newer agents (moxifloxacin, gatifloxacin, and gemifloxacin), levofloxacin should probably be the fluoroquinolone of choice for those infections. Gatifloxacin and moxifloxacin demonstrate moderate in vitro activity against anaerobes and may be considered for the treatment of mixed infections thought to include anaerobes. The exact indications for these agents are currently evolving. Fear of selecting for resistant pathogens has led to their use being restricted in some hospitals.

Oxazolidones (Linezolid)

CHEMISTRY AND MECHANISMS OF ACTION

The oxazolidones have a unique ring structure consisting of a 5-member ring containing an oxygen and a nitrogen. The nitrogen connects to a 6-member ring, and each specific compound has side chains added to both rings at positions A and B (Figure 1.8). These agents bind to the 50S ribosome at a site similar to that used by chloramphenicol. However, unlike chloramphenicol, they do not inhibit the attachment of tRNA, but instead block the initiation of protein synthesis by preventing the nearby 30S subunit from

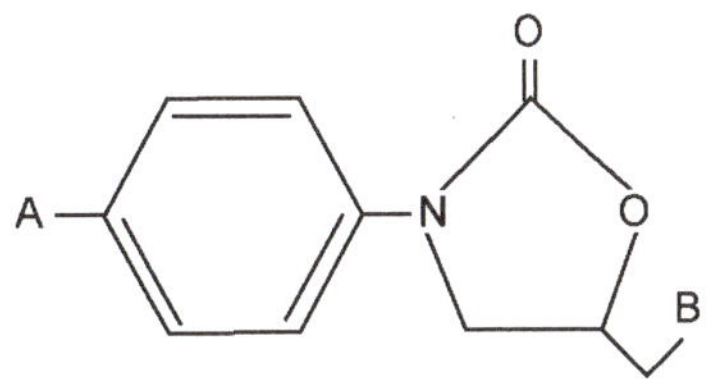

Figure 1–8. Basic structure of the oxazolidones.

KEY POINTS

About the Specific Quinolones

1. Ciprofloxacin:
   a) Excellent coverage of *Pseudomonas*. Also covers many other gram-negative organisms including *Esch. coli*, *Salmonella*, *Shigella*, *Neisseria*, and *Legionella*.
   b) Kills *Mycoplasma*, *Chlamydia*, and *Ureaplasma*.
   c) Recommended for urinary tract infections and prostatitis, gonococcal urethritis, traveler's diarrhea, typhoid fever, and *Salmonella* gastroenteritis; used for cat scratch disease.
2. Levofloxacin, gatifloxacin, moxifloxacin, gemifloxacin
   a) Greater activity against *Streptococcus pneumoniae*, covers highly penicillin-resistant strains.
   b) Also cover methicillin-sensitive *Staphylococcus aureus*.
   c) Recommended for community-acquired pneumonia (levofloxacin preferred).
   d) Levofloxacin, gatifloxacin, and moxifloxacin recommended for mixed skin infections.
   e) Gatifloxacin and moxifloxacin have somewhat improved anaerobic coverage.
   f) Gatifloxacin and moxifloxacin recommended for mixed skin infections.

KEY POINTS

About Linezolid

1. Like chloramphenicol, binds to the 50S ribosome subunit; inhibits the initiation of protein synthesis.
2. Thrombocytopenia common with treatment exceeding 2 weeks; inhibitor of monoamine oxidase; avoid tyramine, pseudoephedrine, serotonin uptake inhibitors.
3. Strictly gram-positive activity; bacteriostatic activity for vancomycin-resistant enterococci (VRE), and methicillin-resistant *Staphylococcus aureus*. Also has activity against penicillin-resistant *Streptococcus pneumoniae*.
4. Recommended for the treatment of VRE.

forming the 70S initiation complex. The oxazolidones are bacteriostatic against staphylococcal species and enterococci.

TOXICITY

Linezolid is the only agent in this class released for use. Reversible thrombocytopenia has been reported in association with prolonged therapy, and monitoring of platelet count is recommended for patients receiving two or more weeks of linezolid. Leukopenia and hepatic enzyme elevations have also been reported. Because this agent is a weak inhibitor of monoamine oxidase, hypertension has been reported in association with ingestion of large amounts of tyramine. Pseudoephedrine and selective serotonin reuptake inhibitors should be prescribed with caution.

PHARMACOKINETICS

Linezolid is well-absorbed orally, and peak serum levels are achieved in 1 to 2 hours. Food slows absorption, but does not lower peak levels. An intravenous preparation is also available. Linezolid achieves excellent penetration of all tissue spaces, including the cerebrospinal fluid. The drug is partly metabolized by the liver and excreted in the urine.

ANTIMICROBIAL ACTIVITY AND TREATMENT RECOMMENDATIONS

Linezolid demonstrates activity only against gram-positive organisms. It has bacteriostatic activity against both vancomycin-resistant *Enterococcus faecium* and *Enterococcus faecalis (VRE)*. This agent is also active against MSSA and MRSA, and has activity against penicillin-resistant *S. pneumoniae*. Linezolid is recommended primarily for the treatment of VRE.

Streptogramins

CHEMICAL STRUCTURE AND MECHANISM OF ACTION

The streptogramins belong to the macrolide family. They are derived from pristinamycin. Quinupristin is a peptide derived from pristinamycin IA and dalfopristin is derived from pristinamycin IIB. A combination of 30:70 quinupristin:dalfopristin has synergistic activity and has been named Synercid. These two agents inhibit bacterial protein synthesis by binding to the 50S bacterial ribosome. Quinupristin inhibits peptide chain elongation, and dalfopristin interferes with peptidyl transferase activity.

TOXICITY

Myalgias and arthralgias are the most common and severe adverse reaction, and they can force discontinuation of the drug (Table 1.10). Administration has also been associated with hyperbilirubinemia.

PHARMACOKINETICS

The streptogramins are administered intravenously, and they are metabolized primarily in the liver (Table 1.14).

ANTIMICROBIAL ACTIVITY AND TREATMENT INDICATIONS

Synercid is active primarily against gram-positive organisms (Figure 5.1). It has proved to be efficacious in the treatment of VRE and MRSA. Synercid or linezolid are the treatments of choice for VRE.

Daptomycin

CHEMICAL STRUCTURE AND MECHANISM OF ACTION

Daptomycin is a large cyclic lipopeptide ($C_{72}H_{101}N_{17}O_{26}$) with a molecular weight of 1620 that was derived from *Streptomyces roseosporus*. Daptomycin has a mechanism of action that is distinctly different from that of other antibiotics. It binds to bacterial membranes and causes rapid depolarization of the membrane potential. As a result, protein, DNA, and RNA synthesis is inhibited. This antibiotic is cidal and causes rapid concentration-dependent killing, but it does not result in the systemic release of cell membrane or cell wall contents. It also demonstrates significant post-antibiotic effect. Synergy with aminoglycosides, β-lactam antibiotics, and rifampin has been observed.

TOXICITY

Muscle pain and weakness are reported in less than 5% of patients. This drug is also associated with a rise

in creatine phosphokinase (CPK; Table 1.10). The patient's CPK levels should be monitored weekly, and the drug should be discontinued if CPK exceeds 1000 in association with symptoms of myopathy, or if CPK exceeds 2000 in the absence of symptoms. Other drugs associated with rhabdomyolysis, specifically HMG-CoA reductase inhibitors (statins), should not be administered with daptomycin. Less commonly, daptomycin administration has resulted in neuropathy associated with a slowing of nerve conduction velocity. The peripheral or cranial nerves can be affected. Patients may experience paresthesia or Bell's palsy. This rare toxicity has also been observed in animal studies.

PHARMACOKINETICS

Daptomycin is given intravenously, and a 4-mg/kg dose achieves peak serum levels of 58 µg/mL (Table 1.14). Daptomycin is 92% protein-bound and is excreted by the kidneys. Its ability penetrate various tissue compartments including the cerebrospinal fluid has not been extensively studied.

SPECTRUM OF ACTIVITY AND TREATMENT RECOMMENDATIONS

Daptomycin kills aerobic and facultative gram-positive organisms, including *Enterococcus faecium* and *faecalis* (including VREs), *S. aureus* (including MRSA), *S. epidermidis* (including methicillin-resistant strains),

S. pyogenes, and *Corynebacterium jeikeium* (Figure 1.5). It is approved for the treatment of complicated skin and soft?tissue infections by susceptible strains and for *S. aureus* (including MRSA) bacteremia and right-sided endocarditis. It is not currently approved for VRE, because of insufficient clinical data. Daptomycin is inactivated by surfactant and should not be used for the treatment of pneumonia.

Metronidazole

CHEMICAL STRUCTURE AND MECHANISM OF ACTION

Metronidazole is a nitroimidazole with a low molecular weight that allows it to readily diffuse into tissues. Within a bacterium, this antibiotic acts as an electron acceptor and is quickly reduced. The resulting free radicals are toxic to the bacterium, producing damage to DNA and to other macromolecules. Metronidazole has significant activity against anaerobes.

TOXICITY

Metronidazole is usually well tolerated, but it can result in a disulfiram (Antabuse–like) reaction with alcohol consumption (Table 1.10). Concern about the mutagenic potential of this agent has resulted in multiple mammalian studies that, overall, have failed to demonstrate significant DNA abnormalities. Metronidazole is not recommended in pregnancy, and it should usually be avoided in patients on Coumadin, because it impairs metabolism of that drug.

KEY POINTS

About Metronidazole

1. Electron acceptor; produces free radicals that damage bacterial DNA.

2. Antabuse-like reaction can occur; mutagenic effects not proven in mammals, but the drug should be avoided in pregnancy. Impairs Coumadin metabolism.

3. Excellent activity against anaerobes, amoebae, *Giardia*, and *Trichomonas*. Penetrates tissues well, including abscesses.

4. Indicated in combination with other antibiotics for mixed bacterial infections. Has no activity against aerobic bacteria.

5. Treatment of choice for *Clostridium difficile*-induced diarrhea. Used as part of combination treatment for *Helicobacter pylori*.

PHARMACOKINETICS

This agent is rapidly and completely absorbed orally, but it can also be given intravenously. Therapeutic levels are achieved in all body fluids, including the cerebrospinal fluid and brain abscess contents. Metronidazole is metabolized primarily in the liver.

SPECTRUM OF ACTIVITY AND TREATMENT RECOMMENDATIONS

Metronidazole was originally used primarily for *Trichomonas* vaginitis, being effective both topically and orally. It is also effective for treating amoebic abscesses and giardiasis. Metronidazole is cidal for most anaerobic bacteria, and it is the antibiotic of choice for covering anaerobes. Because metronidazole has no significant activity against aerobes, it is usually administered in combination with a cephalosporin for aerobic coverage. Metronidazole is the drug of choice for treatment of pseudomembranous colitis attributable to overgrowth of *C. difficile*. Metronidazole is also recommended as part of the regime for *Helicobacter pylori* gastric and duodenal infection.

Sulfonamides and Trimethoprim

CHEMICAL STRUCTURE AND MECHANISMS OF ACTION

The sulfonamides all have a structure similar to para-aminobenzoic acid (PABA), a substrate required for bacterial folic acid synthesis (Figure 1.9). All sulfonamides inhibit bacterial folic acid synthesis by competitively inhibiting PABA incorporation into tetrahydropteroic acid. These agents are bacteriostatic.

A sulfonyl radical is attached to carbon 1 of the 6-member ring, increasing PABA inhibition. Alterations in the sulfonyl radical determine many of the pharmacokinetic properties of the compounds. Trime-thoprim consists of two 6-member rings, one of which has two nitrogens and two amino groups, the other having three methoxybenzyl groups. This agent strongly inhibits dihydrofolate reductase and complements sulfonamide inhibition of folate metabolism (Figure 1.9). Inhibition of bacterial dihydrofolate reductase by trimethoprim is 100,000 times that of the agent's inhibition of the mammalian enzyme, minimizing toxicity to the patient.

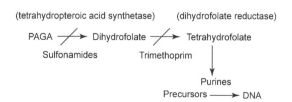

Figure 1–9. Effects of sulfonamides and trimethoprim on the bacterial folate pathway.

Table 1.16. Organisms That May Be Susceptible to Trimethoprim/Sulfa

Usually susceptible	Some susceptible
Streptococcus pyogenes	Staphylococcus aureus
Listeria monocytogenes	(including community-acquired
Bacillus anthracis	methicillin-resistant strains)
Shigella spp.	Strepococcus pneumoniae
Haemophilus influenzae	Proteus mirabilis
Neisseria meningitidis	Klebsiella spp.
Chlamydia trachomatis	Salmonella
Burkholderia cepacia	Neisseria gonorrhoeae
Stenotrophomonas maltophilia	
Yersinia enterocolitica	
Nocardia spp.	

TOXICITY

Hypersensitivity reactions represent the most severe toxicity (Table 1.10). Maculopapular drug rashes, erythema multiforme, Steven–Johnson syndrome, vasculitis (including drug-induced lupus), serum sickness-like syndrome, and anaphylaxis have been reported. Hemolytic anemia can be associated with glucose-6-phosphate dehydrogenase (G6PD) deficiency. Sulfonamides should be avoided in the last month of pregnancy because they displace bilirubin bound to plasma albumin and increase fetal blood levels of unconjugated bilirubin.

PHARMACOKINETICS

Sulfonamides are classified as short-, medium-, or long?acting, depending on half-life. Sulfisoxazole is in the short-acting class, having a half-life of 5 to 6 hours. Sulfamethoxazole and sulfadiazine are medium-acting. All of these agents are generally well absorbed orally. Intravenous preparations are available for some agents. All are metabolized by the liver, undergoing acetylation and glucuronidation, with the metabolites being excreted in the urine. Trimethoprim is excreted primarily by the renal tubules, and very high concentrations of active drug are found in the urine. Some trimethoprim is also excreted in bile. The half-life of trimethoprim is 9 to 11 hours matching the half-life of sulfamethoxazole. The ratio of trimethoprim to sulfamethoxazole supplied is 1:5.

SPECTRUM OF ACTIVITY AND TREATMENT RECOMMENDATIONS

The sulfonamides demonstrate activity against gram-positive and gram-negative organisms; however, resistance in both community and nosocomial strains is widespread (Table 1., Figure 1.5). Sulfonamides have proved to be effective for the empiric treatment of uncomplicated urinary tract infections; however, because of widespread resistance, they are seldom used as empiric therapy in other infections. Sulfonamides are the treatment of choice for *Nocardia asteroides*, and are useful in combination with other agents for the treatment of *M. kansasii*.

Trimethoprim is generally administered in combination with sulfamethoxazole. This combination often

---

KEY POINTS

About Sulfonamides

1. Competitively inhibit para-aminobenzoic acid incorporation, blocking folic acid synthesis; trimethoprim inhibits dihydrofolate reductase, potentiating sulfonamide activity.

2. Hypersensitivity reactions (including Steven–Johnson syndrome) are common; hemolytic anemia seen in G6PD-deficient patients. Agranulocytosis and thrombocytopenia are less common.

3. Broad spectrum of activity for gram-positive and gram-negative organisms, but resistance is common.

4. Used for initial therapy of uncomplicated urinary tract infections. Treatment of choice for *Nocardia*.

5. Trimethoprim–sulfamethoxazole combination is the drug of choice for *Pneumocystis* prophylaxis and treatment.

results in significantly improved activity. Trimethoprim–sulfamethoxazole (TMP-SMX) demonstrates excellent activity against *Listeria monocytogenes*, and it is the antibiotic of choice in the penicillin-allergic patient with listeriosis. It can be used to treat a number of other gram-positive and gram-negative pathogens. However, plasmid-mediated resistance is common, and treatment for most pathogens should be initiated only after sensitivity is confirmed by microbiologic testing. This combination is highly effective for killing *Pneumocystis carinii*, and TMP-SMX is the drug of choice for treatment or prophylaxis of that infection in immunocompromised hosts, including patients with AIDS.

ANTIFUNGAL AGENTS

Fungi are eukaryotes, and they share many of the structural and metabolic characteristics of human cells. As a result, designing agents that affect fungi without harming human cells has proved difficult. One major difference between the two cell types is the primary sterol building block used to form the plasma membrane. The fungal plasma membrane consists of ergosterols; the major sterol component of the human plasma membrane is cholesterol. This difference has been exploited in the development of two classes of drugs. The polyenes act by binding to ergosterol and disrupting the fungal membrane. These agents are fungicidal. The azoles inhibit ergosterol synthesis, and lowered ergosterol levels results in fungal membrane breakdown. These agents are usually fungistatic.

> ### THE MAJOR DIFFERENCE BETWEEN MAMMALIAN AND FUNGAL CELLS
>
> *Like mammals, fungi are eukaryotes. Drug therapy takes advantage of fact that fungi use ergosterols rather than cholesterol as the major building block of their plasma membrane.*

Agents for Treatment of Systemic Fungal Infections

AMPHOTERICIN B

Chemical Structure, Mechanism of Action, and Spectrum of Activity—Amphotericin B is a long, cyclic polyene compound that forms a large rod-like structure. Multiple molecules bind to ergosterol in the fungal membrane, forming pores that result in leakage of

> ### KEY POINTS
>
> ### About the Mechanism of Action and Spectrum of Amphotericin B
>
> 1. Polyene compound forms rod-like structures that bind to ergosterol in the fungal membrane, forming pores that result in a leak of intracellular potassium.
> 2. Rapidly cidal; does not require active growth.

intracellular potassium and in fungal cell death. This fungicidal action is rapid and does not require active growth.

Toxicity—Nephrotoxicity is the major complication associated with the conventional deoxycholate form of amphotericin B. This agent causes vasoconstriction of renal arterioles, resulting in a reduction in glomerular filtration rate. Vasoconstriction also impairs proximal and distal tubular reabsorption, causing potassium, magnesium, and bicarbonate wasting. These effects are reversible. However, permanent loss of nephrons and permanent damage to tubular basement membranes are also observed and correlate with the total dose administered. Renal dysfunction is observed in virtually all patients receiving this drug, and serum creatinine levels of 2 to 3 mg/dL are to be expected. Hydration with normal saline before infusion reduces nephrotoxicity.

Fever is commonly associated with administration of amphotericin B, and fever can be associated with chills and tachypnea, particularly if the drug is infused too rapidly. This agent should be infused slowly [2 to 3 hours for the deoxycholate form (ABD) and under 2 hours for the lipid preparations]. Fever and chills usually diminish with each subsequent dose. However, if those reactions persist, the patient can be premedicated with acetaminophen or 25 to 50 mg hydrocortisone can be added to the solution. This febrile reaction does not represent an allergic reaction and should not be misinterpreted as anaphylaxis. A 1 mg test dose preceding administration of the full dose has not proved to be helpful, and use of a test dose delays achievement of therapeutic antifungal serum and tissue levels. Because of a high incidence of phlebitis, amphotericin B should be administered through a centrally placed intravenous line.

Pharmacokinetics—At physiologic pH, ABD is insoluble in water (Table 1.17). It is stored as a powder that is dispersed as colloidal suspension in a 5% dextrose solution. Following intravenous infusion, amphotericin B is bound to lipoproteins in the serum and then leaves the circulation. The drug is stored in the

Table 1.17. Toxicities of Systemic Antifungal Agents

Key: ● = principle side effect (black); ◐ = less common side effect (dark gray); ○ = rare side effect (light gray); blank = not reported or very rare.

Clinical symptom	Amphotericin B	Amphotericin B lipid	Flucytosine	Fluconazole	Itraconazole	Ketoconazole	Voriconazole	Posaconazole	Caspofungin
Allergic skin rash	○	○	◐	◐	●	◐	◐	○	○
Anaphylaxis	○	○		○	○	○		○	
Stevens–Johnson				○					
Pruritus									○
Hypotension	○	○							
Fever and chills	●	●				○			○
Nausea and vomiting	◐	◐	◐	◐	◐	●	◐	◐	◐
Diarrhea			●	◐		◐		◐	
Headache	◐	◐	◐	◐	◐	◐	◐	◐	
Seizures	○			○					
Visual disturbances			◐	◐		◐	●		
Other neurotoxicity	○		◐	◐		◐	●	○	
Phlebitis	●								
Alopecia (reversible)			●	●					
Adrenal insufficiency						○			
Gynecomastia						◐			
Impotence						◐			
Leg edema					○				
Laboratory tests:									
Renal tubular acidosis	●	○							
Proteinuria									○
Hypokalemia	●	○							
Creatinine↑	●	◐							
Anemia	●								
Other cytopenias	○		◐			○		○	
Eosinophilia	○								
AST/ALT↑	○		○	○	●	●	◐	○	
ALP↑								○	
Drug–drug interactions				○	◐	●	●	◐	

Black = principle side effect; dark gray = less common side effect; light gray = rare side effect; white = not reported or very rare; ↑ = rise; AST/ALT = aspartate aminotransferase/alanine transaminase; ALP = alkaline phosphatase.

liver and other organs and subsequently released into the circulation.

Lipid-associated amphotericin B is ingested by macrophages, resulting in high intracellular levels in that cell type. This drug shows poor penetration of the blood–brain barrier and brain. Therapeutic levels are detectable in inflamed pleural fluid, peritoneum, and joint fluid. Amphotericin B is degraded slowly, and degradation is not affected by hepatic or renal dysfunction. Serum concentrations of the drug are detectable 7 weeks after therapy is discontinued.

Spectrum of Activity—Amphotericin B is effective against most fungal infections and remains the most

effective agent for systemic fungal infections. Clinical resistance to amphotericin B has been demonstrated among *Candida lusitaniae*, *Fusarium* species, and *Pseudalles-cheria boydii*. *C. lusitaniae* initially is susceptible to amphotericin B, but develops resistance during treatment. The alterations in sterol structure required for amphotericin B resistance often reduce tissue invasiveness, such strains being capable of growing only on mucosal surfaces or in the urine.

Efficacy of Various Amphotericin B Preparations—Lipid-associated preparations of amphotericin B are preferred because of their lower nephrotoxicity. However, these preparations are very expensive (Table 1.18) and

Table 1.18. Systemic Antifungal Agents: Half-Life, Dosing, Renal Dosing, and Cost

Antifungal (trade name)	Half-life (h)	Dose	Dose for reduced creatinine clearance (mL/min)	Cost[a]
Amphotericin B deoxycholate (Fungizone)	15 d	0.3–1.0 mg/kg IV q24h (infuse over 4–6 h)	No change required	$
Amphotericin B lipid preparations (Abelcet, Amphotec, AmBisome)	7 d	3–5 mg/kg IV q24h	No change required	$$$$$
Fluconazole (Diflucan)	20–50	100–200 mg PO q12–24h 200–400 mg IV q24h	10–50: Half the dose <10: One quarter to half the dose	$$–$$$
Ketoconazole (Nizoral)	1–4	200–400 mg PO q12–24h	No change required	$–$$$
Itraconazole (Sporanox)	20–60	100–200 mg PO q12–24h 200 mg IV q12h × 4, then 200 mg q24h	<30: Contraindicated	$$$$–$$$$$
Posaconazole (Noxafil)	35	200 mg PO q6h, or 400 mg PO q12h	No change required	$$$$$
Voriconazole (Vfend)	Nonlinear kinetics	200 mg PO q12h 6 mg/kg IV q12h × 2, then 4 mg/kg q12h	<50: IV not recommended; switch to oral	$$$$$
Anidulafungin (Eraxis)	10–15	200 mg IV, then 100 mg q24h	No change required	$$$$
Caspofungin (Cancidas)	9–11	70 mg IV, then 50 mg q24h	No change required	$$$$$
Micafungin (Mycamine)	14–17	150 mg IV q24h	No change required	$$$$$
Flucytosine (Ancobon)	3–6	25–33 mg/kg PO q6h	10–50: 25 mg/kg q12–24h 25 mg/kg q24h (<10)	$$$$$

[a] Intravenous preparations (daily cost dollars): $ = 20–70; $$ >71–110; $$$ = 111–150; $$$$ = 150–200; $$$$$ ≥ 200; oral preparations (10-day course cost dollars): $ = 10–50; $$ = 51–100; $$$ = 101–140; $$$$ = 141–180; $$$$$ ≥ 180.

in most clinical trials have comparable efficacy to amphotericin-B deoxycholate. Liposomal amphotericin B was shown to be superior to ABD for the treatment of pulmonary histoplasmosis. The lipid-associated preparations are recommended in patients with significant preexisting renal dysfunction or in patients who develop progressive renal failure (serum creatinine above 2.5 mg/dl) while being treated ABD. Clinicians also need to be aware of the observation that ABD-related

renal dysfunction (50% increase in baseline creatinine to a minimum of 2 mg/ml) is associated with a 6.6-fold increased risk of death.

AZOLES

Chemical Structure and Mechanism of Action—The azoles are chemically synthesized agents that come in two classes. The first to be synthesized were the imidazoles (miconazole and ketoconazole). Those compounds are now seldom used for systemic infections, being primarily reserved for topical treatment of superficial fungal infections. The second class, the triazoles, are preferred for systemic fungal infection; they are well absorbed orally and have excellent toxicity profiles.

All azoles inhibit a cytochrome P450–dependent demethylation system that results in decreased production of ergosterol and accumulation of intermediate sterols. The loss of ergosterol results in altered fungal membrane permeability, disturbed activity of membrane surface enzymes, and retention of metabolites. These agents have broad antifungal activity, but they demonstrate fungistatic rather than fungicidal activity. Itraconazole can antagonize amphotericin B activity by reducing its binding target, ergosterol.

Toxicity—Ketoconazole not only interferes with fungal sterol metabolism, but at higher doses it also interferes with testosterone and cortisone production (Table 1.17). Gynecomastia and loss of libido are commonly observed. Severe hepatitis can develop during treatment with this agent. As a result of its many toxicities, ketoconazole is rarely prescribed today.

The triazoles (fluconazole, itraconazole, posaconazole, voriconazole) demonstrate minimal toxicity. Side effects include headache, gastrointestinal intolerance, and asymptomatic increases in serum transaminase levels. Voriconazole infusion can be associated with transient loss of light perception. This symptom resolves with subsequent doses. Visual hallucinations less commonly occur.

Pharmacokinetics—Fluconazole is well absorbed orally, and serum levels after ingestion of the oral preparation are comparable to those with intravenous administration. Penetration into tissues and body fluids, including the cerebrospinal fluid, is excellent. Itraconazole is more variable in its oral absorption and requires stomach acidity for adequate absorption. Capsule absorption is enhanced by food and reduced by agents that reduce stomach acidity. Itraconazole penetrates most tissues, but does not cross the blood–brain barrier and enters ocular fluids only minimally. Posaconazole oral absorption is enhanced by food, particularly high-fat meals or liquid nutritional supplements. Voriconazole is well absorbed orally, demonstrating 96% bioavailability, and also can be given intravenously.

All of the azoles are metabolized by the liver via the cytochrome P450 system, and as a consequence, drug–drug interactions are common with these agents. Rifampin, rifabutin, long-acting barbiturates, carbamazepine, and cisapride usually lower azole levels. The azoles slow the metabolism of Coumadin, warfarin, phenytoin, tacrolimus, cyclosporine, certain antihistamines, benzodiazepines, calcium channel blockers, sulfonylureas, prednisolone, digoxin, statins, and anti-HIV protease inhibitors. The doses of these agents usually need to be lowered in the presence of azoles. Drug–drug interactions have proven to be the most problematic with voriconazole. Voriconazole is metabolized primarily by the P450 enzyme CYP2C19, and that enzyme has variable activity depending on the

---

> ## KEY POINTS
>
> ### About the Spectrum of Activity and Indications for Fluconazole
>
> 1. No activity against *Aspergillus*. Active against *Candida albican*, but natural resistance in *C. glabrata* and *C. krusei* is common. Active against Cryptococcus neoformans.
> 2. With prolonged treatment, drug resistance can develop in *Candida* species.
> 3. Treatment of choice for oral candidiasis and *Candida* vulvovaginitis.
> 4. Can be used for uncomplicated *C. albicans* fungemia in the non-immunocompromised patient.
> 5. Can be used to complete therapy of cryptococcal meningitis in HIV patients after an initial course of amphotericin B.
> 6. Prophylaxis reduces *Candida* infections in neutropenic patients. The role of prophylaxis in other settings remains controversial because of the risk of selecting for resistant strains.

patient's genetic background. As a consequence, serum levels can vary by up to a factor of 4 in individuals with rapid as opposed to slow metabolism. In the United States, the co-administration of rifabutin and voriconazole is contraindicated because rifabutin levels may increase by a factor of 3, while voriconazole levels drop below therapeutic levels. Rifampin, carbamazepines, and long-acting barbiturates can also markedly reduce voriconazole levels, and these drugs should probably be discontinued when voriconazole is being administered.

Spectrum of Activity and Treatment Recommendations—Fluconazole—Fluconazole has no activity against *Aspergillus* species, and some strains of *Candida*, including *C. glabrata* and *C. krusei*, demonstrate natural resistance. Because of increased production of demethylase and increased drug efflux, any *Candida* species can develop resistance.

Fluconazole is recommended for the treatment of oropharyngeal and vulvovaginal candidiasis. Intravenous fluconazole has proved therapeutically equivalent to amphotericin B in uncomplicated candidemia in the non-immunocompromised host. However, for the immunocompromised (including neutropenia) host, and for seriously ill patients with deep tissue *Candida* infection, amphotericin B or caspofungin should be used. Fluconazole is also effective for

---

> ## KEY POINTS
>
> ### About Azole Toxicity
>
> 1. Ketoconazole interferes with testosterone and cortisone production, resulting in gynecomastia and loss of libido. Hepatitis can be severe, and the drug should be discontinued when symptoms of hepatitis develop. Liver function tests should be performed.
> 2. Rare side effects of fluconazole, itraconazole, posaconazole, and voriconazole include headache, gastrointestinal intolerance, asymptomatic elevation of serum transaminases.
> 3. Intravenous infusion of voriconazole can be associated with transient loss of light perception.
> 4. Drug–drug interactions with other agents metabolized by the cytochrome P450 system are common, particularly with voriconazole and ketoconazole.

completing the treatment of cryptococcal meningitis in patients with AIDS. After initial therapy with amphotericin B, with or without flucytosine, for 2 weeks, fluconazole (400 mg daily) treatment for 2 months, followed by daily fluconazole maintenance therapy (200 mg daily), is recommended. The role of fluconazole in patients with non-AIDS-related cryptococcal infection has not been defined.

The use of fluconazole for prevention of fungal infections has been explored in neutropenic allogeneic bone marrow transplant patients and was found to reduce mortality and the incidence of invasive *Candida* infections, but no effect on the incidence of *Aspergillus* infections was observed. Fluconazole prophylaxis of leukemia patients also reduced the incidence of invasive *Candida* infections, but had no effect on mortality. Fluconazole is frequently used in the surgical intensive care unit in the hopes of preventing candidemia in patients. To date, such prophylaxis has not been proved to significantly reduce *Candida* infections, and this practice increases the prevalence of fluconazole-resistant fungi, including *C. krusei* and *C. glabrata*. Because of the risk of selecting for resistant fungi, fluconazole prophylaxis is not recommended in patients infected with HIV.

Itraconazole—As compared with fluconazole, itraconazole has demonstrated improved activity against histoplasmosis, coccidiomycosis, blastomycosis, and sporotrichosis. Itraconazole can be used for acute and chronic vaginal candidiasis and HIV-associated oral and esophageal candidiasis, and for consolidation and maintenance therapy for cryptococcal meningitis in patients with AIDS. Itraconazole is the preferred agent for the treatment of lymphocutaneous sporotrichosis and of non-meningeal, non-life-threatening histoplasmosis, blastomycosis, and coccidiomycosis. For disseminated histoplasmosis and coccidiomycosis, amphotericin B remains the treatment of choice. Itraconazole is recommended as primary prophylaxis and for the prevention of relapse of histoplasmosis in patients with AIDS.

Voriconazole and Posaconazole—As compared with amphotericin B deoxycholate, voriconazole demonstrates increased activity against *Aspergillus* and has proven to be superior for the treatment of invasive aspergillosis. Voriconazole is also approved for the treatment of *Fusarium* and *Scedosporium*. Clinical trials exploring the efficacy of voriconazole for invasive candidiasis are currently under way.

The newest azole, posaconazole, has the broadest spectrum in the class. In addition to being effective against *Aspergillus*, this agent has activity against many of the *Zygomycetes*. Posaconazole is currently approved as salvage therapy for mucormycosis.

CASPOFUNGIN/ANIDULAFUNGIN/MICAFUNGIN

Chemical Structure and Mechanism of Action—The echinocandins are all derived from echinocandin B, a semisynthetic lipopeptide that blocks synthesis of β-(1,3)-D-glucan. That polysaccharide is a critical component of the cell wall in many pathogenic fungi.

Toxicity—The echinocandins have proven to be very safe, provoking only the occasional fever, rash, or flushing of the face during infusion (Table 1.17). Serum levels are increased by co-administration of cyclosporin. Agents that may reduce serum levels including efavirenz, nelfinavir, Dilantin, Tegretol, rifampin, and dexamethasone. The echinocandins can reduce serum levels of tacrolimus.

Pharmacokinetics—The echinocandins are not absorbed by the gastrointestinal tract and must be administered intravenously (Table 1.18). They are metabolized by the liver.

Spectrum of Activity and Treatment Indications— The echinocandins are active against *Aspergillus* and *Candida*, including isolates that are resistant to other antifungal agents. They are less effective against *C. parapsilosis* in vitro, and are not active against *Cryptococcus*. They are approved for the treatment of invasive aspergillosis in patients who fail on, or are unable to tolerate, amphotericin B or itraconazole.

Caspofungin can also be used to treat oral candidiasis that is refractory to azole or amphotericin B therapy.

FLUCYTOSINE

Chemical Structure and Mechanism of Action—Flucytosine, or 5-fluorocytosine (5-FC), is a fluorine analog of cytosine. After a multi-step conversion requiring deamination and phosphorylation, the resulting product, 5-fluorouracil (5-FU) acts as an inhibitor of thymidylate synthetase, impairing DNA and RNA synthesis. In humans, 5-FC is not toxic because of a lack of the deaminase required for conversion to 5-FU.

Toxicity—The major toxicity of flucytosine is bone marrow suppression leading to neutropenia, anemia, and thrombocytopenia (Table 1.17). This side effect is dose-related and usually occurs when serum levels exceed 125 μg/mL. Patients with diminished bone marrow reserve such as those with AIDS and those receiving cancer chemotherapy are more likely to suffer this complication. Commonly, 5-FC is administered in combination with amphotericin B. As discussed earlier in this chapter, amphotericin B impairs renal function, and reductions in renal function reduce the clearance of 5-FC. In patients

Table 1.19. Spectrum of the Systemic Antifungals

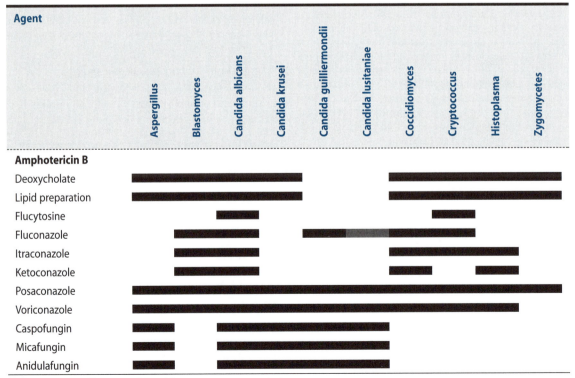

Dark gray = usually susceptible; white = not recommended.

KEY POINTS

About Flucytosine

1. Impairs fungal DNA and RNA synthesis; fungistatic.
2. Cleared by the kidneys; penetrates all tissues and fluids, including the cerebrospinal fluid.
3. High levels cause bone marrow suppression. In patients with renal failure, doses should be adjusted, and serum levels should be monitored.
4. Never use as monotherapy. In cryptococcal meningitis, the combination of amphotericin B and flucytosine sterilize the cerebrospinal fluid faster than does amphotericin B alone. In animal studies, combination therapy is beneficial for *Candida* infections, but efficacy has not be proven in humans.

---

with renal dysfunction, monitoring of peak (2 hours after oral administration) and trough levels (just before the next dose) is recommended. Doses should be adjusted to maintain serum levels between 20 and 100 μg/mL.

Pharmacokinetics—Flucytosine is well absorbed orally (Table 1.18). Because it is a small molecule, 5-FC penetrates tissues well and crosses the blood–brain barrier. Therapeutic levels can be achieved in the cerebrospinal fluid, aqueous humor, joint fluid, and respiratory secretions. The kidneys clear 5-FC.

Spectrum of Activity and Treatment Recommendations—Most strains of *C. albicans* and *Cryptococcus neoformans* are sensitive to 5-FC. Native resistance varies geographically. About 15% of *C. albicans* stains and 3% to 5% of *Cryptococcus neoformans* demonstrate resistance. The effect of 5-FC is usually fungistatic, and it should never be used alone, because resistance rapidly develops with monotherapy. The combination of 5-FC and amphotericin B demonstrates additive or synergistic activity in cryptococcal infections. In cryptococcal meningitis, amphotericin B and 5-FC sterilize the cerebrospinal fluid faster than amphotericin B alone. In vitro and animal testing also suggest that combination therapy for *Candida* may be of benefit; however, efficacy has not been proven in patients.

ANTIVIRAL DRUGS (OTHER THAN ANTIRETROVIRAL AGENTS)

Most antiviral agents target viral nucleic acid synthesis. Because these agents tend to act at a single

---

KEY POINTS

About Antiviral Therapy

1. Usually target viral nucleic acid synthesis.
2. Development of resistance is common and is favored by
   a) high viral load,
   b) high intrinsic viral mutation rate (RNA viruses more than DNA viruses), and
   c) prolonged or intermittent antiviral therapy.

---

step in viral replication, resistance may develop during treatment. The development of resistance is favored by a high viral load, a high intrinsic viral mutation rate (more common in RNA than DNA viruses), and a high degree of selective pressure—that is, prolonged antiviral therapy or repeated courses of treatment. A second method for controlling viral infection is to modify the host immune response. Infusions of antibody preparations and treatment with interferon have proved efficacious in several viral infections.

Antivirals that Block DNA Transcription

ACYCLOVIR, VALACYCLOVIR, FAMCICLOVIR

Chemical Structure and Mechanisms of Action—Acyclovir and valacyclovir are synthetic analogs of guanine in which a side chain has been substituted for a sugar moiety. Famciclovir is a acyclic guanosine analog derived from penciclovir, and this prodrug is quickly converted to penciclovir following oral absorption. These antiviral agents are phosphorylated in virus-infected cells by viral thymidine kinase, forming a monophosphate compound. Host cell kinases then add two additional phosphates, allowing the triphosphate to add to replicating DNA. The acyclic side chain of acyclovir prevents the addition of subsequent nucleic acids to DNA causing premature termination.

Penciclovir is not a DNA chain terminator; it acts primarily as a viral DNA polymerase inhibitor. Acyclovir also selectively inhibits viral DNA polymerase. Because these agents require viral thymidine kinase for their initial phosphorylation step, the concentrations of the triphosphate compounds are 40 to 100 times higher in infected than uninfected cells. Acyclovir and famciclovir resistance are most commonly caused by a reduction in viral thymidine kinase. The loss or reduction in viral thymidine kinase activity impairs acyclovir

Table 1.20. Toxicities of Systemic Antiviral Agents

Clinical symptom	Acyclovir/valacyclovir	Penciclovir/famciclovir	Ganciclovir/valganciclovir	Cidofovir	Foscarnet	Ribavirin	Interferon-α	Oseltamivir	Zanamivir	Rimantadine
Allergic skin rash	■		■							
Pruritus	■		░							
Hypotension	░		░							
Fever and chills			■		■		■			
Nausea and vomiting	■	░	■	■	■			■		■
Fatigue		░				■	■			
Diarrhea										
Headache	■	░	■			■			■	
Dizziness	■							■	░	░
Seizures	░		■		■					
Other neurotoxicity	░		■				■	■		■
Uveitis or retinitis				░			■			
Respiratory problems						░	░		■	
Phlebitis	■									
Alopecia			░							
Laboratory tests:										
Abnormal electrolytes					░					
Creatinine↑	■		░	■	■					
Anemia	░		■		■		■			
Other cytopenias	░		■		░		■			
AST/ALT↑	■		■				■			
Lactic acidosis				░						
Arrhythmias				░						
Drug–drug interactions										■

Black = principle side effect; dark gray = less common side effect; light gray = rare side effect; white = not reported or very rare; ↑ = rise; AST/ALT = aspartate aminotransferase/alanine transaminase.

phosphorylation and also renders the virus resistant to ganciclovir, because that agent also requires activation by viral thymidine kinase.

Toxicity—Toxicity related to these drugs is generally minimal (Table 1.20). Rarely patients develop rash, hematuria, headache and nausea. Neurotoxicity may occur in 1–4% receiving intravenous acyclovir and can result in lethargy, obtundation, coma, hallucinations, seizures, and autonomic instability. Most patients who suffer these complications have renal dysfunction resulting in high acyclovir serum levels. Co-administration of zidovudine and acyclovir increases the risk of developing

Table 1.21. Systemic Antiviral Agents: Half-Life, Dosing, Renal Dosing, and Cost

Antibiotic (trade name)	Half-life (h)	Dose	Dose for reduced creatinine clearance (mL/min)	Cost[a]
Acyclovir (Zovirax)	2–2.5	200–800 mg PO × 3–5 daily 5–10 mg/kg IV q8h <10: 800 mg PO q12h, 2.5–6 mg/kg IV q24h	10–50: 800 mg PO q8h, 5–12 mg/kg IV q12–24h	$–$$$
Valacyclovir (Valtrex)	2.5–3.3	500 mg PO q12h to 1000 mg PO q8h	10–50: 1 g q12–24h <10: 500 mg q24h	$$–$$$$$
Famciclovir (Famvir)	2.3	125 mg PO q12h to 500 mg PO q8h	10–50: q12–24h <10: 125–250 mg q48h	$$$$–$$$$$
Ganciclovir (Cytovene)	2.5–3.6	5 mg/kg IV q12h induction, 5 mg/kg q24h maintenance	50–80: Half the dose, same intervals 10–50: 2.5 mg/kg q24h, or 1.2 mg/kg q24h maintenance <10: 1.2 mg/kg ×3 weekly, or 0.6 mg/kg ×3 weekly maintenance	$
Valganciclovir (Valcyte)	4	900 mg PO q12h × 3 weeks, then 900 mg q24h	10–50: Half the dose <10: 450 mg q48h × 3 weeks, then twice weekly	$$$$$
Cidofovir (Vistide)	17–65	5 mg/kg IV twice weekly	50–80: Usual dose <50: Contraindicated	$
Foscarnet (Foscavir)	3	40–60 mg/kg IV q8h induction, 90–120 mg/kg q24h maintenance	50–80: 40–50 mg/kg q8h induction, 60–70 mg/kg q24h maintenance 10–50: 20–30 mg/kg q8h induction, 50–70 mg/kg q24h maintenance <10: Contraindicated	$$$–$$$$
Ribavirin (Copegus, Rebetol)	0.5–2	<75 kg: 400 mg AM, and 600 mg PO PM >75 kg: 600 mg PO q12h	<50: Not recommended	$$$$–$$$$$
Interferon α 2B (PEG-Intron, Pegasys)		PEG-Intron: 1.5 µg/kg SC weekly Pegasys: 180 mg SC weekly	No changes required	$$$$$
Oseltamivir (Tamiflu)	6–10	Treatment: 75 mg PO q12h Prophylaxis: 75 mg PO q24h	10–50: 75 mg q24h <10: Not recommended	$$–$$$$
Zanamivir (Relenza)	3	5 mg inhalation, 2 inhalations q12h ×5 days	50–80: Usual dose <50: No data	$

(Continued)

Table 1.21. *(Continued)*

Antibiotic (trade name)	Half-life (h)	Dose	Dose for reduced creatinine clearance (mL/min)	Cost[a]
Amantadine (Symmetrel, Symadine)	15–20	<65 years: 100 mg q12h >65 years: 100 mg PO q24h	50–80: 100–150 q24h 10–50: 100 mg × 2–3 weekly <10: 100–200 mg weekly	$
Rimantadine (Flumadine, Rimantid)	24–30	<65 years: 100 mg PO q12h >65 years: 100–200 mg PO q24h	<10: 100 mg q24h	$

[a] Intravenous preparations (daily cost dollars): $ = 20–70; $$ = 71–110; $$$ = 111–150; $$$$ = 150–200; $$$$$ ≥ 200; oral preparations (10-day course cost dollars): $ = 10–50; $$ = 51–100; $$$ = 101–140; $$$$ = 141–180; $$$$$ ≥ 180.

KEY POINTS

About Acyclovir, Valacyclovir, and Famciclovir

1. All require viral thymidine kinase phosphorylation for activity.
2. Acyclovir binds to the replicating viral DNA, causing premature chain termination; acyclovir and famciclovir both inhibit viral DNA polymerase.
3. Resistance is most commonly mediated by a reduction in viral thymidine kinase.
4. Toxicity is minimal. Intravenous administration of acyclovir can cause lethargy, obtundation, hallucinations, and seizures.
5. Valacyclovir is rapidly converted to acyclovir; resulting acyclovir levels are higher than those achieved with oral preparations of acyclovir. Famciclovir is rapidly converted to penciclovir.
6. Excellent activity against herpes simplex 1 and 2. Oral preparations recommended for treatment and prophylaxis of genital herpes and ocular herpes. Intravenous acyclovir recommended for herpes simplex encephalitis.
7. Moderate activity against varicella (intravenous acyclovir recommended for the immunocompromised host), and varicella pneumonia or encephalitis in the normal host. High doses of oral valacyclovir and famciclovir can be used to treat less severe disease.
8. Famciclovir can also be used to treat hepatitis B virus.

lethargy. Intravenous administration can also cause crystalluria and crystalline nephropathy, particularly if the patient is dehydrated. Cyclosporin increases the risk of nephrotoxicity.

Pharmacokinetics—The oral absorption of acyclovir is limited, only 15% to 20% of the drug being bioavailable (Table 1.21). Absorption tends to be even poorer in transplant patients, necessitating higher oral dosing. The prodrug preparation valacyclovir is rapidly and completely converted to acyclovir by hepatic and intestinal valacyclovir hydrolase. Oral valacyclovir achieves acyclovir serum levels that are 3 to 5 times higher than those achieved by oral acyclovir. Similarly, famciclovir is well absorbed orally, and in the liver and intestine, its purine is quickly deacetylated and oxidized to form penciclovir.

Acyclovir and penciclovir are widely distributed in tissues and fluids. Therapeutic levels can be achieved in cerebrospinal fluid, saliva, vaginal secretions, and the aqueous humor. Both drugs are excreted unchanged primarily in the urine. Probenecid reduces renal clearance and increases the half life.

Antiviral Activity and Therapeutic Indications— Acyclovir and famciclovir have excellent activity against herpes simplex viruses 1 and 2. Topical administration of these drugs is of minimal efficacy against herpes simplex labialis, and topical preparations are rarely used. Oral acyclovir and famciclovir are recommended for treatment of genital herpes and are used to prevent recurrent herpes genitalis. Acyclovir is also recommended for the treatment and prevention of recurrent ocular herpes simplex. Intravenous acyclovir has reduced the mortality from herpes simplex encephalitis and is the treatment of choice for that disorder. Acyclovir and famciclovir also have significant activity against varicella; however, higher drug concentrations are required to kill that virus. Intravenous acyclovir is recommended for the treatment of varicella and herpes zoster in the immunocompromised host, and for treatment of varicella pneumonia or encephalitis in the previously healthy adult. Acyclovir demonstrates some activity against Epstein–Barr virus, but is generally not recommended for therapy. This agent also demonstrates modest protection against cytomegalovirus (CMV) when used for prophylaxis in allogeneic bone marrow, renal, and liver transplant recipients; however, ganciclovir has proved to be more efficacious. Famciclovir can reduce levels of hepatitis B viral DNA and serum transaminase in patients with chronic hepatitis B. Its effects are additive when combined with interferon. Famciclovir has also been used to treat recurrent hepatitis B following liver transplantation.

GANCICLOVIR AND VALGANCICLOVIR

Chemical Structure and Mechanisms of Action—Like acyclovir, ganciclovir is a guanine analog. Ganciclovir has an additional hydroxymethyl group on the acyclic side chain. Viral thymidine kinase converts this analog to the monophosphate form, after which host cell kinase phosphorylation produces the active triphosphate form. Ganciclovir triphosphate competitively inhibits viral DNA polymerase incorporation of guanosine triphosphate into elongating DNA, but does not act as a chain terminator.

In infected cells, intracellular concentrations of ganciclovir triphosphate reach levels that are 10 times that of acyclovir triphosphate, and once in the cell, ganciclovir triphosphate persists, having a intracellular half life of 16 to 24 hours. The resulting higher intracellular concentrations may account for the greater activity of ganciclovir against CMV. Ganciclovir is also active against herpes simplex, varicella, and Epstein–Barr virus. Because ganciclovir requires viral thymidine kinase activity for conversion to the active triphosphate form, acyclovir-resistant viral strains with reduced thymidine kinase activity are also less sensitive to ganciclovir. Mutations that alter the structure of the viral DNA polymerase also confer ganciclovir resistance, and these mutants often demonstrate reduced sensitivity to foscarnet and cidofovir.

Toxicity—Significant concentrations of ganciclovir triphosphate accumulate in uninfected cells (Table 1.20). Bone marrow progenitor cells are particularly sensitive to this agent. The triphosphate form can incorporate into cellular DNA and block host cell DNA replication. Neutropenia and thrombocytopenia are commonly observed in patients with AIDS who are receiving ganciclovir, and these patients require close monitoring for WBC and platelet counts during therapy. The risk is lower, but significant, in transplant patients. Co-administration of zidovudine increases the risk of bone marrow suppression. Discontinuation of treatment is recommended if the absolute neutrophil

---

KEY POINTS

About Ganciclovir

1. Guanine analog that primarily inhibits viral DNA polymerase.

2. Like acyclovir and penciclovir, requires viral thymidine kinase for activation. Acyclovir-resistant strains are often resistant to ganciclovir.

3. Bone marrow suppression is a common toxicity, particularly in AIDS patients. The drug should be discontinued if the neutrophil count drops to less than 500 cells/mm^3.

4. Central nervous system complaints—including confusion, psychosis, coma, and seizures—may occur.

5. Most active guanine analog against cytomegalovirus (CMV). Also active against herpes simplex 1 and 2, varicella, and Epstein–Barr virus.

6. Recommended for CMV retinitis, pneumonia, and colitis. Useful for prophylaxis of immunocompromised transplant patients. Following treatment of active infection in AIDS patients with low CD4 counts, oral valganciclovir is given to prevent relapse.

---

count drops below 500 cells/mm3. Central nervous system (CNS) side effects (including headache, confusion, psychosis, coma, and seizures) are also common.

Pharmacokinetics—Valganciclovir is a prodrug that is well absorbed orally and quickly converts to ganciclovir (Table 1.21). With oral administration, excellent serum levels that are nearly comparable to intravenous ganciclovir can be achieved. Ganciclovir readily penetrates all tissues and fluids including the brain and cerebrospinal fluid. The drug is primarily excreted unmodified in the urine.

Spectrum of Activity and Treatment Indications—Of the guanine analogs, ganciclovir has the highest activity against CMV. Ganciclovir is the treatment of choice for CMV infections including retinitis, pneumonia, and colitis. Ganciclovir is also used for prophylaxis of CMV in transplant patients. In patients with AIDS who have persistently low CD4 lymphocyte counts, ganciclovir maintenance therapy is required to prevent relapse of CMV infection after the treatment of active infection has been completed.

CIDOFOVIR

Chemical Structure, Mechanisms of Action, and Pharmacokinetics—Cidofovir (Tables 1.20, 1.21) is an analog of deoxycytidine monophosphate that inhibits viral DNA synthesis. This agent does not require viral kinase for activity, being converted by cellular enzymes to its active diphosphate form. It acts as a competitive inhibitor of viral DNA polymerase and also adds to DNA, substituting for deoxycytidine triphosphate (dCTP), causing premature chain termination. Viral thymidine kinase mutantations do not impair cidofovir activity.

Resistance is conferred through viral DNA polymerase mutations. Such mutations can result in cross-resistance to ganciclovir and, less commonly, to foscarnet. Cidofovir is cleared by the kidneys.

Toxicity—Cidofovir is highly nephrotoxic, causing proteinuria in half of treated patients, and azotemia and metabolic acidosis in a significant number. Vigorous saline hydration and co-administration of probenecid reduces nephrotoxicity. The drug should be discontinued if 3+ proteinuria or higher develops, or if serum creatinine increases by more than 0.4 mg/dL. Neutropenia is also commonly encountered.

Spectrum of Activity and Treatment Indications—Cidofovir has activity against many DNA viruses: CMV; herpes simplex; herpesvirus 6 and 8; varicella; pox viruses, including smallpox; papilloma viruses; polyoma viruses; and adenoviruses. This agent is approved only for the treatment of CMV retinitis in patients with AIDS. Given its highly toxic profile, parenteral use of this drug in other

---

KEY POINTS

About Cidofovir

1. An analog of deoxycytidine monophosphate, it causes premature chain termination of viral DNA and also inhibits viral DNA polymerase.

2. Does not require viral thymidine kinase for conversion to its active form. Acyclovir-resistant strains are usually not resistant to cidofovir.

3. Highly nephrotoxic; causes proteinuria, azotemia, and metabolic acidosis in nearly half of patients. Saline hydration and probenecid reduce nephrotoxicity. Neutropenia also is common.

4. Broad spectrum of antiviral activity including cytomegalovirus (CMV), herpes simplex, herpesvirus 6 and 8, varicella, pox viruses, papilloma virus, polyoma viruses, and adenoviruses.

5. Approved for CMV retinitis in patients with AIDS. Other indications are currently being explored. However, the usefulness of cidofovir is likely to be limited because of renal and bone marrow toxicity.

KEY POINTS

About Foscarnet

1. Blocks binding of deoxynucleotidyl triphosphates to viral DNA polymerase.

2. Nephrotoxicity is common, usually developing during the second week of therapy. Can be reduced by saline hydration. Usually reversible.

3. Also causes abnormalities in serum calcium, magnesium, and phosphate.

4. Active against cytomegalovirus (CMV), herpes simplex, varicella, Epstein-Barr virus, and herpesvirus 8.

5. Approved for the treatment of CMV retinitis and acyclovir-resistant mucocutaneous herpes simplex.

---

viral infections is likely to be limited. Topical therapy may prove efficacious in acyclovir-resistant herpes simplex infections in patients with AIDS, and it is being studied for the treatment of anogenital warts.

FOSCARNET

Chemical Structure and Mechanism of Action—Foscarnet is an inorganic pyrophosphate analog, trisodium phosphonoformate, which reversibly blocks the pyrophosphate binding site of viral DNA polymerase. Foscarnet binding inhibits the polymerase from binding deoxynucleotidyl triphosphates. Mutations to the viral DNA polymerase are primarily responsible for viral resistance; however, resistance among clinical isolates is rare.

Toxicity. Nephrotoxicity is the most common serious side effect of foscarnet, resulting in azotemia, proteinuria, and occasionally acute tubular necrosis (Table 1.20). Renal dysfunction usually develops during the second week of therapy and in most cases reverses when the drug is discontinued. Dehydration increases the incidence of nephrotoxicity, and saline loading is of benefit in reducing this complication. Metabolic abnormalities are frequent. Hypocalcemia is the most common, being the result of chelation by foscarnet. Reductions in ionized calcium can cause CNS disturbances, tetany, paresthesias, and seizures. Other metabolic abnormalities include hypophosphatemia, hypomagnesemia, hypokalemia, hypercalcemia, and hyperphosphatemia. To minimize these metabolic derangements, intravenous infusion should not exceed 1mg/kg per minute. Electrolytes, magnesium, phosphate, and calcium should be closely monitored. Other common side effects include fever, headache, nausea, vomiting, and abnormal liver function tests.

Pharmacokinetics—Foscarnet is poorly absorbed orally and is administered intravenously. This drug penetrates all tissues and fluids, achieving excellent levels in the cerebrospinal fluid and vitreous humor. Foscarnet is excreted unmodified, primarily by the kidneys.

Spectrum of Activity and Treatment Indications. Foscarnet is active against CMV, herpes simplex, varicella, Epstein–Barr virus, and herpesvirus 8. It is approved for the treatment of CMV retinitis and for acyclovir-resistant mucocutaneous herpes simplex.

Other Antiviral Agents

RIBAVIRIN

Chemical Structure and Mechanism of Action—Ribavirin is a guanosine analog that contains the d-ribose side chain. It inhibits DNA and RNA viruses alike. The mechanisms of inhibition are complex and not completely understood. Ribavirin is phosphorylated to the triphosphate form by host cell enzymes, and the triphosphate form interferes with viral messenger RNA formation. The monophosphate form interferes with guanosine triphosphate synthesis, lowering nucleic acid pools in the cell.

Toxicity—Systemic ribavirin results in dose-related red blood cell hemolysis; at high doses, it suppresses the bone marrow (Table 1.20). The resulting anemia reverses when the drug is discontinued. Intravenous administration is not approved in the United States, but is available for patients with Lhasa fever and some other forms of hemorrhagic fever. Aerosolized ribavirin is associated with conjunctivitis and with bronchospasm that can result in deterioration of pulmonary function. A major concern for health care workers exposed to aerosolized ribavirin are teratogenic and embryotoxic effects noted in some animal studies. Pregnant health care workers should not administer this drug.

Pharmacokinetics—Approximately one third of orally administered ribavirin is absorbed. The drug penetrates all tissues and body fluids. Ribavirin triphosphate becomes highly concentrated in erythrocytes (40 times plasma levels) and persists for prolonged periods with red blood cells. The drug is cleared both by the kidneys and by the liver. Aerosolized ribavirin produces high drug levels that have a half life of up to 2.5 h in respiratory secretions. A special aerosol generator is required for proper administration.

Spectrum of Activity and Treatment Recommendations.—Ribavirin is active against a broad spectrum of DNA and RNA viruses including respiratory syncytial virus (RSV), influenza and parainfluenza virus, herpes, adenovirus, pox viruses, Bunyavirus, and arenaviruses. It is approved in the United States for the

KEY POINTS
About Ribavirin

1. Guanosine analog that interferes with viral messenger RNA formation and reduces guanosine triphosphate synthesis, lowering nucleic acid pools in the cell.
2. Systemic drug causes red blood cell hemolysis. Intravenous administration not approved in the United States. Aerosolized form causes conjunctivitis and bronchospasm.
3. Teratogenic and embryotoxic. Pregnant health care workers should not administer.
4. Active against DNA and RNA viruses including respiratory syncytial virus (RSV), influenza and parainfluenza virus, herpes viruses, adenovirus, pox viruses, Bunyavirus, and arenaviruses.
5. Approved for aerosolized treatment of RSV bronchiolitis and pneumonia.
6. Approved for oral administration in combination with interferon for chronic hepatitis C.

aerosol treatment of RSV bronchiolitis and pneumonia in hospitalized patients. Oral ribavirin in combination with interferon is approved for the treatment of chronic hepatitis C.

INTERFERONS

Chemical Structure and Mechanism of Action—The interferons (IFNs) are proteins of 16 to 27,000 Da molecular weight, synthesized by eukaryotic cells in response to viral infections. These cytokines in turn stimulate host antiviral responses. Interferon receptors regulate approximately 100 genes, and in response to INF binding, cells rapidly produce dozens of proteins. A wide variety of RNA viruses are susceptible to the antiviral actions of IFNs; most DNA viruses are only minimally affected.

Toxicity—Side effects tend to mild when doses of less than 5 million units are administered (Table 1.20). Doses of 1 to 2 million units given subcutaneously or intramuscularly are associated with an influenza-like syndrome that is particularly severe during the first week of therapy. This febrile response can be reduced by premedication with antipyretics such as aspirin, ibuprofen, and acetaminophen. Local irritation at injection sites is also frequently reported. Higher doses of INF result in bone marrow suppression, causing granulocytopenia and thrombocytopenia. Neurotoxicity resulting in confusion, somnolence, and behavior disturbances is also common when high doses are administered.

KEY POINTS

About Interferon for Treatment of Viral Infections

1. Binds to host cell interferon receptors, upregulating many genes responsible for the production of proteins with antiviral activity.

2. RNA viruses are more susceptible to the antiviral actions of IFNs.

3. The most common side effect is an influenza-like syndrome. At doses above 5 million units, bone marrow suppression and neurotoxicity may develop. Hepatoxicity and retinopathy are commonly associated with high doses.

4. Approved for chronic hepatitis C, chronic hepatitis B, and Kaposi sarcoma. Intralesional injection approved for condyloma acuminatum.

Hepatoxicity and retinopathy are other common side effects with high dose therapy.

Pharmacokinetics—Intramuscularly and subcutaneously, INF-a is well absorbed; other interferons have more variable absorption (Table 1.21). Assays for biologic effect demonstrate activity that persists for 4 days after a single dose. Pegylated forms result in slower release and more prolonged biologic activity, allowing for once-weekly administration; these forms are preferred in most instances.

Spectrum of Activity and Treatment Recommendations—The effectiveness of INFs has been limited by the frequent side effects associated with effective doses. Treatment approvals have been issued for INFs in chronic hepatitis C, chronic hepatitis B, Kaposi sarcoma and other malignancies, and condyloma acuminatum.

Anti-influenza Viral Agents

AMANTADINE AND RIMANTADINE

Mechanism of Action—Amantadine and rimantadine are effective only against influenza A. They bind to and inhibit the M2 protein. This viral protein is expressed on the surface of infected cells, and it is thought to play an important role in viral particle assembly.

Toxicity—Amantadine causes moderate CNS side effects, especially in the elderly (Table 1.20). Insomnia, inability to concentrate, and dizziness are most commonly reported. Amantadine also increases the risk of seizures in patients with a past history of epilepsy. Rimantadine causes CNS side effects less frequently, and this agent is now preferred over amantadine.

Treatment Recommendations—To be effective, treatment must be instituted within 48 hours of the onset of symptoms (Table 1.21). Efficacy has been proven in healthy adults, but trials have not been performed in high-risk patients.

NEURAMIDASE INHIBITORS

Mechanism of Action—The neuramidase inhibitors have activity against both influenza A and B.

Toxicity—Zanamivir is given by inhaler and commonly causes bronchospasm, limiting its usefulness.

Treatment—To be effective, neuramidase inhibitors must be given within 48 hours of the onset of symptoms.

Amantadine, rimantadine, or oseltamivir can be given for a longer duration as prophylaxis in patients at risk of serious complications from influenza during an epidemic. Influenza vaccine is preferred for prophylaxis.

FURTHER READING

Antibiotic Handbooks

Bartlett JG, Auwaerter PG, and Pham PA. *The ABX Guide: Diagnosis and Treatment of Infectious Diseases.* Montvale, NJ: Thompson PDR; 2005.

Gilbert DN, Moellering RC Jr, Eliopoulos GM, and Sande MA. *The Sanford Guide to Antimicrobial Therapy.* 36th ed. Hyde Park, Vt: Antimicrobial Therapy; 2006.

Electronic Sources

ePocrates and ePocrates ID [software]. San Mateo, Calif: Epocrates, Inc. [Web address: www.epocrates.com; cited:]

The Johns Hopkins University, Division of Infectious Diseases. ABX Guide [Web resource]. Baltimore, Md: The Johns Hopkins University. [Web address: www.hopkins-abxguide.org; cited:]

Other

The choice of antibacterial drugs. *Med Lett Drugs Ther.* 2001;43:69–78.

Bruton L, Lazo J, and Parker K. *Goodman & Gilman's The Pharmacological Basis of Therapeutics.* 11th ed. New York, NY: McGraw–Hill Medical Publishers; 2006.

Mandell GL, Bennett JE, and Dolin R. *Mandell, Douglas, and Bennett's Principles and Practice of Infectious Diseases.* 6th ed. Philadelphia, Pa: Elsevier/Churchill Livingstone; 2005.

Sepsis Syndrome

Time Recommended to complete: 1 day

Reuben Ramphal, M.D.

GUIDING QUESTIONS

1. How is sepsis syndrome defined, and what is SIRS?

2. Do all episodes of bacteremia cause sepsis syndrome, and are all sepsis syndromes the result of bacteremia?

3. Which bacterial products can produce sepsis syndrome?

4. What is a "superantigen," and which bacteria produce them?

5. Which host cells are most important in sepsis syndrome, and how do they mediate it?

6. What are the clinical clues that suggest pre-shock, and why is pre-shock important to recognize?

7. What are the therapeutic measures that need to be instituted in patients with sepsis syndrome?

POTENTIAL SEVERITY

A life-threatening syndrome that must be recognized and treated quickly to prevent progression to irreversible shock.

PREVALENCE

Sepsis—severe infection leading to organ dysfunction—is a problem of increasing magnitude in the United States. Estimates of the occurrence of this syndrome range from 300,000 to 500,000 cases per year. Mortality associated with the syndrome has been reported to be between 15% and 60%, governed by factors such as underlying diseases, age, infecting organism, and the appropriateness of empiric anti-infective therapy. Most cases of sepsis syndrome are the result of bacterial infection, but it should be appreciated that the syndrome is also seen in viral infections (for example, dengue fever), fungal infections for example, candidemia), and certain noninfectious diseases (for example, pancreatitis). For

---

KEY POINTS

About the Prevalence and Definitions of Sepsis Syndrome

1. Prevalence is 300,000–500,000 cases per year in the United States.

2. Mortality ranges from 15% to 60%.

3. Sepsis syndrome is systemic inflammatory response syndrome (SIRS) caused by microbial products.

4. Viruses (dengue fever), fungi (*Candida*), and noninfectious diseases (pancreatitis, tissue ischemia, severe trauma) can also cause SIRS.

5. Severe sepsis is defined as SIRS caused by microbial products that is associated with organ dysfunction.

6. Septic shock is shock associated with sepsis that is unresponsive to volume replacement.

7. Bacteremia does not always cause sepsis syndrome, and sepsis syndrome is not always caused by bacteremia.

the purposes of this chapter, sepsis is presumed to be a result of bacterial agents and their products.

DEFINITIONS

Sepsis represents a continuum that progresses from localized infection to severe sepsis (Figure 2.1). "Sepsis" is best defined as the systemic inflammatory response syndrome (SIRS) caused by microbial products. This definition acknowledges that SIRS may be produced by entities other than infection and that, in the absence of viable organisms, microbial products are capable of producing this clinical picture. "Severe sepsis" is defined as sepsis with organ dysfunction, and it represents progression of SIRS with more severe pathophysiologic disturbances. "Septic shock" is hypotension due to sepsis that has become unresponsive to initial attempts at volume expansion. "Infection," often colloquially called "sepsis," indicates the presence of infection and should not be considered synonymous with sepsis syndrome. Bacteremia is often called sepsis, and although some bacteremias result in sepsis syndrome, not all sepsis syndromes are caused by bacteremia. In fact, in earlier clinical trials of biologic agents in sepsis syndrome, using the best possible definitions and available laboratory studies, fewer than 40% of patients have had proven infection.

PATHOGENESIS

SIRS results from the activation of cellular pathways that lead to a triggering of innate immune responses and coagulation mechanisms. The pathways are linked to ancient mechanisms that defend the host by responding to tissue injury or the presence of microbial products. This innate immune response eventually leads to a classic adaptive immune response characterized by the production of antibodies, activated T cells and memory of antigens.

Much is now known about the microbial triggers of this system, with most of the information having been obtained using a portion of the gram-negative cell wall, the lipopolysaccharide molecule (LPS) or endotoxin. It is clear, however, that gram-positive cell wall material—specifically peptidoglycans and lipoteichoic acid, toxins produced by gram-positive bacteria, and fungal cell walls—is also recognized by a family of molecules on the surfaces of target cells. This recognition leads to the synthesis of molecules that trigger inflammation and coagulation pathways.

Cell Wall Factors

In gram-negative bacteria, the cytoplasmic bilayer is covered with a layer of peptidoglycan. Overlying the peptidoglycan layer is an outer membrane, into which endotoxin is inserted. Endotoxin is the most carefully studied microbial substance implicated in sepsis syndrome and shock. There is compelling evidence that endotoxin plays a key role in the pathogenesis of gram-negative sepsis. Its structural organization is common across all gram-negative bacteria. From the outside going inward, it consists of an "O" side chain that is joined to a core, which is in turn connected to the "business" end of the molecule, the lipid A portion.

Lipid A is anchored into the outer membrane. The triggering of the inflammatory and coagulation systems is believed to begin with the interaction of LPS with cellular receptors on macrophages and mononuclear leukocytes. The structure of lipid A is remarkably well conserved in most common gram-negative bacteria, irrespective of the species from which it is obtained. Indeed, the clinical features of sepsis caused by *Escherichia coli* are similar to those caused by *Klebsiella* or *Enterobacter* species.

The infusion of LPS or lipid A into animals results in a sepsis-like picture. Endotoxin can be found in the blood of patients with gram-negative sepsis. In some cases, such as meningococcemia, there is a good correlation between the plasma level of endotoxin and the outcome; even in more "general" types of gram-negative infection, the presence of endotoxemia correlates with more severe physiologic variables.

In addition to LPS, fungal cells walls, gram-positive cell walls and possibly bacterial flagellins are also capable of interacting with macrophages to trigger the sequence of events leading to sepsis and shock. Endotoxin is not present in gram-positive bacteria. Instead, the cell wall contains a thick layer of peptidoglycan on its surface. In capsular strains the peptidoglycan lies directly beneath the capsule. Embedded in the peptidoglycan are molecules of lipoteichoic acid. Several in vitro studies have demonstrated that these structural components of gram-positive cell walls are able to mimic some of the properties of endotoxin—for example, their ability to induce proinflammatory cytokines from mononuclear cells.

Secreted Factors

In addition to factors that are integral parts of the cell wall, secreted factors from gram-positive bacteria are

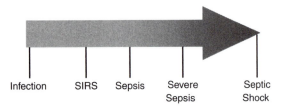

Figure 2–1. Order of progression from infection to septic shock.

believed to cause septic shock. The prototypical factor is toxic shock syndrome toxin 1 (TSST-1), produced by some strains of *Staphylococcus aureus*.

Toxic shock syndrome was first described in menstruation-associated staphylococcal infection of young women. Fever and profound shock were often followed by conjunctival and palmar hyperemia and desquamation. This condition proved to be associated with the production of an exotoxin, TSST-1.

Another secreted factor responsible for shock was discovered in strains of the gram-positive bacteria *Streptococcus pyogenes*. It is called streptococcal pyrogenic exotoxin A (SPEA). Clinically, the action of SPEA has been identified in necrotizing fasciitis due to *Strep. pyogenes* associated with shock. Infection is hypothesized to lead to local or systemic release of toxins, massive lymphocyte activation, and release of cytokines, resulting in cellular injury and organ failure. This mechanism bypasses the macrophage, and the cytokine cascade is triggered at the level of the T cells. This bypassing of the macrophage has given rise to the term "superantigen" to describe toxins that, unlike conventional antigens that require processing by macrophages and dendritic cells are able to directly activate lymphocytes.

KEY POINTS

About the Bacterial Products That Cause Sepsis Syndrome

1. In gram-negative bacteria, lipopolysaccharide (LPS), also called endotoxin, is linked to the outer membrane.
   a) Endotoxin alone can produce the syndrome.
   b) Endotoxin (LPS) is found in the bloodstream of patients with gram-negative bacteremia.
   c) Endotoxin (LPS) blood levels correlate with the clinical severity of sepsis syndrome.
2. Gram-positive bacteria produce peptidoglycans, and lipoteichoic acid can mimic endotoxins.
3. Gram-positive bacteria also secrete exotoxins.
   a) *Staphylococcus aureus* can secrete toxic shock syndrome toxin 1 (TSST-1).
   b) *Streptococcus pyogenes* secretes streptococcal pyrogenic exotoxin A (SPEA).
   c) Called "superantigens," these exotoxins bypass macrophages and directly stimulate T cells.

Host Cell Receptors for Bacterial Products

A detailed discussion of the physiologic host responses to bacteria is beyond the scope of this chapter. Good evidence suggests that, in gram-negative infections, monocyte–macrophage or dendritic cells are the first cells to respond to endotoxin. Endotoxin first binds to LPS-binding protein, an acute-phase protein produced by the liver. The LPS–protein complex acts as the ligand for CD14 (a cell-surface receptor on mononuclear cells) and to toll-like receptor (TLR) 2 or 4 on these cells. There are a number of TLRs that recognize different substances regardless of microbial origin. For example, TLR2 recognizes peptidoglycans, mannans, lipoteichoic acids, and some LPS molecules; TLR4 recognizes LPS; and TLR5 recognizes bacterial flagellin. TLR receptors and co-receptors bind the foreign stimulant and internalize it. Internalization results in signal transduction and cell activation, leading to cytokine release.

Cytokine and Other Inflammatory Mediator Cascades

The activation of monocytes leads to the production of the proinflammatory cytokines (that is, the cytokines that stimulate inflammation), particularly tumor necrosis factor α (TNF-α) and interleukin 1 (IL-1). Infection also activates other host pathways, including the complement and coagulation pathways and the production of reactive oxygen intermediates. Many studies have been conducted in animals in which cytokines have been measured in response to both purified bacterial components and, perhaps more informatively, live bacterial infection. Intravenous injection of live *E. coli* into mice, rabbits, or baboons results in a consistent picture in which proinflammatory cytokines such as IL-1, IL-6, IL-8, and TNF-α, are released in a well-ordered sequence, followed by interferon gamma and then counterregulatory cytokines such as IL-10. This picture is similar to that seen when endotoxin is injected into humans.

How Infection Leads to Septic Shock

Figure 2.2 shows a simple diagram of the pathways leading to septic shock. It must be realized that these events represent a continuum, and they progress at speeds that have not been characterized. However, the general belief is that the larger the inoculum of the challenge molecule, LPS or gram-positive toxins, the more likely the process is to progress rapidly. Additionally the various cell-wall products are likely to differ in their intrinsic potency to stimulate the innate immune system. For example, clinical observation suggests that endotoxin is a more powerful stimulant than are the cells walls of enterococci or coagulase-negative staphylococci, because

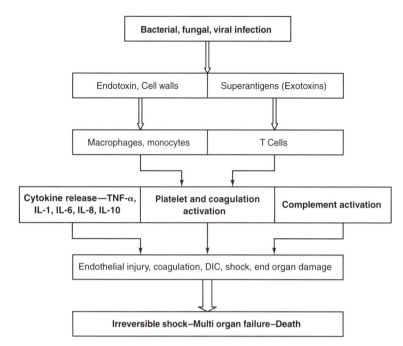

Figure 2-2. Pathophysiology of sepsis syndrome.

humans demonstrate a remarkable tolerance for bacteremia attributable to those organisms.

KEY POINTS

About the Roles of Host Cells in Sepsis Syndrome

1. Monocyte–macrophages or dendritic cells are the first cells to respond to endotoxin (LPS).

2. Endotoxin binds to LPS–protein in serum, and this complex binds to CD14 receptors and to toll-like receptor 4 (TLR4) on mononuclear cells.

3. TLR2 binds peptidoglycans, lipoteichoic acids found in gram-positive bacteria, and mannans found on fungi. It also binds to some forms of LPS. TLR-5 bind bacterial flagellin.

4. Receptor binding stimulates monocyte– macrophages to release
   a) proinflammatory cytokines tumor necrosis factor α and interleukin-1, stimulating inflammation.
   b) toxic oxygen byproducts.
   c) products that activate the complement and coagulation cascades.

CLINICAL MANIFESTATIONS

CASE 2.1

A 66-year-old white woman underwent elective thoracoabdominal aneurysm repair. Three days after surgery, she became confused and developed a new fever. She had no cough, no dysuria, and no abdominal pain. A surgical drain was noted to be leaking increasing amounts of serous fluid. She was receiving vancomycin for operative prophylaxis.

On physical exam, her temperature was 39°C, her pulse was 143 per minute, and her blood pressure was 110/70 mm Hg. She was intubated and on a respirator. She appeared toxic and somewhat lethargic. No skin lesions were noted, and her respiratory, cardiac, and abdominal exams were unremarkable. Her extremities were warm to the touch. Chest X-ray revealed no infiltrates.

Laboratory workup showed that the patient's peripheral white blood cell (WBC) count had dropped to 1400/mm³ from 22,600/mm³ the day before, with 24% polymorphonuclear leukocytes, 37% bands, and 9% metamyelocytes. Her hematocrit was 30%; blood urea nitrogen, 41 mg/dL; serum creatinine, 1.0 mg/dL; and HCO_3, 26 mEq/L. Blood cultures and culture of the surgical drain subsequently grew Escherichia coli. Computed *tomography scan of the abdomen failed to reveal an abscess. She was initially treated with intravenous cefepime and subsequently switched to ceftriaxone. Except for a brief bout of hypotension requiring intravenous saline and dopamine, she fully recovered and was subsequently discharged from the hospital.*

Fever

As noted in case 2.1, fever is usually the first and most common manifestation of sepsis. In general, the higher the temperature, the more likely a patient is to be bacteremic. However, it should be emphasized that hypothermia and normal body temperature are seen in patients who are bacteremic. In fact, there is good reason to believe that hypothermia is a poor prognostic indicator in bacteremic patients, indicating an inability to mount an adequate inflammatory response.

Hemodynamic Changes

Tachycardia is a concomitant finding with fever and is to be expected. Case 2.1 had marked sinus tachycardia associated with her bacteremia. Bradycardia, on the other hand, is unusual, and has been reported in patients with specific bacterial infections, such as typhoid fever and brucellosis. Of the easily measurable hemodynamic changes, hypotension is the most important in determining outcome. Failure to reverse hypotension in its early stages results in serious end-organ damage that may not be reversed by antibiotics or other therapy. The stage at which hypotension is reversible is called pre-shock. The pre-shock stage is often characterized by warm skin, diminished mentation (often worse in the elderly), and oliguria. Persistent hypotension leads to the well-recognized septic shock findings of cool skin, acute renal failure, and, on occasion, hepatic injury.

Acid–Base Disturbances

Reduced tissue perfusion requires a change from aerobic to anaerobic metabolism and causes lactic acid accumulation. Lactic acid and elevated cytokine levels stimulate the respiratory center, resulting in hyperventilation, which initially produces a respiratory alkalosis. This is the first pronounced change that is seen in impending shock. It is diagnostic, and it is usually seen at a time when the hemodynamic changes are reversible with fluid resuscitation. Recognition of this early stage is thus vital to making improvements in the management of a patient with sepsis syndrome. Metabolic acidosis can develop just before or can accompany hypotension, and

---

> ### KEY POINTS
>
> ### About the Clinical Manifestations of Sepsis Syndrome
>
> 1. Fever:
>   a) Fever is the usual presentation. The higher the fever, the more likely the patient is to be bacteremic.
>   b) Hypothermia or normal temperature in association with bacteremia is a bad prognostic sign.
> 2. Hemodynamic changes:
>   a) Tachycardia in association with fever is the rule; pulse is slower in typhoid fever and brucellosis.
>   b) Hypotension is the most important determinant of outcome. Failure to reverse early warm pre-shock leads to irreversible organ damage and death.
> 3. Acid–base balance
>   a) Initially, respiratory alkalosis develops in response to anaerobic metabolism and lactic acid build-up. Recognizing this pre-shock syndrome is critical.
>   b) Failure to treat leads to metabolic acidosis and an increased likelihood of death.
> 4. Respiratory changes
>   a) Hyperventilation occurs early.
>   b) Hypoxia and ARDS are common. Chest X-ray reveals pulmonary edema.

---

it signals the beginning of a fatal downward spiral. Case 2.1 was recognized and treated before the development of acidosis, which explains the patient's rapid recovery.

Respiratory Changes

Tachypnea is a common feature of sepsis, generated by cytokine stimulation of the central nervous system, elevated body temperature, and the accumulation of lactic acid. In addition to hyperventilation, severe depression of oxygenation is often seen. The adult respiratory distress syndrome (ARDS) commonly develops in septic shock and can be experimentally induced by endotoxin. Endotoxin is thought to activate neutrophils that become trapped in the small vessels of the lungs and cause vessel-wall damage and leakage of fluid into the alveoli.

ARDS is diagnosed by chest X-ray changes that mimic cardiac pulmonary edema, and it is accompanied by severe hypoxemia. However, patients with sepsis may also demonstrate pneumonia on chest X-ray, and infection of the lungs can be accompanied by bacteremia and sepsis syndrome (see Chapter 4).

DIAGNOSIS

Diagnosis of sepsis syndrome is perhaps the greatest challenge encountered in designing clinical trials for new therapeutic agents. If fever, tachycardia, and tachypnea with or without leukocytosis are used to define SIRS, then this definition includes other causes in addition to infection. Therefore evidence of actual infection must be sought.

The most prevalent sites of infection are the lungs, bloodstream, abdomen, and wounds. Even with a positive bacterial culture from any of these sites, sepsis in patients fitting the broad definitions of SIRS remains an uncertainty. In fact, most patients with pneumonia would fit this definition of sepsis syndrome, although they rarely require intensive care. The strictest criteria should include the presence of a positive blood culture, preferably two, and should exclude most cases of coagulase-negative staphylococci that are common skin contaminants. Exceptions to a positive blood culture would have to be made in patients presenting clear clinical evidence of an intra-abdominal infection such as peritonitis. Adjunctive information should also include the presence of hypotension that is not a result of hypovolemia or a recent cardiac event.

Critical diagnostic tools that are not currently available include a means to rapidly diagnose the presence of bacteria in the blood and a method to rapidly quantify the inflammatory response. (Infection produces more inflammation than does a noninfectious cause.) Such tests would guide a decision to initiate or not to initiate antibiotics and activated protein C (see "Drotrecogin α" under "Treatment"). A method for detecting early organ damage would also be helpful for determining the severity of SIRS. Currently, reliance must be placed on clinical assessment of illness severity and supportive bacteriologic studies that usually do not become available for 24–48 hours.

The presence of other abnormalities such as thrombocytopenia, evidence of fibrinogen consumption, and clot lysis are helpful, and when accompanied by hypotension, increased cardiac output and changes in peripheral vascular resistance may serve to define infection as the cause of SIRS. However, these findings are more likely to be seen in the more severe cases, where the diagnosis of infection is already clinically apparent.

Case 2.1 had a marked drop in peripheral WBC, with a marked shift to the left and a high percentage of immature granulocyte forms indicating marked consumption of granulocytes. That finding served as a

---

KEY POINTS

About the Diagnosis of Sepsis Syndrome

1. Early diagnosis is difficult and is based on clinical findings.
2. Fever, tachycardia, and hypotension need to be accompanied by documented bacteremia.
3. Tests to quickly demonstrate bacteremia, to accurately assess the extent of inflammation, and to assess organ ischemia are not currently available.
4. Thrombocytopenia and evidence of fibrinogen consumption and clot lysis combined with hypotension, increased cardiac output, and reduced peripheral vascular resistance suggest the diagnosis.

---

useful warning that sepsis had developed, and it precipitated the administration of broad spectrum antibiotic coverage.

These common clinical and laboratory findings are indicative of sepsis:

1. Temperature: <36°C or >38°C
2. Pulse rate: >90/min
3. Respiratory rate: >20 per minute
4. $PaCO_2$: <32, with pH >7.45 (early sepsis)
5. WBC count: <4000/mm³ or >12,000/mm³ with a band count >10%
6. Chills, lethargy, hemorrhagic skin lesions

These laboratory studies are recommended in patients with suspected sepsis syndrome:

1. Two blood cultures, urine culture, and sputum culture if the patient has chest X-ray abnormalities
2. Complete blood count with differential and platelets
3. Coagulation studies to include international normalized ratio, fibrinogen, and D-dimers or fibrin split products
4. Blood gases and metabolic panels

TREATMENT
Antibiotic Therapy

The outcome of patients with sepsis, in particular those with bacteremia, is governed by host and microbial factors alike. In some studies, certain organisms, including *Pseudomonas aeruginosa* and *Candida* species have

Table 2.1. Empiric Antibiotic Therapy for Sepsis Syndrome

Site of infection	Pathogens to be covered	Antibiotics
Lung (hospital acquired)	*Pseudomonas aeruginosa* *Enterobacter*	Cefepime, or ticarcillin–clavulanate Piperacillin–tazobactam, plus aminoglycoside
Abdomen or pelvis	Gram-negative rods Anaerobes	Ticarcillin–clavulanate, or piperacillin–tazobactam, plus aminoglycoside Imipenem or meropenem
Urinary tract	*Escherichia coli* *Klebsiella* *Proteus*	Ciprofloxacin Ceftriaxone
Skin	*Staphylococcus aureus* *Streptococcus pyogenes* Mixed aerobic/anaerobic (necrotizing fasciitis)	Oxacillin, or vancomycin Ticarcillin–clavulanate Piperacillin–tazobactam Imipenem or meropenem
Bacteremia of unknown source (hospital acquired)	Methicillin-resistant *Staph. aureus* (MRSA) Gram negative rods	Cefepime, plus vancomycin
Bacteremia of unknown source (community acquired)	*Staph. aureus* *Strep. pneumoniae* *Esch. coli* *Klebsiella* *Proteus*	Vancomycin, plus ceftriaxone or cefepime

been suggested to carry a higher mortality rate. Polymicrobial bacteremia also carries an increased mortality risk. Therefore, if the clinical situation is epidemiologically consistent with the isolation of more risky pathogens, consideration must be given to covering these possibilities empirically.

The other microbial factor of significance is the susceptibility of the pathogen to empiric therapy. Patients with gram-negative bacteremia treated empirically with antibiotics to which their organism is resistant have significantly higher mortality rates. Therefore, empiric therapy should be embarked upon with a knowledge of local susceptibility patterns, and in situations in which a bacterium was previously isolated from a suspicious site, empiric therapy should cover its susceptibility pattern.

These foregoing considerations aside, other factors may possibly help in choosing empiric therapy for sepsis. In patients presenting with sepsis and a petechial skin rash, consideration must be given to meningococcemia, gonococcemia, *S. aureus* bacteremia or localized *S. aureus* infection, and streptococcal bacteremia or localized *S. pyogenes* infection. The preferred approach is to direct therapy to the most probable site of origin of

the infection and to cover the most likely pathogens from that site (Table 2.1).

It must be recognized that coverage for every possible pathogen is not possible, and certain pathogens in certain locations are unlikely to be responsible for life-threatening sepsis. Such organisms include enterococci at most sites and *S. aureus* in the respiratory tract. These recommendations are made with the assumption that 90% of organisms are sensitive to the drugs chosen, except for hospital-acquired pathogens. Certain hospitals may have specific resistance problems with any given pathogen. In these cases, empiric therapy must be adjusted to reflect antibiotic sensitivities of the local bacterial flora. The regimens suggested in Table 2.1 will cover most other pathogens that are isolated at these sites in significant numbers. In 24–48 hours after blood culture results are available, the antibiotic regimen must be adjusted, with narrower spectrum antibiotics utilized whenever possible to reduce the likelihood of selecting for highly resistant pathogens.

Patient Management

Management of patients with sepsis syndrome requires prompt administration of antibiotics and volume expansion, initially with normal saline. The duration of hypotension before the administration of effective antibiotics has been found to be extremely important in the survival of hypotensive patients. Each hour of delay up to 6 hours resulted in an increase in mortality of 7.9%.

If there is a drainable site of infection in the abdomen or pelvis, or if those locations are the possible sources of infection, immediate surgical consultation must be sought. (See Chapter 8, "Gastrointestinal and Hepatobiliary Infections.") Similarly the presence of gas in soft tissues or clinical evidence of a necrotizing infection mandates surgical consultation and possibly intervention. (See Chapter 10, "Skin and Soft-Tissue Infections.") Any intravascular catheter in place must be removed and cultured. (See Chapter 7, "Cardiovascular Infections.").

The following measurements are suggested in patients who are initially stable and kept on a conventional ward:

1. Hourly measurement of vital signs and urine output
2. Two-hourly measurement of arterial blood pH, $PaCO_2$, and PaO_2

KEY POINTS

About the Treatment of Sepsis Syndrome

1. Empiric antibiotic therapy must take into account
   a) the presumed primary anatomic site of the infection leading to bacteremia.
   b) local hospital antibiotic sensitivities.
   c) sensitivities for bacteria previously grown from possible sites of bacteremia.
2. Empiric therapy must be readjusted based on blood culture results.
3. Volume expansion with normal saline must be initiated emergently.
4. Surgical consultation is required for possible intra-abdominal sepsis and for potential cases of necrotizing fasciitis.
5. Potentially infected intravascular catheters must be removed.
6. Monitoring of patients on conventional wards should include
   a) hourly vital signs.
   b) 2-hourly arterial blood gases.
   c) 4- to 6-hourly serum lactate measurements.
7. Deterioration of these parameters warrants transfer to an intensive care unit.

---

3. Blood lactate and coagulation parameters initially, and perhaps every 4–6 hours until a clear sense develops of how the patient is progressing

Failure of the patient to respond to fluids and antibiotics—as indicated by a persistent fall in blood pressure, accumulation of lactate, increasing hypoxemia, and laboratory signs suggesting a coagulopathy—dictate that the patient be moved to an intensive care unit for closer monitoring and more aggressive hemodynamic support. There are no proven superior therapies at this time. Judicious use of vasopressors is generally recommended, beginning with dopamine and progressing to norepinephrine. Aggressive fluid resuscitation should be continued with specific attention to central venous pressures and pulmonary vascular congestion. Further management needs to be deferred to the intensive care specialists.

Adjunctive Therapies

Many different substances have been used to reverse the persistent hypotension and associated end-organ damage associated with sepsis syndrome. Most of these adjunctive measures have failed to improve mortality in large studies. Given current knowledge of the pathogenesis of sepsis, additional trials are likely to be undertaken in the future. These are some of potential therapies that have not proved beneficial to date:

1. Anti-inflammatory agents such as ibuprofen and even narcotic antagonists have not proven to be of value in large scale studies.
2. Monoclonal antibody against the core of the endotoxin molecule has not been conclusively shown to be beneficial.
3. Antibody against TNF-α and the TNF-α receptor have failed.
4. Studies utilizing IL-1 receptor antagonists have been inconclusive.
5. Platelet activating factor antagonists have failed.

Corticosteroids

The use of corticosteroids in septic shock has been under debate for decades. It is known that some of these patients have or develop adrenal insufficiency. Recent studies have re-examined this question with the startling revelation that, as compared with high doses, low physiologic doses of corticosteroids for 7 days are associated with improved survival. However, debate continues regarding whether only patients with adrenal insufficiency should receive these agents or whether all patients should be so treated. Further studies will be required to clarify the efficacy of low-dose steroids;

however, pending these studies, treatment with 200–300 mg of hydrocortisone or its equivalent daily for 7 days should be strongly considered.

Drotrecogin α

Investigations of sepsis have shown that protein C levels are low and that septic patients are unable to activate this substance. Protein C plays a key role in inhibiting coagulation, and it may be an important inhibitor of monocyte activation. Animal studies have shown that infusion of activated protein C reduces mortality in lethal *E. coli* infections. Clinical trials in humans have subsequently shown a modest reduction of mortality in septic shock when patients are treated with activated protein C. This agent, now called drotrecogin α, has now been approved by the U.S. Food and Drug Administration as an adjunct to standard therapy for the treatment of severe sepsis. Drotrecogin α reduced mortality to 24.7% from 30.8% in placebo-treated patients over 28 days, a statistically significant reduction. Because of the complexity of patient inclusion criteria, very high costs, and potential for bleeding complications, this agent is reserved for use by intensive care and infectious disease specialists. Its major contraindication

is recent surgery, the risk of bleeding complications being prohibitively high in the postoperative patient population.

CONCLUSION

The physician first needs to make an immediate decision about severity of the illness, and with clinical experience, most physicians become skilled at recognizing the sickest patients. Among the severely ill, patients with sepsis syndrome have the highest mortality and morbidity. Early recognition of sepsis and efforts to remove the precipitating cause and to deliver aggressive fluid and vasopressor therapy, optimal supportive care for organ dysfunction, and empiric antimicrobial therapy for the most likely microbial pathogens remain the standard of care.

It is important that the physician reassess empiric antibiotic coverage in 48 hours when culture results have returned. The organisms grown on blood culture can help to identify the site of primary infection. They also often allow the spectrum of antibiotic coverage to be narrowed, reducing the likelihood of patient colonization with highly resistant bacterial flora. (See Chapter 1, "Anti-infective Therapy.") Activated protein C is of modest benefit, but not all patients are candidates for this agent. However, agents of this type that will be more effective are likely to be developed in the future, as more is learned about the mechanisms involved in the progression of sepsis.

KEY POINTS

About Adjunctive Therapies for Sepsis Syndrome

1. Multiple clinical trials have failed to document efficacy for
   a) anti-inflammatory agents.
   b) monoclonal antibody against endotoxin.
   c) anti–tumor necrosis factor α antibodies.
   d) interleukin-1 antagonists.
   e) platelet activating factor antagonists.
2. Corticosteroids is low doses may be beneficial.
3. Activated protein C (drotrecogin α) is of limited efficacy (6% reduction in mortality) and
   a) is extremely expensive;
   b) should only be given by intensive care or infectious disease specialists; and
   c) is contraindicated in postoperative patients because of bleeding complications.

FURTHER READING

Balk RA. Sepsis and septic shock. Definitions, epidemiology, and clinical manifestations. *Crit Care Clin.* 2000;16:179–192.

Bernard GR, Vincent JL, Laterre PF, et al. Efficacy and safety of recombinant human activated protein C for severe sepsis. *N Engl J Med.* 2001;344:699–709.

Kreger BE, Craven DE, McCabe WR. Gram-negative bacteremia. IV. Reevaluation of clinical features and treatment in 612 patients. *Am J Med.* 1980;68:344–355.

Kumar A, Roberts D, Wood KE, et al. Duration of hypotension before initiation of effective antimicrobial therapy is the critical determinant of survival in human septic shock. *Crit Care Med.* 2006;34:1589–1596.

Minneci PC, Deans KJ, Banks SM, Eichacker PQ, Natanson C. Meta-analysis: the effect of steroids on survival and shock during sepsis depends on the dose. *Ann Intern Med.* 2004;141:47–56.

Pittet D, Li N, Woolson RF, Wentzel RP. Microbiological factors influencing the outcome of nosocomial bloodstream infections: a 6-year validated, population-based model. *Clin Infect Dis.* 1997;24:1068–1078.

Russell JA. Management of sepsis. *N Engl J Med.* 2006;355: 1699–1713.

The Febrile Patient

Time Recommended to Complete: 1 day

Frederick Southwick, M.D.

GUIDING QUESTIONS

1. Which region of the brain is primarily responsible for temperature regulation?

2. Does core temperature vary at different times of the day?

3. Is fever beneficial?

4. How and when should fever be treated?

5. How do acetylsalicylic acid and acetaminophen act to reduce fever?

■ TEMPERATURE REGULATION

Body temperature is regulated by the anterior hypothalamus in combination with many other neural structures, including the brain stem, spinal cord, and sympathetic ganglia. The region of the hypothalamus near the optic chiasm is thought to be primarily responsible for maintaining the body's core temperature. A distinct temperature set point is established, and when body core temperature drops below that set point, the nervous system increases body metabolism and stimulates shivering and chills. When core temperature exceeds that set point, the nervous system increases peripheral blood flow and sweating. "Normal" body temperature is 37°C, but it varies from individual to individual, following a normal distribution. Some individuals therefore have a lower set point, and others have a higher set point than the mean "normal" temperature. Furthermore, in each individual's core temperature varies during the day, being lower in the morning and increasing in the evening. Before deciding that a patient has a fever, the physician must be familiar with that patient's normal set point and diurnal core temperature variation.

MECHANISMS UNDERLYING THE FEBRILE RESPONSE

Fever is a consequence of the anterior hypothalamus responding to inflammatory mediators. Among the mediators thought to stimulate a rise in the normal core temperature set point are interleukin 1 (IL-1), tumor necrosis factor α (TNF-α), interleukin 6 (IL-6), and interferon γ (IFN-γ). These cytokines are released primarily by monocytes and macrophages in response to invasion by various pathogens and by other inflammatory stimuli. Investigators speculate that these cytokines stimulate the circumventricular organs near the optic chiasm, activating phospholipase A_2, which in turn stimulates the cyclo-oxygenase pathway to produce increased levels of prostaglandin E_2. This small molecule crosses the blood–brain barrier and stimulates the neurons within the anterior hypothalamus and brain stem responsible for thermal regulation.

BENEFITS AND HARMFUL EFFECTS OF FEVER

In addition to serving as a warning sign for the onset of infection, fever is thought to be beneficial. The growth of some viruses, bacteria, fungi, and parasites are inhibited by a rise in temperature above 37°C. Fever has also been shown to enhance the ability of macrophages and neutrophils to kill foreign pathogens and to improve cell-mediated immune function.

Depending on the individual patient, fever may also have harmful effects. Patients with heart disease may suffer cardiac ischemia because of the increase in heart rate and the oxygen demands associated with fever. Patients with severe pulmonary disease may similarly be

66

unable to compensate for the increased oxygen demands associated with fever. Elderly patients with limited mental capacity may develop confusion and lethargy in response to fever, complicating their care. Children can suffer from seizures in association with high fever—although, to date, there is no proof that reducing fever prevents febrile seizures.

TREATMENT OF FEVER

The primary treatment for fever is to treat the underlying cause. The role of lowering body temperature while trying to determine the primary cause of fever remains controversial.

Based on current understanding of thermal regulation, direct cooling of the body using ice, cold water, or a cooling blanket should be considered only in conjunction with medicines that reset the thermal set point. Otherwise, the central nervous system will respond to such measures by inducing chills and shivering, increasing the patient's discomfort. Use of antipyretics is probably warranted in patients with heart disease, pulmonary disease, and in elderly patients with mental dysfunction in association with fever.

The pharmacologic agents used to reset the thermal set point all inhibit prostaglandin synthetase activity and reduce prostaglandin E_2 production. Acetylsalicylic acid (ASA), nonsteroidal anti-inflammatory drugs (NSAIDs), and acetaminophen are all effective. In children, ASA should probably be avoided because of the increased risk of Reyes syndrome (a deadly syndrome consisting of fatal

hepatic and renal failure), and acetaminophen should be avoided in patients with serious underlying liver disease. Coronary artery vasoconstriction has been associated with NSAIDs, and therefore those drugs probably should not be used in patients with ischemic heart disease. To avoid repeated shifting of the thermal set point and recurrent shivering and chills, antipyretic agents must be administered on a regular schedule until the primary cause of fever has been treated.

■ FEVER OF UNDETERMINED ORIGIN

GUIDING QUESTIONS

1. *What are the criteria used to define FUO?*
2. *Which diseases are most commonly associated with FUO?*
3. *Which diseases are most commonly associated with FUO in the elderly?*
4. *Which basic diagnostic tests should be ordered in cases of FUO?*
5. *What is Sutton's law, and how is this law applied to FUO?*
6. *Should empiric antibiotics be started in cases of FUO?*
7. *What is the prognosis in patients with FUO?*

POTENTIAL SEVERITY

Fever of undetermined origin (FUO) is a chronic disorder that requires a thoughtful diagnostic approach.

DEFINITION OF FUO

At the time that the patient first visits the physician with complaints of fever, the cause is in many cases not apparent. Some physicians label these complaints as FUO. However, the name "fever of undetermined origin" carries with it specific criteria and should not be loosely applied. As first defined in 1961, FUO requires that the patient have

<table>
<tr><td colspan="2" align="center">**KEY POINTS**</td></tr>
</table>

KEY POINTS
About the Definition of Fever of Unknown Origin
1. Fever must persist for more than 3 weeks in order to exclude self-limiting viral illnesses.
2. Temperature must be more than 38.3°C (101°F) to exclude normal variations in core body temperature set point.
3. No diagnosis reached after 3 days of testing.

Table 3.1. Major Causes of Fever of Unknown Origin

"Big 3"	
1.	Infection
2.	Neoplasm
3.	Autoimmune disease
"Little 6"	
1.	Granulomatous disease
2.	Regional enteritis
3.	Familial Mediterranean fever
4.	Drug fever
5.	Pulmonary emboli
6.	Factitious fever

1. an illness that has lasted least 3 weeks,
2. fever of more than 38.3°C on several occasions, and
3. no diagnosis after routine work up for 3 days in hospital or after 3 or more outpatient visits.

A duration of 3 weeks or longer was chosen to eliminate self-limiting viral illnesses that are generally difficult to diagnose and that resolve within that time period. A temperature of more than 38°C was chosen to eliminate those individuals at the far right of the normal temperature distribution curve who normally may have a slightly higher core temperature set point and an exaggerated diurnal temperature variation. Recognizing that, in the present era of managed care, most patients with FUO are now diagnosed and managed as outpatients, the third criterion has been modified to include outpatient diagnostic testing as well as that conducted in hospital.

Before launching a complex and expensive series of diagnostic tests, the physician must carefully document that the patient fulfills the criteria for FUO. Most important is the documentation of true fever. The patient should be instructed to measure both 6 A.M. and 6 P.M. temperature to rule out an exaggerated circadian rhythm. Secondly, an electronic thermometer should always be used to exclude the possibility of factitious fever (discussed in the next subsection). The exact pattern of fever generally is not helpful in identifying the fever's cause.

CAUSES OF FUO

Many diseases can initially present with the primary manifestation of prolonged fever (Table 3.1). The possible causes can be classified into three major categories ("the big three"): infections, neoplasms, and autoimmune disorders. The miscellaneous causes are numerous, the most common being six diseases ("the little six"): granulomatous diseases, regional enteritis, familial Mediterranean fever (FMF), drug fever, pulmonary emboli, and factitious fever.

CASE 3.1

A 19–year-old white male, university sophomore, presented with a 3-week history of fevers to 40°C, fatigue, and anorexia. He was evaluated in the school infirmary and was given intravenous fluids for dehydration. He was treated empirically with penicillin and clarithromycin. Despite this treatment, his fevers persisted.

Epidemiology indicated no recent travel. A review of systems was negative, other than 1 to 2 loose bowel movements daily for the week before admission.

Vital signs included a temperature of 39.2°C, pulse 88 per minute, respirations 20 per minute, blood pressure 122/60 mm Hg. The patient appeared mildly ill. His physical exam was completely normal, including absence of palpable lymph nodes, no skin rashes, no cardiac murmurs, a benign abdominal exam without organomegaly, and a normal joint and extremity exam.

Laboratory workup showed a white blood cell (WBC) count of 11,600/mm³, with 93% polymorphonuclear leukocytes. Hematocrit was 35%; platelets, 228,000/mm³; blood urea nitrogen, 6 mg/dL; serum albumin, 3.0 g/dL; total protein, 6.2 g/dL; alkaline phosphatase (ALP), 327 IU/L; alanine transaminase (ALT), 107 IU/L; and erythrocyte sedimentation rate (ESR), 105 mm/h. Blood cultures were twice negative, and a chest X-ray (CXR) was within normal limits.

Because of the persistent fever and anorexia, the patient underwent an abdominal computed tomography (CT) scan that demonstrated an hepatic abscess 9 cm in diameter in the right lower lobe of the liver. Echinococcal serum titer was negative. Cutaneous aspiration demonstrated thick pus, and culture grew Staphylococcus aureus, *methicillin-sensitive.*

Comment

Other than a mildly elevated ALP level, no clinical clues indicative of liver abscess were seen. On further review of past medical history, the patient reported having intermittent furunculosis. His skin was likely the initial portal of entry, resulting in transient bacteremia and seeding of the liver.

Infection

In patients under the age of 65 years, infection remains the most common cause of FUO (Table 3.2). Common infectious causes of FUO include abscesses, particularly abdominal abscesses that may persist for prolonged periods before being diagnosed. Improvements in imaging techniques have improved on the ability to locate and drain occult pyogenic collections. Osteomyelitis—particularly of the vertebral bodies, mandible, and air sinuses—can also present as FUO. Bone scan is particularly helpful in identifying such infections.

In earlier series, subacute bacterial endocarditis (SBE) was a major cause of FUO. However, improved culture techniques, including prolonged incubation of blood cultures to identify more fastidious slow-growing

Table 3.2. Infectious Causes of Fever of Unknown Origin

1.	Abscesses
2.	Osteomyelitis (vertebrae, mandible, sinuses)
3.	Subacute bacterial endocarditis (murmur usually present, beware of previous antibiotics)
4.	Biliary system infections (may have no right upper quadrant tenderness)
5.	Urinary tract infections (in absence of related symptoms)
6.	Tuberculosis (especially miliary disease)
7.	Spirochetal infection (leptospirosis, *Borrelia*)
8.	Brucellosis (animal exposure, unpasteurized cheese)
9.	Rickettsial infection
10.	*Chlamydia*
11.	Epstein–Barr virus, cytomegalovirus
12.	Fungal infection (*Cryptococcus*, histoplasmosis)
13.	Parasites (malaria, toxoplasmosis, trypanosomiasis)

pathogens such as the HACEK organisms (see Chapter 7 on bacterial endocarditis), and drawing large volumes of blood for culture have improved the sensitivity of blood cultures and reduced the number of undiagnosed cases of SBE. Transesophageal cardiac echo has also improved identification of vegetations. As a result of those advances, SBE has become a less common cause of FUO in recent reports. In almost every case, patients with SBE have an audible murmur, emphasizing the importance of a careful physical exam during the initial evaluation of the patient with FUO.

The physician must also keep in mind that, if the patient has received antibiotics, the utility of blood cultures is markedly reduced. Administration of antibiotics temporarily sterilizes the bloodstream. Antibiotics must be discontinued for 7 to 10 days before blood cultures become positive.

Biliary system infections also can present as FUO. Such patients often have no right upper quadrant pain and no right upper quadrant tenderness. Subacute pyelonephritis can also present with a prolonged fever in the absence of dysuria, frequency, or flank pain.

In cases of FUO, miliary tuberculosis (TB) must always be considered. This potentially lethal disease is most common in elderly and immunocompromised patients, particularly patients with HIV and patients on high-dose glucocorticoids or a TNF inhibitor. Bone marrow culture is particularly helpful in making this diagnosis. A CXR may demonstrate micronodular ("millet seed") interstitial changes; however, this radiologic finding may be absent in elderly individuals. If appropriate antituberculosis therapy is not initiated promptly, these patients usually deteriorate over 2 to 3 weeks and die.

Leptospirosis can cause persistent fever and is difficult to diagnose. A combination of appropriate epidemiology (animal or contaminated soil or water exposure), conjunctival suffusion, aseptic meningitis, liver enzyme abnormalities, and renal dysfunction should alert the clinician to this possibility. Other spirochetal diseases reported to cause persistent fever include Lyme disease and relapsing fever. Animal exposure, particularly the skinning of wild boar, should raise the possibility of brucellosis. Brucellosis can also be contracted by eating unpasteurized cheese.

Rickettsial infections can also cause FUO. Epidemiology plays a critical role in alerting the clinician to this group of pathogens. A history of camping, hunting, or other outdoor activities in areas endemic for these infections should raise the possibility. *Rickettsia* are tick-borne; however, a history of tick bite is not always obtained.

Chlamydia is another intracellular pathogen that on occasion can cause prolonged fever. *Chlamydia psittaci* in particular can result in a mononucleosis-like syndrome. This organism is usually contracted from birds, including pigeons, members of the parrot family (parakeets, macaws, and cockatoos), finches (canaries, goldfinches), and poultry. Epstein–Barr virus and cytomegalovirus can both cause a mononucleosis syndrome resulting in sore throat, lymphadenopathy, splenomegaly, and prolonged fever.

In addition to bacteria and viruses, fungi can occasionally result in FUO, cryptococcosis and histoplasmosis being the two most common fungal diseases reported. Parasites can similarly cause prolonged fever. Malaria (non-falciparum forms), toxoplasmosis, and trypanosomiasis are the most commonly reported parasitic diseases associated with FUO.

Neoplasm

Neoplastic disorders represent the second major category of diseases associated with FUO (Table 3.3). In elderly patients, neoplasia is the most frequent cause, and in this category lymphomas are the most commonly reported cause of fever.

Table 3.3. Neoplastic Causes of Fever of Unknown Origin

1.	Lymphoma (especially Hodgkin, Pel–Ebstein fever)
2.	Leukemia (aleukemic or preleukemic phase)
3.	Hypernephroma (high sedimentation rate)
4.	Hepatoma (generally not metastatic liver disease)
5.	Atrial myxoma

Hodgkin lymphomas intermittently produce pyrogens: one week the patient may be afebrile, and the following week may bring hectic fevers. This fever pattern has been termed Pel–Ebstein fever, which when present, raises the possibility of Hodgkin lymphoma. Patients with non-Hodgkin lymphoma may also present with fever. In some cases, the fever can be high and mimic sepsis.

Patients with leukemia may also present with fever. Older patients in the aleukemic or the preleukemic phase of their disease may have little or no evidence of leukemia on peripheral smear. In earlier series, hypernephroma was noted to cause FUO; however, examination of a large series of patients with hypernephroma has demonstrated that this solid tumor is rarely associated with fever.

The solid tumor most frequently reported as a cause of FUO is primary hepatoma, but tumors that metastasize to liver rarely cause fever. Atrial myxoma is a rare disorder that is associated with fever, and it can mimic subacute bacterial endocarditis. Small pieces of the atrial tumor can break off and embolize to the periphery, causing small infarcts similar to those observed in bacterial endocarditis.

CASE 3.2

A 27–year-old Asian man presented with a chief complaint of fevers of 2 weeks' duration. Two weeks earlier, he had begun to experience fever associated with weakness, malaise, shoulder and neck weakness, and muscle tenderness. He also noted a sore throat. He was admitted to a hospital in Puerto Rico where a CXR demonstrated diffuse pulmonary infiltrates and a sputum Gram stain showed gram-positive cocci. His WBC count was 16,000/mm³. He was treated with intravenous mezlocillin and gentamicin and later switched to ampicillin. He failed to improve, remaining febrile, and he came to the university hospital.

Epidemiology indicated no pets, no allergies, no consumption of unpasteurized milk or raw meat, no swimming in fresh water, no exposure to TB, no history of gonococcus or syphilis.

Social history recorded occasional alcohol use, single status, and employment as a cook. Other than the trip to Puerto Rico, travel was unremarkable. No pets. No exposure to TB or other infectious diseases.

Past medical history indicated that, at age 9, he had an acute febrile episode associated with a rash, severe joint swelling, and high fever. The illness spontaneously subsided.

The patient's physical exam showed a temperature of 38.3°C and a clear chest. Liver edge was palpated 2 cm below the right costal margin, slightly tender. His left upper quadrant was also tender, Skin showed a macular rash over the chest where he had applied rubbing ointment.

Laboratory workup showed a peripheral WBC count of 20,400/mm³, (with 94% polymorphonuclear;eukocytes, 4% lymphocytes, 2% macrophages. Platelet count was 354,000/mm³; hemoglobin, 12.9 g/dL; PaO₂, 69 mm Hg; PaCO₂, 33 mm Hg; HCO₃, 24 mEq/L. A urinalysis was negative. Total bilirubin was 2.8 mg/dL; ALT, 108 IU/L; aspartate aminotransferase (AST) 98 IU/L; and γ-glutamyl transpeptidase (GGT), 42 IU/L.A CXR showed infiltrate in the left lower lobe of the lungs.

Ceftriaxone and erythromycin were started; however, this patient's fevers persisted in the range 38.3°C to 40.6°C.

A subsequent laboratory analysis included an ESR above 100 mm/h, a peripheral WBC count of 35,000/mm³, and a hemoglobin of 9.1 g/dL.

After 4 days of persistent fever, the patient was switched to a tetracycline antibiotic, followed by 3 days of naproxen. Additional tests at that time included a PPD skin test (4 mm), and an acid-fast bacilli stain of sputum (negative). Abdominal ultrasound and CT scans were negative with the exception of consolidation seen in the left and right lung bases. A bronchoscopy was negative for Pneumocystis and Legionella; transbronchial biopsy was consistent with focal pneumonitis. A lumbar puncture showed glucose 89 mg/100 mL, total protein 11 mg/mL, and WBC count 0 in the cerebrospinal fluid. Thick and thin malaria smears were negative; stool samples for ova and parasites were thrice negative. Hepatitis B surface antibody was positive (Ab+), core was Ab+, and surface antigen was negative. He had a 1:185, antinuclear antibodies (ANAs) and rheumatoid factor were negative, and the rapid plasma reagin was also negative. Eight separate blood cultures were negative, and a monospot test was negative. Repeat transaminase values registered ALT 94 IU/L, AST 64 IU/L, ALP 403 IU/L, and GGT 180 IU/L.

The patient continued to have fevers. A liver biopsy demonstrated nonspecific inflammation. Weight loss continued, and the patient's ESR and WBC remained elevated. After 8 days in the hospital, he developed a swollen left wrist and swollen right elbow. He was treated with high-dose oral salicyclates. Within 24 hours of initiation of therapy, he defervesced. Over the next 2 weeks, his symptoms completely resolved. Based on past medical history, clinical presentation, and response to salicyclates, he was discharged with a diagnosis of Still's disease.

Autoimmune Disease

Autoimmune disease is the third major category of diseases that cause FUO (Table 3.4). In early series of FUO cases, systemic lupus erythematosus (SLE) was a frequent cause. However, with improvements in antinuclear and anti-DNA markers, these sensitive tests readily identify cases of SLE. The diagnosis is now usually made within 3 weeks.

Still's disease (adult-onset juvenile rheumatoid arthritis) is one of the most frequent autoimmune diseases resulting in FUO in younger patients. Key clinical features of this disease include an evanescent macular rash, arthralgias, and a sore throat. Patients with

Table 3.4. Autoimmune Diseases That Cause Fever of Unknown Origin

1.	Systemic lupus erythematosus
2.	Still's disease
3.	Hypersensitivity angiitis
4.	Polymyalgia rheumatica, combined with temporal arteritis
5.	Polyarteritis nodosa
6.	Mixed connective tissue disease
7.	Subacute thyroiditis

Table 3.5. Drugs That Cause Fever of Unknown Origin

Antihistamines	Isoniazid
Barbiturates	Nitrofurantoin
Chlorambucil	Penicillins
Dilantin	Procaine amide
Hydralazine	Quinidine
Ibuprofen	Salicyclates
Iodides	Thiouracil
Aldomet	Mercaptopurine

Still's disease often have high fevers associated with a high peripheral WBC counts, and this combination frequently causes the physician to begin antibiotic therapy for a presumed bacterial infection. However, the fever fails to subside after initiation of antibiotics. No specific test is available for Still's disease. Serum ferritin levels are generally markedly elevated, as is the ESR.

In elderly patients, polymyalgia rheumatica is the most common autoimmune disorder to cause FUO. This disease results in proximal muscle weakness and a high ESR. Temporal headaches and visual complaints are present, as is temporal arteritis, a vasculitis commonly associated with polymyalgia rheumatica.

Other autoimmune diseases reported to cause FUO include polyarteritis nodosa, hypersensitivity angiitis, and mixed connective tissue disease. Subacute thyroiditis may present with prolonged fever. On examination, the thyroid is often tender and serum antithyroid antibodies are elevated. Recently, Kikuchi's disease, also called histicytic necrotizing lymphadenitis, has been reported to cause prolonged fever. This self-limiting autoimmune disorder occurs in young Asian females and is associated with generalized lymphadenopathy. Diagnosis is made by lymph node biopsy.

Other Causes of FUO

In addition to the "big 3" categories, clinicians must also consider the "little 6."

The first is granulomatous diseases of unclear causation. This disease group presents with fever and malaise and generally involves the liver. Liver function tests typically demonstrate mild abnormalities in ALP, and liver biopsy reveals granulomas.

The second possibility is regional enteritis. This disease can present with prolonged fever in the absence of gastrointestinal complaints. For this reason, contrast studies of the gastrointestinal tract are generally recommended to exclude this diagnosis.

The third member of the "little 6" is familial Mediterranean fever. As the name implies, this is a genetic disorder associated with recurrent serositis primarily of the abdominal cavity, but it can also result in pleuritis and pericarditis. A family history is critical in raising this possibility.

The fourth disorder in this group is drug fever, one of the most frequently encountered causes of FUO. Table 3.5 lists the drugs that most commonly cause fever. The anti-seizure medication Dilantin is probably the drug that most frequently causes allergic reactions, including fever. Quinidine, procaine amide, sulfonamides, and penicillins are other major offenders. When a patient presents with FUO, all medications should be discontinued or switched to exclude this possibility.

Fifth of the "little 6" diseases is pulmonary emboli. Prolonged bed rest increases the risk of thrombus formation in the calves. When emboli are small, they may not result in respiratory complaints and may simply present as fever. In all patients at risk for thrombophlebitis who present with FUO, pulmonary emboli need to be excluded.

The final disorder in this list is factitious fever. In earlier series, patients often manipulated the mercury thermometer to fool the physician; the advent of the electronic thermometer has made this maneuver impossible. Today, patients usually inject themselves with saliva or stool, causing polymicrobial bacteremia and fever. This disorder occurs almost exclusively in women. A medical background is also the rule. In the absence of

any clear cause for fever, a history of health care training should raise the clinician's suspicion, particularly if the patient takes great interest in her illness and has a medical textbook at the bedside. The diagnostic test of choice is often a search of the patient's room seeking a syringe used for self injection.

Finally, in a recent series, a high proportion of patients (30%) had no explanation for their FUO. In many of these cases, fever spontaneously resolved over 3 to 6 months without harmful consequences.

HISTORY IN FUO

History can play a critical role in narrowing the differential diagnosis and in deciding on the most appropriate diagnostic tests. A review of all symptoms associated with the illness needs to be periodically updated. Symptoms often are transient and are recalled by the patient only after repeated questioning. A patient's past medical history often provides useful clues. History of tuberculosis, tuberculosis exposure, or a positive PPD should be included. Family history must also be thoroughly reviewed to exclude genetic disorders such as cyclic neutropenia and familial Mediterranean fever. Social history needs to include animal exposure (pets, and other domestic or wild animals), home environment, and occupational exposure. Travel history should explore travel to areas endemic for malaria and other parasites, typhoid, coccidiomycosis, histoplasmosis, and tick-borne illnesses. A list of all medications, including over-the-counter and natural organic remedies, must be compiled to exclude the possibility of drug fever.

PHYSICAL EXAM IN FUO

In addition to a careful history, careful repeat physical examination is frequently helpful. Particular attention should be paid to the skin exam, looking for embolic or vasculitic lesions or evidence of physical manipulation. Particular attention should be paid to the nail beds, where small emboli can become trapped in the distal capillaries of the fingers and toes, resulting in small splinter-shaped infarcts. Joint motion and the presence of effusions should be looked for. Careful eye exam should be repeated looking for conjunctival petechiae, conjunctivitis, punctate corneal lesions, uveitis, optic nerve changes, retinal or choroidal abnormalities. Thorough palpation of all lymph nodes needs to be repeatedly performed, documenting the consistency, size, and tenderness. Cardiac exam should be repeated daily, listening for cardiac murmurs and pericardial rubs. The abdomen also should be palpated daily to detect new masses, areas of localized tenderness, and hepato- or splenomegaly.

Table 3.6. Preliminary Tests Recommended for Fever of Unknown Origin

Complete history
Careful physical exam
Complete blood count with differential
Blood smears with Giemsa and Wright stain
Liver function tests
Antinuclear antibodies and rheumatoid factor
Erythrocyte sedimentation rate
Urinalysis
Blood culture
Urine culture
PPD skin test
Chest and abdominal computed tomography scan

LABORATORY STUDIES IN FUO

All patients with FUO should receive a series of basic diagnostic tests (Table 3.6). However, because each case is different, a series of yes-or-no branch points are not possible for guiding the subsequent diagnostic approach to FUO.

In recent years, rather than insufficient studies being the norm, clinicians have erred on the side of excessive and uninformative testing. Each patient's diagnostic workup must be tailored to personal history and physical findings. A cookbook approach subjects the patient to undue costly testing and stress. "Tincture of time" and repeated history and physical exam often allow the physician to apply Sutton's law.

Willy Sutton was a famous bank robber, who, when finally captured, was asked by newspaper reporters, "Willy, why do you rob banks?" Willy replied, "That's where the money is." Clinicians need to focus on diagnostic tests that are likely to have a high yield. They need to "go where the money is."

Classes of Diagnostic Tests

SKIN TESTS

An intermediate-strength PPD should be performed in all patients with FUO who do not have a previously documented positive PPD. The use of skin tests to detect histoplasmosis and coccidiomycosis is not generally recommended.

CULTURES

Blood cultures should be part of the initial workup of all patients with significant prolonged fever. Yield for subacute bacterial endocarditis is usually maximized by drawing blood for three cultures (see Chapter 7). In general no more than six blood cultures should be drawn. They may be repeated periodically or if a significant change occurs in the fever pattern. Because of the possibility of fastidious slow-growing bacteria, all blood cultures should be held for 3 weeks.

Multiple urine samples should be obtained and cultured for tuberculosis in addition to more conventional bacteria. In patients with respiratory complaints or CXR abnormalities, sputum should be cultured, and in patients undergoing bone marrow biopsy, culture is an important component of the marrow analysis. All biopsy specimens need to be cultured. Aerobic, anaerobic, mycobacterial, and fungal cultures should be ordered on virtually all samples. Viral cultures or quantitative polymerase chain reaction (PCR) may also be considered in specific cases in which cytomegalovirus or Epstein–Barr virus is suspected.

SMEARS

Peripheral blood smears with Giemsa and Wright stains are critical for making the diagnosis of malaria, trypanosomiasis, or relapsing fever. In addition to a peripheral WBC count, Wright stain with differential cell count is often helpful in determining the nature of the inflammatory response associated with fever, and it should be performed in all patients with FUO. Stool smears for ova and parasites are usually less helpful, being that gastrointestinal parasites seldom present as FUO.

OTHER PERIPHERAL BLOOD TESTS

Antibody titers should be considered when specific pathogens are part of the differential diagnosis. To prove active infection, rising antibody titers are required. A single titer simply demonstrates a past history of exposure; a rising titer indicates recent infection. Therefore, two samples separated by 3 to 4 weeks need to be drawn. Antibody titers are particularly useful in cytomegalovirus,

---

KEY POINTS

About Diagnostic Workup in Fever of Unknown Origin

1. Physicians usually err by overtesting.
2. A cookbook approach should be avoided.
3. Sutton's law ("Go where the money is") should be applied. Tests should be directed toward specific complaints and abnormalities found on preliminary testing.

Epstein–Barr virus, *Toxoplasma*, *Rickettsia*, *Chlamydia*, and *Brucella* infections. If liver functions are abnormal, hepatitis serology should also be ordered (see Chapter 8). An HIV antibody test should be performed in all patients with potential risk factors (see Chapter 17).

Tests that should be considered to diagnose connective tissue disease in most cases of FUO are antibody titers to human tissue, including ANAs, anti-DNA antibodies, rheumatoid factor, and immune complexes. An ESR assay should be performed in all cases of FUO. A very high ESR is seen in the polymyalgia rheumatica–temporal arteritis combination and in Still's disease. A normal ESR virtually excludes these diagnoses, as well as subacute bacterial endocarditis.

IMAGING STUDIES

Tests That Should Be Ordered in All Patients with FUO—As part of the preliminary workup, a chest CT scan should be ordered. Results to look for are mediastinal enlargement (suggestive of lymphoma), micronodular interstitial changes ("millet seed" pattern, suggestive of miliary tuberculosis), or nodular lesions or infiltrates (can be seen in many infectious diseases, connective tissue diseases, and neoplasms). Abdominal CT scan should also be performed to identify abdominal abscesses, mesenteric nodes, and tumors. Imaging of the chest and abdomen by CT have an approximately 10% yield in patients with FUO who lack specific localizing symptoms.

Tests That Should Be Ordered Depending on the Patient's Symptoms and Signs—In patients who are suspected of having a chronic infection, radionuclide scans may be helpful in localizing the site. Gallium scan may be useful in patients with chronic infection because this agent accumulates in areas of inflammation; however, indium white blood cell scan tends to be more specific. The indium white blood cell scan also has a higher positive yield than abdominal CT scan does for identifying occult intra-abdominal infection.

Another tracer molecule that accumulates in areas of inflammation and in malignant tumors is ^{18}F fluorodeoxyglucose. Unlike other scans, which require that the patient be scanned during a period of 24 to 36 hours, positron emission tomography with ^{18}F fluorodeoxyglucose is completed within a few hours. In preliminary studies, this test has proved more sensitive and specific than gallium scan. For the assessment of osteomyelitis or tumor metastasis to bone (with the exception of prostate cancer and multiple myeloma), technetium scan is the most sensitive and specific technique.

Air sinus films or sinus CT scan can be performed to exclude occult sinus infection and tooth abscess. In patients with a heart murmur and persistent fever, cardiac echo should be considered. Transesophageal echo is the test of choice; it has a greater than 90% sensitivity for detecting cardiac vegetations, and it is also helpful in detecting myocardial abscess and atrial myxoma.

Ultrasound of the lower abdomen may be helpful in cases in which pelvic lesions are suspected. Abdominal CT is not as sensitive in that region because of reflection artifacts generated by the pelvic bones. When other tests are unrevealing, upper gastrointestinal barium study with small bowel follow-through should be ordered to exclude regional enteritis. Barium enema should be considered in older patients; however, yield from this procedure is likely to be low in FUO. Radiographs of all joints should be ordered in any patient with persistent joint complaints to document anatomic defects.

Invasive Procedures—If all noninvasive tests prove to be negative, liver biopsy is recommended to exclude the possibility of granulomatous hepatitis. Laparoscopic guided biopsy improves the yield by allowing biopsies to be taken in areas where abnormalities in the external capsule are seen.

Bone marrow aspiration and biopsy is also recommended as a routine invasive test if all noninvasive studies are negative. Leukemia in its early stages may be detected, as may stage IV lymphoma. It is critical that the bone marrow be appropriately cultured (see the earlier subsection titled "Cultures"), because disseminated tuberculosis, histoplasmosis, coccidiomycosis, and other fungal and mycobacterial infections often seed the bone marrow.

Use of other invasive procedures will depend on the diagnostic findings, history, and physical findings to that point. In elderly patients with a high ESR and persistent fever, temporal artery biopsy is generally recommended. It should be kept in mind that, because skip lesions are common in temporal arteritis, a long sample of the temporal artery should be obtained and multiple arterial sections examined.

In early series of FUO, diagnostic laparotomy was frequently recommended. With the advent of new abdominal imaging techniques, this invasive procedure is now seldom performed; however, it may be considered in selected cases.

In addition to a complete series of cultures, all biopsy specimens should undergo Brown–Brenn, Ziehl–Neelsen, methenamine silver, periodic acid Schiff, and Dieterle silver staining in addition to routine hematoxylin and eosin. Frozen sections should be obtained for immunofluorescence staining, and the remaining tissue block should be saved for additional future studies.

It should be emphasized that, when symptoms, signs, or a specific diagnostic abnormality is found, all other scheduled diagnostic tests should be delayed, and Sutton's law applied. For example, if an abnormal fluid collection is found on abdominal CT, then all other diagnostic procedures can be halted while a needle aspiration of the potential abscess performed. If the result proves to be positive, additional investigations are unnecessary. The "money" has been found.

Ordering tests for completeness' sake is unnecessary. When in doubt about performing additional tests, the wisest course of action is to wait. Over time, the patient's fever may spontaneously resolve, or new manifestations may develop, helping to identify the cause.

TREATMENT OF FUO

In the past, many clinicians discouraged the use of antipyretics in FUO, because these agents mask the pattern of fever. However, as noted earlier in this chapter, with rare exceptions, the pattern of fever has not proved to be helpful in determining the cause of FUO.

Fever is commonly associated with chills, sweating, fatigue, and loss of appetite. Therefore, once true fever has been documented, antipyretics can be administered in most cases of FUO to relieve some of the patient's symptoms while the diagnostic workup is pursued. To avoid repeated shifting of the thermal set point and recurrent shivering and chills, ASA, NSAIDs, or acetaminophen must be administered at the proper time intervals to maintain therapeutic levels. Otherwise, these antipyretics will exacerbate rather than reduce the symptoms of fever.

As was discussed in Chapter 1, physicians often overprescribe antibiotics. In cases of FUO, the temptation to institute an empiric trial of antibiotics is great. This temptation should be avoided. Antibiotics are contraindicated until a specific diagnosis is made. Use of an empiric antibiotic trial often delays diagnosis and is rarely curative. Because infections susceptible to conventional antibiotics represent a small percentage of the diseases that cause FUO, antibiotic treatment will have no effect in most cases. In cases of occult bacterial infection, empiric antibiotics may mask the manifestations of the infection and delay appropriate treatment. Most infections that cause FUO require prolonged antibiotic treatment and surgical drainage. In the absence of a specific diagnosis, clinicians have difficulty justifying a prolonged course of antibiotics, and therefore antibiotics are often discontinued after 1 to 2 weeks, allowing the infection to relapse.

When a connective tissue disorder appears to be the most likely explanation for FUO, empiric use of systemic glucocorticoids is often considered. These agents are very effective in treating temporal arteritis and polymyalgia rheumatica, they may be helpful in Still's disease, and they are used to treat specific complications in lupus erythematosus. However, because these agents markedly reduce inflammation and impair host defense, administration of glucocorticoids can markedly exacerbate bacterial, mycobacterial, fungal, and parasitic infections. Therefore, before considering an empiric trial of glucocorticoids such as prednisone, dexamethasone, or methylprednisone, infection must be convincingly ruled out. The physician must also keep in mind the many potential side effects of prolonged glucocorticoid use (Cushingoid face, osteoporosis, aseptic necrosis of the hip, diabetes mellitus, and opportunistic infections) before committing the patient with FUO to a prolonged course of systemic steroid treatment.

PROGNOSIS

Delay in diagnosis worsens the outcome in cases of intra-abdominal abscess, miliary tuberculosis, disseminated fungal infections, and pulmonary emboli. However, if these diseases are carefully excluded, lack of a diagnosis after an extensive workup is associated a with 5-year mortality of only 3%. The prognosis is somewhat worse in elderly patients because of their increased risk of malignancy. Therefore, once the clinician has completed the FUO diagnostic battery described in this chapter and serious life-threatening diseases have been excluded, additional diagnostic study is not warranted. If fever persists for an additional 4 to 6 months, a complete series of diagnostic studies may then be repeated.

KEY POINTS

About the Treatment of Fever of Unknown Origin

1. Once the pattern of fever has been documented, NSAIDS, acetylsalicyclic acid, or acetaminophen can be used to lower fever.
2. Empiric antibiotics are contraindicated.
3. Glucocorticoids should be used only when infection has been excluded.

■ FUO IN THE HIV-INFECTED PATIENT

Primary HIV infection can present with prolonged fever, and in patients with the appropriate risk profile (see Chapter 17), a diagnosis of HIV needs to be considered. Serum markers are negative in the early stages of HIV infection; quantitative PCR for HIV is therefore the diagnostic test of choice.

In the later stages of HIV infection, fever is a common manifestation of opportunistic infection. In order of

KEY POINTS

About Fever of Unknown Origin in HIV-Infected Patients

1. Can be a manifestation of primary HIV infection.
2. Often the first symptom of an opportunistic infection.
3. Mycobacteria are the most common infectious cause.
4. Cytomegalovirus is also common, as are *Cryptococcus* and *Toxoplasma*.
5. Non-Hodgkin lymphoma is the most common noninfectious cause.

frequency, the most common causes of FUO in patients with AIDS are mycobacterial infections (*Mycobacterium tuberculosis*, *M. avium intracellulare*, other atypical mycobacteria), other bacterial infections, cytomegalovirus, *Pneumocystis*, toxoplasmosis, and *Cryptococcus*, and histoplasmosis. In HIV patients coming from endemic areas, visceral leishmaniasis also needs to be considered. Noninfectious causes include non-Hodgkin lymphoma and drug fever. Additional tests warranted in the HIV patient include mycobacterial blood culture, cryptococcal serum antigen, and cytomegalovirus quantitative PCR. Disseminated histoplasmosis may be difficult to detect and, in our experience, is most readily diagnosed by bone marrow culture.

FEVER IN SURGICAL INTENSIVE CARE AND MEDICAL INTENSIVE CARE PATIENTS

One of the most common problems encountered by the infectious disease consultant is the evaluation of fever in patients residing in the surgical or medical intensive care unit (ICU). These patients are usually severely ill and have multiple potential causes for fever.

In the postoperative patient, wound infection must be excluded. All surgical wounds need to be carefully examined looking for purulent discharge, erythema, edema, and tenderness. In the immediate postoperative period (24 to 48 hours) Streptococcus pyogenes can result septic shock and severe bacteremia with only minimal purulence at the operative site. A Gram stain of serous exudate usually demonstrates gram-positive cocci in chains. In the later postoperative period, *S. aureus* and

nosocomial pathogens such as *Pseudomonas*, *Klebsiella*, and *Escherichia coli* are associated with wound infection.

Appropriate antibiotic therapy is generally guided by culture and Gram stain. Empiric antibiotic therapy should include gram-positive and gram-negative coverage. In patients who have suffered bowel perforation, the development of intra-abdominal abscess is a common cause of fever, and an abdominal CT scan should be ordered to exclude this possibility.

Because most ICU patients are intubated, bacteria colonizing the nasopharynx can more readily gain entry to the bronchi and pulmonary parenchyma, causing bronchitis and pneumonia. As is outlined in more detail in Chapter 4, sputum Gram stain is critical for differentiating colonization from true infection. The presence of a single organism on Gram stain, combined with more than 10 neutrophils per high-power field, strongly suggests infection. Sputum culture identifies the offending organism and sensitivities to antibiotics. Other parameters that are helpful in differentiating colonization from true infection are CXR and arterial blood gases. The presence of a new infiltrate supports the diagnosis of pneumonia, as does a reduction in arterial PaO_2.

Patients in the ICU usually have 1 or 2 intravenous catheters in place, plus an arterial line. These lines are always at risk of becoming infected, and line sepsis is a common cause of fever in the ICU setting. At the onset of new fever, all intravenous and arterial lines should be examined for erythema, warmth, and exudate. Particularly in the patient who has developed shock, all lines should be replaced, and appropriate empiric antibiotic coverage instituted.

S. aureus, *S. epidermidis*, and gram-negative rods are the primary causes of line sepsis. Initial antibiotic coverage should include vancomycin and a 3rd-generation cephalosporin. Empiric antibiotic coverage must be individualized to take into account the prevailing bacterial flora in each ICU and the history of antibiotic use in the patient. Patients who have been in the hospital for prolonged periods and who have received multiple antibiotics are at risk of candidemia, particularly if two or more peripheral site cultures have grown this organism. These patients should be empirically covered with fluconazole or an echinocandin (caspofungin, anidulafungin, or micafungin) pending blood culture results.

Another major infectious cause of fever in the ICU patient is prolonged bladder catheterization. The bladder catheter bypasses the urethra, and despite the use of closed urinary collecting systems, nearly all patients with bladder catheters develop urinary tract infections within 30 days (see Chapter 9). Urinalysis and urine culture therefore need to be part of the fever workup in all patients with urinary catheters.

In patients with nasogastric tubes or those who have been intubated through the nasal passage, the ostia

KEY POINTS

About Fever in the Intensive Care Unit Patient

1. Fever is extremely common in intensive care unit patients.
2. A systematic approach to diagnosis is critical.
3. Key sites of infection include these:
   a) Lungs (critical to differentiate colonization from infection)
   b) Intravenous and intra-arterial lines
   c) Urinary tract (at high risk secondary to prolonged bladder catheterization)
   d) Wounds (particularly in the early postoperative period)
   e) Sinuses (in patients with nasotracheal tubes)
4. Noninfectious causes include pulmonary emboli, drug fever, and old hemorrhage.
5. Empiric antibiotics need to be streamlined based on culture results.
6. Prolonged broad-spectrum antibiotic coverage predisposes to colonization with highly resistant bacteria, fungemia, *Clostridium difficile* colitis, and drug allergies.

draining the air sinuses can become occluded. This condition can lead to sinusitis and fever. Fever work up in these patients therefore needs to include sinus films. If sinusitis is discovered, the tube must be removed from the nasal passage, and appropriate antibiotic coverage instituted (see Chapter 5).

Noninfectious causes of fever also need to be considered. As noted earlier in this chapter, pulmonary emboli may present with fever. Patients in the ICU are usually receiving a large number of medications, and they are therefore at higher risk of developing drug fever. All medications should be reviewed, and when possible, medications should be discontinued or changed.

Another cause of persistent low-grade fever is undrained collections of blood. These collections can be identified by CT scan. Generally, they do not require drainage, but they take time to fully resorb.

Fever in the ICU patient requires a systematic diagnostic approach and the judicious use of antibiotics. Too often, patients are covered unnecessarily for prolonged periods using broad-spectrum antibiotics. This condition leads to the selection of highly resistant bacterial pathogens, and it also predisposes the patient to candidemia and *Clostridium difficile* colitis.

Empiric antibiotic coverage needs to be streamlined once culture data are available. Close communication between the ICU staff and the infectious disease consultant is critical to achieve the best care for the febrile ICU patient.

FURTHER READING

Blockmans D, Knockaert D, Maes A, et al. Clinical value of [(18)F]fluoro-deoxyglucose positron emission tomography for patients with fever of unknown origin. *Clin Infect Dis.* 2001;32:191–196.

Bujak JS, Aptekar RG, Decker JL, Wolff SM. Juvenile rheumatoid arthritis presenting in the adult as fever of unknown origin. *Medicine (Baltimore).* 1973;52:431–444.

de Kleijn EM, Vandenbroucke JP, van der Meer JW. Fever of unknown origin (FUO). I A. prospective multicenter study of 167 patients with FUO, using fixed epidemiologic entry criteria. The Netherlands FUO Study Group. *Medicine (Baltimore).* 1997;76:392–400.

Ghose MK, Shensa S, Lerner PI. Arteritis of the aged (giant cell arteritis) and fever of unexplained origin. *Am J Med.* 1976;60:429–436.

Larson EB, Featherstone HJ, Petersdorf RG. Fever of undetermined origin: diagnosis and follow-up of 105 cases, 1970–1980. *Medicine (Baltimore).* 1982;61:269–292.

Marik PE. Fever in the ICU. *Chest.* 2000;117:855–869.

Mayo J, Collazos J, Martinez E. Fever of unknown origin in the setting of HIV infection: guidelines for a rational approach. *AIDS Patient Care STDS.* 1998;12:373–378.

Mueller PS, Terrell CL, Gertz MA. Fever of unknown origin caused by multiple myeloma: a report of 9 cases. *Arch Intern Med.* 2002;162:1305–1309.

Petersdorf RG, Beeson PB. Fever of unexplained origin: report on 100 cases. *Medicine (Baltimore).* 1961;40:1–30.

Vanderschueren S, Knockaert D, Adriaenssens T, et al. From prolonged febrile illness to fever of unknown origin: the challenge continues. *Arch Intern Med.* 2003;163:1033–1041.

Zenone T. Fever of unknown origin in adults: evaluation of 144 cases in a non-university hospital. *Scand J Infect Dis.* 2006;38:632–638.

Pulmonary Infections

Time Recommended to Complete: 3 days

Frederick Southwick, M.D.

■ ACUTE PNEUMONIAS

GUIDING QUESTIONS

1. What are the factors that predispose the host to develop pneumonia?

2. What are the symptoms, signs, and diagnostic tests that help to differentiate viral from bacterial pneumonia?

3. How useful is sputum Gram stain, and what are the parameters that are used to assess the adequacy of a sputum sample?

4. How should the clinician interpret the sputum culture, and should sputum cultures be obtained in the absence of sputum Gram stain?

5. What are some of the difficulties encountered in trying to determine the cause of acute pneumonia?

6. How helpful is a chest radiograph in determining the specific cause of pneumonia?

7. How often should chest x-ray be repeated, and how long do the radiologic changes associated with acute pneumonia persist?

8. Which antibiotic regimens are recommended for empiric therapy of community-acquired pneumonia and why?

POTENTIAL SEVERITY

Acute pneumonia is a potentially life-threatening illness requiring rapid diagnosis and treatment. A delay in antibiotic treatment increases the risk of a fatal outcome.

GENERAL CONSIDERATIONS IN ACUTE PNEUMONIA

Prevalence

Annually, 2 to 3 million cases of pneumonia are reported in the United States. Estimates suggest that pneumonia is responsible for more than 10 million physician visits, 500,000 hospitalizations, and 45,000 deaths annually. Overall, 258 people per 100,000 population require hospitalization for pneumonia, and that number rises to 962 per 100,000 among those over the of age 65 years. It is estimated that, annually, 1 in 50 people over 65 years of age and 1 in 20 over 85 years will develop a pneumonia. Pneumonia occurs most commonly during the winter months.

Causes

Improved diagnostic techniques have shown that the number of pathogens that cause acute pneumonia is ever expanding (Table 4.1).

The leading cause of acute community-acquired pneumonia remains *Streptococcus pneumoniae*, followed by *Haemophilus influenzae*. *Mycoplasma* and *Chlamydia*

79

Table 4.1. Common Causes of Acute Pneumonia

Organism	Cases (%)[a]
Streptococcus pneumoniae	16–60
Haemophilus influenzae	3–38
Other gram-negative bacilli	7–18
Legionella spp.	2–30
Chlamydia pneumoniae	6–12
Mycoplasma	1–20
Staphylococcus aureus	2–5
Influenza A and B	—
Parainfluenza	—
Respiratory syncytial virus	—
Anaerobes (usually mixed)	—

[a] From published series of bacterial pneumonia.

pneumoniae also account for a significant percentage of acute pneumonias. *Staphylococcus aureus* is an unusual community-acquired pathogen, but it can cause ventilator associated pneumonia. Gram-negative bacteria other than *H. influenzae* are also an uncommon cause of community-acquired pneumonia except in patients with underlying lung disease or alcoholism. Gram-negative pneumonia most commonly develops in hospitals or nursing homes. *Legionella* species vary in importance, depending on the season and geographic area. Anaerobes such as anaerobic streptococci and bacteroids can cause acute pneumonia following aspiration of mouth contents. Common viral pathogens include influenza, parainfluenza, and respiratory syncytial virus.

Pathogenesis and Pathology

Under normal conditions, the tracheobronchial tree is sterile. The respiratory tract has a series of protective mechanisms that prevent pathogens from gaining entry [Figure 4.1(A)]:

1. The nasal passages contain turbinates and hairs that trap foreign particles.
2. The epiglottis covers the trachea and prevents secretions or food from entering the trachea.
3. The tracheobronchial tree contains cells that secrete mucin. Mucin contains a number of antibacterial compounds including immunoglobulin A antibodies, defensins, lysozymes, and lactoferrin. Mucin also is sticky, and it traps bacteria or other foreign particles that manage to pass the epiglottis.
4. Cilia lining the inner walls of the trachea and bronchi beat rapidly, acting as a conveyer belt to move mucin out of the tracheobronchial tree to the larynx.
5. When significant volumes of fluid or large particles gain access to the trachea, the cough reflex is activated, and the unwanted contents are quickly forced out of the tracheobronchial tree.
6. If pathogens are able to bypass all of the above protective mechanisms and gain entry into the alveoli, they encounter a space that, under normal circumstances, is dry and relatively inhospitable. The presence of an invading pathogen induces the entry of neutrophils and alveolar macrophages that ingest and kill infecting organisms. Immunoglobulins and complement are found in this space. Surfactants also have a protective function.
7. The lymphatic channels adjacent to the alveoli serve to drain this space and transport fluid, macrophages, and lymphocytes to the mediastinal lymph nodes.

Bacterial pathogens usually gain entry into the lung by aspiration of mouth flora or by inhalation of small aerosolized droplets (<3 μm in diameter) that can be transported by airflow to the alveoli. Once the pathogen takes hold, a series of inflammatory responses is triggered. These responses have been most carefully studied in pneumonia attributable to *S. pneumoniae*.

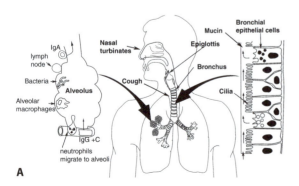
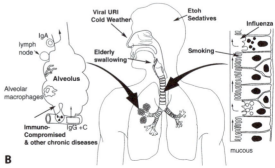

Figure 4–1. **A.** Host defense in the respiratory tract. **B.** Factors that interfere with host defense of the respiratory tract.

KEY POINTS

About the Protective Mechanisms of the Lung

1. Normally the tracheobronchial tree is sterile.
2. The nasal turbinates trap foreign particles, and the epiglottis covers the trachea.
3. Mucin has antibacterial activity, and cilia transport mucin out of the lung.
4. Coughing expels foreign material that enters the tracheobronchial tree.
5. Alveoli can deliver polymorphonuclear leukocytes (PMNs), macrophages, immunoglobulins, and complement to destroy invading pathogens.
6. Lymphatics drain macrophages and PMNs to the mediastinal lymph nodes.

First, an outpouring of edema fluid into the alveoli occurs, serving as an excellent culture media for further bacterial growth. As fluid accumulates, it spills over to adjacent alveoli through the pores of Kohn and the terminal bronchioles, resulting in a centrifugal spread of infection. Coughing and the physical motion of respiration further enhance spread.

KEY POINTS

About the Pathogenesis of Pneumonia

1. Pathogens are aspirated or inhaled as small aerosolized droplets.
2. Bacterial invasion of the alveoli induces
   a) edema fluid that spreads to other alveoli through the pores of Kohn, and
   b) infiltration by polymorphonuclear leukocytes and red blood cells, followed by macrophages.
3. Infection spreads centrifugally:
   a) Newer regions in the periphery appear red ("red hepatization").
   b) Older regions are central and appear gray ("gray hepatization").
4. Streptococcal pneumonia does not cause permanent tissue destruction.
5. *Staphylococcus aureus*, gram-negative rods, and anaerobes cause permanent damage.

Next, polymorphonuclear leukocytes (PMNs) and some red blood cells begin to accumulate in the alveolar space. Eventually, they fill the region and form a zone of consolidation.

Macrophages then enter the lesions and assist the PMNs in clearing the infection. Histopathology reveals zones of varying age. The most distal regions represent the most recent areas of infection. There, edema fluid, PMNs, and red blood cells predominant. On lower power microscopy, this region has an appearance similar to the architecture of the liver—an effect termed "red hepatization." Older central regions have more densely packed PMNs and macrophages. This region has a grayer color and forms the zone of "gray hepatization."

Pulmonary pathogens demonstrate marked differences in their invasiveness and ability to destroy lung parenchyma. *S. pneumoniae* causes minimal tissue necrosis and is associated with little or no scar formation. Full recovery of pulmonary function is the rule. *S. aureus* releases a number of proteases that permanently destroy tissue. Gram-negative rods and anaerobic bacteria also cause permanent tissue destruction.

Predisposing Factors

Most bacterial pneumonias are preceded by a viral upper respiratory infection [Figure 4.1(B)]. Influenza virus is well known to predispose to *S. pneumoniae* and *S. aureus* pneumonia. Viral infections of the upper respiratory tract can damage the bronchial epithelium and cilia.

Virus-mediated cell damage also results in the production of serous fluid that can pool in the pulmonary alveoli, serving as an excellent culture media for bacteria. The low viscosity of this fluid, combined with depressed ciliary motility, enables the viral exudate to carry nasopharyngeal bacteria past the epiglottis into the lungs. Smoking also damages the bronchial epithelial cells and impairs mucociliary function. As a consequence, smokers have an increased risk of developing pneumonia. Congenital defects in ciliary function (such as Kartagener's syndrome) and diseases resulting in highly viscous mucous (such as cystic fibrosis) predispose patients to recurrent pneumonia.

An active cough and normal epiglottal function usually prevent nasopharyngeal contents from gaining access to the tracheobronchial tree. However, drugs such as alcohol, sedatives, and anesthetics can depress the level of consciousness and impair these functions, predisposing the patient to pneumonia. Elderly individuals, particularly after a cerebrovascular accident, often develop impairments in swallowing that predispose them to aspiration. In addition, elderly people demonstrate reduced humoral and cell-mediated immunity, rendering them more susceptible to viral and bacterial pneumonia.

Patients with impairments in immunoglobulin production, T- and B-cell function, and neutrophil and macrophage function are also at greater risk for developing pneumonia. Organ-transplant patients on immunosuppressive agents and AIDS patients have a greater likelihood of developing pneumonia. Chronic diseases, including multiple myeloma, diabetes, chronic renal failure, and sickle cell disease have been associated with an increased risk of pneumonia.

Cold weather is thought to contribute to the development of pneumonia. Cold, dry weather can alter the viscosity of mucous and impair bacterial clearance. Cold weather also encourages people to remain indoors, a situation that enhances person-to-person spread of respiratory infections.

Symptoms and Signs

CASE 4.1

A 55-year-old woman was first seen in the emergency room in December complaining of a nonproductive cough, nasal stuffiness, and fever. She also noted diffuse severe muscle aches and joint pains and a generalized headache. In her epidemiologic history, she noted that she had recently seen her grandchildren, who all had high fevers and were complaining of muscle aches.

Physical exam showed these positive findings: temperature, 39°C; throat, erythematous; nasal discharge, clear; muscles, diffusely tender. A chest x-ray (CXR) was within normal limits.

Three days into the clinical course of her illness, the patient noted some improvement in her cough, muscle aches, and joint pains; however, on the 4th day, she developed a high fever (40°C) preceded by a teeth-chattering chill. That day, her cough became productive of rusty-colored opaque sputum, and she began feeling short of breath.

A repeat physical exam showed a temperature of 40.6°C and a respiration rate of 36 per minute. In general, this was a very ill-appearing, anxious woman, gasping for air. Lungs were mildly dull to percussion, with E-to-A changes, and rales and rhonchi localized to the left lower lobe.

A peripheral white blood cell (WBC) count measured 16,000/mm³, with 68% PMNs, 20% immature forms (bands and metamyelocytes), 8% lymphocytes,

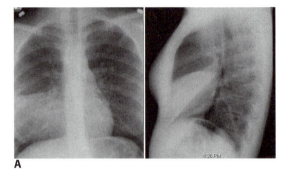

A

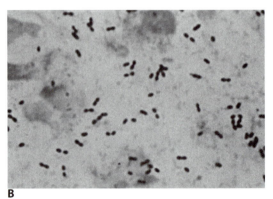

B

Figure 4–2. Pneumococcal pneumonia: **A.** Chest radiograph demonstrates classical lobar infiltrate (Courtesy of Dr. Pat Abbitt, University of Florida); and **B.** sputum Gram stain shows *Streptococcus pneumoniae*. Note that the cocci come to a slight point, explaining the term "lancet-shaped." *See color image on color plate 1*

and 4% monocytes. Sputum Gram stain showed many gram-positive lancet-shaped diplococci, many PMNs (>10/high-power field), and no squamous epithelial cells. A CXR revealed a dense left lower lobe and lobar infiltrate (Figure 4.2).

In case 4.1, the patient's initial symptoms suggested a viral illness involving the upper respiratory tract (rhinitis and nonproductive cough); central nervous system (CNS) or air sinuses, or both (headache); and musculoskeletal system (myalgias and arthralgias). Such symptoms are generally attributed to an influenza-like illness. A number of viruses can explain these symptoms, including influenza, parainfluenza, adenovirus, respiratory syncytial virus (more common in children, but also found in elderly individuals and transplant patients), rhinoviruses (usually less severe), and enteroviruses.

Subsequently, within a 24-hour period, this patient experienced the abrupt onset of a new constellation of symptoms. The onset of the new illness can be classified as acute. An illness is termed "acute" when symptoms and signs develop over 24 to 48 hours. Symptoms that develop over 3 days to 1 week are generally classified as subacute, and symptoms that progress more slowly (over 3 weeks to several months) are classified as chronic.

In generating a potential list of causative agents, the infectious disease specialist frequently uses the pace of the illness to narrow the possibilities. Pneumonias are generally classified into two groups: acute and chronic. Most bacterial and viral pneumonias develop quickly; fungal and mycobacterial pulmonary infections tend to develop at a slower pace. Acute pneumonia can be further classified as "typical" or "atypical." Typical pneumonia is characterized by the more rapid onset of symptoms, more severe symptomatology, a productive cough, and dense consolidation on CXR, as observed in case 4.1. Atypical pneumonia tends to be slower in onset (often subacute), symptoms tend to be less severe, cough is productive of minimal sputum, and CXR usually reveals a patchy or interstitial pattern. Finally, pulmonary infections are separated into community-acquired or nosocomial. "Community–acquired" is defined as an infection developing in a patient who has not recently (>14 days) been hospitalized or resided in a chronic care facility.

Although considerable overlap in symptoms, signs, and CXR findings are observed in cases of acute community-acquired pneumonia, certain key clinical characteristics are helpful in guiding the determination of the most likely causes (Table 4.2). Generation of a logical differential list of potential pathogens guides the choice of diagnostic tests and narrows the possible treatment regimens.

Important symptoms that need to be reviewed include these:

KEY POINTS

About the Classification of Pneumonia

Pneumonias are classified by

1. pace of illness:
   a) Acute—symptoms develop over 24 to 48 hours.
   b) Chronic—symptoms progress over 3 weeks or longer.
2. specific constellations of symptoms:
   a) Typical—rapid onset, more severe symptoms, productive cough, dense consolidation on chest X-ray (CXR).
   b) Atypical—somewhat slower onset, less severe symptoms, nonproductive cough, patchy interstitial pattern on CXR.
3. environment in which the pneumonia was acquired:
   a) Community-acquired—patient not recently (>14 days) in a hospital or chronic care facility.
   b) Nosocomial—patient in a hospital at the time the infection developed.

---

1. **Cough.** Frequency of the cough, production of sputum, and color of the sputum should be documented. A nonproductive cough or a cough productive of scanty sputum suggests an atypical pneumonia; a cough productive of rusty-colored sputum raises the possibility of *S. pneumoniae.* Thick, "red current jelly" sputum has been reported in cases of *Klebsiella pneumoniae*; green-colored sputum is more frequently encountered in patients with *H. influenzae* and *Pseudomonas aeruginosa* pneumonia (typically a nosocomial pathogen, or found in patients cystic fibrosis). Frank hemoptysis is observed in cavitary tuberculosis, lung abscess, and lung carcinoma. It should be emphasized that considerable overlap occurs in the sputum characteristics of the various forms of pneumonia, and these observations cannot be considered specific.

2. **Chest discomfort.** Pleuritic chest pain (pain associated with deep inspiration) is classically described in patients with *S. pneumoniae.* Pain is usually sharp and stabbing. Because the pulmonary parenchyma has no pain-sensing nerves, the presence of chest pain indicates inflammation of the parietal pleura. When the diaphragm becomes inflamed, the pain can mimic cholecystitis or appendicitis, and on occasion this sort of pain has precipitated exploratory laparotomy. Anaerobes, *S. pyogenes*, and *S. aureus* are

Table 4.2. Clinical Characteristics of Acute Community-Acquired Pneumonia Classified by Cause

Causative agent	Classical symptoms	Typical radiographic findings
Streptococcus pneumoniae	Rusty-colored sputum, rigor, pleuritic chest pain	Lobar infiltrate, air bronchograms
Haemophilus influenzae	More gradual onset; seen in smokers with COPD	Lobar or patchy infiltrates
Staphylococcus aureus	Follows influenza pneumonia, rapidly progressive acute disease	Bronchopneumonia, lung abscess, pneumothorax, and empyema
Aspiration pneumonia	Follows from loss of consciousness, poor gag reflex, abnormal swallowing; foul-smelling sputum	Dense consolidation (more in the right lower lobe than in the left lower lobe, or in posterior segment of upper lobes); later, lung abscess and empyema
Legionella pneumophila	Nonproductive cough, gastrointestinal symptoms, confusion	Lobar pneumonia, cavities in immunocompromised patients
Atypical pneumonia	Mild-to-moderate symptoms, nonproductive cough, pulmonary exam often normal	Patchy lower lobe bronchopneumonia

COPD = chronic obstructive pulmonary disease.

other pathogens that can also spread to the pleura and cause chest pain. Pleuritic pain is also characteristic of pleurodynia, a pain syndrome caused by the enteroviruses coxsackievirus and echovirus.

3. **Rigor.** Mild chills are encountered in most febrile illnesses. However, a teeth-chattering, bed-shaking chill indicative of a true rigor is usually associated with bacteremia. This symptom is very prominent, and patients often can report the exact time of their first rigor. A single rigor is the rule in *pneumococcal infection; multiple rigors are more typical of S. aureus, anaerobes, Klebsiella* species, and *S. pyogenes. H. influenzae* seldom causes rigors.

4. **Shortness of breath.** A report of increased shortness of breath suggests poor alveolar oxygen exchange, indicative of severe infection. Some patients experience shortness of breath as a result of pleuritic chest pain that limits the ability to breath deeply. To avoid pain, patients may breath quickly and shallowly, and this breathing pattern may be interpreted as shortness of breath.

5. **Epidemiology.** A careful epidemiologic history is often helpful. A number of environmental factors predispose to pneumonia. Animal exposure must be carefully reviewed, including contact with wild game, birds, bats, and rodents (see Chapter 13). Exposure to outside air conditioning units or construction sites should be identified (legionnaires' disease). Travel history may be helpful. For example, travel to the Southwest raises concerns about coc-

cidiomycosis, and travel to the Ohio River valley raises the possibility of histoplasmosis. Because many respiratory illnesses spread from person to person, a history of exposure to family members or friends with illnesses should be ascertained. Occupational and sexual history should also be elicited.

KEY POINTS

About the History in Pneumonia

1. **Cough.** Frequency, production of sputum, color and thickness of sputum.
2. **Chest pain.** Pain on deep inspiration, usually sharp, suggests pleural involvement. Seen in *Streptococcus pneumoniae*, *Staphylococcus aureus*, *Streptococcus pyogenes*, anaerobes, and coxsackievirus and echovirus.
3. **Rigor.** Bed-shaking chills, 1 rigor in *S. pneumoniae*, more than 1 in *S. aureus*, *Klebsiella* spp., *S. pyogenes*, and anaerobes.
4. **Shortness of breath.** A worrisome symptom, may be the result of pleuritic chest pain rather than poor gas exchange.
5. **Epidemiology.** Travel history, animal exposure, exposure to people with respiratory illnesses, occupational and sexual history.

KEY POINTS

About the Physical Exam in Pneumonia

1. A respiratory rate >30/min, a blood pressure <90 mm Hg, a pulse >125/min, and a temperature <35°C or >40°C are bad prognostic findings.

2. Depressed mental status and stiff neck suggest bacterial meningitis.

3. Pulmonary auscultation often underestimates the extent of pneumonia:
   a) Bronchial breath sounds and egophony suggest consolidation.
   b) Dullness to percussion indicates consolidation or a pleural effusion.
   c) Pleural effusion is accompanied by decreased breath sounds and, in some cases, a friction rub.

A thorough physical examination should be performed during the initial evaluation for possible pneumonia. Vital signs are helpful in determining the severity of illness. A respiratory rate of more than 30 breaths per minute, a systolic blood pressure under 90 mm Hg, a pulse above 125 beats per minute, and a temperature below 35°C (95°F) or above 40°C (104°F) are all bad prognostic signs. Depressed mental status is also associated with a poor prognosis.

Ear, nose, and throat examination may reveal vesicular or crusted lesions consistent with *Herpes labialis*, an infection that may reactivate as a consequence of the stress of the primary illness. Neck stiffness in association with depressed mental status may indicate the development of bacterial meningitis, a potential complication of pneumococcal pneumonia.

Pulmonary auscultation often fails to detect the extent of infection, and when pneumonia is being considered, the physical exam should be followed by a CXR. Asymmetry of chest movements may be observed, movement being diminished on the side with the pneumonia. When infection has progressed to consolidation, as in case 4.1, filling of the lung parenchyma with exudate alters sound conduction. Air flow from the bronchi is conducted through this fluid to the chest wall, resulting in bronchial or tubular breath sounds. When the patient is asked to say "E," an "A" is heard on auscultation (egophony). Percussion of the chest wall also demonstrates dullness in the areas of consolidation. Dullness to percussion in association with decreased breath sounds suggests the presence of a pleural effusion. A "leathery" friction rub may be heard over the site of consolidation, indicating pleural inflammation.

Laboratory Findings

Physical examination is unreliable for making the diagnosis of pneumonia. If pneumonia is a potential diagnosis, CXR must to be performed to confirm or exclude the disease. The radiologic pattern can serve as a rough guideline to possible causative agents; however, the use of immunosuppressive agents (resulting in neutropenia, decreased cell-mediated immunity, and depressed macrophage function) can greatly alter the typical radiologic appearance of specific pathogens. Patients with AIDS also present with atypical CXR.

Five classical patterns have been described:

1. **Lobar pneumonia.** "Lobular pneumonia" refers to a homogeneous radiologic density that involves a distinct anatomic segment of the lung (Figure 4.2). Infection originates in the alveoli. As it spreads, this form of infection respects the anatomic boundaries of the lung and does not cross the fissures. Lobar pneumonia is most commonly seen with *S. pneumoniae, H. influenzae,* and *Legionella.*

2. **Bronchopneumonia.** The bronchopneumonia form of pulmonary infection originates in the small airways and spreads to adjacent areas (Figure 4.3). Infiltrates tend to be patchy, to involve multiple areas of the lung, and to extend along bronchi. Infiltrates are not confined by the pulmonary fissures. Bronchopneumonia is commonly observed with *S. aureus,* gram-negative bacilli, *Mycoplasma, Chlamydia,* and respiratory viruses.

3. **Interstitial pneumonia.** Infections causing inflammation of the lung interstitium result in a fine diffuse granular infiltrate (Figure 17.2). Influenza and cytomegalovirus commonly present with this CXR pattern. In AIDS patients, *Pneumocystis jirovecii* infection results in interstitial inflammation combined with increased alveolar fluid that can mimic cardiogenic pulmonary edema. Miliary tuberculosis commonly presents with micronodular interstitial infiltrates.

4. **Lung abscess.** Anaerobic pulmonary infections often cause extensive tissue necrosis, resulting in loss of lung tissue and formation of cavities filled with inflammatory exudate (Figure 4.4). *S. aureus* also causes tissue necrosis and can form cavitary lesions.

5. **Nodular lesions.** Histoplasmosis, coccidiomycosis, and cryptococcosis can present as nodular lung lesions (multiple or single) on CXR. Hematogenous pneumonia resulting from right-sided endocarditis commonly presents with "cannonball" lesions that can mimic metastatic carcinoma.

> ## KEY POINTS
>
> ### About Chest X-Ray in Pneumonia
>
> 1. If pneumonia is being considered, a chest X-ray (CXR) should always be performed.
> 2. Radiographic patterns may be atypical in patients receiving immunosuppressants and in patients with AIDS.
> 3. Five typical CXR patterns have been described:
>   a) **Lobar pattern.** *Streptococcus pneumoniae*, *Haemophilus influenzae*, and *Legionella*.
>   b) **Bronchopneumonia pattern.** *Staphylococcus aureus*, gram-negative organisms, *Mycoplasma*, *Chlamydophila*, and viral.
>   c) **Interstitial pattern.** Influenza and cytomegalovirus, *Pneumocystis*, miliary tuberculosis.
>   d) **Lung abscess.** Anaerobes, *S. aureus*.
>   e) **Nodular lesions.** Fungal (histoplasmosis, coccidiomycosis, cryptococcosis) and right-sided endocarditis.
> 4. Patterns on chest radiographs are only rough guides. Considerable overlap between the various pathogens has been observed.

The role of high-resolution chest CT scan is evolving, and this test has proved helpful for more clearly demonstrating interstitial infiltration, pulmonary cavities, nodules, and pleural fluid collections.

Patients with an infiltrate, who are under age 65, have a normal mental status, and normal or only mildly deranged vital signs can be treated as outpatients (Figure 4.5). Sputum Gram stain and culture are optional in these patients, as are any additional tests.

In more severely ill patients who are being considered for hospitalization, additional tests to assess the severity of the illness need to be ordered.

A complete and differential blood cell count should be obtained. Patients with bacterial pneumonia usually have an elevated peripheral WBC count and a left shift. When pneumococcal pneumonia is accompanied by a low peripheral WBC count (<6000), a fatal outcome is more likely. The finding of anemia (hematocrit <30%), usually indicative of chronic underlying disease, is also associated with a worse prognosis.

Blood oxygenation also needs to be assessed. The O_2 saturation should be determined, and if it is at all depressed, an arterial blood gas should be obtained. Systemic acidosis (pH <7.35) and an arterial partial pressure below 60 mm Hg are bad prognostic signs. A significant depression in oxygenation reflects loss of alveolar function and lack of oxygen transfer to alveolar capillaries. Deoxygenated blood passes from the right side of the heart to the left side, creating a physiologic right-to-left shunt.

Other metabolic parameters also need to be assessed. A blood urea nitrogen level above 30 mg/dL reflects hypoperfusion of the kidneys or dehydration (or both) and is a negative prognostic finding. A serum sodium reading below 130 mEq/L reflects increased antidiuretic hormone secretion in response to decreased intravascular volume in addition to severe pulmonary disease. Such a reading is another negative prognostic finding, as is a serum glucose level exceeding 250 mg/dL. Two blood cultures should be drawn before antibiotics are started. Positive blood cultures definitively identify the cause of the disease. Blood cultures are positive in 1% to 16% of cases of community-acquired pneumonia.

Sputum requires careful analysis and frequently provides helpful clues to the probable diagnosis. Sputum samples often become contaminated with bacteria and cells from the nasopharynx, making interpretation of the cultures difficult. Ideally, acquisition of sputum should be supervised by a physician to ensure that the patient coughs deeply and brings up the sample from the tracheobronchial tree and does not simply expectorate saliva from the mouth. The adequacy of the sample should be determined by low-power microscopic analysis of the sputum Gram stain. The presence of more than 10 squamous epithelial cells per low-power field indicates significant contamination from the nasophar-

> ## KEY POINTS
>
> ### About Blood Tests in Pneumonia
>
> 1. With the exception of patients under the age of 50 years, without underlying disease, and with normal vital signs, multiple blood tests are used to assess the severity of disease.
> 2. A peripheral white blood cell count below 6000/mm^3 in *Streptococcus pneumoniae* is a bad prognostic finding.
> 3. Anemia (hematocrit <30%), blood urea nitrogen above 30 mg/dL, serum sodium below 130 mEq/L, and glucose above 250 mg/dL are associated with a worse prognosis.
> 4. Arterial blood o_2 below 60 mm Hg and pH below 7.35 worsen prognosis.
> 5. Two blood samples should be drawn before antibiotics are stated; blood cultures are positive in up to 16% of patients.

ynx, and the sample should be discarded. The presence of more than 25 PMNs per low-power field and the presence of bronchial epithelial cells provide strong evidence that the sample originates from the tracheo-bronchial tree.

Despite originating from deep within the lungs, sputum samples usually become contaminated with some normal throat flora as they pass through the nasopharynx. Gram stain can be helpful in differentiating normal flora (mixed gram-positive and gram-negative rods and cocci) from the offending pathogen. When a single bacterial type predominates, that bacterium is likely to be the primary pathogen. For example, the presence of more than 10 lancet-shaped gram-positive diplococci per high-power field provides strong evidence that *S. pneumoniae* is the cause of the pneumonia (approximately 85% specificity and 65% sensitivity, Figure 4.2).

In reviewing bacterial morphology, the observer must assess the adequacy of decolorization. In ideally stained regions, the nucleus and cytoplasm should be gram-negative, and a mixture of gram-positive and gram-negative organisms should be seen. A gram-positive nucleus indicates underdecolorization, and the presence of gram-negative bacteria only (including cocci) suggests overdecolorization.

Sputum Gram stain is also helpful for assessing the inflammatory response. The presence of many PMNs suggests a bacterial cause for the disease; a predominance of mononuclear cells is more consistent with *Mycoplasma*, *Chlamydia*, or a viral infection.

Sputum culture is less helpful than Gram stain, because normal flora contaminating the sample frequently overgrow, preventing identification of the true pathogen. To reduce overgrowth, samples should be quickly inoculated onto culture media. Rapid processing has been shown to increase the yield for *S. pneumoniae*. Sputum cultures are falsely negative approximately half the time. Because of the potential problems with sampling error, and the inability to accurately quantify bacteri by standard culture, sputum should never be cultured in the absence of an accompanying Gram stain.

Culture is most helpful in determining the antibiotic sensitivities of potential pathogens. The combination of sputum Gram stain and antibiotic sensitivity testing may allow the clinician to narrow the spectrum of antibiotic coverage, reducing the likelihood of selecting for highly resistant pathogens. In the intubated patient, sputum culture alone should never be the basis for initiating antibiotic therapy. Sputum culture will almost always be positive, a result that often simply represents colonization and not true infection (see Chapter 1).

Additional methods for sputum analysis are being developed. Polymerase chain reaction (PCR) is being used to amplify specific strands of DNA from

---

> ### KEY POINTS
>
> ### About Sputum Gram Stain and Culture
>
> 1. Ideally the sputum collection should be supervised by a physician.
> 2. Adequacy of the sample is assessed by low-power microscopic analysis:
>   a) More than 10 squamous epithelial cells indicates extensive contamination with mouth flora.
>   b) More than 25 polymorphonuclear leukocytes (PMNs) or bronchial epithelial cells (or both) per low-power field indicate an adequate sample.
> 3. Sputum Gram stain should be performed in all seriously ill patients with pneumonia.
>   a) Decolorization should be assessed for adequacy.
>   b) Predominance of a single organism suggests that the probable pathogen has been found.
>   c) Predominance of PMNs suggests bacterial pneumonia.
>   d) Predominance of mononuclear cells suggests *Mycoplasma*, *Chlamydophila*, or a virus.
> 4. Sputum culture
>   a) Should never be ordered without an accompanying Gram stain.
>   b) Should not be the sole basis for antibiotic treatment.
>   c) Often represents colonization rather than infection when positive in the intubated patient.
>   d) Is insensitive, because mouth flora can overgrow the pathogen.
>   e) Is helpful for determining the antibiotic sensitivity of pathogens identified by Gram stain.

---

pathogens. This method will be particularly helpful in identifying organisms that are not normally part of the mouth flora and that are difficult to culture: *L. pneumophila*, *Mycoplasma pneumoniae*, *Chlamydia pneumoniae*, and *P. jirovecii*.

When *Legionella* pneumonia is a consideration (see specific discussion later in this chapter), urinary antigen for *L. pneumophila* serogroup 1 (the most common pathogenic serogroup) should be performed. This test is moderately sensitive and highly specific. A positive test is therefore diagnostic; a negative test does not exclude the diagnosis, however. A urinary antigen test for *S. pneumoniae* is also available and is recommended as potentially useful in adults (80% sensitivity for bacteremic patients, 97% specificity). This test is frequently positive in children colonized with *S. pneumoniae*, and is therefore not recommended for that patient population.

More invasive procedures are usually not required in community-acquired pneumonia, but may be considered in the severely ill patient when an adequate sputum sample cannot be obtained. Invasive procedures such as fiberoptic bronchoscopy with protected brushing or lavage are more commonly required in the immunocompromised patient (see Chapter 16). The sheath surrounding the brush reduces, but does not eliminate, contamination by mouth flora.

Quantitative cultures are required to differentiate infection from contamination, with growth of more than 10^3 to 10^4 organisms per milliliter indicating infection. Lavage of a lung segment with sterile fluid samples a larger volume of lung and is particularly useful for diagnosing *P. jirovecii* pneumonia in AIDS patients (see Chapter 17). Bronchoscopy has been shown to be useful in diagnosing not only *P. jirovecii*, but also mycobacterial infections and cytomegalovirus.

The use of bronchial lavage to assist in the diagnosis of ventilator-associated pneumonia (VAP) is controversial. Contamination of samples by organisms colonizing the endotracheal tube can result in misinterpretation of the quantitative cultures. As compared to samples derived from endotracheal suction, samples obtained by bronchoscopy offer no benefit in regard to morbidity, mortality, or reduction in antibiotic use in VAP.

DECIDING ON HOSPITAL ADMISSION IN ACUTE PNEUMONIA

The Pneumonia Patient Outcome Research Team developed useful criteria called the pneumonia severity index (PSI) for assessing pneumonia severity; however, that index proved to be complex and difficult to use. A simpler index called the CURB-65 (confusion, urea nitrogen, respiratory rate, blood pressure, age 65 years or older) has been shown to have sensitivity and specificity nearly equal to that of the PSI. Both indexes can be used to guide decisions on admission to a hospital ward or intensive care unit. As shown in Figure 4.5, patients with a score of 0 or 1 can be treated as outpatients; those with a score of 2 or more warrant hospitalization. A patient with a score of 4 to 5 generally requires placement in an intensive care unit.

Empiric Treatment

The mainstay of treatment is administration of antibiotics (Table 4.3). Antibiotic treatment should not be delayed because of difficulties with sputum collection. Therapy should be started within 4 hours of diagnosis.

Delays beyond this period have been associated with increased mortality.

In patients requiring hospitalization for acute community-acquired pneumonia, cefotaxime or ceftriaxone (covers *S. pneumoniae*, *H. influnezae*, *S. aureus*, *Klebsiella* spp, some gram-negative organisms, and aerobic mouth flora), combined with an advanced macrolide [azithromycin or clarithromycin (covers *Legionella*, *Mycoplasma*, *Chlamydia*)] is recommended for empiric therapy. If aspiration pneumonia is suspected, metronidazole can be added.

In ambulatory patients, either a macrolide in the form of azithromycin or clarithromycin, or a respiratory fluoroquinolone (gatifloxacin, moxifloxacin, or levofloxacin) possessing good gram-positive activity is considered efficacious. Concerns have been raised about the development of resistance to fluoroquinolones, and many experts recommend that this class of antibiotics be reserved for older patients with underlying disease. These patients are not only exposed to the standard causes of community-acquired pneumonia, they also experience an increased incidence of gram-negative bacilli that will be covered by those agents.

The appropriate duration of treatment has not been systematically studied. For *S. pneumoniae*, patients are generally treated for 72 hours after they become afebrile. For infections with bacteria that cause necrosis of lung (*S. aureus*, *Klebsiella*, and anaerobes), therapy should probably be continued for more than 2 weeks. Treatment for 2 weeks is generally recommended for *Mycoplasma pneumoniae*, *Chlamydia pneumoniae*, and *Legionella* in the immunocompetent patient. Patients on intravenous antibiotics can generally be switched to oral antibiotics when their clinical condition is improving, they are hemodynamically stable, their gastrointestinal tract is functioning normally, and they are capable of taking medications by mouth. In many cases, those criteria are met within 3 days. When possible, the oral antibiotic should be of the same antibiotic class as the intravenous preparation. If staying within the class is not possible, then the oral agent should have a spectrum of activity similar to that of the intravenous agent.

Response to treatment can be assessed by monitoring temperature, respiratory rate, PaO_2 and oxygen saturation, peripheral white blood cell count, and frequency of cough. The changes seen on CXR often persist for several weeks despite clinical improvement. Although CXR is not helpful for assessing improvement, conventional films can be combined with pulmonary CT scan to assess the development of complications such as pneumothorax, cavitation, empyema, and adult respiratory distress syndrome (ARDS), and to document continued progression of infiltrates despite therapy.

Table 4.3. Empiric Treatment of Pneumonia, Infectious Diseases Society of America, 2003

Disease characteristics	Drug	Dose	Comments
Community-acquired pneumonia			
No comorbidity No previous antibiotics Outpatient	Clarithromycin[a] or azithromycin[a] or erythromycin or doxycycline	500 mg PO q12h 500 mg PO, followed by 250 mg PO q24h 500 mg q6h 100 mg PO q12h	Low serum levels, high levels in macrophages, preferred for *Haemophilus influenzae* Gastrointestinal toxicity is common Bacteriostatic agent
No comorbidity Previous antibiotics, or nursing home resident	Respiratory fluoroquinolone: gatifloxacin or levofloxacin or moxifloxacin Advanced macrolide, plus β-lactam antibiotic: cefuroxime axetil or cefpodoxime or cefprozil or amoxicillin–clavulanate	400 mg PO q24h 500 mg PO q24h 400 mg PO q24h Doses as above 500 mg PO q12h 400 mg PO q12h 500 mg PO q12h 2 g PO q12h	Levofloxacin-resistant *Streptococcus pneumoniae* reported in Canada If aspiration suspected, amoxicillin or amoxicillin–clavulanate recommended.
Comorbidity (CHF, COPD, DM, cancer, renal disease) Inpatient, medical ward No recent antibiotics	Advanced macrolide Respiratory fluoroquinolone Respiratory fluoroquinolone Clarithromycin or azithromycin, plus ceftriaxone or cefotaxime	Doses as above Doses as above Doses as above Dose PO as above 500 mg IV q24h 1 g IV or IM q24h 1 g IV q8h	
Inpatient, medical ward Recent antibiotics	Advanced macrolide, plus β-lactam antibiotic (preferred) or respiratory fluoroquinolone	Doses as above Doses as above	Regimen depends on the previous antibiotic
Inpatient, ICU *Pseudomonas* not an issue	IV β-lactam antibiotic, plus advanced macrolide or respiratory fluoroquinolone	Doses as above	

Continued

Table 4.3. (Continued)

Disease characteristics	Drug	Dose	Comments
Inpatient, ICU *Pseudomonas* an issue	Piperacillin–tazobactam or imipenem or meropenem or cefepime	4 g/0.5 g IV q6h 0.5–1 g IV q6h 1 g IV q8h 1–2 g IV q8h	
Aspiration pneumonia			
Community	Penicillin G Clindamycin	2 × 10⁶ U IV q4h 600 mg IV q8h	Covers usual mouth flora Slightly more effective than penicillin for lung abscess
In hospital	Ceftriaxone plus metronidazole Respiratory fluoroquinolone plus metronidazole Piperacillin–tazobactam or ticarcillin–clavulanate	1 g IV q24h 500 mg IV q8h Doses as above 500 mg IV q8h 3 g/0.375 g IV q6h 3.1 g IV q4–6h	 Regimen used by the author Requires a large fluid load

ᵃ Advanced macrolides.

CHF = congestive heart failure; COPD = chronic obstructive pulmonary disease; DM = diabetes mellitus; ICU = intensive care unit.

Outcome

In the United States, 45,000 deaths are attributed to pneumonia annually. In hospitalized patients, overall mortality ranges from 2% to 30%. Mortality from pneumonia and influenza is particularly high in individuals over the age of 65 years, causing 150 to 250 deaths per 100,000 population annually. Mortality is also higher in individuals with underlying diseases. Five comorbid illnesses have been identified that result in statistically significant increases in mortality:

- Neoplastic disease
- Liver disease
- Congestive heart failure
- Cerebrovascular disease
- Renal disease

SPECIFIC CAUSES OF ACUTE COMMUNITY-ACQUIRED PNEUMONIA

Great overlap occurs among the clinical manifestations of the pathogens associated with acute community-acquired pneumonia. However, constellations of symptoms, signs, and laboratory findings serve to narrow the possibilities. By developing an ability to focus on a few pathogens or to identify a specific pathogen, clinicians can better predict the clinical course of pneumonia and can narrow antibiotic coverage.

Streptococcus pneumoniae

PATHOGENESIS

Pathogenic strains of *S. pneumoniae* have a thick capsule that prevents PMN binding and that blocks phagocytosis. Certain capsular types (1, 3, 4, 7, 8, and 12 in adults, and 3, 6, 14, 18, 19, and 23 in children) account for most pneumonia cases. Type 3 has the thickest polysaccharide capsule, and it is the most virulent strain, being associated with the worst prognosis. Immunoglobulins that specifically recognize the capsule are able to link the bacterium to the PMN surface through Fc receptors, enabling PMNs and macrophages (classified as phagocytes) to efficiently ingest and kill the pneumococci. The complement product C3b enhances phagocytosis of the bacteria by the same mechanism. Immunoglobulins and C3b are called "opsonins," which are products that enhance foreign particle ingestion by phagocytes.

In addition to its polysaccharide capsule, *S. pneumoniae* possesses a number of other virulence factors that enhance adherence to epithelial cells, resist phagocytosis,

KEY POINTS

About Treatment and Outcome of Pneumonia

1. Treatment must be instituted within 4 hours of diagnosis.
2. Delays are associated with increased mortality.
3. Appropriate triage should be guided by the CURB-65 classification.
4. Empiric therapy depends on the patient and disease characteristics:
   a) **Outpatient with no comorbidity and no previous antibiotics.** Use a macrolide (azithromycin or clarithromycin). If previous antibiotics or elderly nursing home patient, add a β-lactam antibiotic, or use a respiratory fluoroquinolone.
   b) **Hospitalized patient.** Use a 3rd-generation cephalosporin (ceftriaxone or cefotaxime) combined with a macrolide (azithromycin or clarithromycin). If *Pseudomonas* is a concern, use piperacillin–tazobactam, imipenem, or meropenem.
   c) **Aspiration outpatient.** Use penicillin or clindamycin.
   d) **Aspiration inpatient.** Use a 3rd-generation cephalosporin or a respiratory fluoroquinolone plus metronidazole; or use ticarcillin–clavulanate or piperacillin–tazobactam.
5. Using chest radiographs to monitor improvement is not recommended. (They can take several weeks to clear.) They are useful for documenting worsening of disease or development of complications.
6. Mortality ranges from 2% to 30%. Mortality higher with age more than 65 years, neoplastic disease, liver disease, congestive heart failure, cerebrovascular accident, and renal disease.

KEY POINTS

About the Pathogenesis of *Streptococcus pneumoniae*

1. The thick outer capsule blocks phagocytosis. Type 3 has the thickest capsule.
2. Immunoglobulins and complement are important opsonins that allow phagocytes to ingest invading pneumococci.
3. *Strep. pneumoniae* does not produce protease and seldom destroys lung parenchyma.
4. It does not cross anatomic barriers such as lung fissures.
5. Disease manifestations are caused primarily by the host's inflammatory response to the organism.

identified. Because opsonins are required for efficient phagocytosis of the encapsulated organism, patients with hypogammaglobulinemia and multiple myeloma are at increased risk for developing this infection, as are patients with deficiencies in complement (C1, C2, C3, C4). Patients with HIV infection also have defects in antibody production, and they have a higher incidence of pneumococcal infection. Patients with splenic

KEY POINTS

About *Streptococcus pneumoniae* Prevalence and Predisposing Factors

1. *S. pneumoniae* is the most common form of community-acquired bacterial pneumonia.
2. The risk is higher in patients with deficiencies in opsonin production:
   a) Hypogammaglobulinemia
   b) Complement deficiency
   c) HIV infection
3. Splenic dysfunction increases the risk of fatal pneumococcal bacteremia.
4. Risk is increased in patients with chronic diseases:
   a) Cirrhosis
   b) Alcoholism
   c) Nephrotic syndrome
   d) Congestive heart failure
   e) Chronic obstructive pulmonary disease

and activate complement. *S. pneumoniae* does not produce significant quantities of proteases, and disease manifestations are primarily the consequence of the host's inflammatory response. As a result, permanent tissue damage is rare, and spread of the disease across anatomic boundaries, such as lung fissures, is uncommon.

PREVALENCE AND PREDISPOSING FACTORS

S. pneumoniae remains the most common cause of acute community-acquired pneumonia; it represents two thirds of the cases in which a specific pathogen is

About Clinical Manifestations and Diagnosis of Pneumococcal Pneumonia

1. Three classic features may be found:
   a) Abrupt onset accompanied by a single rigor
   b) Rusty-colored sputum
   c) Pleuritic chest pain
2. Sputum Gram stain is often helpful: more than 10 gram-positive lancet-shaped diplococci per high-power field indicate pneumococcal pneumonia.
3. Sputum culture is insensitive; specimens (alpha hemolytic, optochin sensitive) should be plated quickly.
4. Blood samples for culture should always be drawn; up to 25% may be positive.
5. A urine pneumococcal antigen test may prove helpful, but may be positive in patients who are simply colonized with Streptococcus pneumoniae.
6. A chest radiograph shows a classical lobar pattern; small pleural effusions are common, true empyema rare. Abnormalities persist for 4 to 6 weeks after cure.

dysfunction have a higher risk of overwhelming *S. pneumoniae* sepsis because the spleen plays a vital role in clearing this bacteria from the bloodstream, particularly in the absence of specific anti-pneumococcal capsule antibody. Other chronic diseases, including cirrhosis, nephrotic syndrome, congestive heart failure, chronic obstructive pulmonary disease, and alcoholism, are also associated with greater risk of pneumococcal infection.

UNIQUE CLINICAL CHARACTERISTICS

Classically, pneumococcal pneumonia has a very abrupt onset that begins with a single severe rigor. Because *S. pneumoniae* invasion of the lung leads to capillary leakage of blood into the alveolar space, sputum can become rusty in color. Furthermore, pneumococcal infection frequently infects the peripheral lung and spreads quickly to the pleura. As a result, pleuritic chest pain is a common complaint.

DIAGNOSIS

Sputum Gram Stain—A careful analysis of the sputum is best performed by a knowledgeable physician. Areas with significant numbers of PMNs per high-power field and a predominance of gram-positive lancet-shaped

diplococci suggest the diagnosis [Figure 4.2(B)]. A finding of pneumococci within the cytoplasm of a PMN strongly supports invasive infection.

Sputum Culture—*S. pneumoniae* is catalase negative, bile soluble, and, like *S. viridans*, demonstrates alpha (green) hemolysis on blood agar plates. The propensity of normal mouth flora, in particular *S. viridans*, to overgrow frequently interferes with the identification of *S. pneumoniae*. The optochin disk inhibits growth *of* S. *pneumoniae*, but not of *S. viridans*, and this test is used to differentiate the two organisms. Another problem with sputum culture arises from the fact that *S. pneumoniae* can be present as normal mouth flora in up to 60% of healthy people. A positive sputum culture in the absence of a positive Gram stain or a positive blood culture may therefore simply represent contamination of the sputum with saliva.

Blood Cultures—Some reports have claimed that 25% of patients with pneumococcal pneumonia develop positive blood cultures; however, the denominator required to calculate this percentage is uncertain. Even in the absence of a positive sputum Gram stain, a positive blood culture in combination with the appropriate symptoms and CXR findings is interpreted as true infection. A urine test for pneumococcal polysaccharide antigen is available and is positive in 80% of adults with bacteremia.

Chest X-Ray—The CXR usually reveals a single area of infiltration involving one or more segments of a single lobe. Involvement of the entire lobe is less common. This organism respects the confining fissures of the lung and rarely extends beyond those boundaries, which explains the classical lobar radiologic pattern [Figure 4.2(A)].

Air bronchograms are found in a few cases. This radiologic finding is the consequence of the alveoli filling with inflammatory fluid and outlining the air-containing bronchi. When found, bronchograms are associated with a higher incidence of bacteremia.

Pleural fluid may be detected in up to 40% of cases. In most instances, the volume of fluid is too small to sample by thoracentesis, and if antibiotic treatment is prompt, only a small percentage go on to develop true empyema.

The radiologic improvement of pneumococcal pneumonia is slow. Despite rapid defervescence and resolution of all symptoms, radiologic changes often persist for 4 to 6 weeks. If the patient is improving clinically, follow-up CXRs are therefore not recommended during this period.

TREATMENT AND OUTCOME

In the early antibiotic era, *S. pneumoniae* was highly sensitive to penicillin [minimum inhibitory concentration (MIC)< 0.06 μg/mL]. However, since the late 1990s, isolates in the United States have become increasingly resistant, with 40% demonstrating intermediate resistance (MIC = 0.1–1 µg/mL), and a small percentage demonstrating high-level resistance (MIC > 2 µg/mL). In some areas of Europe and South Africa, higher percentages of resistant strains have been observed. In the Netherlands and Germany, where strictly limited antibiotic use is the standard of care, the prevalence of resistant strains is lower.

Currently, many intermediate strains remain sensitive to the 3rd-generation cephalosporins ceftriaxone and cefotaxime (MIC < 1 µg/mL); however, resistance to these antibiotics is increasing. For intermediately resistant strains, amoxicillin is more active than is penicillin VK, and amoxicillin is therefore the preferred oral antibiotic. Because penicillin resistance results from a decrease in the affinity of penicillin-binding proteins, intermediate (but not high–level) resistance can be overcome by raising the concentration of penicillin.

With the exception of the CNS, where the blood–brain barrier limits antibiotic penetration, standard doses of penicillin are effective in curing infections attributable to intermediately resistant pneumococci. Penicillin resistance is usually associated with resistance to many other classes of antibiotics, including the tetracyclines, macrolides, and clindamycin. Imipenem is also inactive against highly resistant strains. The respiratory fluoroquinolones that possess good gram-positive activity (levofloxacin, gatifloxacin, moxifloxacin) and vancomycin usually retain excellent activity against all resistant strains. Several cases of pneumonia attributable to levofloxacin-resistant *S. pneumoniae* have recently been reported; however, the overall percentage of pneumococcal strains that are resistant to fluoroquinolones remains low.

TREATMENT RECOMMENDATIONS

For doses of the drugs discussed here, see Table 4.3.

For penicillin-sensitive strains, penicillin G or amoxicillin remain the preferred treatment. Ceftriaxone is also effective. If the patient fails to improve within 48 hours, the possibility of a resistant strain must be considered, and coverage with a respiratory fluoroquinolone is recommended. For cases in which meningitis is suspected, a fluoroquinolone should not be used because of poor penetration of the cerebrospinal fluid, and the patient should be covered with vancomycin. In the penicillin-allergic patient, a respiratory fluoroquinolone can be used.

In the pre-antibiotic era, the mortality rate for pneumococcal pneumonia was 20% to 40%. In the antibiotic era, the mortality rate was reduced to approximately 5%. Prognosis is adversely influenced by

1. Age (patients above 65 years of age and infants have worse outcomes)
2. Delayed treatment
3. Infection with capsular type 2 or 3

KEY POINTS

About the Treatment, Outcome, and Prevention of Pneumococcal Pneumonia

1. A significant percentage of *Streptococcus pneumoniae* are resistant to penicillin:
   a) 25% to 35% are intermediately resistant (MIC = 0.12–1 µg/mL).
   b) a smaller percentage demonstrate high-level resistance (MIC > 2 µg/mL).
2. Penicillin or ampicillin remain the treatment of choice for penicillin-sensitive strains.
3. High-dose parenteral penicillin, a 3rd-generation cephalosporin or an oral amoxicillin used for intermediate-sensitivity strains, except for meningitis.
4. A respiratory fluoroquinolone (gatifloxacin, moxifloxacin, levofloxacin) is used for strains with high-level resistance. Avoid fluoroquinolones in meningitis, and cover with vancomycin.
5. Mortality is approximately 5%; prognosis is worse for infants and for patients older than 65 years of age, and for those whose treatment is delayed or who have capsular types 2 or 3, multilobar pneumonia, bacteremia or meningitis, or jaundice, or who are pregnant, have an underlying disease, or alcohol intoxication.
6. The 23-valent pneumococcal vaccine is safe and efficacious. It should be given to patients who are over 65 years of age, who have a chronic disease, and who are asplenic, immunocompromised, or alcoholic.

---

4. Involvement of more than one lobe of the lung
5. WBC count less than 6000/mm^3
6. Bacteremia, shock, or the development of meningitis
7. Jaundice
8. Pregnancy
9. Presence of other underlying diseases (heart disease, cirrhosis, diabetes)
10. Alcohol intoxication

PREVENTION

Despite the use of antibiotics, mortality during the first 36 hours of hospitalization has not changed. To prevent early mortality and to reduce the incidence of *S. pneumoniae* infection—the penicillin-sensitive and penicillin-resistant strains alike—vaccination is strongly recommended for all patients with chronic illnesses or those over the age of 65 years.

Generation of specific antibodies directed against the bacterial cell wall confer, prevent, or reduce the severity of disease. Polyvalent vaccine containing antigens to 23 capsular types is available and is effective (approximately 60% reduction of bacteremia in immunocompetent adults). Efficacy decreases with age and is not measurable in immunocompromised patients. The vaccine has proved to be safe and inexpensive, and should be widely used.

Haemophilus influenzae

Group B and non-typable *H. influenzae* can both cause community-acquired pneumonia. Infection with non-typable *H. influenzae* is more common in elderly individuals and in smokers with chronic obstructive pulmonary disease. The onset of symptoms tends to be more insidious than that seen with *S. pneumoniae*, but the clinical pictures are otherwise indistinguishable. A CXR can demonstrate lobar or patchy infiltrates, and sputum Gram stain reveals small gram-negative pleomorphic coccobacillary organisms.

Because of their small size and their color, which is similar to background material, *H. influenzae* may be missed by an inexperienced diagnostician. For the patient requiring hospitalization, intravenous ceftriaxone or cefotaxime is recommended. For oral antibiotic treatment, amoxicillin–clavulanate is effective. However, a number of other oral antibiotics, including trimethoprim–sulfamethoxazole, the newer macrolides (azithromycin and clarithromycin), the fluoroquinolones, and the extended-spectrum cephalosporins (cefpodoxime, cefixime) are also active against this organism.

Staphylococcus aureus

Fortunately, community-acquired pneumonia attributable to *S. aureus* is rare. The most common predisposing factor is a preceding influenza infection. An increase in the incidence of *S. aureus* pneumonia is often a marker for the onset of an influenza epidemic. *S. aureus* pneumonia is also more common in intravenous drug users and in AIDS patients, in association with *P. jirovecii* pneumonia.

In a few communities, community-acquired methicillin-resistant *S. aureus* (cMRSA) pneumonia has been described in addition to methicillin-sensitive *S. aureus* (MSSA). The clinical manifestations of this infection are similar to other forms of bacterial pneumonia. However the illness is often severe, being associated with high fever and a slow response to conventional therapy. A CXR can demonstrate patchy infiltrates or dense diffuse opacifications. *S. aureus* produces multiple proteases that allow this bacterium to readily cross the lung fissures and simultaneously involve multiple lung segments. This broader involvement explains the typical bronchopneumonia pattern on CXR [Figure 4.3(A)]. The rapid spread and aggressive destruction of tissue also explains the greater tendency of *S. aureus* to form lung abscesses and induce a pneumothorax. Spread of this infection to the pleural space can result in empyema (seen in 10% of patients). Sputum Gram stain reveals sheets of PMNs and an abundance of gram-positive cocci in clusters and tetrads [Figure 4.3(B)], and culture readily grows *S. aureus*. Blood cultures may also be positive.

The treatment of choice for MSSA is high-dose intravenous nafcillin or oxacillin. For MRSA

KEY POINTS

About Haemophilus influenzae Pneumonia

1. This small, gram-negative, pleomorphic coccobacilli is aerobic. It may be mistaken for the background material on sputum Gram stain.
2. Non-typable strains are more common in eledderly people and in smokers with COPD.
3. Clinically, *Haemophilus influenzae* is similar to *S. pneumoniae*, with a somewhat slower onset.
4. Parenteral ceftriaxone or cefotaxime should be used to treat hospitalized patients. Multiple oral regimens–amoxicillin-clavulanate, newer macro-lides, fluoroquinolones, and extended-spectrum cephalosporins are useful in outpatients.

KEY POINTS

About Staphylococcus aureus Pneumonia

1. These large gram-positive aerobic cocci form tetrads and clusters.
2. The disease most commonly follows influenza, and is seen in patients with AIDS and in IV drug abusers.
3. Destructive bronchopneumonia is complicated by
   a) lung abscesses,
   b) pneumothorax, and
   c) empyema.

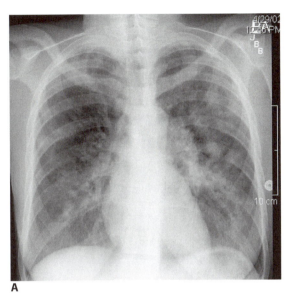

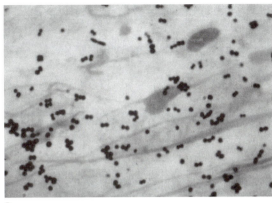

Figure 4–3. *Staphylococcus aureus* pneumonia: **A.** Chest radiograph demonstrates a classic bronchopneumonia (Courtesy of Dr. Pat Abbitt, University of Florida), and **B.** sputum Gram stain shows gram-positive cocci in clusters and tetrads. *See color image on color plate 1*

pneumonia, vancomycin is generally recommended. The dose of vancomycin should be adjusted to maintain a trough level of 15 to 20 μg/mL to assure therapeutic levels in the lung. Linezolid is an expensive alternative that has equivalent efficacy.

Legionella pneumophila

Legionella species are gram-negative bacilli found throughout the environment in standing water and soil. Infection most commonly results from inhalation of water droplets contaminated with *Legionella*. Cooling towers or shower heads are most often responsible for aerosolizing contaminated water. Less commonly, nosocomial infection has resulted from the use of unsterilized tap water in respiratory therapy devices. Outbreaks of *Legionella* pneumonia have also been associated with soil excavation. Immunocompromised patients, smokers, and elderly people are more susceptible to this infection.

Clinically, *Legionella* infection causes symptoms typical of other acute community-acquired pneumonias, including high fever, cough, myalgias, and shortness of breath. As compared with other bacterial pneumonias, cough usually produces only small amounts of sputum. Gastrointestinal symptoms, confusion, and headache are more frequently encountered in patients with *Legionella*. Laboratory findings are similar to other acute pneumonias. The only distinctive finding may be hyponatremia, which is noted in approximately one third of patients. A CXR frequently demonstrates lobar

pneumonia. In the immunocompromised host, cavitary lesions may be seen. Small pleural effusions are also commonly found.

Diagnosis requires a high index of suspicion, because sputum Gram stain reveals only acute inflammatory cells. The microbiology laboratory must be alerted to the possibility of *Legionella* species to assure that sputum samples are cultured on buffered-charcoal yeast-extract agar with added suppressive antibiotics. *Legionella* can also be identified by direct fluorescent antibody staining, although the sensitivity of this technique is low (30% to 50%). Amplification of *Legionella* DNA from sputum samples by PCR is available in certain reference laboratories, but not commercially. For *L. pneumophila* serogroup 1, the most common cause of *Legionella* pneumonia in the United States (>80% of cases), a highly sensitive and specific urinary antigen test is commercially available. The antigen is excreted early in the illness and persists for several weeks.

For mild disease, an oral macrolide, fluoroquinolone, or tetracycline may used. However, in more severe disease, high doses of intravenous azithromycin or a fluoroquinolone (ciprofloxacin or levofloxacin) are recommended. In transplant patients, a fluoroquinolone is preferred because the macrolides interfere with cyclosporin or tacrolimus metabolism. In the immunocompetent patient, therapy should be continued for 5 to 10 days with azithromycin and for 10 to 14 days with a fluoroquinolone. In the immunocompromised patient, therapy needs to be prolonged for 14 to 21 days to prevent relapse. Mortality is high in legionnaires' disease, being

---

KEY POINTS

About *Legionella* Pneumonia

----

1. These aerobic gram-negative bacteria do not take up Gram stain well.
2. Found in soil and standing water. Aerosolized by cooling towers and shower heads. Also contracted after soil excavation.
3. Elderly people, smokers, and immunocompromised patients are at increased risk.
4. Similar to other acute pneumonias. Somewhat unique characteristics include
   a) minimal sputum production,
   b) confusion and headache,
   c) gastrointestinal symptoms, and
   d) hyponatremia.
5. Diagnostic techniques include
   a) culture on buffered-charcoal yeast-extract agar,
   b) direct fluorescent antibody stain (low sensitivity),
   c) polymerase chain reaction (still experimental), and
   d) urinary antigen to serotype I (causes 80% of infections), which is sensitive and specific, and persists for several weeks.
6. Azithromycin or a fluoroquinolone are the treatments of choice. In transplant patients, fluoroquinolones are preferred. Mortality is high: 16% to 50%.

16% to 30% in community-acquired disease and up to 50% in hospitalized patients.

Atypical Pneumonia

The atypical forms of pneumonia tend to be subacute in onset, with patients reporting up to 10 days of symptoms before seeking medical attention. Atypical pneumonia is associated with a nonproductive cough, and clinical manifestations tend to be less severe. It is important to keep in mind that significant overlap occurs in the clinical manifestations of this group of infections and the more typical forms of pneumonia associated with purulent sputum production.

Mycoplasma pneumoniae is one of the most frequent causes of "walking pneumonia." This infection is seen primarily in patients under age 40 years; it is an uncommon cause of pneumonia in elderly individuals. The disease is seasonal, with the highest incidence of Mycoplasma being seen in the late summer and early fall. Sore throat is usually a prominent symptom, and bullous myringitis is seen in 5% of cases. Presence of this abnormality is highly suggestive of *Mycoplasma*. Tracheobronchitis results in a hacking cough that is often worse at night and that persists for several weeks. Physical exam may reveal some moist rales, but classically, radiologic abnormalities are more extensive than predicted by the exam. Findings on CXR consist of unilateral or bilateral patchy lower-lobe infiltrates in a bronchial distribution. The clinical course is usually benign. Fever, malaise, and headache usually resolve over 1 to 2 weeks, but cough can persist for 3 to 4 weeks. Peripheral WBC is usually less than 10,000. And sputum Gram stain and culture reveal only normal mouth flora and a moderate inflammatory response.

Diagnosis is made by history and clinical manifestations. Epidemiologic history of contact with a person having similar symptoms is particularly helpful. Currently, no definitive test is available. Sputum PCR has been found to be sensitive and specific, but that test is not commercially available. Cold agglutinin titers in excess of 1:64 support the diagnosis and correlate with severity of pulmonary symptoms, but are not cost effective. Complement fixation antibody titers begin to rise 7 to 10 days after the onset of symptoms.

Because a reliable, rapid diagnostic test is not currently available, therapy is usually empiric. A macrolide or tetracycline is the treatment of choice; alternatively, a fluoroquinolone can be administered. Azithromycin is the preferred agent when *Mycoplasma* is suspected, and a standard 5-day course is effective in most cases.

Chlamydia pneumoniae (Taiwan acute respiratory agent) is another important cause of atypical pneumonia. This pathogen is a common cause of community-acquired pneumonia, representing 5% to 15% of cases. The disease occurs sporadically and presents in a manner similar to *Mycoplasma*, with sore throat, hoarseness, and headache in addition to a nonproductive cough. Radiologic findings are also similar to those with *Mycoplasma*. No rapid diagnostic test is widely available, and treatment is empiric. A tetracycline is considered the treatment of choice, but macrolides and fluoroquinolones are also effective.

The final major group of organisms that cause atypical pneumonia is the respiratory viruses: influenza A and B, adenovirus, parainfluenza virus, and respiratory syncytial virus. The respiratory syncytial virus infects primarily young children, elderly people, and the immunocompromised host. These viruses can all present with a nonproductive cough, malaise, and fever.

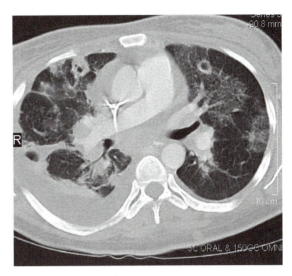

Figure 4–4. Empyema following aspiration pneumonia. CT scan showing a large right pleural effusion as well as discrete rounded cavitary lesions in the lung parenchyma of both the left and right lower lobes. (Courtesy of Dr. Pat Abbitt, University of Florida)

Auscultatory findings are minimal, and lower lobe infiltrates are generally observed on CXR. The clinical virology laboratory can culture each of these viruses from sputum or a nasopharyngeal swab. Rapid commercial tests (10 to 20 minutes) are available for detection of influenza (Quick View, Flu O1A, and Zstatflu). These tests have a sensitivity of 57% to 77%, and all three can distinguish between types A and B.

If influenza A virus is diagnosed, early treatment of the virus with amantadine or rimantadine is recommended. Neuramidase inhibitors are also available, and these agents have activity against both influenza A and B. The influenza vaccine is safe and efficacious, and should be given annually in October through early November to patients over 65 years of age, individuals with serious underlying diseases, nursing home residents, and health care workers (see Chapter 15).

Aspiration Pneumonia

CASE 4.2

A 35–year-old white man arrived in the emergency room complaining of left-sided chest pain during the preceding 4 days. He had begun drinking large quantities of alcohol 8 days earlier. He vaguely recalled passing out on at least two occasions. He developed a persistent cough, productive of green sputum, 4 days before admission. At that time, he also began experiencing left-sided chest pain on deep inspiration (pleuritic pain). Initially these pains were dull; however, over the next few days, they became increasingly sharp.

Physical exam showed a temperature of 38°C and a respiratory rate of 42 per minute. This was a disheveled man, looking older than his stated age, breathing shallowly and rapidly, in obvious pain.

A check of the throat revealed a good gag reflex, extensive dental caries, several loose teeth, severe gingivitis, and foul-smelling breath and sputum. Decreased excursion of the right lung was noted, and the right lower lung field was dull to percussion. Bronchovesicular breath sounds were heard diffusely (inspiratory and expiratory breath sounds of equal duration); moist, medium rales were heard in the right lower and left lower lung fields. Egophony and whispered pectoriloquy were also heard in these areas.

Laboratory workup showed a hematocrit of 50%; a WBC count of 21,400/mm³, with 79% PMNs, 7% bands, 1% lymphocytes, and 13% monocytes. Blood gasses showed a pH of 7.46, PaO_2 of 56 mm Hg, and a PaCO_2 of 36 mm Hg. Sputum Gram stain revealed many PMNs and a mixture of gram-positive cocci, gram-positive rods, and gram-negative rods. A CXR demonstrated dense right lower lobe infiltrate.

While on antibiotics, this patient continued to complain of chest pain and developed decreased breath sounds in the right lower lobe associated with dullness to percussion. A repeat CXR and CT scan demonstrated a large right pleural effusion [see Figure 4-4(A)], and thoracentesis revealed more than 100,000 PMNs/mm³, pleural fluid pH of 7.0, and total protein 3.4 mg/mL. Gram stain showed a mixture of gram-positive cocci and gram-positive and gram-negative rods.

Aspiration pneumonia should be suspected in patients with a recent history of depressed consciousness and in patients with a poor gag reflex or an abnormal swallowing reflex. The elderly patient who has suffered a stroke is particularly susceptible to aspiration. In case 4.2, the patient's heavy consumption of alcohol led to depression in consciousness.

Three major syndromes are associated with aspiration:

1. **Chemical burn pneumonitis.** Aspiration of the acidic contents of the stomach can lead to a chemical burn of the pulmonary parenchyma. Aspiration of large quantities of fluid can result in the immediate opacification of large volumes of lung. Acid damage causes pulmonary capillaries to leak fluid, release cytokines, and permit infiltration by PMNs. In some patients, noncardiogenic pulmonary edema or ARDS develops. Onset of symptoms occurs immediately after aspiration.

2. **Bronchial obstruction resulting from aspiration of food particles.** The inhalation of solid particles results in mechanical obstruction and interferes with ventilation. The patient immediately becomes tachypneic.

3. **Pneumonia resulting from a mixture of anaerobic and aerobic mouth flora.** This form of pneumonia develops several days after aspiration of mouth flora. Patients with severe gingivitis have higher bacterial colony counts in the mouth, and they aspirate a higher inoculum of organisms, increasing the likelihood of a symptomatic pneumonia.

Case 4.2 had poor dental hygiene and severe gingivitis, predisposing him to the latter form of pneumonia. Often, the sputum is putrid-smelling as a result of the high number of anaerobes. Necrosis of tissue is common in this infection, resulting in the formation of lung abscesses. Infection often spreads to the pleura, resulting in pleuritic chest pain as experienced in case 4.2. Pleural effusions filled with bacteria and PMNs can develop as observed in this case. Effusions containing bacteria and large numbers of PMNs are called empyemas. Necrosis of the pleural lining and lung parenchyma can result in formation of a fistula tracking from the bronchus to the pleural space. Development of a bronchopleural fistula prolongs hospitalization and may eventually require surgical repair.

DIAGNOSIS

Sputum is often foul-smelling as a result of the high numbers of anaerobic bacteria. Sputum Gram stain reveals many PMNs and a mixture of gram-positive and gram-negative organisms. Sputum culture usually grows normal mouth flora. When aspiration occurs in the hospitalized patient, the mouth often is colonized with more resistant gram-negative organisms plus *S. aureus*. In these patients, a predominance of gram-negative rods or gram-positive cocci in clusters may be seen on Gram stain, and gram-negative rods or *S. aureus* may be cultured from the sputum.

A CXR reveals infiltrates in the dependent pulmonary segments. When aspiration occurs in the upright position, the lower lobes are usually involved, more commonly the right lower lobe than the left. This difference has an anatomic explanation. The right bronchus divides from the trachea at a straighter angle than does the left mainstem bronchus, increasing the likelihood that aspirated material will flow to the right lung. When aspiration

---

KEY POINTS

About Aspiration Pneumonia

1. Can occur in cases of loss of consciousness, poor gag reflex, or difficulty swallowing.

2. Three forms of aspiration:
   a) **Aspiration of gastric contents** leads to pulmonary burn and noncardiogenic pulmonary edema.
   b) **Aspiration of an obstructing object** causes atelectasis and immediate respiratory distress.
   c) **Aspiration of mouth flora**, when associated with poor dental hygiene and mixed mouth aerobes and anaerobes, can lead to foul smelling sputum and eventually lung abscess and empyema. Hospital-acquired aspiration causes gram-negative and *Staphylococcus aureus* pneumonia.

3. Treatment depends on the form of the disease:
   a) Penicillin or clindamycin for community-acquired infection.
   b) Third-generation cephalosporin and metronidazole for hospital-acquired infection.
   c) Bronchoscopy for obstructing foreign bodies.

occurs in the recumbent position, the superior segments of the lower lobes or the posterior segments of the upper lobes usually become opacified.

TREATMENT

Clindamycin or penicillin are both effective antibiotic coverage for community-acquired aspiration pneumonia because they kill both aerobic and anaerobic mouth flora (Table 4.3). In cases in which lung abscess has developed, clindamycin has been shown to be slightly superior.

In nosocomial aspiration, broader coverage with a 3rd-generation cephalosporin combined with metronidazole is generally recommended. Alternatively, a semisynthetic penicillin combined with a β-lactamase inhibitor (ticarcillin–clavulanate or piperacillin–tazobactam) or a carbapenem (imipenem or meropenem) can be used.

If aspiration of a foreign body is suspected, bronchoscopy is required to remove the foreign material from the tracheobronchial tree.

Rarer Causes of Community-Acquired Pneumonia

ACTINOMYCOSIS

Actinomyces species are microaerophilic or anaerobic gram-positive rods that can be part of the polymicrobial flora associated with aspiration pneumonia, particularly in patients with poor oral hygiene. Disease is most commonly caused by *Actinomyces israelii*.

Actinomycosis pulmonary infection is often indolent and slowly progressive. Lung parenchymal lesions are usually associated with pleural infection, resulting in a thickened pleura and empyema. This organism can break through fascial planes. Sponta-

neous drainage of an empyema through the chest wall should strongly suggest the possibility of actinomycosis. "Sulfur granules" are often found in purulent exudate; they consist of clusters of branching *Actinomyces* filaments.

Gram stain reveals branching forms that are weakly gram-positive. These forms can be differentiated from *Nocardia* by modified stain for acid-fast bacilli (AFB), *Actinomyces* being acid-negative and *Nocardia* being acid-positive. The organism should be cultured under anaerobic conditions, and grows slowly, with colonies usually requiring a minimum of 5 to 7 days to be identified. Growth can take up to 4 weeks.

High-dose intravenous penicillin (18 to 24×10^6 U daily) is recommended for 2 to 6 weeks, followed by oral penicillin therapy for 6 to 12 months. Therapy must be continued until all symptoms and signs of active infection have resolved. Other antibiotics that have been successfully used to treat actinomycosis include erythromycin, tetracyclines, and clindamycin.

NOCARDIOSIS

Nocardia is an aerobic gram-positive filamentous bacterium that often has to be differentiated from *Actinomyces*. *Nocardia* is ubiquitous in the environment, growing in soil, organic matter, and water. Pneumonia occurs as a consequence of inhaling soil particles. The number of species causing human disease is large and

---

KEY POINTS

About Actinomycosis

1. These branching gram-positive bacteria are microaerophilic or anaerobic, slow growing, modified acid-fast negative.
2. Infection is associated with poor oral hygiene.
3. Slowly progressive infection, breaks through fascial planes, causes pleural effusions and fistula tracks, forms "sulfur granules."
4. Alert clinical microbiology to hold anaerobic cultures.
5. Treatment must be prolonged: high-dose intravenous penicillin for 2 to 6 weeks, followed by 6 to 12 months of oral penicillin.

KEY POINTS

About Nocardiosis

1. *Nocardia* are gram-positive branching bacteria, aerobic, slow growing, modified acid-fast.
2. Ubiquitous organism found in the soil.
3. Inhalation of soil particles leads to pneumonia.
4. The organism infects
   a) immunocompromised patients (causing disseminated disease in AIDS),
   b) normal hosts, and
   c) patients with alveolar proteinosis.
4. Pulmonary infection can lead to bacteremia and brain abscess that can mimic metastatic lung carcinoma.
5. Alert clinical microbiology to use selective media and to hold cultures.
6. Treatment must be prolonged. High-dose parenteral trimethoprim–sulfamethoxazole for at least 6 weeks, followed by oral treatment for 6 to 12 months.

includes *N. abscessus, N. brevicatena/paucivorans* complex, *N. nova* complex, *N. transvalensis* complex, *N. farcinica, N. asteroides* complex, *N. brasiliensis*, and *N. pseudobrasiliensis*.

Infection more commonly develops in patients who are immunocompromised; however, 30% of cases occur in otherwise normal individuals. Patients with AIDS, organ transplant, alcoholism, and diabetes are at increased risk of developing nocardiosis. In addition to pulmonary disease, these patients are at increased risk for developing disseminated infection. Patients with chronic pulmonary disorders, in particular patients with alveolar proteinosis, have an increased incidence of pulmonary *Nocardia* infection.

Onset of pulmonary disease is highly variable. In some cases, onset is acute; in others, onset is gradual. Symptoms are similar to other forms of pneumonia. A CXR may reveal cavitary lesions, single or multiple nodules, a reticular nodular pattern, interstitial pattern, or a diffuse parenchymal infiltrate. *Nocardia* pulmonary infection often seeds the bloodstream and forms abscesses in the cerebral cortex. The combination of a lung infiltrate with a CNS lesion or lesions is often mistaken for lung carcinoma with CNS metastasis.

Diagnosis is made by sputum examination or lung or cerebral cortex biopsy. Gram stain demonstrates weakly gram-positive branching filamentous forms that are acid-fast on modified AFB stain. On tissue biopsy, organisms are demonstrated on Brown–Brenn or methenamine silver stain. The organism is slow growing and is frequently overgrown by mouth flora on conventional plates. The clinical laboratory should be alerted to the possibility of *Nocardia* so that they can incubate bacteriologic plates for a prolonged period and use selective media.

Most *Nocardia* are sensitive to sulfonamides and trimethoprim. Trimethoprim–sulfamethoxazole is generally accepted as the treatment of choice, with a daily dose of 2.5 to 10 mg/kg of the trimethoprim component. High-dose therapy should be continued for at least 6 weeks, followed by lower doses for 6 to 12 months. Some *Nocardia* species are resistant to sulfonamides, but they are sensitive to amikacin, imipenem, 3rd-generation cephalosporins, minocycline, dapsone, and linezolid. Whenever possible, culture and antibiotic sensitivities should be used to guide antibiotic therapy.

NOSOCOMIAL (HOSPITAL-ACQUIRED) PNEUMONIA

Pneumonia is the second most common form of nosocomial infection. It accounts for 13% to 19% of all nosocomial infections. Hospital-acquired pneumonia is defined as a pneumonia that develops 48 hours or longer after hospitalization and that was not developing at the time of admission. Nosocomial pneumonia is a very serious complication and represents the leading infectious-related cause of death in the hospital, the mortality being roughly 1 of every 3 cases. Development of pneumonia in the hospital prolongs hospitalization by more than 1 week.

The condition that most dramatically increases the risk of nosocomial pneumonia is endotracheal intubation. Endotracheal tubes bypass the normal protective mechanisms of the lung, and they increase the risk of pneumonia by a factor of between 6 and 21. It has been estimated that the risk of pneumonia while on a ventilator is 1% to 3% daily. Other factors that increase the risk of pneumonia include age greater than 70 years; CNS dysfunction, particularly coma, leading to an increased likelihood of aspiration; other severe underlying diseases; malnutrition; and metabolic acidosis. Patients on sedatives and narcotics have depressed epiglottal function and are also at increased risk of aspiration. Corticosteroids and other immunosuppressants reduce normal host defenses and allow bacteria to more readily invade the lung parenchyma.

Aerobic gram-negative bacteria account for more than half the cases of nosocomial pneumonia.

KEY POINTS

About Nosocomial Pneumonia

1. Pneumonia is one of the most common nosocomial infections.
2. Risk factors include
   a) endotracheal intubation (20 times the baseline risk, 1% to 3% incidence daily),
   b) age greater than 70 years,
   c) depressed mental status,
   d) underlying disease and malnutrition, and
   e) metabolic acidosis.
3. Primary causes are gram-negative bacilli and *Staphylococcus aureus*.
4. Colonization is difficult to differentiate from infection. Bronchoscopy is not helpful. Factors that favor infection include:
   a) worsening fever and leukocytosis with left shift;
   b) sputum Gram stain with increased PMNs, predominance of one organism;
   c) decreasing Pao_2 indicative of pulmonary shunting; and
   d) expanding infiltrate on chest radiographs.
5. Broad-spectrum empiric therapy can be initiated after samples are obtained for culture, but coverage should be adjusted based on culture results and clinical response.

Escherichia coli, Klebsiella, Serratia, Enterobacter, and *Pseudomonas* species represent the most common gram-negative rods. *S. aureus* is the most common gram-positive pathogen, causing 13% to 40% of nosocomial pneumonias. The risk of *S. aureus* infection is higher in patients with wound infections or burns, and it is also higher in intubated patients with head trauma or neurosurgical wounds. Anaerobes are often isolated in nosocomial pneumonia, but they are thought to be the primary agent in only 5% of cases. *S. pneumoniae* is seldom the cause of pneumonia in the patient who has been hospitalized for more than 4 days.

Diagnosis of true pneumonia is often difficult in the intubated patient. In elderly patients with chronic bronchitis and congestive heart failure or ARDS, definitively proving that the patient has or does not have an infection is often impossible. Differentiating infection from colonization represents a critical branch point in the appropriate management of antibiotics (see case 1.0). Within 3 to 5 days of antibiotic initiation, the mouth flora and the flora colonizing the tracheobronchial tree change. A change in the organisms growing from sputum culture is therefore to be expected and does not in itself indicate that the patient has a new infection. The change simply documents colonized of the patient with resistant flora. For example, in a high percentage of patients receiving broad-spectrum antibiotics, *Candida albicans* begins to grow in sputum cultures because of the reduction in the competing bacterial mouth flora. However, that organism does not invade the lung and almost never causes airborne pneumonia. Antifungal coverage is therefore not required unless the patient develops symptomatic thrush.

Evidence supporting the onset of a new infection includes

- a new fever or a change in fever pattern;
- a rise in the peripheral WBC count, with a increase in the percentage of PMNs and band forms (left shift);
- Gram stain demonstrating increased number of PMNs in association with a predominance of bacteria that are morphologically consistent with the culture results;
- increased purulent sputum production from the endotracheal tube;
- reduced arterial PaO_2, indicating interference with alveolar–capillary oxygen exchange; and
- enlarging infiltrate on CXR.

Multiple studies have used bronchoscopy with protected brushings or bronchial lavage and quantitative cultures and Gram stains. A randomized trial found that that samples obtained by bronchoscopy provide no advantage over endotracheal suction, and therefore that procedure is not recommended in ventilation-associated pneumonia.

When infection is likely or the patient is extremely ill, and when a new pulmonary infection cannot be convincingly ruled out, antibiotics should be quickly started; or, if the patient is receiving antibiotics, the regimen should be changed to cover for antibiotic-resistant bacteria. In the absence of specific findings indicative of infection, colonization is more likely, and the antibiotic regimen should not be changed.

Indiscriminate modifications of antibiotic therapy eventually select for highly resistant pathogens that are difficult—or in some cases impossible—to treat. Switches to broader-spectrum, more powerful antibiotics should be undertaken cautiously, and should be initiated only when convincing evidence for a new infection is present. In the patient who is deteriorating clinically, broader-spectrum coverage can be temporarily instituted once blood, urine, and sputum samples for culture and Gram stain have been obtained. The 3-day rule should then be applied (see Chapter 1), with the antibiotic regimen being modified within 3 days, based on the culture results, so as to prevent colonization with even more highly resistant bacteria.

These regimens (see Table 4.3) are recommended for nosocomial pneumonia:

1. Third-generation cephalosporin (ceftriaxone, cefotaxime, ceftizoxime, or ceftazidime)
2. Cefepime
3. Ticarcillin–clavulanate or piperacillin–tazobactam
4. Imipenem or meropenem

An aminoglycoside (gentamicin, tobramycin, or amikacin) may or may not be added. If *P. aeruginosa* is suspected, ciprofloxacin, piperacillin–tazobactam, ticarcillin–clavulanate, cefepime, aztreonam, imipenem, or meropenem should be used. Many experts recommend administration of two agents from different classes to prevent development of resistance. Aminoglycosides should never be used alone to treat *Pseud. aeruginosa* because the antibiotic levels achievable in the lung are low. Aerosolized tobramycin (80 mg twice daily) has proven to be useful adjunctive therapy. If *Staph. aureus* is suspected, vancomycin should be added pending culture and sensitivity results. Specific anaerobic coverage is usually not required in the absence of clear aspiration.

Empyema

CAUSATION

Infection of the pleural space is most commonly the consequence of spread of pneumonia to the parietal pleura. More than half of empyema cases are associated with pneumonia. The most common pathogens in this setting are *S. pneumoniae, S. aureus, S. pyogenes*, and anaerobic mouth flora. Empyema is also a complication of trauma and surgery, and when those are the inciting factors,

---

KEY POINTS

About Empyema

1. Suspect empyema if fever persists despite appropriate antibiotic treatment of pneumonia.
2. The condition is most common with *Streptococcus pneumoniae*, *Staphylodcoccus aureus*, *S. pyogenes*, and mouth anaerobes.
3. A chest radiograph with lateral decubitus is sensitive; computed tomography scan is also helpful.
4. If empyema is being considered, an ultrasound guided thoracentesis should be performed.
5. When pH is less than 7.2, glucose is less than 40 mg/dL, and lactate dehydrogenase exceeds 1000 IU/L, empyema is strongly suggested.
6. Use tube drainage initially; if loculation continues, urokinase can be given. May require surgical intervention.
7. Early diagnosis and drainage prevents lung and pleura compromise.
8. Mortality associated with empyema is high: 8% to 15% in young patients, and 40% to 70% in elderly ones.

S. aureus and aerobic gram-negative bacilli predominate. In the immunocompromised patient, fungi and gram-negative bacilli are most commonly encountered.

PATHOPHYSIOLOGY

Pleural effusions occur in approximately half of all pneumonias; however, only 5% of pneumonias develop true empyema. Because pleural fluid is deficient in the opsonins, immunoglobulin G, and complement, bacteria that find a way to this culture medium are only ineffectively phagocytosed by PMNs. As PMNs break down in the closed space, they release lysozyme, bacterial permeability-increasing protein, and cationic proteins. These products slow the growth of bacteria, lengthening doubling times by a factor of 20 to 70. The slow growth of the bacteria renders them less sensitive to the cidal effects of antibiotics. In the empyema cavity, pH is low, impairing WBC function and inactivating some antibiotics—in particular, the aminoglycosides.

CLINICAL MANIFESTATIONS

Persistent fever despite appropriate antibiotic treatment for pneumonia should always raise the possibility of an enclosed pleural infection. Fever is often accompanied by chills and night sweats. Pleuritic chest pain is a common complaint, as is shortness of breath. Physical exam is helpful in detecting large effusions. As noted in case 4.2, the area in which fluid is collecting is dull to percussion, and breath sounds are decreased. At the margin between fluid and aerated lung, egophony and bronchial breath sounds are commonly heard, reflecting areas of pulmonary consolidation or atelectasis.

On CXR, fluid collections as small as 25 mL can alter the appearance of the hemidiaphragm on posterior–anterior view, and on lateral views, 200 mL of fluid is generally required to blunt the posterior costophrenic angle. A lateral decubitus view with the pleural effusion side down can demonstrate layering of 5 to 10 mL of free fluid. Contrast-enhanced chest CT is particularly helpful in differentiating lung abscess from empyema, and it demonstrates the full extent of the effusion and the degree of pleural thickening.

Ultrasound is very useful in determining the dimensions of the effusion, and it is the most effective method for guiding thoracentesis. Septations are readily visualized by this technique and indicate the development of a loculated collection that requires drainage. Ultrasound guidance of thoracentesis is strongly recommended because of the associated decreased incidence of complicating pneumothorax. The fluid should be analyzed for cellular content, and Gram stain, fungal stain, AFB stain, and aerobic and anaerobic cultures should be obtained. If the fluid is frankly purulent, the pleural space should be completely drained. If the fluid is not overtly purulent, the fluid should also be analyzed for pH, glucose, lactate dehydrogenase, and total protein. A pleural fluid pH below 7.2, a glucose level below 40 mg/dL, and a lactate dehydrogenase level above 1000 IU/L are consistent with empyema and justify pleural fluid drainage to prevent loculation, pleural scarring, and restrictive lung disease.

TREATMENT

Antibiotic therapy for the offending pathogen is of primary importance, and antibiotic coverage depends on the pathogen identified by sputum or pleural fluid Gram stain and culture. When a significant pleural fluid collection is apparent, a more prolonged course of antibiotics (2 to 4 weeks) is generally required.

Parapneumonic effusions that move freely and that are less than 1 cm in width on lateral decubitus film can be managed medically; thoracentesis is not required. If the collection is larger or does not flow freely, thoracentesis should be performed. If biochemical evidence for empyema is present, drainage by chest tube is recommended. Repeated thoracentesis is rarely successful in completely draining the pleural fluid collection unless the fluid has a thin viscosity and is present in small volumes. Drainage by closed chest tube is usually successful with smaller effusions occupying up to 20% of the hemithorax, but it is often ineffective when the volume of fluid occupies more than 40% of the hemithorax. Interventional radiology is required to precisely place French catheters at sites of loculation and to break up areas of adhesion under CT guidance. If tube drainage proves ineffective after 24 hours, intrathoracic urokinase (125,000 U diluted in 50 to 100 mL sterile normal saline) should be instilled to break down intrapleural fibrin and encourage free drainage of infected fluid. If thoracentesis and urokinase are unsuccessful, operative intervention is required.

Empyema is a serious complication, with an associated 8% to 15% mortality in young, previously healthy patients and 40% to 70% mortality in patients who are elderly or have significant underlying disease. Patients with nosocomial pathogens and polymicrobial infection also have a worse prognosis. Delay in diagnosis and appropriate drainage increases the need for surgical resection of the pleura and manual re-expansion of the lung.

■ CHRONIC PNEUMONIAS

GUIDING QUESTIONS

1. How is tuberculosis contracted, and how can this disease be prevented?

2. What is primary tuberculosis?

3. What is secondary tuberculosis?

4. Why are the apices of the lung the most common location for tuberculosis?

5. What are the typical symptoms and findings in miliary tuberculosis?

6. How is tuberculosis diagnosed?

7. Why should combination antituberculous therapy always be prescribed in active tuberculosis?

8. What does having a positive PPD mean, and how should an individual with a positive test be treated?

9. In which areas of the country is histoplasmosis most commonly encountered, and why?

10. In which areas of the country is coccidiomycosis most commonly encountered, and why?

TUBERCULOSIS

POTENTIAL SEVERITY

The miliary form of the tuberculosis can be fatal. Clinicians must maintain a high index of suspicion for tuberculosis in immigrants, indigent and elderly patients, and patients with AIDS.

CASE 3.3

A 73-year-old black man, a retired bartender, came to the emergency room complaining of increasing shortness of breath and worsening cough over the preceding 3 weeks. About 5 months earlier, he had begun to notice night sweats that drenched his pajamas. That symptom was followed by development of a nonproductive cough. He began bringing up small quantities of yellow sputum 1 month before presentation at the emergency room. At the time that he noticed the sputum production, he began experiencing increased shortness of breath, even after mild exertion (walking 2 blocks to the grocery store). During the past few months, he felt very tired, and he has lost 10 pounds despite a "good" diet.

Epidemiologic history indicated city residence and visits with a number of old drinking buddies. The patient denied exposure to anyone with tuberculosis, and he had no family history of tuberculosis.

Past medical history revealed an abnormal CXR 20 years earlier and treatment at New York City's Bellevue Hospital with isoniazid (INH) and para-aminosalicylic acid for 1 year.

Social history indicated that the patient had recently retired after 35 years of tending bar. He lives alone in a 1-bedroom apartment and supports himself on Social Security. He is a former smoker (half a pack daily for 28 years) and drinks half a pint daily.

On physical exam, his temperature was 38°C and his respiratory rate was 18 per minute, presenting a picture of a thin male breathing comfortably. Aside from mild clubbing of his nail beds, the physical findings (including lung exam) were within normal limits.

The laboratory workup showed a hematocrit of 39% and a WBC count of 6000/mm³, with 55% PMNs, 30% lymphocytes, and 15% monocytes.

Sputum Gram stain revealed many PMNs, few gram-positive cocci, and rare gram-negative rods.

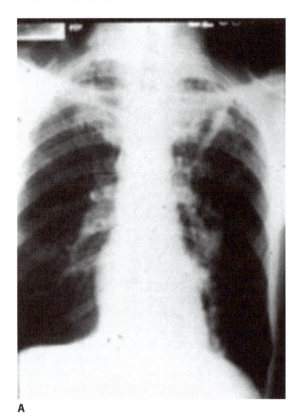

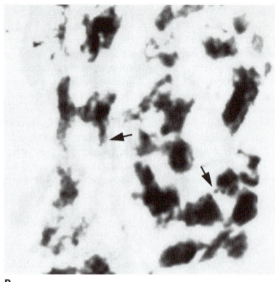

B

A

Figure 4–5. Cavitary pulmonary tuberculosis: **A.** Chest radiograph demonstrates bilateral upper lobe cavitary lesions, and **B.** sputum smear for acid-fast bacilli confirms the presence of those organisms. *See color image on color plate 1*

Bilateral upper lobe cavitary lesions were observed on CXR [see Figure 4.5(A)]. Acid-fast stain of the sputum revealed multiple acid-fast bacilli per high-power field [see Figure 4.5(B)].

Pathogenesis

Mycobacterium tuberculosis is an aerobic, nonmotile bacillus with a waxy lipid-rich outer wall containing high concentrations of mycolic acid. This waxy outer wall fails to take up Gram stain. Visualization of mycobacteria requires heating to melt the outer wall, which allows for penetration and binding of the red dye fuchsin. The lipids in the cell wall bind this dye with high affinity and resist acid–alcohol decolorization. This acid-fast bacillus is small in size and appears beaded [Figure 4.5(B)]. Genomic analysis reveals that, as compared with other bacteria, *M. tuberculosis* has a large number of genes encoding for enzymes that regulate

lipogenesis and lipolysis. The resulting high lipid content of this pathogen accounts for many of its unique clinical characteristics, including its ability to resist killing by macrophages and PMNs and to survive for many years within the body. Rate of growth in *M. tuberculosis* is very slow, being about 1/20th the growth rate of most conventional bacteria. The slow rate of growth may also be explained by the waxy cell wall, which limits access to nutrients.

Mycobacteria survive and grow in macrophages, and they therefore induce a profound chronic inflammatory response. On gaining entry to the lungs, these organisms are ingested by alveolar macrophages and transported to the hilar lymph nodes. Here macrophages and dendritic cells present tubercular antigens to T cells, inducing a cell-mediated immune response. Helper T cells (CD4+) then activate macrophages to kill the mycobacteria and control the infection. Accumulation of one of the cell wall waxes, cord factor, stimulates the formation of granulomas that contain clusters of epithelioid cells, giant cells, and lymphocytes. Over time, the centers of the granulomas become necrotic, forming cheesy debris called caseous necrosis. Caseating granulomas are the hallmark lesion of tuberculosis. This pathologic finding is only rarely found in other diseases. If intracellular growth of *M. tuberculosis* continues, increasing numbers of macrophages are activated to produce multiple cytokines. Interleukin 1 stimulates the hypothalamus to raise core body temperature, causing fever. Tumor necrosis factor interferes with lipid metabolism and causes severe weight loss. These cytokines are primarily responsible for the symptoms of fever, night sweats, and weight loss described in case 4.3.

Epidemiology

Humans are the only reservoir for *M. tuberculosis*. Person-to-person spread of infection is almost exclusively caused by inhalation of droplet nuclei that have been aerosolized by coughs or sneezes. The likelihood of inhaling infectious droplets is greatly increased in a closed, crowded environment. A single cough has been estimated to form 3000 infectious droplets, with a sneeze producing even higher numbers.

The infectiousness of an individual patient can be estimated by AFB smears. The higher the number of organisms per microscopic field, the greater the infectious potential. Patients with laryngeal tuberculosis are particularly infectious and can release large numbers of organisms while speaking. Patients with AIDS and

tuberculosis often harbor a large organism burden. Patients with large pulmonary cavities tend to intermittently release large numbers of infectious particles.

Repeated exposure and close contact are generally required to contract this disease. Respiratory isolation and rapid treatment of infected individuals are the primary ways to prevent spread of infection.

Despite the availability of antituberculous agents, tuberculosis remains a leading cause of death worldwide. Crowded living conditions and the existence of immunologically naive populations continue to allow rapid person-to-person spread, particularly in underdeveloped countries. After a surge in cases in the United States during the mid-1980s because of the AIDS epidemic, the case rate has steadily declined. In 2002, it reached the lowest level ever recorded: 5.2 cases per 100,000. This steady decline among permanent U.S. residents contrasts with the steady increase in the percentage of tuberculosis cases among people immigrating to the United States. Immigrants now account for half of all reported cases in the United States. Individuals immigrating from underdeveloped countries have higher rates of infection. For example, the rate among Vietnamese immigrants is 120 per 100,000

KEY POINTS

About the Pathogenesis of Tuberculosis

1. Slow-growing aerobic rod, not seen on Gram stain. The lipid-rich outer wall binds the red dye fuchsin, which is not removed by acid, making the bacterium acid-fast.
2. The lipid wall also allows the bacterium to resist drying and many disinfectants. It further allows the bacterium to survive within macrophages for years.
3. Macrophages carry the mycobacterium to the lymph nodes, where a cell-mediated immune response is generated.
4. Caseating granulomas are formed as a consequence of the cell-mediated immune response and the accumulation of lipid-rich bacteria.
5. Increased levels of interleukin 1 cause fever, and increased levels of tumor necrosis factor cause weight loss.

KEY POINTS

About the Epidemiology of Tuberculosis

1. Humans are the only reservoir of this disease.
2. Person-to-person spread occurs via aerosolized infectious droplets from sneezes or coughs.
   a) Laryngeal tuberculosis is highly infectious.
   b) Patients with HIV release large numbers of organisms.
   c) Large cavitary lesions are also highly infectious.
3. People with these characteristics are at increased risk:
   a) Immigrants from developing countries
   b) Alcoholics
   c) Urban poor
   d) Single men
   e) Intravenous drug abusers
   f) Migrant farm workers
   g) Prison inmates
   h) People infected with HIV
   i) Elderly people
4. A genetic predisposition is found in people who are black, Hispanic, Asia Pacific Islanders, and Native Americans (5 to 10 times the incidence seen in caucasians)

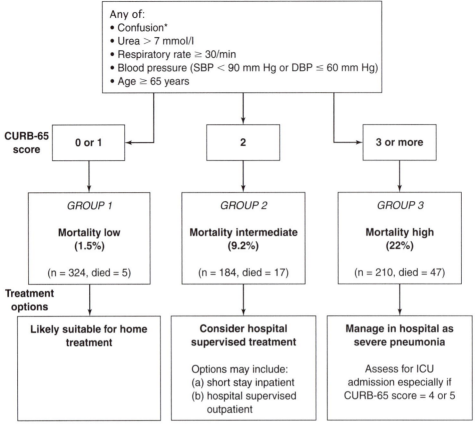

Figure 4–6. CURB-65 (confusion, urea, respirations, blood pressure, age 65) criteria for the management of community-acquired pneumonia (30-day mortalities in parenthesis). Adapted from Lim WS, van der Eerden MM, Laing R, et al. Defining community acquired pneumonia severity on presentation to hospital: an international derivation and validation study. *Thorax.* 2003;58:377–382.

person–years, and among Haitian immigrants it is 133 per 100,000. Immigrants from established market economies such as those of Western Europe have rates similar to those in the United States.

Tuberculosis occurs more frequently in single men, alcoholics, intravenous drug abusers, the urban poor (particularly homeless people), migrant farm workers, and prison inmates. Elderly people are more likely to develop secondary tuberculosis because cell-mediated immunity wanes with age.

A genetic predisposition to the development of active tuberculosis is known. People with European heritage tend to be more resistant, probably as a consequence of the devastating effects of the tuberculosis epidemic during the Industrial Revolution. At that time, tuberculosis was responsible for one fourth of the deaths in Europe, killing off a significant percentage of the population that had a reduced immune

---

KEY POINTS

About Primary Tuberculosis

1. Represents the first exposure to inhaled infectious particles.
2. Followed by a flu-like illness.
3. Spread is controlled over 4 to 8 weeks by the development of cell-mediated immunity.
4. Ghon foci are calcified lung lesions at the site of the primary infection.
5. Bacteremia develops and seeds the kidneys, epiphyses of the long bones, and vertebral bodies (areas with high oxygen content). The infection can later reactivate.

response to mycobacteria. As compared with white people, people who are black or Hispanic, or who are Asia Pacific Islanders or Native Americans experience a 5 to 10 times higher incidence of tuberculosis. Patients with AIDS are particularly susceptible to tuberculosis, and this population has spread the infection to others. Areas and demographic groups in which AIDS is more prevalent therefore have a higher incidence of tuberculosis.

The patient in case 4.3 has a number of epidemiologic characteristics that increase his risk for tuberculosis. He is a single male, black, possibly alcoholic, and elderly.

Clinical Manifestations

There are two forms of human tuberculosis infection: primary tuberculosis and secondary tuberculosis.

PRIMARY TUBERCULOSIS

Primary disease occurs when a patient inhales infectious *M. tuberculosis* droplets for the first time. A flu-like illness usually follows; however, some people experience no symptoms. Within 4 to 8 weeks of exposure, the human host usually mounts a cell-mediated immune response. Activated macrophages control the spread and growth of the organism. Pulmonary lesions heal spontaneously and form areas of fibrosis or calcification called Ghon lesions or foci. A Ghon lesion in combination with hilar adenopathy is called a Ranke complex.

In addition to transporting organisms to the hilum and mediastinum, infected macrophages may gain access to the thoracic duct, enter the bloodstream, and spread throughout the body. *M. tuberculosis* grows best in regions with high oxygen tension, including the kidneys, long-bone epiphyses, and vertebral bodies. It most commonly infects the apices of the lung, the regions with the highest oxygen content and reduced lymphatic flow.

Although the infection is brought under control, the bacilli are not usually completely eradicated. Organisms can survive for decades, being held in check by the host immune response. But any condition that subsequently depresses cell-mediated immunity can free *M. tuberculosis* to grow and cause symptomatic secondary tuberculosis.

MILIARY TUBERCULOSIS

In some individuals, initial exposure to *M. tuberculosis* fails to induce cell-mediated immunity, or the immune response is not robust enough to control the infection. Under these conditions, the mycobacteria continue to multiply and disseminate, causing miliary tuberculosis. Very young and very old patients are at higher risk of developing disseminated disease, as are patients receiving immunosuppressants and those

---

KEY POINTS

About Miliary Tuberculosis

1. The disease develops in very young, very old, and HIV-infected patients.
2. It is also associated with alcoholism, malignancy, connective tissue diseases, renal failure, and pregnancy.
3. In children, it presents with high fever, night sweats, weight loss, hepatosplenomegaly, and lymphadenopathy.
4. Adults usually show moderate- to low-grade fever, night sweats, malaise, anorexia, weakness, and weight loss.
5. Look for choroid tubercles in the fundi (present in up to 50% of cases).
6. Provokes leukemoid reaction, anemia, hyponatremia, abnormal liver function tests. May also produce adrenal insufficiency.
7. Micronodular interstitial pattern on chest radiographs; may be negative in elderly and HIV-infected patients.
8. Blood samples, transbronchial biopsy, bone marrow samples, and liver biopsy may all yield positive cultures.
9. Provide early treatment for all suspected cases, using isoniazid, rifampin, ethambutol, and pyrazinamide.

---

with HIV infection. Underlying medical conditions often associated with miliary tuberculosis include alcoholism, malignancy, connective tissue diseases, renal failure, and pregnancy. However, it must be emphasized that absence of an underlying disease does not exclude the possibility of miliary tuberculosis.

Children usually present to the physician with high fever, night sweats, weight loss, hepatosplenomegaly, and lymphadenopathy. However in adults, particularly elderly people, the clinical manifestations may be subtle. Patients usually have nonspecific complaints of fever, malaise, anorexia, weakness, and weight loss. Night sweats are also common.

Physical exam usually reveals a chronically ill patient with no specific findings. In some patients, lympha-denopathy may be detected. In all patients, fundoscopic exam should be carefully performed following pupillary dilation and may reveal choroid tubercles in up to 50% of cases. The diagnosis is often missed, and in up to 20% cases, it is made postmortem.

The peripheral WBC count is usually normal; however, some patients develop extremely high WBC counts (30,000 to 40,000/mm^3), also termed a "leukemoid reaction," that can be mistaken for leukemia. Pancytopenia can also develop. Liver function abnormalities are common. Elevated alkaline phosphatase and moderate increases in transaminase values are found in most patients. Serum sodium may be low as a consequence of adrenal insufficiency (a well-known complication of miliary tuberculosis) or inappropriate antidiuretic hormone secretion. Morning and evening serum cortisol levels should be measured to exclude adrenal insufficiency. In approximately two thirds of patients, CXR reveals small nodules (0.05 to 1 mm in diameter) that resemble millet seeds (the basis for the designation "miliary"); however, a negative CXR in elderly patients and in patients with HIV does not exclude this diagnosis. In a few patients, ARDS may develop, causing complete opacification of the lungs.

The key to the diagnosis of miliary tuberculosis is a high index of suspicion. Sputum smears are positive in only a few patients. Samples from enlarged lymph nodes, liver biopsy, and bone marrow should therefore be sought for histopathology (seeking granulomas and acid-fast bacilli) and culture. Transbronchial biopsy can yield the diagnosis in many patients. Blood samples for culture should be drawn; in AIDS patients, cultures are commonly positive. If CNS symptoms are noted, a lumbar puncture should also be performed, although the resulting smears are usually negative.

A delay in treatment can have fatal consequences. Therefore, if miliary tuberculosis is high on the differential diagnosis, empiric antituberculous therapy should be initiated as soon as samples for culture have been obtained. A 4-drug combination consisting of INH, rifampin, pyrazinamide, and ethambutol is the preferred regimen. Patients usually defervesce within 7 to 14 days.

SECONDARY TUBERCULOSIS

Reactivation of tuberculosis after primary disease occurs in 10% to 15% of patients. In half of these cases the infection reactivates within 2 years of exposure. In past decades, reactivation occurred most commonly in elderly patients, but in the United States today, most secondary cases are now reported in middle-aged adults (30 to 50 years of age). Early in the course of reactivation, patients are often asymptomatic, and evidence of reactivation is found only on CXR. However if the infection is not detected, symptoms slowly develop and worsen over several months. The gradual nature of symptom onset often causes patients to delay seeing a physician. The patient in case 4.3 has the typical symptoms of secondary tuberculosis: a progressively worsening cough with sputum production, low-grade fever, night sweats, fatigue, and weight loss. Symptoms that suggest more advanced disease are hemoptysis (indicating erosion of a tuberculous cavity into an arteriole) and pleuritic chest pain (suggesting pleural involvement and probable tuberculous pleural effusion).

Physical exam is often unrevealing, as observed in case 4.3. Despite the presence of extensive pulmonary disease, auscultation may be normal. Fine rales may be heard in the apices after a short cough and quick inspiration or after full expiration followed by a cough and rapid inspiration (post-tussive rales).

The hallmark of secondary pulmonary disease is the presence of apical cavitary lesions on CXR. Lesions usually develop in posterior segments of the upper lobes just below the clavicle. Less frequently, infiltrates are noted in the apex of the lower lobe (usually obscured by the heart shadow). In addition to routine posterior–anterior and lateral chest films, an apical lordotic view is often helpful in visualizing upper lobe apical lesions. A chest CT scan can be helpful for assessing the extent of disease and for defining the size of the cavities. Unlike conventional lung abscesses, tuberculous cavities

---

KEY POINTS

About Secondary Tuberculosis

1. Reactivation occurs in 10% to 15% of patients, half within 2 years of primary disease.

2. Reactivation is most common in men 30 to 50 years of age.

3. Apical infection is most common. The high oxygen content and reduced lymphatic flow favor *M. tuberculosis* survival in this region.

4. Symptoms progress slowly over several months: worsening cough with sputum production, low-grade fever, night sweats, fatigue, and weight loss.

5. Hemoptysis or pleuritic pain indicate severe disease.

6. Physical exam usually produces minimal findings; post-tussive rales may be seen.

7. Chest radiograph shows apical cavities (without fluid); order apical lordotic. A computed tomography scan is often helpful.

8. Cavitary disease is highly infectious; cavities contain between 10^9 and 10^{10} organisms. Isolate all patients. In HIV infection, the chest radiograph often does not show cavities. All pneumonias in patients with AIDS are considered to involve tuberculosis until proven otherwise.

rarely have air fluid levels. In patients with AIDS, infiltrates may be in any region of the lung and may not cavitate. Any HIV-infected patient with a new pulmonary infiltrate should therefore be considered to have tuberculosis until proven otherwise. In fact, in some instances, HIV-infected patients with active respiratory tuberculosis may have a negative CXR.

Individuals with cavitary disease are potentially highly infectious. Cavities may contain between 10^9 and 10^{10} organisms. Patients should be placed in respiratory isolation while sputum AFB smears and cultures are obtained. The number of organisms seen on smear directly correlates with infectiousness—that is, the higher the number of organisms per microscopic field, the higher the likelihood of disease spread.

Diagnosis

The classic test for making the diagnosis of pulmonary tuberculosis is the Ziehl–Nielson acid-fast sputum smear. Morning sputum samples tend to have the highest yield. A single negative smear should not delude the clinician into a false sense of security. Three sputum smears are recommended, because in cavitary disease, the release of infectious droplets is intermittent. Only after three smears are negative should the patient be declared to be at low risk for spreading infection. Negative smears do not definitively exclude tuberculosis.

To be positive, the sputum smear must contain 10^4 organisms per milliter. A fluorochrome stain using auramine–rhodamine is more sensitive and allows sputum to be examined at low magnification (20x or 40x magnification) as compared with conventional AFB smears that must be examined at high magnification (100x). Sputum smear has only a 60% sensitivity as compared with sputum culture. The PCR technique can effectively detect as few as 10 organisms in a clinical specimen. Two assays, one using mycobacteria RNA as its initial template, and the other using mycobacterial DNA, are commercially available. Sensitivity and specificity are greater than 95% in smear-positive cases, and specificity in smear-negative cases is high. False negative and false positive results are common in less experienced laboratories, and nucleic acid amplification assays are recommended only to complement traditional methods. In patients on antituberculous therapy, PCR cannot differentiate killed from actively growing organisms.

Culture remains the most accurate method for diagnosing *M. tuberculosis*. In patients that fail to produce sputum, aspiration of the gastric contents in the morning before the patient arises from bed is useful for obtaining samples for culture. In patients with suspected disseminated disease, blood samples in which all cells are lysed to release intracellular mycobacteria should be collected. The bacterium grows at about 1/20th the rate of more conventional bacteria, taking 3 to 6 weeks to grow on Lowenstein–Jensen medium. Living mycobacteria can be more quickly detected in blood, sputum, pleural fluid, or CSF using the Bactec radiometric or fluorometric culture system, which is designed to detect mycobacteria metabolism within 9 to 16 days. Drug susceptibilities can also be reliably tested using this method.

Treatment

The principal strategies for treating mycobacteria differ somewhat from more conventional bacteria. Because mycobacteria are intracellular and grow very slowly, and because dormant tuberculous organisms found in necrotic cavitary lesions are difficult to kill, antituberculous therapy must be prolonged—a period of months.

Secondly, because the number of mycobacterial organisms in the host is usually high, the potential for selecting for resistant mycobacteria is high. To reduce this risk, treatment with two or more antimycobacterial medications is recommended. Generally, 1 in 10^6 organisms is resistant to INH. Cavitary lesions often contain between 10^9 and 10^{10} organisms, assuring the survival and replication of resistant organisms. Administration of two drugs reduces the probability of selecting for a resistant organism because only 1 in 10^{12} organisms ($10^6 \times 10^6$) would be expected to be resistant to both antimicrobial agents.

A third major consideration is advent of multidrug-resistant *M. tuberculosis* (MDR-TB). These mycobacteria

---

KEY POINTS

About the Diagnosis of Tuberculosis

1. Ziehl–Nielson acid-fast stain can detect 10^4 organisms per milliter with 60% sensitivity.
2. Release of acid-fast bacilli from cavitary lesions is intermittent. To ensure low infectivity, three negative smears are needed.
3. Culture remains the most sensitive and specific test.
   a) Mycobacterium tuberculosis grows at 1/20th the rate of conventional bacteria.
   b) Automated techniques can detect bacteria within 9 to 16 days.
   c) Growth in conventional Lowenstein–Jensen medium takes 3 to 6 weeks.
4. Polymerase chain reaction is available, but should be performed only by experienced laboratories.

Table 4.4. Toxicities of Antibtuberculousis Medications

Clinical symptom	Isoniazid	Rifampin	Pyrazinamide	Ethambutol	Streptomycin	Quinolones	Cycloserine	Para-aminosalicylic acid	Ethionamide
Allergic skin rash	dark gray	light gray	light gray	light gray	light gray	light gray	light gray	dark gray	dark gray
Fever	dark gray		light gray		light gray				
Photosensitivity			light gray			light gray			
Anaphylaxis		light gray							
Diarrhea (*Clostridium difficile*)		light gray				light gray			
Gastrointestinal intolerance		dark gray	dark gray	dark gray		dark gray		black	black
Behavior changes	light gray			dark gray		black	dark gray	light gray	
Neuropathy	black			light gray			dark gray		dark gray
Hearing or balance problems					dark gray				
Vision problems				dark gray	dark gray				
Seizures	light gray					light gray			
Musculoskeletal problems		light gray	black			black		light gray	light gray
Orange urine and tears		black							
Laboratory tests:									
Hyperuricemia		light gray	black						
Creatinine↑		light gray			black	light gray		light gray	
Cytopenias	light gray			light gray			dark gray		
Eosinophilia		light gray							
AST/ALT↑	black						dark gray	light gray	dark gray
Bilirubin↑		light gray							dark gray
Glucose↑ or ↓	light gray							light gray	
Prolonged QT						dark gray			
Drug interactions	light gray	black							

Black = principal side effect; dark gray = less common side effect; light gray = rare side effect; white = not reported or very rare; ↑ = rise; AST/ALT = aspartate aminotransferase/alanine transaminase.

are resistant to isoniazid and rifampin, and they must be treated with three or more other antimycobacterial agents. In the early 1990s in the United States, MDR-TB was major concern; however, with improved infection control measures, the use of four drug regimens, and directly observed therapy, the incidence of MDR-TB has been reduced to less than 2%, and resistance to INH alone is approximately 8%.

Resistance is classified as either secondary or primary. Primary resistance is defined as infection with a resistant strain in a patient who has never received antituberculous drugs. When a resistant strain is cultured from a patient who were previously treated for drug-sensitive tuberculosis, the infection is said to be secondarily resistant. Secondary resistance is a major problem among homeless people, illicit drug users, and patients with AIDS.

Table 4.5. Antituberculous Medications: Half-Life, Dosing, Renal Dosing, and Cost

Antituberculous agent (trade name)	Half-life (h)	Dose	Dose for reduced creatinine clearance (mL/min)	Cost[a]
First line				
Isoniazid (Tubzid, Nydrazid)	0.5–4 2–5	300 mg PO or IM q24h	No change required No change required	$ $
Rifampin (Rifadin, Rimactane)	early 2 late	600 mg PO q24h	No change required	$
Pyrazinamide	10–16	15–30 mg/kg PO q24h, divided into 2–4 doses		
Ethambutol (Myambutol)	3–4	15–25 mg/kg PO q24h	50–80: 15 mg/kg q24h 10–50: 15 mg/kg q24–36h <10: 15 mg/kg q48h	$
Streptomycin	2–5	1–2 g IM or IV q24h	50–80: 15 mg/kg q24–48h 10–50: 15 mg/kg q72–96h <10: 7.5 mg/kg q72–96h	$
Second line				
Ciprofloxacin (Cipro)	4	750 mg PO q12h	10–50: q18h/<10: q24h	$$$
Amikacin (Amikin)	2	7–10 mg/kg IM or IV q24h (not to exceed 1 g), 5 ×/week	Renal dosing based on serum levels	$$
Capreomycin (Capastat)	4–6	1 g IM q24h	10–50: 7.5 mg/kg q24–48h <10: 7.5 mg/kg ×2 weekly	$$$$$
Cycloserine (Seromycin)	8–12	250–500 mg PO q12h	10–50: 250–500 mg q24h <10: 250 mg q24h	$$$$
Para-aminosalicylic acid	2	10–12 g PO q24h in 3–4 divided doses	Obtain from the U.S. Centers for Disease Control and Prevention	
Ethionamide (Trecator)	4	0.5–1 g PO q24h in 1–3 doses	<10: 5 mg/kg q48h	$$– $$$

[a] 10-Day course cost dollars: $ = 10–50; $$ = 51–100; $$$ = 101–140; $$$$ = 141–180; $$$$$ ≥180.

Table 4.6. Typical Course of Direct Observed Therapy for Tuberculosis

Timing	Frequency	Regimen
Weeks 1–2	Once daily	Isoniazid 300 mg Rifampin 600 mg Pyrazinamide 1.5 g (<50 kg), 2 g (51–74 kg), 2.5 g (>74 kg) Streptomycin 750 mg (<50 kg) or 1 g (>50 kg)
Weeks 3–8	Twice weekly	Isoniazid 15 mg/kg Rifampin 600 mg Pyrazinamide 3 g (<50 kg), 3.5 g (51–74 kg), 4.0 g (>74 kg) Streptomycin 1 g (<50 kg), 1.25g (51–74 kg), 1.5 g (>74 kg)
Weeks 9–26	Twice weekly	Isoniazid 15 mg/kg Rifampin 600 mg

Outside of the United States, the percentages of MDR-TB and INH-resistant strains vary widely. The worldwide median frequency of primary INH resistance is estimated to be 7.3%, with higher levels being observed in Asia, Africa, and Latin America, and lower levels in Europe and Oceania. The worldwide incidence of primary MDR-TB is 1.4%; however, rates of MDR-TB as high as 14% have been reported in countries inwhich tuberculosis control programs have deteriorated (Latvia, South Korea, and Russia, for example). Extensively drug resistant tuberculosis (XDR) has recently been reported in South Africa. XDR TB fails to respond to nearly all drugs. The mortality can exceed 90%.

The various antituberculous agents have been classified as first-line and second-line drugs. First-line medications include INH, rifampin, pyrazinamide, streptomycin, and ethambutol. These agents are more efficacious and less toxic than the second-line drugs. With the exception of ethambutol, first-line agents are also bactericidal. Whenever possible, first-line drugs should be employed for the treatment of *M. tuberculosis*. Tables 4.4 and 4.5 summarize the toxicities and recommended doses of each of these agents.

KEY POINTS

About Antieuberculous Therapy

1. A four-drug regimen (pending sensitivity testing) is recommended.
   a) Of every 10^6 organisms, 1 is naturally resistant to one drug.
   b) Cavitary lesions contain between 10^9 and 10^{10} organisms.
   c) A minimum of two effective drugs are needed to prevent resistance ($10^6 \times 10^6 = 10^{12}$).
   d) Primary isoniazid (INH) resistance is common; to reliably prevent resistance, treat with INH, rifampin, pyrazinamide, and ethambutol (pending sensitivities).
2. INH-resistance is 8% in the United States, 7.3% worldwide. Higher in Asia, Africa, and Latin America.
3. Multidrug resistance is below 2% in the United States, but up to 14% in parts of Eastern Europe.
4. Secondary resistance occurs in patients who don't reliably take their medications.
5. Directly observed therapy (DOT) is now recommended for unreliable patients, and for patients with INH- or rifampin-resistant strains.

The recommended treatment for presumed drug-sensitive pulmonary tuberculosis (pending sensitivity tests) is a four-drug regimen: INH, rifampin, pyrazinamide, and ethambutol or streptomycin. This regimen is recommended for 2 months, to be followed by INH, rifampin, and pyrazinamide for 4 months. If MDR-TB is suspected, extensive susceptibility testing should be performed, and expert advice sought to design an appropriate regimen. Treatment should consist of at least three drugs to which the organism is proven to be susceptible. Fluoroquinolones combined with aminoglycosides are particularly useful for treating MDR-TB.

In patients who are deemed to be unreliable, directly observed therapy (DOT) should be instituted. Poor adherence greatly increases the risk of secondary MDR-TB, and with the institution of DOT in these patients, the emergence of resistance is minimized. DOT is recommended for all patients with INH- or rifampin-resistant organisms. One commonly accepted DOT regimen is outlined in Table 4.6.

Prevention

Tuberculosis is spread strictly from person to person. Identifying and preventing individuals who have been exposed to tuberculosis from developing active disease is a major public health goal. The purified protein derivative (PPD) test is a very helpful skin test that assesses exposure to tuberculosis. The test is produced by acid precipitation of tubercle bacilli proteins, and the 5-tuberculin unit dose has been standardized and is administered as a 0.1-mL subcutaneous injection on the volar aspect of the forearm. Deeper injection is ineffective because tuberculous proteins can be removed by blood flow, producing a false negative result.

The injection should produce a discrete raised blanched wheal. The test is read 48 to 72 hours after injection; however, the reaction usually persists for 1 week. The diameter of induration is measured, and a diameter of more than 10 mm is defined as positive. A positive test indicates high risk for contracting tuberculosis. Of people with a PPD reaction 10 mm in diameter, 90% are infected with tuberculosis. If the reaction measures more than 15 mm, 100% are infected. The 15-mm diameter is defined as a positive reaction in individuals with no risk factors for tuberculosis. In individuals who are immunocompromised (HIV-positive, organ transplant patients receiving more than 15 mg prednisone daily) or who are recent household contacts of a patient with active tuberculosis, more than 5 mm is considered a positive reaction.

A positive test simply indicates that, sometime in the past, the individual was exposed to active tuberculosis; however, this finding does not indicate active

KEY POINTS

About Tuberculosis Testing and Prophylaxis

1. The purified protein derivative (PPD) test is carefully standardized, and induration at 48 hours is considered positive at
   a) more than 5 mm in people who are HIV-positive or immunocompromised, or who have had recent household exposure;
   b) more than 10 mm in people at overall risk for exposure; and
   c) more than 15 mm in people with no risk factors.
2. A positive result indicates exposure sometime in the past; negative to positive conversion indicates exposure during the period between tests.
3. Prophylaxis with isoniazid (300 mg daily for 6 months) if
   a) conversion within the last two years and negative chest radiograph (CXR).
   b) positive PPD and negative CXR (recommendation of the Centers for Disease Control and Prevention).
   c) abnormal CXR, and three follow-up sputum smears for acid-fast bacilli are negative.
4. If prophylaxis recipient is older than 35 years, a consumer of alcohol or other hepatotoxic drugs, pregnant, or HIV-positive, risk of INH hepatitis requires monthly monitoring of hepatic enzymes.

disease. The conversion from negative to positive in an individual who is tested annually indicates exposure to tuberculosis during the time interval between tests. Tuberculin skin tests are useful in otherwise healthy individuals, but cannot be relied upon to determine exposure in HIV patients with low CD4 counts, in patients receiving immunosuppressants, or in patients with severe malnutrition.

Individuals with a positive PPD should have a CXR, and if pulmonary lesions are noted, three sputum samples should be obtained for culture and smear. Prophylaxis should be given only if all sputum samples prove negative for tuberculosis. Because the risk of developing active disease is highest within 2 years of exposure, all individuals who have converted from a negative to a positive test within 2 years should receive INH prophylaxis. Preventive therapy is also warranted when a positive test is associated with other specific risk factors (HIV infection, known recent exposure to tuberculosis, abnormal CXR, intravenous drug abuse, and certain underlying diseases).

In other individuals with a positive PPD, the risk of INH hepatotoxicity must be balanced against the likelihood of preventing the development of active disease.

The U.S. Centers for Disease Control and Prevention currently recommends that all individuals with a positive PPD receive prophylaxis. However, in individuals 35 years of age or older, the risk of hepatotoxicity may outweigh the potential benefit of INH prophylaxis. Hepatic enzymes should be monitored at monthly intervals in HIV-positive patients, pregnant women, patients with underlying liver disease, and in those receiving other potentially hepatotoxic drugs or drinking alcohol daily. Prophylaxis should be discontinued if transaminase levels rise exceed 3 times the normal values in association with symptoms consistent with hepatitis.

The recommended prophylactic regimen is INH 300 mg daily for 6 months. For HIV-infected patients, 12 months of INH prophylaxis is recommended.

Atypical Mycobacteria

Atypical mycobacteria are found throughout the environment in soil and water. These organisms have a low virulence, and they do not usually cause pulmonary disease in otherwise healthy individuals. In patients with underlying pulmonary disease, these organisms can be inhaled and cause pulmonary infection.

M. avium complex is the most common of the atypical mycobacteria to infect the lung. A cavitary upper lobe lesion is the usual manifestation of this disease. The cavities tend to be somewhat smaller and thinner walled than those with *M. tuberculosis*. Pulmonary infection with *M. avium* complex is seen

KEY POINTS

About Atypical Mycobacteria Pulmonary Infection

1. Atypical mycobacteria are found in soil and water.
2. Infects males over the age of 50 years, who are also alcoholic, smokers with chronic lung disease. Often presents as upper lobe cavitary disease.
3. Infects women over the age of 60 years without apparent underlying disease. Presents as right middle lobe or lingular disease.
4. *M. avium* is the most common pathogen; *M. kansasii, M. fortuitum,* and *M. abscessus* are rarer.
5. Management is complex and requires a pulmonary or infectious disease specialist.

primarily in male smokers in their early fifties who abuse alcohol. Infection of the lungs is also seen in women 60 year of age or older with no apparent underlying disease, most commonly involving the right middle lobe or lingula.

M. kansasii, *M. fortuitum*, and *M. abscessus* can also infect the lungs, causing chronic cavitary disease. Because these organisms are found throughout the environment and may colonize as well as infect patients with chronic lung diseases, elaborate criteria for differentiating colonization from infection have been established. Therapy for atypical mycobacterial infection must be prolonged and is based on sensitivity testing. Often these organisms respond poorly to therapy, and resection of the infected lung segment may be required for cure. Management of these patients is complex and requires the supervision of an experienced pulmonary or infectious disease specialist.

Fungal Pneumonias

The most common forms of fungal pneumonia in the normal host are histoplasmosis and coccidiomycosis. In the immunocompromised host, *Cryptococcus* and *Aspergillus* can also cause pneumonia (see Chapter 15).

HISTOPLASMOSIS

Epidemiology. *Histoplasma capsulatum* is one of the more common causes of chronic pneumonia in the Midwestern and Southeastern United States. This organism survives in moist soil in temperate climates and is most commonly reported in the Ohio and Mississippi River valleys. The development of histoplasmosis is generally associated with construction or excavation of soil contaminated with *H. capsulatum*. Infection is also reported in spelunkers, who contract the infection by disturbing dried bat guano containing high concentrations of infectious particles. Exposure to infectious particles can also occur after the renovation of old buildings previously inhabited by birds or bats.

Pathogenesis. *H. capsulatum* is a fungus and exists in two forms: mycelia or yeast. In the moist soil of temperate climates, the organism exists in the mycelial form as macroconidia (8 to 15 μm in size) and microconidia (2 to 5 μm in size). When infected soil is disturbed, microconidia float in the air and can be inhaled into the lung. Once in the lung, microconidia are ingested by alveolar macrophages and neutrophils. In the intracellular environment of these phagocytes, the mycelia transform to rounded, encapsulated yeast cells. During this transformation, multiple genes are upregulated, including a gene that increases production of a calcium-binding protein important for acquiring calcium (an essential ion for yeast survival) from the intracellular environment. The

> **KEY POINTS**
>
> **About the Epidemiology and Pathogenesis of Histoplasmosis**
>
> 1. Found primarily in the Midwest and Southeast United States.
> 2. Grows in moist soil in temperate zones, mainly Ohio and Mississippi River valleys.
> 3. Found in caves and old buildings; bat guano is a concentrated source.
> 4. Mycelial form in soil, as macro- and microconidia. Microconidia readily aerosolized.
> 5. Inhaled microconidia ingested by macrophages and neutrophils convert to yeast forms and upregulate many genes, including a gene for calcium binding.
> 6. Yeast forms are transported to hilar nodes, where cell-mediated immunity is induced.

expression of this calcium-binding protein may explain the frequent finding of calcifications in infected tissues.

As is observed in tuberculosis, infected macrophages transport the yeast forms to the hilar lymph nodes where *Histoplasma* antigens are presented to T cells. Within several weeks, cell-mediated immunity develops, and CD4 T cells activate macrophages to produce fungicidal products.

Clinical Manifestations. In more than 90% of patients, infection is controlled. In many patients, primary exposure is asymptomatic or results in a mild influenza-like illness. Very young people, elderly people, and patients with compromised immune systems are more likely to develop active disease. Symptoms usually develop within 14 days of exposure and may include high fever, headache, nonproductive cough, and dull nonpleuritic chest pain. This form of chest pain is thought to be the result of mediastinal node enlargement. In other patients, chest pain may be sharper and may worsen upon lying down, reflecting the development of pericarditis (observed in approximately 6% of cases).

On CXR, patchy infiltrates may be seen during acute disease that subsequently calcify producing a "buckshot" appearance. Healed histoplasmosis is also the most common cause of calcified lesions in the liver and spleen. In acute disease, mediastinal lymphadenopathy may be prominent and may mimic lymphoma or sarcoidosis. A history of exposure to a site where soil was excavated is particularly important in trying to

---

KEY POINTS

About the Clinical Manifestations of Histoplasmosis

1. In 90% of cases, a brief self-limiting flu-like illness occurs or the person remains asymptomatic.

2. Disease can develop in elderly, very young, and immunocompromised individuals.

3. At 14 days post exposure, the individual may have
   a) high fever, headache, nonproductive cough, and dull, nonpleuritic chest pain.
   b) a CXR with patchy infiltrates that later convert to "buckshot" calcifications.
   c) mediastinal lymphadenopathy that may mimic lymphoma or sarcoidosis.
   d) progressive mediastinal fibrosis (a rare complication).

4. Cavitary disease is clinically similar, with men older than 50 years who have chronic obstructive pulmonary disease at higher risk.

5. Disseminated disease occurs in 10% of symptomatic primary disease.
   a) Likelihood of dissemination occurs in people who are very old, very young, or immunosuppressed (because of AIDS or transplantation).
   b) Meningitis with lymphocytosis and low glucose may develop.
   c) Reticulonodular pattern on CXR in most cases, but CXR normal in one third.

Progressive disseminate histoplasmosis occurs in about 10% of symptomatic primary infections. Progressive dissemination also develops as a consequence of reactivation of old disease. In the immunosuppressed individual, reactivation is the most likely pathway for disseminated disease. Onset of symptoms is usually abrupt. Fever and malaise are followed by nonproductive cough, weight loss, and diarrhea. Hepatosplenomegaly usually develops, and lymphadenopathy may be detected. Anemia, thrombocytopenia, and leukopenia are observed in a high proportion of patients. Meningitis may develop, resulting in lymphocytosis and low glucose in the cerebrospinal fluid. A CXR may show a reticulonodular pattern or scattered nodular opacities; however, the CXR is normal in nearly one third of cases. Mortality is high if treatment is not initiated.

Diagnosis. *H. capsulatum* can be readily grown from tissue samples and body fluids using brain–heart infusion media containing antibiotics and cycloheximide (inhibits the growth of saprophytic fungi). Mycelial growth can usually be detected within 7 days and confirmed using a DNA probe. The clinical microbiology

---

KEY POINTS

About the Diagnosis of Histoplasmosis

1. Sputum culture is often positive.
   a) Requires selective media (brain–heart infusion with antibiotics and cycloheximide).
   b) Not a routine method; clinical microbiology must be notified.
   c) Bronchoscopy improves yield (90% in HIV patients).

2. Bone marrow positive in 50% of cases.

3. Lysis–centrifugation method positive in up to 50% of blood samples.

4. Polysaccharide urine and serum antigen test is the most sensitive, being positive for
   a) 90% of disseminated disease,
   b) 40% cavitary disease, and
   c) 20% acute pulmonary disease

5. Method can also be used to test bronchoscopic lavage fluid.

6. Histopathology shows noncaseating or caseating granulomas. Silver stain best for identifying the yeast forms. Hematoxylin–eosin is not useful; periodic acid Schiff may help with identification.

7. Urine antigen test positive in 90% of disseminated histoplasmosis

---

differentiate between these various possibilities. Occasionally, mediastinal nodes can become massively enlarged, reaching diameters of 8 to 10 cm. Severe mediastinal fibrosis is rare, but it can lead to impingement and obstruction of the superior vena cava, bronchi, and esophagus.

Chronic cavitary histoplasmosis develops in about 8% of patients. This complication is more common in men over the age of 50 years who have chronic obstructive pulmonary disease. The symptoms and CXR findings associated with chronic pulmonary histoplasmosis are indistinguishable from cavitary tuberculosis. In fact, in the past, patients in the Midwestern and Southeastern United States with chronic pulmonary histoplasmosis were frequently misdiagnosed as having pulmonary tuberculosis and were mistakenly confined to tuberculosis sanatoriums. Spontaneous resolution of cavitary disease occurs in 10% to 60% of cases.

lab must be notified that *H. capsulatum* is the possible pathogen, because the necessary culture methods are not employed on routine samples.

A single sputum culture has only a 10% to 15% yield; collection of multiple sputum cultures increases the yield. Bronchoscopy has proved useful for providing good sputum samples yielding positive cultures in 90% of HIV patients with pulmonary histoplasmosis. Bone marrow and blood cultures should also be obtained and are positive in up to 50% of cases. The lysis–centrifugation blood culture technique (also used to culture mycobacteria) is the most sensitive method. The most effective method for detecting progressive disseminated histoplasmosis is the urine and serum polysaccharide antigen test. Antigen is detected in up to 90% of patients with disseminated disease. The antigen test is also positive in 40% of patients with cavitary pulmonary diseases and 20% with acute pulmonary histoplasmosis. Pulmonary lavage fluid can also be tested in this manner. A PCR method is available only on an experimental basis.

Histopathologic examination of infected tissue also allows for rapid diagnosis. Noncaseating or caseating granulomas may be seen. An excessive fibrotic reaction may be seen in some patients. Silver stains are most effective for identifying the typical yeast forms in tissue biopsies. Organisms are poorly visualized by hematoxylin–eosin staining, but can often be seen on periodic acid Schiff stain.

Treatment. Itraconazole is the most effective azole for oral treatment. In patients with acute pulmonary histoplasmosis who fail to improve over the first week, itraconazole 200 mg daily for 4 to 6 weeks is recommended. If the patient is unable to tolerate azoles or cannot take oral medications, amphotericin B 0.4 to 0.5 g/kg

can be administered intravenously until symptoms subside. In patients with extensive mediastinal involvement, itraconazole 200 mg daily, can be given for 3 to 6 months. If rapid resolution of symptoms is necessary, amphotericin B is preferred.

Patients with severe mediastinal fibrosis may also require surgical intervention to correct vascular and airway obstruction. In cavitary pulmonary disease, progression of lesions over 2 to 3 months or persistent cavities associated with declining respiratory function warrant treatment with itraconazole 200 mg twice daily for a minimum of 6 months. Amphotericin B may be required if lesions fail to improve on itraconazole therapy. In acute, life-threatening progressive disseminated histoplasmosis, amphotericin B should be given in high doses: 0.7 to 1 mg/kg daily. Once the patient has defervesced, the dosage can be lowered to 0.4 to 0.5 mg/kg, or the patient can be switched to itraconazole 200 mg twice daily.

COCCIDIOMYCOSIS

Epidemiology—Like *H. capsulatum*, *Coccidioides immitis* survives and grows in soil. The ideal conditions for survival of *C. immitis* are dry, alkaline soil, hot summers, and winters with few freezes. These conditions exist in central California's San Joaquin Valley and in the southern regions of Arizona, New Mexico, and Texas. *C. immitis* is also found in Mexico, Central America, and South America. Infections are most commonly reported in the summer months when dry soil more readily forms dust particles. Epidemics have been associated with disruption of soil by archeological excavation, earthquakes, and dust storms. In recent years, the incidence of coccidiomycosis has increased as a consequence of the increased numbers of people living in endemic areas.

Pathogenesis. Also like *H. capsulatum*, *C. immitis* is a dimorphic fungus. It exists in soil as mycelia that can form small arthroconidia (5-µm barrel-shaped structures). Arthroconidia can become airborne, whereupon they are inhaled by humans and become lodged in the terminal bronchioles. In the warm moist environment of the lung, the arthroconidia transform into spherules. As the spherules mature, their outer walls thin, and they release endospores that are ingested by macrophages. As is observed in histoplasmosis and tuberculosis, macrophages transport the infectious particles to the hilar lymph nodes, the lymphatic system, and the bloodstream, resulting in dissemination. Cell-mediated immunity is critical for control of the infection.

Clinical Manifestations. Approximately two thirds of patients exposed to arthroconidia experience minimal symptoms. When symptoms are noted, they usually develop 7 to 21 days after exposure. Nonproductive cough and fever are the most frequent symptoms. Pleuritic chest pain, shortness of breath, headache, and fatigue are also commonly reported. Skin manifestations may include erythema nodosum (red, painful nodules on the anterior shins), erythema multiforme (target-like lesions involving the entire body, including the palms and soles) or a nonpruritic papular rash. Arthralgias may develop in association with erythema nodosum. Eosinophilia is commonly observed on peripheral blood smear.

In about half of patients, a CXR is abnormal, most commonly demonstrating unilateral infiltrates, pleural effusions, and hilar adenopathy. In patients with depressed cell-mediated immunity (primarily patients with AIDS and CD4 counts below 100/mm^3), the infection can disseminate, causing diffuse opacification of the lungs and severe respiratory failure. Meningitis, skin lesions, bone infection and arthritis may also develop as a consequence of dissemination.

In some patients pulmonary infection can persist, causing progressive destruction of lung parenchyma associated with a productive cough, chest pain, weight loss. A CXR may demonstrate areas of fibrosis, nodules, cavitary lesions, or a combination. An isolated nodule can persist in approximately 4% of pulmonary cases and can be differentiated from neoplasm only by biopsy. These lesions seldom calcify as the lesions of histoplasmosis do. A chronic pleural

---

KEY POINTS

About the Clinical Manifestations of Coccidiomycosis

1. Symptoms (nonproductive cough, fever, pleuritic chest pain, shortness of breath, headache, and fatigue) occur in about one third of exposed individuals 7 to 21 days after inhalation.

2. Skin manifestations are common: erythema nodosum, erythema multiforme, nonpruritic papular rash.

3. Eosinophilia may be noted on peripheral blood smear.

4. Abnormal CXR findings are frequent: unilateral infiltrates, pleural effusions, hilar adenopathy.

5. In patients with AIDS whose CD4 counts fall below 100/mm^3, the disease can disseminate, causing diffuse lung opacification, meningitis, bone infection, and arthritis.

6. Chronic lung disease can lead to fibrosis, nodules, or cavities.

7. Isolated pulmonary nodules are not calcified, can be differentiated from neoplasm by biopsy.

8. Chronic pleural effusions most commonly develop in young, healthy, athletic males.

---

effusion can result from the rupture of a peripheral cavitary lesion into the pleural space. This complication is most commonly reported in young, otherwise healthy, athletic males.

Diagnosis. Travel to, or past residence in, an endemic area should alert the clinician to the possibility of coccidiomycosis. Examination of induced sputum or sputum obtained by bronchoscopy may reveal spherules. The fungus is not seen on Gram stain, but can be detected by silver stain. Biopsies of infected tissue should be obtained; they usually reveal caseating or noncaseating granulomas and spherules. The organism grows readily as a white mold on routine mycology media and on bacterial media under aerobic conditions.

Multiple serologic tests are available. These tests are often required to make the diagnosis, because of unavailability of sputum and biopsy specimens. Immunoglobulin M (IgM) serum titers against *C. immitis* are usually positive within the first week of disease. Immunoglobulin G (IgG) levels are most commonly tested by complement fixation or immunodiffusion. Levels of IgG increase after IgM and often persist for years. A correlation has been observed

KEY POINTS

About the Diagnosis of Coccidiomycosis

1. Spherules may be seen on induced sputum or after bronchoscopy.
2. The organisms are readily cultured on routine bacterial and mycology culture plates.
3. Histopathology shows noncaseating and caseating granulomas; Gram stain is not useful, silver stain is best.
4. Multiple serology tests are available to measure immunoglobulin G (IgG) and M (IgM) antibody titers.
   a) The IgM titer is elevated in acute disease.
   b) The IgG level often persists for years. A rising titer exceeding 1:32 signals dissemination; a falling titer is indicative of a favorable prognosis.

between the IgG serum titer and severity of disease. A rising titer that exceeds 1:32 may signal disseminated disease; a falling titer indicates a favorable prognosis. Patients with no detectable lesions can have titers below 1:8 for many years after exposure.

Treatment. Most infections with this organism spontaneously resolve. Treatment is reserved for patients with disseminated disease and patients with persistent

KEY POINTS

About the Treatment of Coccidiomycosis

1. Treatment usually reserved for disseminated disease.
2. Amphotericin B given for severe disease.
3. Fluconazole or itraconazole given for less-severe disease.
4. Treatment continues for a minimum of 6 months.
5. Complement fixation immunoglobulin G titers should decline to a stable low tier.
6. For meningitis, triazole therapy should be continued indefinitely.
7. Surgical resection can be used to expand lung lesions.

or progressive coccidioidal pneumonia with hypoxia. Treatment needs to also be considered in patients with pulmonary disease who are at increased risk for dissemination, including people that are black, Philippino, pregnant, diabetic, and immunosuppressed (including patients with AIDS).

Amphotericin B remains the preferred initial therapy for life-threatening disseminated disease or severe pulmonary disease until the infection is under control. High doses of amphotericin B (0.7 to 1 mg/kg daily) are recommended. In less severe disease, fluconazole (400 to 800 mg daily) or itraconazole (200 mg twice daily) are used. These agents are preferred because of their low toxicity and suitability for prolonged therapy. Treatment should be continued until symptoms and signs of infection have resolved. A minimum of 6 months' therapy is recommended. In patients with meningeal involvement, triazole therapy should be continued indefinitely.

Surgical debridement of large purulent collections is recommended. Resection of rapidly expanding pulmonary cavities should be performed to prevent rupture into the pleural space. Surgical resection is also recommended to prevent bronchopleural fistula formation and to correct life-threatening pulmonary hemorrhage.

FURTHER READING

General

File TM. Community-acquired pneumonia. *Lancet.* 2003;362: 1991–2001.

Hageman JC, Uyeki TM, Francis JS, et al. Severe community-acquired pneumonia due to *Staphylococcus aureus,* 2003-04 influenza season. *Emerg Infect Dis.* 2006;12:894–899.

Heyland D, Dodek P, Muscedere J, Day A. A randomized trial of diagnostic techniques for ventilator-associated pneumonia. *N Engl J Med.* 2006;355:2619–2630.

Jackson ML, Neuzil KM, Thompson WW, et al. The burden of community-acquired pneumonia in seniors: results of a population-based study. *Clin Infect Dis.* 2004;39:1642–1650.

Mandell LA, Wunderink RG, Anzueto A, et al. Infectious Diseases Society of America/American Thoracic Society consensus guidelines on the management of community-acquired pneumonia in adults. *Clin Infect Dis.* 2007;44(suppl 2):S27–S72.

Lim WS, van der Eerden MM, Laing R, et al. Defining community acquired pneumonia severity on presentation to hospital: an international derivation and validation study. *Thorax.* 2003;58:377–382.

Marrie TJ, Wu L. Factors influencing in-hospital mortality in community-acquired pneumonia: a prospective study of patients not initially admitted to the ICU. *Chest.* 2005;127:1260–1270.

Mortensen EM, Restrepo M, Anzueto A, Pugh J. Effects of guideline-concordant antimicrobial therapy on mortality among patients with community-acquired pneumonia. *Am J Med.* 2004; 117:726–731.

Oosterheert JJ, van Loon AM, Schuurman R, et al. Impact of rapid detection of viral and atypical bacterial pathogens by real-time polymerase chain reaction for patients with lower respiratory tract infection. *Clin Infect Dis.* 2005;41:1438–44.

Spindler C, Ortqvist A. Prognostic score systems and community-acquired bacteraemic pneumococcal pneumonia. *Eur Respir J.* 2006;28:816–823.

Pneumococcal Pneumonia

Bauer T, Ewig S, Marcos MA, Schultze-Werninghaus G, Torres A. *Streptococcus pneumoniae* in community-acquired pneumonia. How important is drug resistance? *Med Clin North Am.* 2001;85:1367–1379.

Marrie TJ. Pneumococcal pneumonia: epidemiology and clinical features. *Semin Respir Infect.* 1999;14:227–236.

Musher DM, Alexandraki I, Graviss EA, et al. Bacteremic and non-bacteremic pneumococcal pneumonia. A prospective study. *Medicine (Baltimore).* 2000;79:210221.

Musher DM, Montoya R, Wanahita A. Diagnostic value of microscopic examination of Gram-stained sputum and sputum cultures in patients with bacteremic pneumococcal pneumonia. *Clin Infect Dis.* 2004;39:165–169.

Haemophilus influenzae Pneumonia

Sarangi J, Cartwright K, Stuart J, Brookes S, Morris R, Slack M. Invasive *Haemophilus influenzae* disease in adults. *Epidemiol Infect.* 2000;124:441–447.

Aspiration Pneumonia

Marik PE. Aspiration pneumonitis and aspiration pneumonia. *N Engl J Med.* 2001;344:665–671.

Legionnaires' Disease

Akbas E, Yu VL. Legionnaires' disease and pneumonia. Beware the temptation to underestimate this "exotic" cause of infection. *Postgrad Med.* 2001;109:135–138,141–142,147.

Murdoch DR. Diagnosis of *Legionella* infection. *Clin Infect Dis.* 2003;36:64–69.

Waterer GW, Baselski VS, Wunderink RG. *Legionella* and community-acquired pneumonia: a review of current diagnostic tests from a clinician's viewpoint. *Am J Med.* 2001;110:41–48.

Atypical Pneumonia

Schneeberger PM, Dorigo-Zetsma JW, van der Zee A, van Bon M, van Opstal JL. Diagnosis of atypical pathogens in patients hospitalized with community-acquired respiratory infection. *Scand J Infect Dis.* 2004;36:269–273.

Actinomycosis and Nocardiosis

Heffner JE. Pleuropulmonary manifestations of actinomycosis and nocardiosis. *Semin Respir Infect.* 1988;3:352–361.

Yildiz O, Doganay M. Actinomycoses and *Nocardia* pulmonary infections. *Curr Opin Pulm Med.* 2006;12:228–234.

Tuberculosis

Campbell IA, Bah-Sow O. Pulmonary tuberculosis: diagnosis and treatment. *BMJ.* 2006;332:1194–1197.

Packham S. Tuberculosis in the elderly. *Gerontology.* 2001;47: 175–179.

Palomino JC. Newer diagnostics for tuberculosis and multi-drug resistant tuberculosis. *Curr Opin Pulm Med.* 2006;12:172–178.

Small PM, Fujiwara PI. Management of tuberculosis in the United States. *N Engl J Med.* 2001;345:189–200.

Histoplasmosis

Hage CA, Davis TE, Egan L, et al. Diagnosis of pulmonary histoplasmosis and blastomycosis by detection of antigen in bronchoalveolar lavage fluid using an improved second-generation enzyme-linked immunoassay. *Respir Med.* 2007;101:43–47.

Restrepo A, Tobon A, Clark B, et al. Salvage treatment of histoplasmosis with posaconazole. *J Infect.* 2007;54:319–327.

Wheat LJ. Histoplasmosis: a review for clinicians from non-endemic areas. *Mycoses.* 2006;49:274–282.

Coccidiomycosis

Crum-Cianflone NF, Truett AA, Teneza-Mora N, et al. Unusual presentations of coccidioidomycosis: a case series and review of the literature. *Medicine (Baltimore).* 2006;85:263–277.

Fish DG, Ampel NM, Galgiani JN, et al. Coccidioidomycosis during human immunodeficiency virus infection. A review of 77 patients. *Medicine (Baltimore).* 1990;69:384–391.

Valdivia L, Nix D, Wright M, et al. Coccidioidomycosis as a common cause of community-acquired pneumonia. *Emerg Infect Dis.* 2006;12:958–962

Eye, Ear, Nose, and Throat Infections

5

Time Recommended to Complete: 1 day

Frederick Southwick, M.D.

■ EYE INFECTIONS

GUIDING QUESTIONS

1. *What is the most common cause of conjunctivitis?*

2. *What is the greatest risk factor for development of keratitis?*

3. *Which symptom is most helpful for differentiating conjunctivitis from keratitis?*

4. *Which infection is associated with unsterilized tap water?*

5. *What is the most likely diagnosis in the patient with a recurrent history of a red eye?*

6. *What are the three most common ways in which patients develop endophthalmitis?*

Many eye infections are managed by the ophthalmologist, who possesses the specialized equipment and skills required for optimal diagnosis and treatment. However, infectious disease consultants and primary care physicians need to be familiar with these forms of infection to be able to initiate preliminary empiric therapy pending referral.

CONJUNCTIVITIS

> POTENTIAL SEVERITY
>
> *Usually responds rapidly to therapy and does not threaten vision.*

Predisposing Factors

The conjunctiva is a mucous membrane that covers the globe of the eye up to the cornea and the lid of the eye.

The surface of this transparent membrane is normally protected from infection by tears, which contain numerous antibacterial agents, including lysozyme and immunoglobulins A and G. Patients with decreased tear production—for example those, with scleroderma with infiltration of the lacrimal duct—often experience recurrent conjunctivitis and also keratitis.

Causes and Clinical Manifestations

Inflammation of the conjunctiva is called conjunctivitis. It is accompanied by dilatation of vessels within the membrane, causing the underlying white sclera to appear red. In addition to redness, pus formation accompanies conjunctivitis. Purulent discharge is commonly associated with swelling of the eyelids, pain, and itching. Upon awakening in the morning, the patient may find that dried exudate has glued the eyelid shut. Vision is usually unimpaired, and the cornea and pupil appear normal.

Bacteria, viruses, *Chlamydia*, fungi, and parasites can all cause conjunctivitis (Table 5.1). Allergic reactions and toxic substances can also produce inflammation of the

Table 5.1. Infectious Causes of Conjunctivitis

Type of Infection	General Symptoms, Comments	Infecting Agent	Specific Symptoms, Comments
Bacterial	Thick purulent exudate	*Staphylococcus aureus*	
		Streptococcus pneumoniae	Petechial hemorrhages
		Haemolphilus influenzae	Petechial hemorrhages
		Moraxella catarrhalis	
		Neisseria gonorrhoeae	More severe, sexual transmission
		Neisseria meningitidis	More severe
		Serratia marcescens	Found in chronic care facilities
		Pseudomonas aeruginosa	Found in chronic care facilities
Viral	Serous exudate	Adenoviruses	Common
		Enteroviruses	Common
		Herpes simplex	Rare, blisters on eyelid
		Varicella	Rare, skin lesions
		Measles	Rare, skin lesions
Chlamydial		*Chlamydia trachomatis*	Mucopurulent, corneal involvement
Fungal	Rare, granulomatous	*Candida*	Usually after use of steroid drops
		Blastomyces	
		Sporothrix schenckii	
Parasitic	Developing countries	*Trichinella spiralis*	
		Taenia solium	
		Schistosoma haematobium	
		Onchocerca volvulus	
		Loa loa filariasis	

conjunctiva. The specific findings on eye exam vary depend on the particular cause:

1. **Bacterial.** Bacterial conjunctivitis is highly contagious, particularly among children. Copious quantities of pus usually exude from the eye, and when pus is removed, it is quickly replaced by new exudate. The discharge is usually thick and globular.

2. **Viral.** Viral infection is the most common cause of conjunctivitis, representing approximately 14% of diagnosed cases. The exudate in viral infection is less purulent and more serous in nature. In viral, chlamydial, and toxic conjunctivitis, the lymphatic tissue in the conjunctiva can become hypertrophied, forming small, smooth bumps called follicles. Viral conjunctivitis is highly contagious; the second eye commonly becomes involved within 24 to 48 hours. Unilateral involvement does not exclude the diagnosis, however. The infection is self-limiting, resolving over a period of 1 to 3 weeks.

3. **Chlamydial.** *Chlamydia trachomatis* conjunctivitis is a leading cause of blindness worldwide. In the United States, this infection is most commonly seen in indigent Native Americans. Another form of *C. trachomatis* infection, inclusion conjunctivitis, is transmitted to adults by genital secretions from an infected sexual partner. This form of conjunctivitis is also common in neonates who pass through an infected birth canal.

4. **Fungal.** Fungal conjunctivitis is rare. *Candida* conjunctivitis is usually associated with prolonged use of corticosteroid eye drops.

5. **Parasitic.** The parasites listed in Table 5.1 have all been associated with conjunctivitis.

6. **Allergic and toxic.** Pollens can induce allergic conjunctivitis that usually involves both eyes and is accompanied by itching. Almost any topical solution applied to the eye can also result in an allergic conjunctivitis. Hard and soft contact lenses and cosmetics are also frequent offenders. This form of conjunctivitis is usually accompanied by itching.

7. **Other.** Other clinical conditions in which conjunctivitis is a component of the disease include Reiter's syndrome, keratoconjunctivitis sicca, graft-versus-host disease, and pemphigoid.

Diagnosis

Cultures are not usually obtained in routine cases of conjunctivitis. In more severe cases, conjunctival scrapings are obtained for culture and Gram stain. An abundance of polymorphonuclear leukocytes (PMNs) are found in bacterial and chlamydial conjunctivitis. Viral conjunctivitis usually results in a mononuclear cell exudate, and allergic conjunctivitis is associated with a predominance of eosinophils. Follicular inflammation combined with an exudate containing PMNs strongly suggests chlamydial infection.

Treatment

In severe bacterial and chlamydial conjunctivitis, systemic treatment is recommended. For milder forms, topical antimicrobial agents usually are sufficient. Fluoroquinolone eye-drop preparations are preferred because they treat both gram-positive and gram-negative pathogens (see "Corneal infections," later in this chapter, for dosing). Alternative topical agents include gentamicin or tobramycin for gram-negative infections, and polymyxin B/bacitracin, neomycin/polymyxin, polymyxin B–trimethoprim, or erythromycin for gram-positive infections.

CORNEAL INFECTIONS

Corneal infections cause inflammation of the cornea, which is also termed keratitis. Any corneal inflammation must be considered sight-threatening and should be treated promptly. Corneal perforation can lead to blindness. Because of the potential subtleties of diagnosis and treatment, and the potential consequences of misdiagnosis, all patients with significant corneal lesions should be referred to an ophthalmologist experienced in the management of keratitis.

Predisposing Conditions

A small break in the cornea is usually required for bacteria and fungi to gain entry into the cornea. Trauma to the eye, contact lens abrasions, eye surgery, and defective tear production can all result in damage to corneal epithelium. Defective eye closure in comatose patients receiving respiratory support puts those patients at increased risk for keratitis. Immunosuppression and diabetes mellitus also increase the risk of keratitis.

CASE 5.1

A 28-year-old white man had been spending long hours at work and was somewhat sleep deprived. Three days earlier he had gone to the beach for the afternoon. The night before seeing the doctor, he noted a sensation of a foreign body in his left eye. Every time he blinked, he noted pain. When he awoke in the morning, his left eye was glued shut with yellow exudate. On prying the lid open, he noted that the eye was extremely red and sensitive to light. His vision in that eye was blurred and images were outlined by halos. In the ophthalmologist's office later that day, a slit-lamp exam revealed a large dendritic lesion that stained with fluorescein, indicative of herpes simplex keratitis (Figure 5.1).

Causes and Clinical Manifestations

The primary symptom of keratitis is eye pain. The rich enervation of the corneal surface transmits the pain sensation each time the eyelid migrates across the corneal ulcer. As described in case 5.1, patients often complain of a foreign body sensation in their eye. Unlike conjunctivitis, corneal edema usually impairs vision. Photophobia and reflex tearing are also common. Slit-lamp examination can identify the corneal break and the degree of inflammation. Loss of corneal substance (which can lead to perforation or corneal scar formation) may be apparent. Intraocular inflammation is commonly seen. Severe inflammation can lead to the

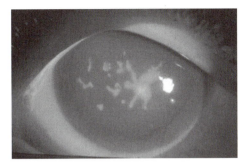

Figure 5–1. Herpes keratitis. Fluorescein stain shows the typical dendritic corneal lesions of herpes simplex. Picture courtesy of Dr. William Driebe, University of Florida College of Medicine. *See color image on color plate 1*

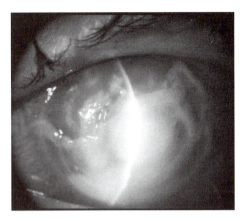

Figure 5–2. *Pseudomonas aeruginosa* keratitis. Note the large hypopyon that accompanies the severe corneal opacification in this patient who used tap water to wash hard contact lenses. Picture courtesy of Dr. William Driebe, University of Florida College of Medicine.

collection of inflammatory cells in the anterior chamber. These cells then settle by gravity at the bottom of the chamber, forming a hypopyon (Figure 5.2).

Clinical manifestations in keratitis, including the eye findings, vary with the cause of the condition:

1. **Bacterial.** Bacterial infection (Table 5.2) is the leading cause of keratitis, accounting for 65% to 90% of cases. Several bacteria produce toxins and enzymes that allow them to penetrate intact corneal epithelium; most other bacteria require a break in the epithelial lining to invade the cornea. Gram-positive organisms are most frequently cultured, *Staphylococcus aureus* being the most common pathogen in this group. However, a number of other gram-positive cocci and bacilli have also been associated keratitis. One of the most destructive bacteria is *Pseudomonas aeruginosa*. Infection with this gram-negative rod is commonly associated with hard contact lenses. Pain is severe, and the corneal ulcer spreads rapidly as a consequence of the production of bacterial proteases. Development of a large hypopyon is the rule (Figure 5.2). Perforation can occur quickly. The exudate is often greenish in color, and the infiltrate appears soupy. Other gram-negative rods also produce a soupy infiltrate. In addition to *Neisseria*, other gram-negative coccobacilli can also cause bacterial keratitis.

2. **Viral.** Patients with a history of a recurrent red eye most commonly have recurrent herpes simplex keratitis. Latent virus in the Vth cranial nerve reactivates and migrates down the nerve to the corneal surface. Ultraviolet light exposure, menstruation, fever, and other acute stresses can induce viral reactivation. In the hospitalized patient with unilateral red eye, herpes simplex keratitis should always be considered. Corneal anesthesia may develop initially, minimizing pain. Erythema and a foreign body sensation associated with tearing are frequently noted. A classic dendritic lesion that stains with fluorescein dye is readily seen on slit-lamp exam (Figure 5.1). Other forms of viral keratitis are less common (Table 5.2).

3. **Fungal.** Corneal ulcers caused by hyphae-forming fungi such as *Aspergillus* most commonly follow an eye injury from organic material (such as a tree branch). Use of chronic glucocorticoid eye drops also increases the risk of fungal keratitis. Ulcers tend to be superficial and are often elevated above the corneal surface. The infiltrate tends to be irregular, and an immune ring is often apparent. Smaller satellite lesions are commonly seen surrounding the main infiltrate. A severe anterior-chamber reaction associated with a hypopyon is commonly observed. Yeast-like fungi such as *Candida* can also cause corneal ulcers. These infections tend to be more indolent, but they can have all the characteristics described for hyphae-forming fungi.

4. **Protozoal.** Protozoa are a rare but very serious cause of corneal ulcers. *Acanthamoeba* species most commonly develop in contact lens wearers, particularly those that use unsterilized tap water in their cleaning solutions. Acanthamoeba ulcers are painful, progress slowly, and fail to respond to topical antibiotics.

Diagnosis and Treatment

Slit-lamp examination is helpful in identifying the potential cause of an eye infection. If a bacterial or fungal cause is suspected, corneal scrapings for culture,

Table 5.2. Infectious Causes of Keratitis

Type of Infection	General Symptoms, Comments	Infecting Agent	Specific Symptoms, Comments
Bacterial		*Neisseria gonorrhoeae, Neisseria meningitidis, Corynebacterium diphtheriae, Listeria, Shigella*	Contain toxins and enzymes that permit penetration of the cornea
		Staphylococcus aureus	Common
		Streptococcus pneumoniae	Ulcer has sharp margins, early hypopyon
		S. epidermidis, S. viridans, S. pyogenes, Enterococcus, Peptostreptococcus	Less common, gram-positive cocci
		C. diphtheriae, Bacillus, Clostridium	Uncommon gram-positive bacilli
		Pseudomonas aeruginosa	Most destructive, large hypopyon, green exudate
		Proteus mirabilis, Klebsiella pneumoniae, Serratia marcescens, Escherichia coli, Aeromonas hydrophila	Less common gram-negative bacilli
		Pasteurella multocida, Acinetobacter spp.	Less common, gram-negative coccobacilli
		Moraxella spp.	Chronic ulcers, debilitated patients, including alcoholics
Viral		Herpes simplex	Recurrent red eye, dendritic lesions
		Varicella, zoster	Involves ophthalmic branch of the Vth cranial nerve
		Epstein–Barr virus	
		Measles	
Fungal	Elevated ulcers, immune ring, Hypopyon	*Aspergillus,* other hyphae-forming fungi	Eye injury, organic matter, steroid eye drops
		Candida	More indolent
Protozoal		*Acanthamoeba* spp.	Contact lenses cleaned with tap water, painful, progresses slowly

gram stain, Giemsa stain, and methenamine silver stain should be performed. A surgical blade is gently scraped across the surface of the ulcer, and the resulting samples are inoculated onto solid media. Aerobic bacteria grow readily on standard media within 48 hours. Special processing may be required if *Acanthamoeba*, a fungus, *Mycobacteria*, or *Chlamydia* is the suspected pathogen. Viral keratitis can usually be diagnosed by appearance and generally does not require culturing.

Treatment must be instituted emergently. Because of the potential risk of perforation and visual loss, patients with bacterial keratitis and significant ulceration are often hospitalized for close observation.

Initially, therapy can be based on Gram stain in 75% of patients. In cases in which a cause is not clearly identified or the patient has already received antibiotic therapy, broader antibiotic coverage is warranted. Antibiotics are commonly given topically and, in some instances, also subconjunctivally. Systemic therapy in addition to topical therapy is recommended for patients with imminent perforation.

Topical regimens include bacitracin 5000 U/mL and gentamicin (13 mg/mL) for *Streptococcus pneumoniae*; cephalothin (50 mg/mL), plus bacitracin for other gram-positive cocci such as *S. aureus*; tobramycin (13.6 to 15 mg/mL) or gentamicin for *Pseudomonas* species; gentamicin for other gram-negative bacilli; amphotericin B (1.5 to 3 mg/mL), plus flucytosine (1%) for yeast-like fungi; natamycin (5%) for hyphal fungi; and neomycin (5 to 8 mg/mL), plus pentamidine isethionate (0.15%)

for *Acanthamoeba* species. Topical fluoroquinolones are also efficacious and have been recommended as empiric therapy for non-sight-threatening bacterial keratitis. Ofloxacin 0.3% is effective, and it is the least toxic regimen. This fluoroquinolone is often combined with topical cephalothin.

Eye drops need to be administered every half hour during the day and hourly during sleep for 7 to 10 days. Subconjunctival injections should repeated every 12 to 24 hours for a total of 3 to 6 doses. For herpes simplex keratitis, trifluridine ophthalmic solution or topical acyclovir are recommended for 7 to 10 days. Oral acyclovir 400 mg twice daily is often given for several months or, in some cases, for years to prevent recurrence.

ENDOPHTHALMITIS

Endophthalmitis is an inflammatory disease involving the ocular chamber and adjacent structures. When the inflammation involves all of the ocular tissue layers and chambers, the disease is called panophthalmitis.

Predisposing Conditions and Causes

Endophthalmitis has three major causes, each associated with distinctive pathogens. In order of frequency, they are

1. **Posttraumatic endophthalmitis.** Mixed infections are common. *Staphylococcus epidermidis* and *S. aureus*, *Streptococcus* species, and *Bacillus* species are the most frequently cultured. Although *Bacillus cereus* is usually a minimally invasive organism, this bacteria causes rapidly progressive endophthalmitis when it gains entry into the eye. Fungi are encountered in penetrating injuries caused by organic matter. The likelihood of infection is increased when a foreign body is retained in the eye.

2. **Hematogenous endophthalmitis.** Any source of bacteremia can seed the choroid, with subsequent spread to the retina and vitreous humor. Two thirds of blood-borne infections arise in the right eye, and one quarter involve both eyes. The most common blood-borne pathogens to cause endophthalmitis are fungi, in particular, *Candida albicans*. *B. cereus* is the most common cause of hematogenous endophthalmitis in intravenous drug abusers. Patients with bacterial meningitis caused by *S. pneumoniae*, *Neisseria meningitidis*, and *Haemophilus influenzae* may also develop endophthalmitis. In neonates, Group B streptococcus is most common, and in elderly patients, Group G streptococcus. In the immunocompromised host with pulmonary infiltrates, *Nocardia asteroides* can gain entry into both the eye and the cerebral cortex. If the primary source of bacteremia is not apparent, subacute bacterial endocarditis should be considered.

3. **Endophthalmitis resulting from the contiguous spread of uncontrolled bacterial or fungal keratitis.**

4. **Endophthalmitis associated with ocular surgical procedures.** Acute postoperative endophthalmitis generally originates from endogenous flora in the eye. The most common pathogens are gram-positive cocci (*S. epidermidis* being most common), followed by *S. aureus*, and *Streptococcus* species. Infection most frequently develops within 24 hours after surgery, but can develop up to 5 days postoperatively. Delayed postoperative endophthalmitis usually arise weeks to months after surgery and is caused by opportunistic pathogens. Endophthalmitis can also develop after creation of a filtering bleb. This surgical procedure allows bacteria to gain entry into the chamber of the eye; it is frequently preceded by conjunctivitis.

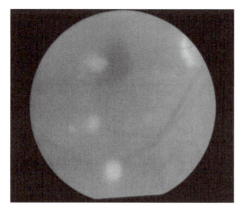

Figure 5–3. *Candida* retinitis. The typical rounded white exudates are caused by seeding from the bloodstream. Picture courtesy of Dr. William Driebe, University of Florida College of Medicine. *See color image on color plate 1*

Clinical Manifestations

Eye pain, photophobia, reduced vision, and redness are the primary symptoms of bacterial endophthalmitis. In cases of hematogenous spread, sudden onset of blurred vision without pain, photophobia, or redness is the most common complaint. On exam, eyelid edema, chemosis of conjunctiva, and moderate-to-severe anterior or chamber inflammation with a hypopyon are often seen. Retinal hemorrhages, venous sheathing, and loss of the red reflex are noted on retinal exam. In fungal endophthalmitis, the symptoms and signs tend to be less severe. The patient often complains only of blurry vision or spots in the visual field. In the comatose patient, *Candida* endophthalmitis is commonly missed unless frequent fundoscopic examinations are performed. Monitoring of the fundi is recommended in all patients who have developed candidemia. Findings of focal areas of inflammation, particularly gray-white fluffy exudates in the retina, chorioretina, or inferior vitreous strongly suggest *Candida* endophthalmitis (Figure 5.3).

Diagnosis and Treatment

Cultures and smears must be obtained promptly from the aqueous and vitreous, the vitreous giving the highest positive yield. Specimens of exudate from the conjunctiva are often misleading. Cultures of the site of foreign body penetration should be obtained in cases of traumatic endophthalmitis. In patients suspected of hematogenous endophthalmitis, cultures of blood, urine, and cerebrospinal fluid often reveal the causative agent. In patients with vision better than light perception, vitreous sampling should be followed by intravitreal antibiotic

---

injection. In patients with only light perception, vision is improved by immediate vitrectomy, followed by intravitreal antimicrobials.

Initially, broad-spectrum antibiotic intravitreal injection is recommended—for example, vancomycin 0.1 mL of a 10 mg/mL solution, plus gentamicin 0.1 mL of a 1 mg/mL solution. Systemic therapy must be instituted in cases of hematogenous endophthalmitis, but is not of benefit in other forms of the disease. For *Candida* endophthalmitis, intravenous amphotericin B is recommended, and in more severe cases, intravitreous amphotericin B (5 to 10 μg) is also administered. About half of all patients with endophthalmitis retain 20/400 visual acuity or better. One in 10 patients requires enucleation.

■ THROAT INFECTIONS

GUIDING QUESTIONS

1. *What is the most common cause of pharyngitis?*

2. *Which disease is suggested by the presence of a gray pseudomembrane?*

3. *What complication should be considered when unilateral tonsillar swelling develops?*

4. *Which infection should be considered in the patient with inspiratory stridor and sore throat?*

PHARYNGITIS

POTENTIAL SEVERITY

Usually a self-limiting disease. One exception is the rare, life-threatening complication of peritonsillar abscess.

Causes and Clinical Manifestations

Pharyngitis is one of the most common infectious diseases that presents to the primary physician, and it has many causes. Viruses are most common: rhinoviruses and coronaviruses (common cold viruses), adenoviruses, herpes simplex, parainfluenza viruses, influenza viruses, coxsackievirus A, Epstein–Barr virus, cytomegalovirus, and HIV. The most common bacterial cause is group A streptococci (GAS), also called *Streptococcus pyogenes*. GAS accounts for more than 50% of all cases of pharyngitis in children, but only about 10% of the cases in adults. Other forms of streptococci, groups B and G, have also been associated with pharyngitis in adults. Mixed anaerobic flora can cause a severe form of pharyngitis called Vincent's angina that extends under the tongue and into the neck.

In recent decades, *Corynebacterium diphtheriae* has become an occasional cause of pharyngitis in the United States. With the waning immunity of the elderly population, recrudescence of this dangerous infection is now an increasing risk. Classically, a grayish pseudomembrane that tightly adheres to the pharyngeal wall develops. This finding should alert the clinician to the possibility of diphtheria.

Neisseria gonorrhoeae and *Treponema pallidum* are two rarer causes of pharyngitis that need to be included as part of the differential diagnosis in sexually promiscuous patients. And when pharyngitis is accompanied by pneumonia, *Mycoplasma* and *Chlamydia* are the most likely causes.

Diagnosis and Treatment

Antibiotics are over-utilized in the management of pharyngitis and criteria for differentiating group A streptococcal pharyngitis from other forms have been established. The Centor clinical criteria are the most widely accepted:

1. Tonsillar exudates
2. Tender anterior cervical adenopathy
3. Fever by history
4. Absence of cough

If three to four of these criteria are met, the positive predictive value is only 40% to 60%, but the absence of three to four of the criteria has a negative predictive value of 80%. Patients with positive criteria should receive a rapid antigen test for GAS. The tonsillar area should be extensively swabbed to assure diagnostic accuracy, with the sample being acid- or enzyme-extracted for rapid antigen testing. Several different tests are available. All have a better than 90% specificity, but their sensitivity is variable (35% to 95% depending on the study). The recommended practice is therefore to perform a throat swab for culture in patients with positive Centor criteria and a negative rapid antigen test. Most clinicians use a dual-tip pharyngeal swab and send the second tip for culture if the antigen test is negative.

If medial displacement of one or both tonsils is observed, the possibility of a peritonsillar abscess must always be considered. In the antibiotic era, this complication is rare, and it can be readily diagnosed by computed tomography (CT) of the neck with contrast. This study clearly delineates the location and size of the abscess. Delay in appropriate surgical intervention can result in spread of the infection to the retropharyngeal

KEY POINTS

About Pharyngitis

1. Viruses are the most common cause. With severe prolonged pharyngitis, keep in mind primary HIV and Epstein–Barr virus.
2. *Streptococcus pyogenes* is also common (50% in children, 10% adults).
3. A grayish pseudomembrane should suggest *Corynebacterium diphtheriae*.
4. Keep *Neisseria gonorrhoeae* in mind in the sexually promiscuous patient.
5. If asymmetric tonsillar swelling is seen, consider a peritonsillar abscess
6. Centor criteria (tonsillar exudates, cervical adenopathy, fever, lack of cough) suggest, but do not prove a bacterial cause,
7. The rapid antigen test for *S. pyogenes* is specific, but varies in sensitivity. A negative rapid antigen test should be followed by a throat culture.
8. Avoid antibiotics in viral pharyngitis. Penicillin remains the drug of choice for *S. pyogenes*, and its use reduces the risk of post-streptococcal glomerulonephritis and rheumatic heart disease.

Table 5.3. Antibiotic Therapy for Ear, Nose, and Throat Infections

Infection	Drug	Dose	Relative Efficacy	Comments
Pharyngitis (viral most frequent)				
	Penicillin VK	500 mg PO q6h × 10 days	First line	Avoid antibiotics Administer only if *Streptococcus pyogenes* infection proven
	Benzathine penicillin	1.2 × 10⁶ U IM × 1		
	Erythromycin	500 mg q6h × 10 days	First line	For penicillin-allergic patients
Epiglottitis				
	Ceftriaxone, or	1 g IV or IM q24h	First line	Intubation recommended for children
	Cefotaxime	1 g IV q8h		
Malignant otitis externa				
	Ciprofloxacin	750 mg IV or PO q12h	First line	Prolonged therapy, × 6 weeks
	Ceftazidime	2 g IV q8h		
	Cefepime	2 g IV q12h		
Otitis media				
	Amoxicillin (or)	500 mg–1 g PO q8h	First line	Amoxicillin more cost effective; if no improvement, switch to amoxicillin–clavulanate
	Amoxicillin–clavulanate	875/125 mg PO q12h		
	2nd generation cephalosporin:		First line	If failure to improve on amoxicillin, can also use one of these regimens
	Cefuroxime	500 mg PO q12h		
	Cefpodoxime	400 mg PO q12h		
	Cefprozil	500 mg PO q12h		
Mastoiditis (acute)				
	Ceftriaxone, or	1 g IV or IM q24h	First line	Therapy × 4–6 wks
	Cefotaxime	1 g IV q8h		
Mastoiditis (chronic)				
	Piperacillin–tazobactam	3/0.375 g IV q6h		Polymicrobial, including anaerobes. Intraoperative cultures helpful
	Ticarcillin–clavulanate	3.1 g IV q4–6h		
	Imipenem	500 mg IV q6h		
Sinusitis (outpatient)				
	Amoxicillin–clavulanate	875/125 mg PO q12h	First line	
	Cefuroxime	400 mg PO q12h	First line	
	Gatifloxacin	400 mg PO q24h	Second line	Danger of selecting for resistant *Streptococcus pneumoniae*; use for penicillin-allergic patients
	Levofloxacin	500 mg PO q24h		
	Moxifloxacin	400 mg PO q24h		
Sinusitis (inpatient)				
	Ceftriaxone, or	1 g IV or IM q24h	First line	
	Cefotaxime +	1 g IV q8h		
	metronidazole +	500 mg IV q8h		
	nafcillin or oxacillin	2 g IV q4h		

and pretracheal spaces. Entry into the retropharyngeal area can result in spread to the danger space, which extends to the posterior mediastinum. The result can be the development of potentially fatal purulent pericarditis (see Chapter 7).

Treatment depends on the cause of the illness (Table 5.3). Too often, the primary care physician administers antibiotics for viral pharyngitis, a practice that is thought to have contributed to the increasing incidence of penicillin-resistant *S. pneumoniae* infections (see Chapters 4 and 6). Antibiotics should not be administered to patients who lack between three and four of the Centor criteria, nor to patients with three or four positive criteria who have a negative rapid antigen test and a negative throat culture. In patients with positive Centor criteria and a negative antigen test, 2 days of antibiotics may be prescribed while awaiting throat culture results. In cases of proven *S. pyogenes*, the treatment of choice continues to be penicillin: for adults, oral penicillin VK or a single injection of long-acting benzathine penicillin (1.2×10^6 U intramuscularly). For penicillin-allergic patients, a 10-day course of erythromycin is recommended. Although antibiotic treatment of *S. pyogenes* shortens the symptomatic period by only 24 to 48 hours, eradication of the organism from the pharynx markedly reduces the incidence of post-streptococcal glomerulonephritis and rheumatic heart disease.

EPIGLOTTITIS

POTENTIAL SEVERITY

An infectious disease emergency because of the risk of a fatal respiratory arrest.

In the past, epiglottitis occurred most commonly in children, but with the advent of the *H. influenzae* B vaccine (HIB), adults now constitute a higher proportion of the cases seen. Patients present with a sore throat that subsequently results in drooling and difficulty swallowing, followed by difficulty breathing. Patients often sit in an upright position leaning forward and may or may not have inspiratory stridor. Indirect laryngoscopy reveals a swollen, cherry-red epiglottis. Swelling at this site can be confirmed by lateral neck radiography. The risk of respiratory arrest secondary to airway obstruction is high, and in children, this event is associated with an 80% mortality. Therefore, in pediatric cases, a tentative

KEY POINTS

About Epiglottitis

1. Usually a disease of children, but increasingly common in adults.
2. Sore throat combined with drooling and inspiratory stridor suggest the diagnosis.
3. Indirect laryngoscopy demonstrates a cherry-red epiglottis.
4. Respiratory arrest is a danger, and pediatric patients should be electively intubated.
5. *Haemophilus influenzae* is the most common cause, but streptococcal and staphylococcal cases are increasing in frequency.
6. Ceftriaxone or cefotaxime are the treatments of choice.

diagnosis should made based on clinical presentation, and emergent laryngoscopy and nasotracheal intubation performed under anesthesia. Adult patients can be closely observed in an intensive care setting until respiratory distress resolves. An endotracheal tube should be placed at the bedside in those cases.

The primary cause of this infection is *H. Influenzae*. However streptococcal pneumonia, other *Streptococcus* species and *S. aureus* are increasing in frequency in children and adults alike. Treatment with intravenous cefotaxime or ceftriaxone for 7 to 10 days is recommended (see Table 5.3).

■ EAR INFECTIONS

GUIDING QUESTIONS

1. Which organism is responsible for malignant otitis externa?
2. Why do children develop otitis media more commonly than adults do?
3. What are the two most common pathogens that cause otitis media?
4. Untreated mastoiditis can result in which two complications?

OTITIS EXTERNA

POTENTIAL SEVERITY

In the normal host, usually an annoying, but not serious disease; however, in the diabetic or immuno-compromised host, can be life-threatening.

Otitis externa is also called "swimmer's ear," and it originates with water trapped in the external auditory canal, producing irritation, maceration, and infection. This infection can follow swimming, but it also follows irrigation of the ear to remove cerumen. Symptoms include local itching and pain. Physical findings may include redness and swelling of the external canal. Tenderness of the pinna is often noted.

Gram-negative bacilli are most commonly cultured, with *P. aeruginosa* being the major pathogen. Polymyxin drops combined with hydrocortisone (Corticosporin Otic) are used to treat localized disease. Oral fluoroquinolones should be avoided to prevent the selection of quinolone-resistant gram-negative pathogens.

A more invasive form of otitis externa called malignant otitis externa can develop in diabetics and immunocompromised patients. In this disease, pain tends to be more severe and can spread to the temporomandibular joint. Granulation tissue is often found in the external canal. This necrotizing infection can spread to the cartilage, blood vessels, and bone. Infection can involve the base of the skull, meninges, and brain, resulting in death. Multiple cranial nerves can be damaged, including cranial nerves VII, IX, X, and XII.

This infection is usually accompanied by an elevated erythrocyte sedimentation rate. Diagnosis is made by CT scan or magnetic resonance imaging and can be confirmed by gallium scan. *P. aeruginosa* is almost always the cause. Systemic therapy for *Pseudomonas* must be instituted for a minimum of 6 weeks, and necrotic tissue surgically debrided (see Table 5.3). As a consequence of the overuse of fluoroquinolones, infections with ciprofloxacin-resistant *Pseudomonas* are now being reported, necessitating prolonged treatment with intravenous ceftazidime or cefepime.

OTITIS MEDIA

POTENTIAL SEVERITY

Rapid treatment and close follow-up reduce the risk of serious complications. Delay in therapy can lead to potentially fatal complications.

Otitis media occurs most commonly in childhood, and by the age of 3 years, two thirds of children have had at least one attack. Otitis media with effusion is the consequence of obstruction of the eustachian tube. In younger children, the eustachian tube tends to be smaller and more susceptible to obstruction. Loss of drainage results in accumulation of serous fluid and resorption of air in the middle ear.

The initial precipitating event is usually a viral upper respiratory infection. Five to 10 days later, the sterile fluid collection becomes infected with mouth flora, resulting in ear pain, ear drainage, and occasionally, hearing loss. Fever, vertigo, nystagmus, and tinnitus are other associated symptoms. In infants, other accompanying symptoms include irritability and loose stools.

The finding of redness of the tympanic membrane is consistent with, but not proof of, otitis media. It can be the result of diffuse inflammation of the upper respiratory tract. Presence of fluid in the middle ear should be determined by pneumatic otoscopy. More recently, acoustic reflectometry has become available as a method for monitoring ear effusions.

The American Academy of Pediatrics recommends these criteria for a diagnosis of otitis media:

1. Recent, usually abrupt onset of signs and symptoms of middle-ear inflammation and effusion; AND
2. presence of middle-ear effusion that is indicated by any of
   a. bulging of the tympanic membrane,
   b. limited or absent mobility of the tympanic membrane,

KEY POINTS

About Otitis Media

- -

1. Results from obstruction of the eustachian tube in association with a viral upper respiratory tract infection. More common in children who have narrow eustachian tubes.

2. Infants may present with irritability and diarrhea.

3. Diagnosis is made by demonstrating the presence of fluid behind the tympanic membrane and inflammation of that membrane.

4. *Streptococcus pneumoniae, Haemophilus influenzae,* and *Moraxella catarrhalis* are the most common causes.

5. Amoxicillin to start; follow with amoxicillin–clavulanate or cefuroxime if no response within 72 hours.

c. air–fluid level behind the tympanic membrane, OR

d. otorrhea; AND

3. signs or symptoms of middle-ear inflammation as indicated by either

a. distinct erythema of the tympanic membrane OR

b. distinct otalgia (discomfort clearly referable to either or both ear) that interferes with or precludes normal activity or sleep.

Patients more than 2 years of age who do not meet the foregoing criteria should be observed for at least 24 hours before antibiotic therapy is considered. One exception is the patient with conjunctivitis and symptoms suggestive of otitis media. These patients have a high likelihood of infection with *H. influenzae* and should receive antibiotic therapy.

The cause of otitis media can be determined by needle aspiration of the tympanic membrane; however, this procedure is generally recommended only for immunocompromised patients. Culture of the nasopharynx is not helpful in predicting the bacterial flora in the middle ear. The pathogens that primarily cause otitis media are *S. pneumoniae*, *H. influenzae* (usually non-typable strains not covered by HIB vaccine), *Moraxella catarrhalis*, and less commonly, *S. pyogenes*, and *S. aureus*.

Amoxicillin is inexpensive and covers most cases of bacterial otitis media. Many experts recommend starting with amoxicillin, recognizing that patients with β-lactamase producing organisms (some strains of *H. influenzae* and

Moraxella catarrhalis) will not respond. If improvement is not seen within 72 hours, the patient should be switched amoxicillin–clavulanate and cefuroxime. Treatment for 10 days is recommended (see Table 5.3)

MASTOIDITIS

POTENTIAL SEVERITY

A rare consequence of otitis media that can lead to fatal complications.

CASE 5.2

Five months before presenting to the emergency room, a 44-year-old white man had noted purulent drainage from his right ear. The drainage was associated with fever and a shaking chill. He received no medical treatment at that time, and the symptoms spontaneously resolved. Three weeks before presentation, he again noted increased purulent drainage from the same ear, associated with earache and dizziness. One week before presentation, he developed a severe right-sided headache, and he experienced difficulty walking because of dizziness. Dizziness was accompanied by nausea and vomiting.

Past medical history revealed chronic right otitis media since the age of 13 years. Physical examination found a temperature of 38.9°C (102°F), foul-smelling purulent discharge from a perforated right tympanic membrane, and tenderness behind the right ear, with localized erythema and swelling. Laboratory workup showed a white blood cell (WBC) count of 8900, with 68% PMNs. Analysis of fluid from a lumbar puncture found a WBC count of 950 (with 92% mononuclear cells), protein 275 mg/dL, and glucose 45 mg/dL. The sample was culture-negative. Mastoid radiographs uncovered extensive destruction of the right mastoid air cells, the attic, and the aditus. Mastoidectomy was performed, and infection of the temporal bone, epidural space, and mastoid were noted. An intraoperative culture found Proteus mirabilis.

With the advent of antibiotics, mastoiditis is now a rare complication of otitis media. However, as described in case 5.2, infection can occasionally spread to the mastoid air cells. Swelling, redness, and tenderness can develop directly behind the ear in the area of the mastoid bone. Chronic mastoid disease can spread to the temporal bone and cause temporal lobe brain abscess. The infection can also spread by epiploic veins to the lateral and sigmoid venous sinuses, causing septic thrombosis. As seen in case 5.2, radiographs of the mastoid area may show increased density with loss of mastoid trabeculae, bony sclerosis, and lytic lesions of the temporal and parietal bones (Figure 5.4). Treatment is similar to that given for otitis media (see Table 5.3); however, therapy must be prolonged for 3 to 4 weeks. Chronic mastoid infections can be associated with gram-negative aerobic bacteria (as in case 5.2).

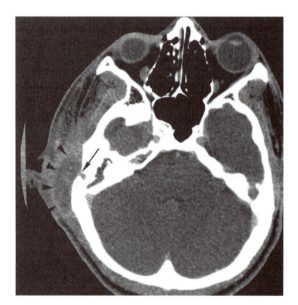

Figure 5–4. Computed tomography scan with contrast of mastoiditis. This axial view shows marked soft-tissue swelling in the area of the mastoid, surrounded by an enhancing ring (arrowheads). The arrow points to the otic canal. Picture courtesy of Dr. Ilona Schamalfus, University of Florida College of Medicine.

If an abscess has formed within the mastoid, or if temporal lobe abscess or septic lateral sinus thrombosis has developed, surgical drainage and mastoidectomy need to be performed. Case 5.2 had headache, and the severe destruction demonstrated by the mastoid radiographs warranted mastoidectomy and surgical exploration of the temporal region.

■ SINUS INFECTIONS

GUIDING QUESTIONS

1. *Infection of which air sinus is the most difficult to evaluate by physical exam?*

2. *Which physical findings are helpful in evaluating bacterial sinusitis?*

3. *What is the most common complication associated with ethmoid sinusitis?*

4. *What are the complications associated with frontal sinusitis?*

5. *What are the complications associated with sphenoid sinusitis?*

6. *How can orbital cellulitis be differentiated from septic cavernous sinus thrombosis?*

> ### POTENTIAL SEVERITY
>
> *Delays in therapy can result in spread of infection outside of the air sinus, with possibly fatal complications.*

SINUSITS
Predisposing Factors

Viral upper respiratory infections caused by rhinoviruses, influenza viruses, parainfluenza viruses, and adenoviruses cause inflammation of the sinuses and production of serous exudate. About 0.5% to 1% of viral upper respiratory infections progress to bacterial sinusitis.

Anatomic obstruction increases the likelihood of bacterial sinusitis. Causes of obstruction include septal deformities, nasal polyps, foreign bodies, chronic adenoiditis, intranasal neoplasms, and indwelling nasal tubes. Patients undergoing nasotracheal intubation or those who have a large-bore nasogastric tube are at increased risk for developing bacterial sinusitis. These tubes interfere with normal drainage of the sinus ostia. Nasal allergies are associated with edema, obstruction, and the accumulation of serous fluid; they are another predisposing factor for bacterial sinusitis. Dental abscesses of the upper teeth can spread to the maxillary sinuses and can result in recurrent bacterial sinusitis. Two genetic disorders, cystic fibrosis (associated with abnormally viscous mucous) and Kartagener's syndrome (which causes defective mucous cell ciliary function) are rarer predisposing factors for bacterial sinusitis.

Clinical Manifestations

CASE 5.3

A 15-year-old white female developed an upper respiratory infection 3 weeks before admission to hospital. Nasal discharge was clear, but after 10 days, she developed a severe left retro-orbital and left occipital headache, associated with left-eye tearing. She saw her physician 3 days later, complaining of persistent headache and nausea. Tenderness over the left maxillary sinus was noted. She was treated with Neo-Synephrine nose drops and Gantrisin (a sulfa antibiotic). She failed to improve, and 2 days later, she developed swelling of both eyes. Tetracycline was started, but she became confused and uncooperative.

Physical examination showed a temperature of 39.4°C, with a pulse of 140 per minute, and a respiratory rate of 40 per minute. The patient was toxic, disoriented, and lethargic.

An ear, nose, throat exam revealed dry, crusted purulent secretions in the left middle turbinate. Proptosis, chemosis, and complete ocular paralysis of the left eye was noted. Proptosis and chemosis of the right eye was less severe, with lateral gaze palsy (deficit of the VIth cranial nerve). Left disc blurred margin indicated papilledema. Tenderness was elicited over the left maxillary and frontal sinuses. Sensation on the left side of the face in the ophthalmic and maxillary branches of the Vth cranial nerve was decreased. The patient's neck was very stiff. The remainder of the exam unremarkable.

A laboratory workup showed a WBC count of 18,700/mm³, with 78% PMNs and 10% bands. An analysis of the cerebrospinal fluid showed a WBC count of 18,000/mm³, with 95% PMNs, protein 400 mg/dL, and glucose 25 mg/dL. Sinus radiographs revealed opacification of the left frontal, ethmoid, maxillary, and sphenoid sinuses. Six days after admis-

sion, the patient died. Autopsy revealed pansinusitis (including the left sphenoid sinus), bilateral cavernous sinus thrombosis, and bacterial meningitis. Culture of the meninges grew group H. streptococci.

Although case 5.3 is unusually severe, it does illustrate many of the potential clinical manifestations of sinusitis. The most common initial symptom is a pressure sensation over the involved sinus or sinuses. Pressure subsequently progresses to pain in the area of the infected sinus. Infection of the sphenoid sinus, which is located deep within the skull, does not cause an easily recognizable pain syndrome. As described in case 5.3, sphenoid sinusitis is associated with retro-orbital pain and/or severe pain extending to the frontal, temporal, and occipital regions. Pain is frequently unilateral and severe; it interferes with sleep and is not relieved by asparin. Sphenoid sinus pain is often misdiagnosed as a migraine headache, resulting in delayed treatment.

In addition to pain, patients usually experience nasal blockage, and they often note drainage of thick, discolored, purulent material. However, some deny nasal drainage, instead complaining of a foul taste or smell. As a consequence of chronic postnasal drainage, recurrent coughing is a frequent complaint, particularly in the

KEY POINTS

About the Clinical Manifestations of Sinusitis

1. Pressure sensation and headache are the primary symptoms.
2. Retro-orbital and hemicranial headache suggest sphenoid sinusitis.
3. Drainage from the infection is purulent, foul-smelling, and bad-tasting.
4. Fever is rare in adults.
5. Sinus tenderness can be elicited in maxillary and frontal, but not sphenoid, sinusitis.
6. Transillumination can be helpful in maxillary and frontal sinusitis; extensive experience required.
7. Look for purulent drainage from the ostia and posterior nasopharynx.
8. Hypo- or hyperesthesia of the ophthalmic amd maxillary branches of the Vth cranial nerve found in maxillary, ethmoid, and sphenoid disease.

nighttime, when the patient is lying in a recumbent position. Surprisingly, despite extensive inflammation in the sinuses, few adults experience fever. Fever develops more commonly in children with sinus infection.

As noted in case 5.3, physical examination can readily elicit localized sinus tenderness over the maxillary and frontal sinuses. In maxillary sinus infection, tooth tenderness may appear. Infection of the sphenoid sinus is not associated with tenderness. Transillumination can be performed in a darkened room using a flashlight tightly sealed to the skin. Marked reduction in light transmission correlates with active purulent infection in maxillary sinusitis. Light reduction may also be helpful for diagnosing frontal sinusitis; however, accurate performance of the exam requires experience. Examination of the nose reveals edema and erythema of the nasal mucosa, and if the ostia are not completely obstructed, a purulent discharge may be seen in the nasal passage and posterior pharynx. Inflammation of the Vth cranial nerve is often associated with sphenoid sinusitis, posterior ethmoid sinus infection, cavernous sinus thrombosis, and, less commonly, with maxillary sinusitis. Hypo- or hyperesthesia in the regions enervated by the ophthalmic and maxillary branches may be detected on sensory exam. That finding was noted in case 5.3, and in combination with oculomotor paralysis, proptosis, papilledema of the left eye, and meningitis, it indicated that the patient's bacterial sinusitis was complicated by cavernous sinus thrombosis (see "Complications," later in this section).

Diagnosis

Despite extensive inflammation of the sinuses, the peripheral WBC count is often within normal limits. Case 5.3 had meningitis, which explains her peripheral leukocytosis. Cultures of the nasopharynx correlate poorly with intra-sinus cultures and are not recommended. Direct sampling of the infected sinus is required for accurate microbiologic assessment. Fiberoptic cannu-

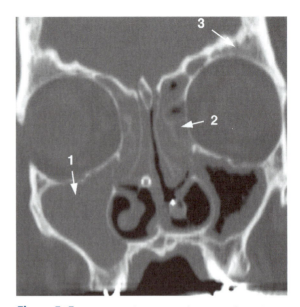

Figure 5–5. Computed tomography scan of pansinusitis, coronal view of the air sinuses. **1.** Maxillary sinus; **2.** Ethmoid sinus; **3.** Frontal sinus. Note the marked opacification of the right maxillary sinus and the marked mucosal thickening of the left maxillary sinus. Both ethmoid sinuses are opaque, as are the frontal sinuses. Picture courtesy of Dr. Ilona Schamalfus, University of Florida School of Medicine.

lation can be performed, but such cultures are often contaminated by normal mouth flora. In children, needle aspiration of the infected maxillary sinuses has produced accurate sampling, but this procedure is not recommended in routine cases.

Sinus radiographs are helpful for assessing maxillary sinusitis; they should include a Waters' view. If sphenoid sinusitis is being considered, an overpenetrated lateral sinus film should be ordered, or the diagnosis may be missed. Positive radiographic findings include one or more of sinus opacification, air fluid levels, and mucosal thickening (>8 mm). Computed tomography scan is the diagnostic study of choice for assessing sinus infections, and a limited CT scan of the sinuses is a cost-effective alternative to conventional sinus films (Figure 5.5). The integrity of the bony sinus walls can be assessed in more detail with a CT scan. Such a study can readily detect extension of the infection from the ethmoid sinuses to the orbit and development of an orbital abscess (Figure 5.6). Computed tomography scan is also useful for assessing extension of frontal sinus infection to the epidural or subdural space, and for diagnosing frontal brain abscess, a rare complication of frontal sinusitis. In

---

KEY POINTS

About the Diagnosis of Sinusitis

1. Nasopharyngeal cultures are not helpful.
2. A limited computed tomography scan of the sinuses is preferred over routine sinus radiographs in sphenoid, ethmoid, and frontal sinusitis.
3. A computed tomography scan allows for assessment of bony erosions and extension of infection beyond the sinuses.

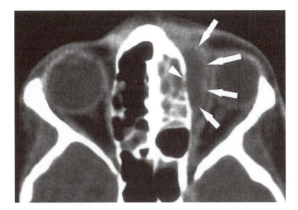

Figure 5–6. Computed tomography scan with contrast of orbital cellulitis with accompanying orbital abscess. This axial view shows the break in the ethmoid sinus wall (arrowhead) and the ring enhancing orbital abscess (arrows) that is pushing the eye laterally. Picture courtesy of Dr. Ilona Schamalfus, University of Florida College of Medicine.

KEY POINTS

About the Complications of Ethmoid Sinusitis

- -

1. Ethmoid sinusitis can easily spread medially through the lamina papyracea to cause periorbital cellulitis, orbital cellulitis, orbital abscess, or septic cavernous sinus thrombosis (rare).

2. Orbital cellulitis is usually unilateral; cavernous sinus thrombosis is bilateral. Papilledema, deficits of the Vth cranial nerve, and pleocytosis of the cerebrospinal fluid are also found with septic cavernous sinus thrombosis.

3. Orbital computed tomography scan with contrast delineates the extent of infection.

4. Surgical drainage of the sinus is recommended if loss of visual acuity, proptosis, or ophthalmoplegia develop.

---

sphenoid sinusitis, CT with contrast injection is the study of choice for detecting early extension to the cavernous sinuses. It can also readily detect development of sinus mucocele.

Complications

Distinct complications are associated with ethmoid, frontal, and sphenoid sinusitis. To be able to make the proper diagnostic evaluation and begin prompt therapy, the primary care physician and the infectious disease specialist must both be able to recognize the early clinical manifestations associated with spread of infection beyond the sinuses. Complicated air sinus infection can be life-threatening and frequently leads to permanent neurologic deficits.

The ethmoid sinus is separated from the orbit by the lamina papyracea. This thin layer can easily be breached by infection, particularly in children. Infection in the ethmoid sinus can also spread to the orbit via the ethmoid veins. The extent of orbital involvement varies and can cause four different syndromes:

1. **Periorbital cellulitis.** Infection of the skin in the periorbital area results in swollen eyelids, but eye movements are normal and no displacement of the eye is seen.

2. **Orbital cellulitis.** When infection spreads to the orbital tissue, not only are the eyelids swollen, but the eye becomes tender to palpation. Ophthalmoplegia with reduction of all eye movements occurs

as a consequence of inflammation of the extraocular muscles. Chemosis (marked swelling and erythema of the conjunctiva) develops—a reflection of the intense inflammation within the orbit. Finally, proptosis (outward displacement of the eye) is usually seen as a consequence of edematous tissue within the orbit pushing the eye out of its socket. This infection is usually unilateral.

3. **Orbital abscess.** A discrete abscess can develop in the periosteum or soft tissue of the orbit. This complication cannot be detected by exam, the diagnosis being made by CT scan of the orbit. Abscess formation usually warrants surgical drainage (Figure 5.6).

4. **Cavernous sinus thrombosis and meningitis.** Orbital infection can spread via the superior ophthalmic veins to the cavernous sinus. Because the cavernous sinuses are connected by the intercavernous sinuses, and because the superior ophthalmic veins have no valves, infection usually spreads quickly from one cavernous sinus to the other. As a consequence, bilateral eye involvement is the rule. The finding of bilateral eye involvement makes orbital cellulitis less likely. Other findings that favor a diagnosis of cavernous sinus thrombosis are abnormal sensation in the Vth cranial nerve, development of papilledema, and inflammatory cells in the cerebrospinal fluid. High-resolution CT scan with contrast is now the diagnostic study of choice.

Surgical intervention should be considered if progression on antibiotics, loss of visual acuity below 20/60,

<table>
<tr><td>

KEY POINTS

**About the Complications
of Frontal Sinusitis**

1. Infection can spread anteriorly, causing Pott's puffy tumor.
2. Infection can spread posteriorly and cause epidural, subdural, or brain abscess.
3. Posterior spread leads to severe headache, but frontal cerebral cortex lesions are usually neurologically silent.
4. Contrast enhanced computed tomography scan is recommended in cases of severe frontal sinusitis.

</td><td>

KEY POINTS

**About the Complications
of Sphenoid Sinusitis**

1. Sphenoid sinusitis is the most dangerous form of sinusitis.
2. Most patients require hospitalization and intravenous antibiotics.
3. The sphenoid is close to many vital neurologic structures.
4. The major complication is septic cavernous sinus thrombosis.
5. Computed tomography scan with contrast defines the sites of involvement, including cavernous sinus thrombosis.
6. Surgical drainage of the sinus is often required to prevent spread outside its walls.

</td></tr>
</table>

proptosis, or ophthalmoplegia occurs. The ethmoid sinuses should be drained, further debridement being guided by the findings of a CT scan.

Frontal sinusitis can also be life-threatening if not properly managed. Infection can spread anteriorly into the frontal bone, causing a subperiosteal abscess that can result in pitting edema of the forehead. This complication has been termed "Pott's puffy tumor."

Infection can also spread posteriorly. Particularly in teenage males, the posterior wall of the frontal sinus may be thin, allowing infection to spread to the epidural or subdural space. Infection can also reach the cerebral cortex, forming a brain abscess. These complications are usually associated with a severe frontal headache that interferes with sleep and that is not relieved by asparin. In some cases, seizures may develop, but in most instances, frontal brain abscess is neurologically silent. Abscess formation in the subdural or epidural space and brain abscess are readily diagnosed by contrast-enhanced CT scan.

Sphenoid sinusitis is the most dangerous sinus infection. If a patient with sphenoid sinusitis does not respond rapidly to oral antibiotics and decongestants, intravenous antibiotics should be initiated. Nafcillin and a third-generation cephalosporin are generally adequate coverage (see the "Treatment" subsection).

A low threshold should be set for surgical drainage. The sphenoid sinus lies deep in the skull. Its walls are adjacent to the pituitary gland, optic canals, dura mater, and cavernous sinuses. The thickness of the lateral walls of the sphenoid sinuses varies. If infection extends beyond these walls, patients can present with cavernous sinus infection which causes impairment of function in the IIIrd, IVth, and VIth cranial nerves, causing ophthalmoplegia, Vth nerve dysfunction [ophthalmic and maxillary branches (hypo or hyperesthesia)], proptosis, and chemosis. Case 5.3 had all of those characteristics and had sphenoid sinusitis and septic cavernous sinus thrombosis. The intercavernous sinuses allow infection to spread from one sinus to the other, usually within 24 hours. Diagnosis is most readily made by contrast-enhanced CT scan. The early venous phase following administration of contrast demonstrates regions of reduced or irregular enhancement, thickening of the lateral walls, and bulging of the sinus. Anticoagulation with heparin in the very early stages of infection may be helpful, although intravenous antibiotics (covering *S. aureus*, other gram-positive organisms, and gram-negative organisms as indicated) are the mainstay of treatment.

Microbiology

These major pathogens are associated with bacterial sinusitis:

1. *S. pneumoniae* and *H. influenzae* (50% to 70% in maxillary sinusitis)
2. Other gram-positive aerobic mouth flora (*S. pyogenes*, *S. viridans*)
3. Occasionally, other gram-negative aerobic mouth flora (*Moraxella catarrhalis*)
4. *S. aureus* more frequent in ethmoid and sphenoid disease
5. Anaerobic mouth flora (*Bacteroides melanogenicus* and anaerobic streptococci) more frequent in adults and in patients with chronic sinusitis

KEY POINTS

About the Microbiology and Treatment of Sinusitis

1. *Streptococcus pneumoniae* and *Haemophilus influenzae* are most common. Anaerobes are seen in adults and in chronic disease. *Staphylococcus aureus* is most frequent in sphenoid disease.
2. Gram-negative organismss (*Pseudomonas aeruginosa*) are seen in patients with AIDS.
3. Fungi (*Aspergillus*) often infects neutropenic patients.
4. The threshold for antibiotic treatment must be low. Use Amoxicillin–clavulanate; cefuroxime axetil; fluoroquinolones (concerns about resistance). Azithromycin is no better than amoxicillin, and amoxicillin is no longer recommended for initial therapy.
5. Patients with frontal, ethmoid, or sphenoid sinus infection often require hospitalization and intravenous antibiotics (oxacillin plus a third-generation cephalosporin plus metronidazole).

6. Gram-negative organisms rare in the normal host, most frequent in chronic sinusitis
7. *Pseudomonas aeruginosa* frequent in patients with AIDS
8. Fungal sinusitis, particularly *Aspergillus*, becoming an increasing problem in immunocompromised patients, being most frequently associated with neutropenia

Treatment

Nasal decongestants are helpful for preventing sinus obstruction during acute viral upper respiratory tract infections. Neo-Synephrine nose drops, 0.25% to 0.5%, every 4 hours are effective, but treatment that lasts longer than 3 to 4 days results in tachyphylaxis or rebound nasal congestion. Pseudoephedrine may also be used, but concern has been raised that the treatment may unduly dry out the nasal passages and increase the viscosity of the nasal discharge. Inhalation of steam theoretically should improve nasal drainage by clearing the ostia; however, no studies are available that support the treatment.

The efficacy of antibiotic treatment is poorly studied, but given the risk of complications, most experts maintain a low threshold for treatment with antibiotics. Patients with acute bacterial sinusitis may become asymptomatic despite the persistence of pus and active infec-

tion. Persistent infection may result in irreversible mucosal damage of the sinus wall and chronic sinusitis.

The timing of antibiotic therapy remains controversial. A reasonable guideline is to institute antibiotics if symptoms of sinusitis persists for 7 to 10 days after the initial onset of a viral upper respiratory infection. The presence of purulent, foul-smelling exudate or severe headache should also encourage the initiation of antibiotics. No single antibiotic will treat all possible pathogens. Treatment should be continued for a minimum of 10 days. Table 5.3 lists the recommended oral regimens.

1. Amoxicillin plus clavulanic acid (Augmentin) is probably the drug of choice. It covers *S. pneumoniae*, *H. Influenzae* (including ampicillin-resistant strains), *Moraxella catarrhalis*, and *S. aureus*.
2. The second-generation cephalosporin cefuroxime axetil has a spectrum of activity that is similar to that of Augmentin. Several third-generation oral cephalosporins have also been recommended.
3. The fluoroquinolones—levofloxacin, gatifloxacin, or moxifloxacin—cover all of the major pathogens that cause acute bacterial sinusitis. The development of fluoroquinolone-resistant *S. pneumoniae* is a major concern. These antibiotics should therefore be reserved for the penicillin-allergic patient.
4. Amoxicillin is a cheaper alternative, but it has a narrower spectrum. This antibiotic was previously considered the drug of choice for initial therapy, but more recent bacteriologic studies have revealed a high percentage of β-lactamase–producing organisms capable of degrading amoxicillin.
5. Azithromycin is no more efficacious then amoxicillin, but it is more costly.

Patients with frontal, ethmoid, and sphenoid sinusitis frequently require hospitalization and intravenous antibiotic therapy to prevent spread of the infection to vital organs beyond the sinus walls. High-dose intravenous antibiotics directed at the probable organisms (see the "Microbiology" subsection) should be instituted emergently. Empiric therapy should include a penicillinase-resistant penicillin (either nafcillin or oxacillin) at maximal doses, plus a third-generation cephalosporin (either ceftriaxone or cefotaxime). Anaerobic coverage should also be instituted with intravenous metronidazole (see Table 5.3).

FURTHER READING

Eye Infections

Benson WH, Lanier JD. Current diagnosis and treatment of corneal ulcers. *Curr Opin Ophthalmol.* 1998;9:45–49.

Callegan MC, Engelbert M, Parke DW, Jett BD, Gilmore MS. Bacterial endophthalmitis: epidemiology, therapeutics, and bacterium–host interactions. *Clin Microbiol Rev.* 2002;15:111–124.

Leibowitz HM. The red eye. *N Engl J Med.* 2000;343:345–351.

Shields SR. Managing eye disease in primary care. Part 2. How to recognize and treat common eye problems. *Postgrad Med.* 2000;108:83–6,91–6.

Sheikh A, Hurwitz B. Topical antibiotics for acute bacterial conjunctivitis: a systematic review. *Br J Gen Pract.* 2001;51:473–477.

Pharyngitis

Ebell MH, Smith MA, Barry HC, Ives K, Carey M. The rational clinical examination. Does this patient have strep throat? *JAMA.* 2000;284:2912–2918.

Hayes CS, Williamson H. Management of group A beta-hemolytic streptococcal pharyngitis. *Am Fam Physician.* 2001;63: 1557–1564.

Humair JP, Revaz SA, Bovier P, Stalder H. Management of acute pharyngitis in adults: reliability of rapid streptococcal tests and clinical findings. *Arch Intern Med.* 2006;166:640–644.

Epiglottitis

Berger G, Landau T, Berger S, Finkelstein Y, Bernheim J, Ophir D. The rising incidence of adult acute epiglottitis and epiglottic abscess. *Am J Otolaryngol.* 2003;24:374–383.

Faden H. The dramatic change in the epidemiology of pediatric epiglottitis. *Pediatr Emerg Care.* 2006;22:443–444.

Malignant Otitis Externa

Ismail H, Hellier WP, Batty V. Use of magnetic resonance imaging as the primary imaging modality in the diagnosis and follow-up of malignant external otitis. *J Laryngol Otol.* 2004;118:576–579.

Rubin Grandis J, Branstetter BF 4th, Yu VL. The changing face of malignant (necrotising) external otitis: clinical, radiological, and anatomic correlations. *Lancet Infect Dis.* 2004;4:3439.

Otitis Media

American Academy of Pediatrics Subcommittee on Management of Acute Otitis Media. Diagnosis and management of acute otitis media. *Pediatrics.* 2004;113:1451–1465.

Garbutt J, Jeffe DB, Shackelford P. Diagnosis and treatment of acute otitis media: an assessment. *Pediatrics.* 2003;112:143–149.

Rovers MM, Schilder AG, Zielhuis GA, Rosenfeld RM. Otitis media. *Lancet.* 2004;363:465–473.

Schwartz LE, Brown RB. Purulent otitis media in adults. *Arch Intern Med.* 1992;152:2301–2304.

Stool S, Carlson LH, Johnson CE. Otitis media: diagnosis, management, and judicious use of antibiotics. *Curr Allergy Asthma Rep.* 2002;2:297–303.

Sinusitis

Erkan M, Aslan T, Ozcan M, Koc N. Bacteriology of antrum in adults with chronic maxillary sinusitis. *Laryngoscope.* 1994;104:321–324.

Gwaltney JM, Wiesinger BA, Patrie JT. Acute community-acquired bacterial sinusitis: the value of antimicrobial treatment and the natural history. *Clin Infect Dis.* 2004;38:227–233.

Piccirillo JF. Clinical practice. Acute bacterial sinusitis. *N Engl J Med.* 2004;351:902–910.

Scheid DC, Hamm RM. Acute bacterial rhinosinusitis in adults: part I. Evaluation. *Am Fam Physician.* 2004;70:1685–1692.

Tami TA. The management of sinusitis in patients infected with the human immunodeficiency virus (HIV). *Ear Nose Throat J.* 1995;74:360–363.

Lew D, Southwick FS, Montgomery WW, Weber AL, Baker AS. Sphenoid sinusitis. A review of 30 cases. *N Engl J Med.* 1983;309:1149–1154.

Complications of Ear, Nose, and Throat Infections

Ramsey PG, Weymuller EA. Complications of bacterial infection of the ears, paranasal sinuses, and oropharynx in adults. *Emerg Med Clin North Am.* 1985;3:143–160.

Southwick FS. Septic thrombophlebitis of major dural venous sinuses. *Curr Clin Top Infect Dis.* 1995;15:179–203.

Central Nervous System Infections

Time Recommended to Complete: 2 days

Frederick Southwick, M.D.

GUIDING QUESTIONS

1. *What layers of the brain make up the meninges?*

2. *Where is the subdural space?*

3. *What is the blood-brain barrier and why is it important to consider when treating central nervous system infections?*

■ CENTRAL NERVOUS SYSTEM INFECTIONS

POTENTIAL SEVERITY

Often life-threatening, infections of the central nervous system are infectious disease emergencies. They require immediate treatment.

Central nervous system (CNS) infections are fortunately rare, but they are extremely serious. The cerebral cortex and spinal cord are confined within the restricted boundaries of the skull and bony spinal canal. Inflammation and edema therefore have devastating consequences, often leading to tissue infarction that in turn results in permanent neurologic sequelae or death.

To understand the pathogenesis and clinical consequences of CNS infections, a working knowledge of basic neuroanatomy and neurophysiology is important.

The cerebral cortex and spinal cord are suspended in and bathed by cerebrospinal fluid (CSF), which is produced by the choroid plexus lining the walls of the cerebral ventricles and resorbed by. The arachnoid villi drain into a large midline vein, the superior sagittal sinus. The cortex and spinal cord are surrounded by three tissue layers called the meninges. The two layers closest to the cortex are called the pia mater (directly overlying the cerebral cortex) and the arachnoid. These layers make up the leptomeninges. The third layer, the dura mater (pachymeninges), serves as the outer layer (Figure 6.1). The CSF flows between the pia mater and arachnoid in the subarachnoid space.

Central nervous system infections are classified by the site of the infection. Infection of the cerebral cortex is called encephalitis, and infection of the meninges is called meningitis. Abscesses usually form in three locations within the central nervous system: the cerebral cortex, where they are termed brain abscesses; between the dura and arachnoid, where they are called subdural abscesses; or immediately outside the dura, where they form epidural abscesses.

The capillaries of the brain and spinal cord differ from those in other regions of the body. The tight junctions linking the endothelial cells of the vessels in this region are less permeable than they are in vessels elsewhere. The limited permeability of the CNS vessels forms a physiologic barrier that is commonly called the blood–brain barrier. This barrier protects the CNS from invading pathogens and toxic substances. However, the impermeability of the CNS capillaries not only confers a protective effect, it also prevents the entry of immunoglobulins, complement, and antibiotics. Therefore, if a pathogen breaches the blood–brain barrier, the host's initial defense mechanisms are impaired, which partly explains the rapid progression and serious consequences of CNS infections. Antibiotics used to treat central nervous system infections must be capable of penetrating the blood–brain barrier,

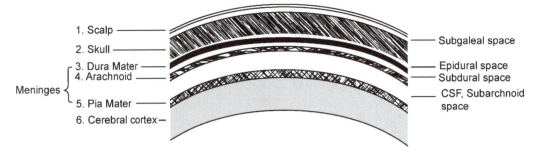

1. Scalp
2. Skull
3. Dura Mater
4. Arachnoid
Meninges
5. Pia Mater
6. Cerebral cortex

Subgaleal space
Epidural space
Subdural space
CSF, Subarchnoid space

Figure 6–1. Schematic depiction of the subgaleal, epidural, subdural, and subarachnoid spaces in the central nervous system.

and because penetration of all antibiotics is impeded, maximal doses (sometimes termed "meningeal doses") are required to cure CNS infections.

MENINGITIS

BACTERIAL MENINGITIS

Bacterial meningitis remains one of the most feared and dangerous infectious diseases that a physician can encounter. This form of meningitis constitutes a true

GUIDING QUESTIONS

1. *What are the primary infections that lead to bacterial meningitis?*

2. *What are the symptoms and signs that raise the possibility of meningitis?*

3. *If a diagnosis of meningitis is being considered, what key test must be performed?*

4. *Which characteristics of the cerebrospinal fluid are helpful in differentiating viral from bacterial meningitis?*

5. *What are the complications associated with bacterial meningitis?*

6. *In addition to rapid administration of antibiotics, what therapeutic modality may improve outcome in bacterial meningitis?*

infectious disease emergency. It is important that the physician quickly make the appropriate diagnosis and initiate antibiotic therapy. Minutes can make the difference

between life and death in bacterial meningitis. The rapid progression of disease leaves no time to look through textbooks to decide on appropriate management. To assure the best outcome, every clinician needs a basic understanding of bacterial meningitis and its management.

Epidemiology and Causes

With the advent of the *Haemophilus* influenza B (HiB) vaccine, the incidence of bacterial meningitis in children declined dramatically in the United States. Bacterial meningitis is now primarily an adult disease. The wider use of pneumococcal vaccine in patients older than 65 years of age and in patients with chronic underlying diseases also promises to reduce the incidence in adults.

Bacterial meningitis is not a reportable disease in the United States, and so an exact incidence is not available, but an estimate places the number at about 3 to 4 per 100,000 population. In underdeveloped countries, the incidence is at least 10 times higher, reflecting crowded conditions, and a lack of vaccination programs as well as other preventive public health measures.

Community-acquired bacterial meningitis in children and adults is caused mainly by four major pathogens (Table 6.1):

1. **Streptococcus pneumoniae.** *S, pneumoniae* is the most common cause of community-acquired meningitis in the United States. In other parts of the world, *Neisseria meningitidis* predominates. *S. pneumoniae* first causes infection of the ear, sinuses, or lungs, and then spreads to the bloodstream, where it seeds the meninges. *S. pneumoniae* is also the most common cause of recurrent meningitis in patients with a CSF leak following head trauma.

2. **Neisseria meningitidis.** *N. meningitidis* can cause isolated, sporadic infection or an epidemic. *N. meningitidis* first infects the nasopharynx, causing sore throat. In individuals lacking anti-meningococcal antibodies, nasopharyngeal carriage may be followed by bacteremia and seeding of the meninges. Crowded

Table 6.1. Causes of Bacterial Meningitis in Adults

	Community (%)	Nosocomial (%)
Streptococcus pneumoniae	38	8
Gram-negative bacilli	4	38
Neisseria meningitidis	14	1
Listeria spp.	11	3
Streptococci	7	12
Staphylococcus aureus	5	9
Haemophilus influenzae	4	4

KEY POINTS

About the Epidemiology and Causes of Bacterial Meningitis

1. Primarily a disease of adults.
2. Community-acquired disease is associated with four major pathogens:
   a) *Streptococcus pneumoniae* is the most common. Meningitis follows bacteremia from ear, sinus, or lung infection. Also associated with chronic leaks of cerebrospinal fluid.
   b) *Neisseria meningitidis* begins with colonization of the nasopharynx. Sporadic cases are often associated with terminal complement defects. Epidemics occur in crowded environments such as dormitories and military training camps.
   c) *Listeria monocytogenes* occurs in neonates, pregnant women, and immunocompromised patients. It is contracted by eating contaminated refrigerated foods.
   d) *Haemophilus influenzae* was the most common form of meningitis in children. Following widespread administration of the *H. influenzae* B vaccine, it is now rare.
3. Neonates develop gram-negative and group B streptococcus meningitis.
4. Nosocomial meningitis is usually associated with neurosurgery or placement of a ventriculostomy tube. It is caused by gram-negative rods, *Staphylococcus aureus*, enterococci, *S. epidermidis*, *Bacillus subtilis*, and corynebacteria.

environments, such as college dormitories or military training facilities, increase the risk of *N. meningitidis* spread. Epidemics usually occur in the winter months when person-to-person transmission by respiratory secretions is most frequent. Patients with defects in terminal complement components are also at increased risk of contracting sporadic meningococcal infection.

3. **Listeria monocytogenes.** *L. monocytogenes* infects primarily individuals with depressed cell-mediated immunity, including pregnant woman, neonates, patients on immunosuppressive drugs, or individuals infected with HIV. People over the age of 60 may also have an increased risk of developing *Listeria*. This form of meningitis is contracted by ingesting contaminated food. Heavy contamination with *Listeria* can occur when foods are stored for prolonged periods at 4°C, because the organism can grow in a cool environment. *Listeria* can contaminate unpasteurized soft cheeses and other improperly processed dairy products. High counts of this organism have also been found in defectively processed hot dogs and fish. When *Listeria* enters the gastrointestinal tract, it is able to silently invade the gastrointestinal lining, enter the bloodstream, and infect the meninges.

4. **Haemophilus influenzae.** Before administration of the HIB vaccine became common place, *H. influenzae* was the most common pathogen to cause meningitis in children; however, meningitis resulting from this organism is now rare.

The causes of bacterial meningitis in neonates reflect the organisms with which they come into contact during passage through the birth canal. *Escherichia coli* is the most common cause of neonatal meningitis. followed by group B streptococci.

Nosocomial bacterial meningitis has increased in frequency since the late 1980s. This increased incidence can be explained by the increased numbers of patients undergoing neurosurgical procedures and having hardware placed in the cerebral ventricles. The bacteriology of nosocomial meningitis is very different from that of the community-acquired disease. Gram-negative rods predominate, *E. coli* and *Klebsiella* being the most common. *Staphylococcus aureus* and streptococci are other frequent pathogens (see Table 6.1). Patients undergoing ventricular shunt placement can develop meningitis from contaminated plastic shunt tubing. *S. epidermidis*, *S. aureus*, enterococci, *Bacillus subtilis*, and corynebacteria (previously called diphtheroids) are most commonly encountered.

PATHOGENESIS OF BACTERIAL MENINGITIS

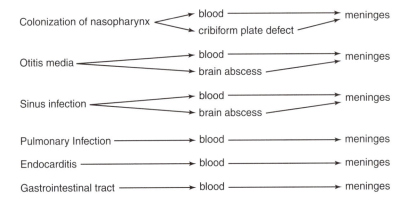

Figure 6–2. Routes for bacterial invasion of the meninges.

Pathogenesis

Bacterial meningitis is most commonly blood-borne. Primary infections of the ears, sinuses, throat, lungs, heart, and gastrointestinal tract can all lead to bacteremia and, on rare occasion, the blood-borne bacteria gain entry into the subarachnoid space (Figure 6.2). Blood-borne bacteria may gain entry through the large venous sinuses in the brain. Bacteria can settle along these slow-flowing venous channels, then escape and penetrate the dura and arachnoid, infecting the CSF. Less commonly, bacteria can enter the CSF through a break in the cribriform plate or a defect in the base of the skull following basilar skull fracture. Patients with head trauma can develop CSF leakage at these sites, and bacteria from the nasopharynx or middle ear, primary *S. pneumoniae*, can track up through the leak into the subarachnoid space. Patients who develop brain abscesses secondary to otitis media and mastoiditis or bacterial sinusitis on rare occasion can develop meningitis because of direct spread of bacteria from the abscess to the subarachnoid space.

Because the blood–brain barrier blocks entry of immunoglobulins and complement, bacteria are able to grow unimpeded by the host's immune system in the early phases of infection. As the number of organisms increases, polymorphonuclear leukocytes (PMNs) are attracted to the site. As they attempt to kill organisms, PMNs often lyse, releasing toxic oxygen products, proteolytic enzymes, and inflammatory cytokines. These products lead to necrosis and edema of the surrounding tissue.

The marked inflammatory response in the subarachnoid space damages the cerebral microvasculature, increasing the permeability of the blood–brain barrier. Leakage of serum from the damaged vessels increases the protein level in the CSF. Inflammation at the surface of the cerebral cortex can induce vasculitis and occlusion of small arteries and cortical veins alike, causing cerebral infarction. Inflammation of the arachnoid and pia matter alters glucose transport into this region, lowering glucose levels in the CSF. Inflammation of the subarachnoid space may impair CSF flow and cause hydrocephalus. Inflammation damages neural cells in the cerebral cortex and causes cerebral edema. The ultimate consequences of intense inflammation and bacterial invasion of the meninges are increased intracranial pressure, decreased cerebral blood flow, and cerebral cortex hypoxia, leading to irreversible ischemic damage.

KEY POINTS

About the Pathogenesis of Bacterial Meningitis

1. Infectious organisms gain entry to the subarachnoid space and cerebrospinal fluid (CSF)
   a) most commonly by bacteremia, gaining entry through the large venous channels;
   b) by nasopharyngeal spread through a CSF leak caused by a cribriform plate defect or basilar skull fracture; or
   c) direct spread from a brain abscess or air sinus infection.
2. Rapid growth occurs in the CSF because the blood–brain barrier blocks entry of immunoglobulins and complement.
3. Inflammation damages the blood–brain barrier, increasing permeability, allowing entry of serum protein, and impairing glucose transport.
4. Progressive cerebral edema, increased CSF pressure, and decreased cerebral blood flow lead to irreversible ischemic damage.

CASE 6.1

A 47-year-old sales manager and father of two arrived in the emergency room in deep coma. He had a history of recurrent ear infections since age 12. Three days before admission to the hospital, the patient had complained of a severe left earache. He took the ear drops prescribed by his local physician, and the pain disappeared during the night. The evening before he presented to the emergency room, the patient began complaining of headache and feeling "sort of disoriented." An hour after onset of the headache, he began vomiting, and he vomited five times during the night. The morning of admission, his wife reported that he appeared drowsy. He stayed home from work, sleeping most of the morning. About noon he awoke, but he did not recognize his wife. He began speaking incoherent sentences and became very restless. By 4 P.M., he was failing to respond when his wife called his name, and he was brought to the emergency room.

A physical examination recorded a temperature of 40°C, a blood pressure of 140/100 mm Hg, a pulse of 140 per minute, and a respiratory rate of 20 per minute. This was a very ill-appearing man who did not respond to his name, and who moved all limbs only in response to deep pain.

The patient's ears were bilaterally blocked with cerumen. The pupils of his eyes were dilated to 8 mm, but reacted to light. Optic disc margins were flat. The neck was very stiff, with both Kernig's and Brudzinski's signs present. Coarse diffuse rhonchi were evident throughout all lung fields. No skin lesions were seen. A neurologic exam showed no cranial nerve abnormalities. Reflexes were symmetrical, and the patient moved all limbs.

Laboratory workup found a peripheral WBC count of 19,500/mm³, with 39% polymorphonuclear leukocytes (PMNs), 50% band forms, 6% lymphocytes, and 5% monocytes. Hematocrit was 35.5%, and chest X-ray (CXR) showed no infiltrates.

A lumbar puncture was performed in the emergency room. Opening CSF pressure was found to be 560 mm H₂O (normal: 70 to 180 mm). A CSF analysis showed a WBC count of 9500/mm³ (95% PMNs), protein 970 mg/dL (normal: 14 to 45 mg/dL), and glucose 25 mg/dL, with a simultaneous serum glucose level of 210 mg/dL (normal: 50 to 75 mg/dL, generally two thirds of serum glucose). Gram-stain of the CSF revealed gram-positive lancet-shaped diplococci. Cultures of CSF and blood grew S. pneumoniae.

Clinical Manifestations of Bacterial Meningitis

Understanding that meningitis is usually the consequence of hematogenous spread from a primary infection, the clinician needs to inquire about antecedent symptoms of ear, nose, and throat infections, as well as about symptoms of pneumonia. The meningitis in case 6.1 was preceded by otitis media.

Case 6.1 had many of the typical symptoms of meningitis. Classically, patients with bacterial meningitis have symptoms of an upper respiratory tract or ear infection that is abruptly interrupted by worsening fever accompanied by one or more "meningeal" symptoms.

Headache is usually severe and unremitting, often being reported as the most severe headache ever experienced. Generalized pain is the rule, reflecting diffuse inflammation of the meninges. Pain may radiate down the neck. Asparin and other over-the-counter pain medications are usually ineffective.

Neck stiffness is frequently noted and is a consequence of meningeal inflammation precipitating muscle spasms in the back of the neck.

As experienced in case 6.1, vomiting is a frequent symptom. The cause of vomiting is unclear, but may be secondary to brain stem irritation and/or elevated intracerebral pressure.

Altered consciousness usually develops within hours of the onset of headache. As noted in case 6.1, the patient may become difficult to rouse and often becomes confused and disoriented. Family members often wait surprising long before becoming concerned enough to bring the patient to the hospital. Unfortunately, such delays dramatically worsen the prognosis of bacterial meningitis. In more severe cases, loss of consciousness may be accompanied by grand mal or focal seizures.

Physical examination usually demonstrates high fever or hypothermia. Two maneuvers in addition to a simple test of neck stiffness are commonly used to test for meningeal inflammation:

1. Brudzinski's nape-of-the-neck sign is elicited by flexing the neck forward. This movement stretches the meninges and is resisted by the patient with meningeal inflammation, because the maneuver causes severe pain.

2. Kernig's sign requires that the knee be bent at a 45-degree angle as the patient lies supine. As the leg is straightened, the patient with meningeal irritation will resist straightening, complaining of lower back and hamstring pain.

Although emphasized in most textbooks as key physical findings, neck stiffness and Kernig's and Brudzinski's signs have not proved to be sensitive indicators of meningitis. Exacerbation of headache by sudden head movement (head jolt) may be a more sensitive finding.

A careful ear, nose, and throat examination should be performed. Findings of otitis media (dull tympanic membrane, fluid behind the ear drum) may be discovered in cases of *S. pneumoniae* and *H. influenzae* or pharyngeal erythema may be noted in cases of *N. meningitidis*. The nose should be carefully examined looking for a clear nasal discharge suggestive of a CSF leak. Usually, however, meningeal inflammation temporarily closes the CSF leak at the time of presentation, such leakage becoming apparent only after the patient recovers. The nasal passage and posterior pharynx may also reveal a purulent discharge suggestive of sinusitis, an infection that less commonly leads to meningitis.

Auscultation of the heart may reveal a diastolic murmur suggesting aortic insufficiency, which would strongly suggest bacterial endocarditis as the primary infection leading to meningitis. Most cases of endocarditis complicated by meningitis are the result of infection with *S. aureus*.

Lung exam may reveal findings of pneumonia (asymmetrical lung expansion, bronchovesicular breath sounds, rales, egophony, and dullness to percussion), making *S. pneumoniae* the most likely cause. In all patients with meningitis, a CXR should also be performed to exclude pneumonia.

A thorough examination of the skin needs to be performed looking for purpuric lesions. Petechiae and purpura are most commonly encountered in patients with meningococcemia, but they may also may be found in *S. aureus* endocarditis and echovirus 9 and rickettsial infections (see Chapter 13). In patients who are asplenic, pneumococcal or *H. influenzae* sepsis is commonly associated with disseminated intravascular coagulation and petechial lesions. The finding of petechiae or purpura is usually a bad prognostic sign.

Finally, and most importantly, a neurologic exam must be performed.

First, mental status must be carefully described. The exact level of neurologic function should be documented by determining a Glasgow score (Table 6.2). The level of consciousness on admission is an important criterion for the use of corticosteroids and is also a useful prognostic indicator. The patient who is unresponsive to deep pain (Glasgow score 3) has a much higher mortality than the patient who responds to voice (Glasgow score 10 to 15).

Next, the cranial nerves should be assessed. Lateral-gaze palsy as a result of VIth nerve dysfunction can result from increased intracranial pressure. Focal findings such as hemiparesis, asymmetric pupillary response to light, or other unilateral cranial nerve deficits are uncommon in bacterial meningitis, and they raise the possibility of a space-occupying lesion such as a brain

Table 6.2. Glasgow Coma Score[a]

E: Eye opening	Spontaneous	4
	Responds to verbal command	3
	Response to pain	2
	No eye opening	1
V: Best verbal response	Oriented	5
	Confused	4
	Inappropriate words	3
	Incomprehensible sounds	2
	No verbal response	1
M: Best motor response	Obeys commands	6
	Localizing response to pain	5
	Withdrawal response to pain	4
	Flexion to pain	3
	Extension to pain	2
	No motor response	1

[a] Worst possible score is 3; best possible score is 15. Each category should be scored individually—for example, E4V5M6. Interpretation: ≥13 = mild brain injury; 9–12 = moderate brain injury; ≤8 = severe brain injury.

KEY POINTS

About Clinical Manifestations in Bacterial Meningitis

1. Upper respiratory or ear infection interrupted by the abrupt onset of meningeal symptoms:
   a) Generalized, severe headache
   b) Neck stiffness
   c) Vomiting
   d) Depression of mental status

2. Physical findings:
   a) Brudzinski's (neck flexion) and Kernig's (straight leg raise) signs are insensitive; "head jolt" maneuver may have higher sensitivity
   b) Abnormal ear exam (*Streptococcus pneumoniae* or *Haemophilus influenzae*), pharyngeal erythema (*Neisseria meningitidis*), or clear nasal discharge resulting from a cerebrospinal fluid leak (*S. pneumoniae*)
   c) Petechial or purpuric skin lesions most common with *N. meningitidis*, also seen with rickettsial infection, echovirus 9, *Staphylococcus aureus*, and asplenic sepsis.
   d) Neurologic exam should look for focal findings (suggests a space-occupying lesion) and assess mental status (Glasgow score is an important prognostic factor).

abscess or tumor. The finding of papilledema on fundoscopic exam is rare in meningitis and usually indicates the presence of a space-occupying lesion.

It is important to keep in mind that meningitis in very young and very old individuals does not present with these classic symptoms and signs. In elderly people, the onset of meningitis is often more insidious. The earliest symptoms are usually fever and alterations in mental status. Meningeal signs are less commonly reported, and many elderly patients have neck stiffness as a consequence of osteoarthritis, an old cerebrovascular accident, or Parkinson's disease. The physician must have a high index of suspicion and must aggressively exclude the possibility of bacterial meningitis in an elderly patient with fever and confusion. In very young patients, neonatal and infant meningitis presents simply as fever and irritability. No history is obtainable, and as a consequence, lumbar puncture should be included in the fever work-up of the very young patient.

Diagnosis

The critical test for making a diagnosis of meningitis is the lumbar puncture. If the clinician has included meningitis as part of the differential diagnosis, a lumbar puncture needs to be performed. Too often, clinicians order a computed tomography (CT) scan before performing a lumbar puncture, needlessly delaying the appropriate diagnostic study.

If no focal neurologic deficits are apparent, and if papilledema is not seen on fundoscopic examination, a lumbar puncture can be safely performed (Figure 6.3). The major exception is patients with AIDS or those receiving immunosuppressants. These patients have a higher frequency of cortical space-occupying lesions.

At the time of lumbar puncture, CSF pressure should be documented by manometry. In cases of bacterial meningitis, CSF pressure is almost always elevated, and high elevation suggests severe cerebral edema or defective CSF resorption, or both.

Cellular and biochemical analysis of the CSF is very helpful in deciding on the most likely cause of meningitis (Table 6.3).

Patients with bacterial meningitis who have not received prior antibiotics have increased numbers of WBCs with more than 90% PMNs in their CSF. Patients with *L. monocytogenes* can have a lower percentage of PMNs. *Listeria* grows and survives within the cytoplasm of host cells, a condition that can stimulate a monocytic CSF response in some patients. Patients who have received antibiotic therapy before their lumbar puncture may also have a reduced percentage of PMNs.

Because bacterial meningitis causes marked inflammation of the meninges, glucose transport is impaired, and CSF glucose is usually low ("hypoglycorrhachia"). Normally, the CSF glucose concentration is about two thirds that of serum glucose; a blood sample for serum glucose should therefore be drawn at the time of the

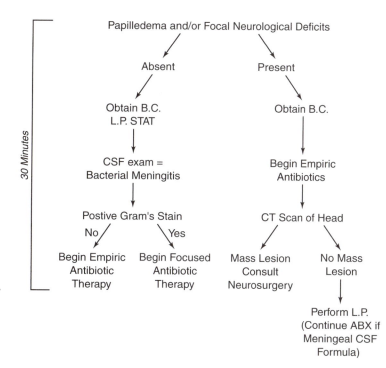

Figure 6–3. Initial management of suspected bacterial meningitis adapted from Mandell GL, Bennett JL, Dolin R. *Mandell, Douglas, and Bennett's Principles and Practice of Infectious Diseases.* Philadelphia, Pa: Churchill Livingstone; 2000.

Table 6.3. Profiles of Cerebrospinal Fluid in Central Nervous System Infections

Type of infection	WBC type	Glucose[a]	Protein
Untreated bacterial	Polymorphonuclear leukocytes	Low (often <25 mg/dL)	Elevated (150–1000 mg/dL)
Tuberculous, fungal, treated bacterial	Lymphocytes	Low	Moderately elevated (80–500 mg/dL)
Viral	Lymphocytes	Normal (low in early mumps)	Moderately elevated (usually <150 mg/dL)
Parameningeal (brain abscess)	Polymorphonuclear leukocytes or lymphocytes	Normal	Normal or slightly elevated

[a] Usually about two thirds of the level in the patient's serum.
WBC = white blood cell.

lumbar puncture to more accurately assess the CSF glucose level. In patients with pneumococcal meningitis, a CSF glucose level below 25 mg/dL is associated with worse clinical outcome.

As a consequence of inflammatory damage to blood vessels within the meninges, serum leaks into the cerebrospinal fluid, causing a rise in protein concentration.

Concentrations can reach 1000 mg/dL in some cases, and the CSF protein almost always exceeds the normal adult concentration of 50 mg/dL in cases of bacterial meningitis.

The combination of PMNs, low glucose, and high protein in the CSF is almost always caused by bacterial meningitis, and the finding of this CSF formula warrants treatment with antibiotics.

In addition to CSF cell, glucose, and protein levels, Gram stain and culture of the CSF are needed. In more than 75% of bacterial meningitis cases, the Gram stain is positive. The exception is cases involving *L. monocytogenes*. Because this organism usually remains intracellular, Gram stain is positive in only 25% of cases. Latex agglutination tests for *H. influenzae*, *S. pneumoniae*, and *N. meningitidis* are available, and may be ordered in patients with a negative Gram stain. However, it must be emphasized that the sensitivity of these tests is somewhat variable, and a negative latex agglutination test does not exclude the possibility of bacterial meningitis. The CSF culture should be planted immediately after lumbar puncture, and in the absence of prior antibiotics, it remains the most sensitive test for diagnosis. In addition, a positive culture allows for antibiotic sensitivity testing, which is particularly important for guiding treatment of *S. pneumoniae* and enteric pathogens.

KEY POINTS

About the Diagnosis of Bacterial Meningitis

1. If meningitis is a consideration, a lumbar puncture must be performed.
2. If focal neurologic deficits and papilledema are absebt, a lumbar puncture can be performed before computed tomography scan.
3. Opening pressure of the cerebrospinal fluid (CSF) should be measured; it is often elevated.
4. The CSF formula is very helpful in deciding whether a patient has bacterial meningitis. Bacterial meningitis is suggested in the presence of
   a) more than 90% polymorphonuclear leukocytes (except with *Listeria*),
   b) elevated CSF protein (usually 150 to 1000 mg/dL), and
   c) low CSF glucose [less than two thirds the serum value (less than 25 mg/dL is prognostic of poor outcome)].
5. Gram stain of CSF is positive in more than 75% of cases (except 25% with *Listeria*).
6. Blood and CSF cultures allow for antibiotic sensitivity testing.

Treatment

Evaluation and institution of antibiotic therapy should occur within 30 minutes if bacterial meningitis is being strongly considered. In cases in which a focal neurologic deficit is evident or papilledema is found, empiric antibiotic therapy should be instituted *before* sending the patient for CT scan (Figure 6.3). Blood samples for culture should be drawn before antibiotics are started; they often yield the cause of the illness. Empiric antibiotic treatment is also required if Gram stain of the CSF proves negative.

Empiric therapy depends on the age and immune status of the patient and on whether infection is nosocomial or community-acquired (Table 6.1). For community-acquired meningitis in patients aged 3 months to 60 years, maximal doses of a third-generation cephalosporin (ceftriaxone or cefotaxime) is recommended. (For doses, see Table 6.4.) If the patient is severely ill, vancomycin should be added to this regimen to cover for the possibility of penicillin-resistant *S. pneumoniae* (see Chapter 4, for a full discussion of penicillin-resistant *S. pneumoniae*). In the patient with an immediate hypersensitivity reaction to penicillin or a history of allergy to cephalosporins, vancomycin is recommended. In patients over the age of 60 years, maximal doses of ampicillin are added to the third-generation cephalosporin to cover for *L. monocytogenes*. This organism is not sensitive to cephalosporins, and penicillin or ampicillin are the treatment of choice. For the immunocompromised host, a third-generation cephalosporin, ampicillin, and vancomycin are recommended for empiric therapy. In patients post neurosurgery or in patients who have a cerebrospinal fluid shunt, vancomycin and ceftazidime or cefepime are recommended.

Once a specific bacterium is identified, the antibiotic regimen can be focused. Table 6.4 outlines the recommended regimens for each major pathogen.

Penicillin-resistant *S. pneumoniae* is a particular concern, given the high prevalence of these strains and the poor penetration of antibiotics across the blood–brain barrier. Intermediately resistant stains (penicillin MIC = 0.1 to 1 µg/mL) may initially improve on penicillin therapy; however, as the integrity of the blood–brain barrier improves, the patient may relapse as a consequence

Tabel 6.4. Antibiotic Treatment for Bacterial Meningitis

Organism	Antibiotic	Dose	Alternative
Streptococcus pneumoniae (penicillin MIC < 0.1 µg/mL)	Penicillin Ceftriaxone Cefotaxime	20–24 × 10⁶ U daily, divided q4h 2–4 g daily, divided q12h 12 g daily, divided q6h	Chloramphenicol: 4–6 g daily, divided q6h
Streptococcus pneumoniae (MIC > 0.1 µg/mL)	Vancomycin, plus rifampin 300 mg q12h	2 g daily, divided q12h	Chloramphenicol
Neisseria meningitidis	Penicillin	20–24 × 10⁶ U daily, divided q4h	Ceftriaxone Cefotaxime
Listeria monocytogenes	Ampicillin, with or without gentamicin	12 g daily, divided q4H 4–8 mg intrathecal 5 mg/kg daily systemic	Trimethoprim–sulfamethoxazole 15–20 mg/kg daily (trimethoprim, divided q6h)
Haemophilus influenzae	Ceftriaxone Cefotaxime	2–4 g daily, divided q12h 12 g daily, divided q6h	Chloramphenicol
Enterobacteriaceae	Ceftriaxone, with or without gentamicin	2–4 g daily, divided q12h 4–8 mg intrathecal	Aztreonam 6–8 g daily, divided q6h
	Cefotaxime, with or without gentamicin	5 mg/kg daily, systemic 12 g daily, divided q6h	Trimethoprim–sulfamethoxazole
Pseudomonas aeruginosa	Ceftazidime, plus gentamicin	6–12 g daily, divided q8h 4–8 mg intrathecal 5 mg/kg daily systemic	Antipseudomonal penicillin: 18–24 g daily, divided q4h, plus gentamicin
Staphylococcus aureus (methicillin-sensitive)	Nafcillin, or Oxacillin, with or without rifampin	9–12 g daily, divided q4h 9–12 g daily, divided q4h 600 mg daily, divided q12h	Vancomycin, plus rifampin Trimethoprim–sulfamethoxazole, plus rifampin
S. aureus (methicillin-resistant)	Vancomycin, plus rifampin	2 g daily, divided q12h 600 mg daily, divided q12h	
S. epidermidis	Vancomycin, plus rifampin	2 g daily, divided q12h 600 mg daily, divided q12h	

$20\text{--}24 \times 10^6$

of reduced levels of penicillin in the CSF. For this reason, high-dose ceftriaxone or cefotaxime is recommended for intermediately penicillin-resistant *S. pneumoniae* meningitis, because these cephalosporins achieve higher levels in CSF.

For infections with highly penicillin-resistant *S. pneumoniae* (penicillin MIC >2 μg/mL), vancomycin needs to be added to the third-generation cephalosporin to assure adequate inhibitory concentrations in the CSF. Vancomycin penetrates the intact blood–brain barrier poorly, and in some patients, therapeutic levels may not be achieved in the CSF without intrathecal administration. Rifampin combined with vancomycin may also be effective for the treatment of highly resistant *S. pneumoniae*. This regimen has been recommended for patients receiving high-dose dexamethasone (see discussion of treatment for inflammation that follows), because corticosteroid therapy reduces meningeal inflammation and improves the integrity of the blood–brain barrier, decreasing vancomycin levels in the CSF. The antibiotic response should be monitored in patients infected with highly penicillin-resistant pneumococci. In these patients, the lumbar puncture should be repeated 24 to 36 hours after the initiation of therapy.

Aminoglycosides, erythromycin, clindamycin, tetracyclines, and first-generation cephalosporins should not be used to treat meningitis, because these drugs do not cross the blood–brain barrier.

Neurologic damage is primarily a consequence of an excessive inflammatory response. Corticosteroids reduce inflammation, and in children with *H. influenzae* bacterial meningitis, dexamethasone (0.15 mg/kg q6h × 4 days) has been shown to reduce CSF pressure, CSF PMNs, and protein, to increase CSF glucose, and to improve cerebral blood perfusion. Dexamethasone also significantly reduces the incidence of deafness. In adults with pneumococcal meningitis and Glasgow coma scores of 8 to 11, dexamethasone administration (10 mg q6h × 4 days) was also found to reduce morbidity and mortality. Dexamethasone should be given just before or simultaneously with antibiotics, because inflammatory mediators are released in response to the lysis of bacteria induced by antibiotic treatment. Other inhibitors of inflammation, such as monoclonal antibodies directed against the adherence receptors of leukocytes, are potentially promising, but remain experimental.

Additional therapeutic measures are primarily directed at reducing cerebral edema and controlling seizures. Administration of hypotonic solutions should be avoided. The airway must be protected, and hypoventilation with associated hypercarbia should be avoided, because elevated $PaCO_2$ levels cause cerebral vessel dilation and may increase intracranial pressure. Hyperventilation can also be harmful for the opposite reason: reductions in $PaCO_2$ may reduce cerebral perfusion and increase the risk of infarction. When intracranial pressure is documented by lumbar puncture to be markedly elevated, intravenous 20% mannitol can be administered to remove free water from the cerebral cortex and to quickly reduce cerebral edema. Oral glycerol may also reduce cerebral edema, and its efficacy is presently being investigated. Seizures develop in 20% to 30% of patients with meningitis, but anti-seizure medications (Dilantin and diazepam are most commonly used) are not recommended for prophylaxis. These agents are administered only after the first seizure.

Complications

Mortality remains high in patients with bacterial meningitis. *L. monocytogenes* is associated with the highest mortality, 26%; followed by *S. pneumoniae*, 19%; and

---

KEY POINTS

**About the Treatment
of Bacterial Meningitis**

1. Antibiotics should be given within 30 minutes if bacterial meningitis is suspected.

2. Blood samples for culture should be drawn and antibiotics given before a computed tomography scan is done.

3. Maximal doses of antibiotics must given because of limited passage through the blood–brain barrier.

4. Empiric therapy for
   a) community-acquired disease, patient 3 months to 60 years is ceftriaxone or cefotaxime. If severely ill, add vancomycin. If more than 60 years or immunocompromised, use ceftriaxone or cefotaxime, plus ampicillin and vancomycin.
   b) nosocomial disease, is vancomycin and ceftazidime or cefepime.

5. Give dexamethasone 30 minutes before antibiotics in
   a) children (shown to be efficacious in *Haemophilus influenzae*).
   b) adults (efficacious in *Streptococcus pneumoniae* with Glasgow coma score of 8 to 11).

6. Maintain ventilation, prevent increase in $PaCO_2$ or decrease in PaO_2.

7. Avoid hypotonic solutions, consider mannitol or glycerol for increased cerebrospinal fluid pressure.

8. Anti-seizure medications after first seizure.

N. meningitidis, 13% mortality. *H. influenzae* meningitis tends to be less severe, being now associated with an average mortality of 3%. Mortality is higher in very young and elderly individuals. Neurologic sequelae in surviving patients are common. The young patient whose brain is developing often suffers mental retardation, hearing loss, seizure disorders, or cerebral palsy. Older patients may develop hydrocephalus, cerebellar dysfunction, paresis, a seizure disorder, and hearing loss.

Prevention

Given the high mortality and high incidence of permanent neurologic sequelae associated with bacterial meningitis, the medical community must strive to reduce the incidence of these devastating infections.

VACCINES

Three of the primary pathogens that cause community-acquired bacterial meningitis are encapsulated organisms, and therefore opsonins [immunoglobulin G (IgG) and complement] play a critical role in allowing host macrophages and PMNs to ingest these pathogens and clear them from the bloodstream. Reduced time in the bloodstream reduces the likelihood of seeding the meninges. The remarkable reduction in invasive *H. influenzae* type B following the widespread administration of the HIB vaccine illustrates the power of this preventive measure. Protective levels of immunoglobulin are achieved when the PedvaxHIB vaccine is administered at 2 and 4 months of age. Two other HIB vaccines are also available that should be administered at 2, 4, and 6 months of age.

A quadrivalent meningococcal vaccine directed against serogroups A, C, Y, and W135 is now available and is recommended for high-risk groups, including military recruits, college students, asplenic patients, and patients with terminal complement deficiencies. This vaccine is also useful for controlling epidemics and should be administered to travelers going to areas where the prevalence of meningococcal disease is high, (Visit www.CDC.gov for current recommendations for travelers.)

A major problem with the current vaccine is the lack of a suitable immunogen against serogroup B. Serogroups B and C are primarily responsible for meningococcal meningitis in the United States. A second problem with the vaccine is the fact that immunity tends to be short-lived, with antibody titers decreasing after 3 years following a single dose of the vaccine. The incidence of meningococcal disease remains low in the United States (approximately 1 in 100,000 population), and therefore this vaccine is not recommended for routine immunization.

A safe, inexpensive, and efficacious 23-valent pneumococcal vaccine is available and has been underutilized. The mortality attributable to pneumococcal infection is higher than that attributable to any other vaccine-preventable disease (approximately 40,000 annually in the United States), and about half of these deaths could be prevented by vaccination. Individuals more than 65 years of age are at higher risk for developing invasive pneumococcal infection including meningitis and should be vaccinated. Other groups that warrant vaccination include patients with chronic cardiovascular, pulmonary, or liver disease, diabetes mellitus, and sickle cell disease, and patients with functional asplenia or those who have had a splenectomy. A single intramuscular or subcutaneous injection is protective for 5 to 10 years. For most patients, revaccination

---

KEY POINTS

About the Outcome and Prevention of Bacterial Meningitis

1. Mortality is high: 26% for Listeria, 19% for Streptococcus pneumoniae, 13% for Neisseria meningitidis, and 3% for Haemophilus influenzae.

2. Permanent sequelae are common:
   a) In children: mental retardation, hearing loss, seizure disorders, cerebral palsy
   b) In adults: hydrocephalus, cerebellar dysfunction, paresis, seizure disorder, hearing loss

3. Efficacious vaccines are available:
   a) *S. pneumoniae*: 23-valent vaccine; safe, inexpensive. Recommended in individuals more than 65 years of age; those with chronic cardiovascular, pulmonary, or liver disease, diabetes mellitus, sickle cell disease, and asplenia; heptavalent conjugated vaccine for all children under 2 years of age.
   b) *H. influenzae*: PedvaxHIB vaccine at age 2 and 4 months; safe, inexpensive.
   c) *N. meningitidis*: quadrivalent meningococcal vaccine for serogroups A, C, Y, and W135; misses group B. Recommended in military recruits, college students, and individuals with asplenia and terminal complement defects.

4. Chemoprophylaxis use:
   a) *H. influenzae*: Rifampin within 6 days for household contacts with unvaccinated child under 2 years of age, and for children under 2 years of age exposed in a daycare center.
   b) *N. meningitidis*: Single-dose ciprofloxacin within 5 days for household and daycare contacts, and for those exposed to oral secretions from the index case.

is not recommended. Exceptions are the immunocompromised host and patients over 65 years of age who often develop a more rapid decline in protective antibody levels. Revaccination may considered after at least 5 years have passed since initial vaccination. A heptavalent conjugated vaccine that is immunogenic in children under the age of 2 years is recommended for routine pediatric immunization. This vaccine has significantly reduced invasive pneumococcal disease in children. It is given in four doses at 12 to 15 months, and ages 2, 4, and 6.

CHEMOPROPHYLAXIS

Brief antibiotic treatment has been used to prevent secondary cases of *H. influenzae* and *N. meningitidis*. Secondary cases generally occur within 6 days of an index case of *H. influenzae* and within 5 days of an index case of *N. meningitidis* meningitis. Both organisms are carried in the nasopharynx and, in a person lacking specific humoral immunity, these organisms can become invasive. Choice of the individuals to target for prophylaxis has been carefully delineated by epidemiologic data, but fear plays a major role in determining who eventually receives prophylaxis. For *H. influenzae*, household contacts with at least one unvaccinated child under the age of 2 years require prophylaxis. Data on daycare exposure remains controversial; however, most experts agree that children under the age of 2 who may have been exposed in a daycare should receive chemoprophylaxis.

The recommended agent for *H. influenzae* prophylaxis is rifampin 20 mg/kg daily (maximum dose in adults: 600 mg q24h) for 4 days is recommended. Rifampin prophylaxis is not recommended for pregnant woman because of the potential risk of rifampin to the fetus. For *N. meningitidis*, a single dose of ciprofloxacin 500 mg is the preferred prophylactic regimen, and this regimen is recommended for close contacts including household members, daycare contacts, and people who may have been directly exposed to the index patient's oral secretions (kissing, mouth-to-mouth resuscitation, endotracheal tube intubation). Given the potential severity of this disease and the minimal harm of a single dose of antibiotic, physicians should probably maintain a low threshold for using prophylaxis. This brief treatment may help to alleviate the extreme anxiety associated with meningococcal disease.

VIRAL MENINGITIS

CASE 6.2

A 45-year-old woman was admitted to the hospital with a chief complaints of severe headache and neck stiffness over 8 days. Ten days prior to admission, she had noted some mild stiffness of the back of her neck,

associated with fever and mild shivering. Two days later, she developed a sharp, throbbing bi-temporal headache that radiated to the vertex. Her headache was made worse by sitting up or moving. Bright light bothered her eyes. She also noted some muscle stiffness in other areas in particular her lower back. She felt very tired and lost her appetite. Although she felt lethargic at times, she never lost touch with reality.

An epidemiologic history revealed that during the fall (several weeks before admission), she had administered psychometric tests to a large number of students (ages 10 to 20 years).

Physical examination found a temperature of 38°C. This mildly ill-appearing middle-aged woman was alert but sitting in a dark room complaining of severe headache. Eyes showed mild conjunctival erythema with normal discs. Neck was mildly stiff and negative for Kernig's and Brudzinski's signs. The remainder of the exam, including ear, nose, and throat and neurologic exams, was within normal limits.

Laboratory workup showed a hematocrit of 40%; a WBC count of 6000/mm³, with 45% PMNs, 50% lymphocytes, and 5% monocytes. Lumbar puncture showed an opening pressure (OP) of 100 mm H_2O, and CSF analysis found a WBC count of 180/mm³ (50% PMNs, 48% lymphocytes, 2% monocytes), protein 59 mg/dL, and glucose 61 mg/dL, with simultaneous serum glucose 84 mg/dL. A Gram stain of the CSF was negative for organisms. A repeat lumbar puncture 8 hours later revealed an OP of 100 mm H_2O, and a WBC count of 170/mm³ (2% PMNs, 95% lymphocytes, 3% monocytes), protein 58 mg/dL, and glucose 61 mg/dL. (No blood for serum glucose was drawn at this time.) Gram stain of the CSF remained negative.

During this patient's hospital course, her headache persisted, as did her low-grade fever. She remained alert and continued to have photophobia and a mildly stiff neck. She was discharged on the third hospital day, and her symptoms resolved over the next week.

Viral meningitis is the most common form of meningitis. It is caused primarily by the non-polio enteroviruses, echoviruses, and coxsackieviruses. In temperate climates, infections occur mainly in the warmer months of the year, usually during the summer and early fall. In tropical climates, the infection occurs year round.

Enteroviruses are spread by the fecal–oral route, and small epidemics are frequently reported. Herpes simplex virus type 2 (HSV-2) is the second most common cause, and this form of viral meningitis is often accompanied by vesicular skin lesions in the genital area. This virus is also the most common cause of recurrent Mollaret's aseptic meningitis. Varicella virus is the third most common cause, and aseptic meningitis usually is not accompanied by skin lesions.

In the nonimmune patient, mumps virus is often associated with aseptic meningitis that may occur in the absence of salivary gland swelling. The peak incidence of this virus is seen in children 5 to 9 years of age. Less commonly, herpes simplex virus type 1 (HSV-1) causes meningitis. And the mononucleosis syndromes caused by Epstein–Barr virus and cytomegalovirus can be accompanied by meningitis.

Lymphocytic choriomeningitis virus was previously thought to be a common cause of aseptic meningitis, but recent studies have found this virus to be rare. It is transmitted in the urine of rodents, and a diagnosis of lymphocytic choriomeningitis should be considered in individuals who potentially have had contact with rodents or rodent excreta. This infection occurs most commonly in the winter, when rodents are more likely to take up residence in human dwellings.

Finally, at the time of initial HIV infection, 5% to 10% of patients may experience symptoms of aseptic meningitis. In some of these cases, HIV has been isolated from the CSF (see Chapter 17).

As illustrated in case 6.2, severe headache is the most common complaint. Headache is usually generalized, but may localize bilaterally to the frontal, temporal, or occipital regions. Photophobia is another very common complaint, and patients usually request that their room remain darkened. Neck stiffness and diffuse myalgias are also common. On physical examination, the skin should be carefully viewed for maculopapular rashes (found in some strains of echovirus). Eye exam may reveal conjunctivitis, frequently associated with enteroviral infections. Significant nuchal rigidity is found in more than half of all cases of aseptic meningitis. Patients may be slightly lethargic; however. unlike patients with bacterial and fungal meningitis, patients with viral meningitis rarely exhibit significant depression in mental status. Focal neurologic findings should not be observed in this disease.

Lumbar puncture usually reveals a predominance of lymphocytes, a normal glucose level, and mildly elevated CSF protein (Table 6.2). The CSF leukocyte count usually ranges between 100 and 1000 /mm^3. In some forms of viral meningitis (mumps and lymphocytic choriomeningitis), CSF glucose may be lowered early in the disease. Also early in the disease, PMNs may predominate in the CSF, making it impossible to safely exclude bacterial meningitis. These patients should therefore not be sent home, but covered with empiric antibiotics pending CSF and blood cultures and follow-up lumbar puncture. In most cases, a repeat lumbar puncture 12 to 24 hours later reveals a predominance of lymphocytes, and the patient can be dis-

charged. However, in some patients, PMNs may persist for up to 48 hours, necessitating continued observation in the hospital and antibiotic administration. A negative CSF culture after 48 hours greatly reduces the probability of bacterial meningitis, but the threshold for antibiotic coverage must be low to prevent inadvertent delays in the treatment of a bacterial meningitis.

Polymerase chain reaction (PCR) for HSV-1 and HSV-2 in CSF is sensitive and specific, and available in most hospital laboratories. Enterovirus PCR has also been shown to be sensitive and specific, but the test is not usually available in hospitals. Proof of enterovirus CSF infection would allow the patient to discharged home, because, with the exception of patients with severe immunoglobulin deficiency, viral meningitis is a self-limiting disease that usually resolves spontaneously within 7 to 10 days. In

---

KEY POINTS

About Viral Meningitis

1. Viral meningitis is most commonly caused by
   a) enteroviruses, echovirus, and coxsackievirus (most frequent, seen in summer and early fall).
   b) mumps in the nonimmune (may be no parotid gland swelling, ages 5 to 9 years).
   c) herpes simplex type 2 (primary disease, also Mollaret's recurrent meningitis).
   d) Epstein–Barr virus and cytomegalovirus (rare).
   e) lymphocytic choriomeningitis virus (excreted in rodent urine, rare).
   f) HIV (can be the initial presentation of infection).

2. Primary clinical manifestations include
   a) headache and photophobia, stiff neck;
   b) no loss of consciousness; and
   c) conjunctivitis, maculopapular rash, and occasionally with echovirus, petechial rash.
   d) Epstein–Barr virus and cytomegalovirus (rare).

3. The cerebrospinal fluid (CSF) shows a predominance of lymphocytes, early polymorphonuclear leukocytes (PMNs), normal glucose, mild protein increase.

4. Polymerase chain reaction can make the diagnosis of HSV-1 or -2 and enterovirus, but diagnosis is often presumptive.

5. Treatment consists mainly of observation, with antibiotics if CSF contains PMNs; self-limiting disease, lasts 7 to 10 days.

patients with agammaglobulinemia, a chronic enteroviral meningitis ("meningoenchephalitis") can develop that continues for years. This condition is often fatal. Treatment with systemic and intraventricular pooled IgG preparations has been successful in some of these patients.

TUBERCULOUS MENINGITIS

Tuberculous meningitis arises most commonly in association with miliary tuberculosis. Meningitis can also develop if a tubercle ruptures into the subarachnoid space. About 25% of patients have no evidence of an extracranial site of tuberculous infection.

The symptoms and signs of tuberculous meningitis vary. In some patients, it can mimic other forms of acute bacterial meningitis; in others, the disease is more indolent and presents with a mild headache and malaise. Because tuberculous meningitis involves primarily the basilar meninges, inflammation often involves the pons and optic chiasm, leading to dysfunction of the IIIrd, IVth, and VIth cranial nerves, causing abnormalities in extraocular movements and the pupillary response. Changes in mental status need to be carefully documented; outcome correlates closely with the neurologic findings. Patients who are stuporous or have hemiplegia have a nearly 50% risk of dying or suffering severe neurologic sequelae.

KEY POINTS

About Tuberculous Meningitis

1. Usually develops during miliary tuberculosis.
2. No pulmonary disease is evident in 25% of cases.
3. Clinically similar to other forms of meningitis:
   a) Basilar process involving the pons and optic chiasm
   b) Deficits of the IIIrd, IVth, and VIth cranial nerves
   c) Non-communicating hydrocephalus a possibility
   d) Development of coma a bad prognostic sign
4. The cerebrospinal fluid (CSF) obeys the "500 rule": fewer than 500 white blood cells, usually lymphocytes; protein less than 500 mg/dL; glucose often less than 45 mg/dL.
5. Culture should use large volumes of CSF; smear for acid-fast bacilli is positive in one third of cases; polymerase chain reaction is a sensitive test.
6. Fatal if not treated within 5 to 8 weeks.
7. Treatment with isoniazid, rifampin, and pyrazinamide; add corticosteroids for hydrocephalus.

In most children, but in only 50% of adults, a CXR demonstrates changes consistent with tuberculosis. A PPD test is helpful and is usually positive. However, a negative PPD does not exclude the diagnosis.

Lumbar puncture is the key to diagnosis, usually obeying the "500 rule." That is, the leukocyte count is usually below 500/mm^3 (usual range: 100 to 500/mm^3), and protein is usually below 500 mg/dL (range: 100 to 500 mg/dL). In addition, a moderate depression in CSF glucose is usually encountered (below 45 mg/dL); however, in a significant number of cases, CSF glucose may exceed this value. A predominance of mononuclear leukocytes is the usual cellular response; however, early in tuberculous meningitis, PMNs may predominate in up to one quarter of patients. A CSF smear for acid-fast bacilli is positive in slightly more than one third of cases, but repeat examination of multiple samples that have been centrifuged increases the sensitivity. Large volumes of CSF should be collected for culture to increase the culture yield. Amplification tests using PCR for tuberculosis are now available. They are highly specific, but their sensitivity does not match culture. A negative CSF PCR therefore does not exclude the diagnosis. A CT or magnetic resonance imaging (MRI) scan with contrast may reveal rounded densities indicative of tuberculomas, basilar arachnoid inflammation, and hydrocephalus. Flow of CSF may be impaired as a consequence of basilar inflammation that blocks travel through the aqueduct of Sylvius.

After appropriate cultures are obtained, treatment should be initiated immediately. Untreated tuberculous meningitis is fatal within 5 to 8 weeks of the onset of symptoms. Prognosis is worse in patients under the age of 5 year or over the age of 50 years. A three-drug regimen consisting of isoniazid, rifampin, and pyrazinamide is recommended. Ethambutol or streptomycin can be added if infection with a resistant organism is suspected. In addition to antituberculous agents, a glucocorticoid (adults: 60 mg prednisone daily; children: 2 to 4 mg/kg daily) or dexamethasone (adults: 10 mg intravenously every 6 hours; children: 0.4 mg/kg daily given intravenously every 6 hours) is recommended in patients with hydrocephalus so as to reduce basilar inflammation.

CRYPTOCOCCAL MENINGOENCEPHALITIS

Cryptococcus neoformans is found predominantly in pigeon droppings. High concentrations of this yeast-like fungus are found in pigeon nesting areas and on ledges where pigeons perch. The organism is inhaled and subsequently gains entry into the bloodstream, where it seeds the brain and meninges, causing a meningoencephalitis.

Cryptococcus has a thick capsule consisting of negatively charged polysaccharides that are immunosup-

KEY POINTS

About Cryptococcal Meningoencephalitis

1. Transmitted by pigeon excreta.
2. Inhaled, infects the lung, bloodstream, meninges, and brain.
3. Yeast, with a thick capsule that is immunosuppressive. Produces melanin and mannitol.
4. Symptoms wax and wane, and diagnosis often delayed for more than 1 month.
   a) Headache is the most common symptom.
   b) Personality change and confusion develop as disease progresses.
   c) Stiff neck is uncommon.
   d) Deficits of the IIIrd, IVth, VIth, and VIIIth cranial nerves can occur.
5. A lumbar puncture is required for diagnosis; increased cerebrospinal fluid (CSF) pressure often associated.
   a) White blood cells (WBCs) 20 to 200/mm^3, with a predominance of mononuclear cells
   b) Mildly elevated protein and moderately depressed glucose
   c) Positive India ink preparation in 25% to 50% of cases, and positive cryptococcal antigen in approximately 90%
   d) Culture usually positive in 5 to 7 days
6. Computed tomography or magnetic resonance imaging scan with contrast may show hydrocephalus, cerebral edema, and ring-enhancing lesions (cryptococcomas).
7. Treat with amphotericin B and flucytosine for 2 weeks, fluconazole for 3 to 6 months.
8. Mortality is 25% to 30%; prognosis is worse if CSF produces a positive India ink preparation, an antigen titer higher than 1:32, a WBC count below 20/mm^3, or increased opening pressure; or if extraneural infection is present.

pressive, blocking both cell-mediated immune responses and leukocyte migration. These effects explain the minimal inflammatory response elicited by invading cryptococci. Strains that produce melanin demonstrate increased virulence, and this cell wall product is thought to provide protection against oxidants. The high concentrations of dopamine in the CNS serve as a substrate for melanin production. *Cryptococcus* also produces mannitol, a product that may induce cerebral edema and inhibit phagocyte function.

Cryptococci infect immunocompromised hosts most commonly, but infections in normal hosts are also reported. This form of meningitis is the most common in patients with AIDS (see Chapter 17). In the non-HIV-infected patient, cryptococcal CNS infection usually has a slowly progressive, waxing and waning course, characterized by severe intermittent headache, followed by mild confusion and personality changes that can progress to stupor and coma. The subacute onset and nonspecific nature of this illness often delay the diagnosis. On average, the diagnosis is determined 1 month after the onset of symptoms. The progression of this illness tends to be more rapid in HIV-infected patients, and the larger burden of organisms results in marked inhibition of the inflammatory response (see Chapter 17).

Like *Mycobacterium tuberculosis*, *Cryptococcus* produces a basilar meningitis that can cause oculomotor palsies because of dysfunction in the IIIrd, IVth, VIth cranial nerves, hearing loss, and hydrocephalus. Patients may experience decreased visual acuity and diplopia. Neck stiffness is often minimal, and the possibility of meningoencephalitis may not be considered. Papilledema is noted in up to one third of cases. Focal motor deficits and seizures are rare.

The diagnosis is made by lumbar puncture. Pressure of the CSF is often elevated above 200 mm H$_2$O, reflecting disturbances in CSF flow and resorption. The CSF formula typically has 20 to 200 WBCs/mm^3, with a predominance of mononuclear cells, mildly elevated protein, and moderately decreased glucose.

The CSF can be mixed one-to-one with India ink, and this preparation reveals encapsulated rounded particles in 25% to 50% of infected patients without HIV. Lymphocytes and starch granules can be mistaken for yeast forms. True cryptococcal forms have a double refractile wall, a distinctly outlined capsule, and refractile inclusions within their cytoplasm (Figure 6.4). The most useful finding is a budding yeast form, which, when encountered, provides strong proof of a true cryptococcal infection.

Cryptococcal polysaccharide antigen latex agglutination is highly sensitive and specific. The CSF antigen titer is determined by serially diluting the CSF. In most cases of HIV-associated cryptococcal meningitis, cryptococcal antigen can also be detected in the serum. However, a negative serum antigen test does not exclude cryptococcal meningitis in the normal host. A CSF culture is positive in 90% of patients, and culturing large volumes of CSF (10 to 15 mL) can increase the yield. The organism usually grows within 5 to 7 days on standard media, and use of birdseed agar can enhance growth. In addition to CSF analysis, brain CT or MRI scan with contrast is recommended to assess the degree of hydrocephalus and the extent of cerebral edema, and

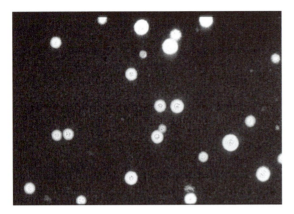

Figure 6–4. India ink preparation of cerebrospinal fluid shows cryptococcal yeast forms. Two examples of budding yeast are seen, a finding that is highly specific for these organisms.

to look for the presence of discrete, ring-enhancing masses called cryptococcomas.

In the patient who does not have AIDS, the goal of therapy is to eradicate the infection. Conventional amphotericin B (0.5 to 0.7 mg/kg daily) or lipid preparations (5 mg/kg daily) and flucytosine (100 to 150 mg/kg daily given in four divided doses) are recommended for a minimum of 2 weeks (see Chapter 1). If the patient has improved clinically, therapy can be switched to oral fluconazole (400 mg daily), with consolidation therapy continued for 3 to 6 months. In patients who respond poorly to therapy, a lumbar puncture should be repeated at 2 weeks. Amphotericin B and flucytosine should be continued until CSF cultures are sterile.

Mortality for cryptococcal meningitis is 25% to 30% in patients who do not have AIDS. Poor prognostic factors include a positive CSF India ink preparation, a CSF cryptococcal antigen titer in excess of 1:32, a CSF WBC count below 20/mm^3, elevated CSF opening pressure, and extraneural infection.

■ ENCEPHALITIS

POTENTIAL SEVERITY

An acute and severe illness associated with a high mortality.

VIRAL ENCEPHALITIS

CASE 6.3

A 74-year-old white man with a history of chronic steroid use (10 mg prednisone daily) and stage I chronic lymphocytic leukemia presented at the emergency room with confusion and fever. Four days before admission, he complained of being increasingly tired. Two days before admission, he became increasingly lethargic, sleeping on floor. His wife had difficulty rousing him, and she noted that he was no longer interested in any activity.

The morning of admission, he displayed bizarre behavior (putting underwear on top of his pajama bottoms, for example). He also became unsteady, requiring help from his wife to walk. His temperature at home was 38.9°C (102°F). On arrival at the ER, he was mildly lethargic, but was talking and answering simple questions.

The man was living in Florida with his wife. His wife reported that he spent considerable time outside and had been bitten by multiple mosquitoes.

Physical examination showed a temperature of 39.8°C (103.6°F). No lesions in the mouth were noted, and the sclera lacked erythema. The neck showed some increased tone, but lacked Kernig's or Brudzinski's sign. A few rhonchi were heard in the lungs, but no murmurs or rubs in the heart, and the abdomen was unremarkable. No skin lesions were noted.

A neurologic exam revealed an ataxic gait, all extremities moving, some diffuse hyperreflexia, and generalized increased muscle tone.

By hospital day 2, the patient's mental status had deteriorated. He only groaned and winced with painful stimuli.

Laboratory –workup included CT and MRI scans of the head that were within normal limits. A lumbar puncture showed a WBC count in the CSF of 100/mm^3 (40% PMNs, 47% lymphocytes, 13% monocytes), with protein 106 mg/dL and glucose 68 mg/dL. Serum immunoglobulin M (IgM) for West Nile virus was markedly elevated.

Outbreaks of West Nile viral illness in North America, starting in the 1990s, have raised the public's awareness and concern about viral encephalitis. The causative encephalitides fall into two major groups: those that are arthropod–borne, and those that are caused by viruses that spread person-to-person.

Table 6.5. Encephalitis Caused by Arboviruses

Disease	Virus	Locations	Hosts	Clinical Remarks
Eastern equine encephalitis	Alphavirus	Eastern United States, Canada, Central and South America, Caribbean, Guyana	Birds, horses	Severe disease, high mortality
Western equine encephalitis	Alphavirus	United States, Canada, Central and South America, Guyana	Birds, small mammals, snakes, horses	Mild disease, primarily in children
Venezuelan equine encephalitis	Alphavirus	Northern South America, Central America, Florida, Texas	Horses, rodents, birds	Febrile illness, encephalitis uncommon
St. Louis encephalitis	Flavivirus	Western, central, and southern United States, Central and South America, Caribbean	Birds	Attacks people over 50 years of age
West Nile encephalitis	Flavivirus	Eastern United States (New York, Florida)	Birds	Usually mild disease, severe disease in elderly people
Japanese encephalitis	Flavivirus	Japan, Siberia, Korea, China, Southeast Asia, India	Birds, pigs, horses	Can cause severe encephalitis
California group encephalitis	Bunyavirus	United States, Canada	Small mammals	School-age children, permanent behavior changes

Mosquito-borne disease is caused by arboviruses that include the alphaviruses, flaviviruses, and the bunyaviruses (Table 6.5). These infections occur in the summer months when mosquitoes are active. The responsible viruses often infect birds and horses in addition to humans. In the case of West Nile virus, crows are particularly susceptible, and the finding of a dead crow warrants increased surveillance. To document disease activity, public health officials frequently set out sentinel chickens in areas heavily infested with mosquitoes. The various arboviruses tend to be associated with outbreaks in specific areas of the country, and these organisms have somewhat different host preferences (Table 6.5). Prevention is best accomplished by avoiding mosquito bites. Long-sleeved shirts and long pants should be worn outdoors. During times of increased viral encephalitis activity, people should avoid the outdoors in the early evening when mosquitoes prefer to feed. Insect repellants are another important protective measure.

Encephalitis-causing viruses that spread from person-to-person include mumps, measles, Varicella virus, human herpesvirus 6, and the most common form of sporadic encephalitis, HSV-1. These forms of viral encephalitis can occur at any time during the year. Other, rarer causes of viral encephalitis include cytomegalovirus, Epstein–Barr virus, and enteroviruses. A particularly deadly form of encephalitis, rabies, is caused by the rabies virus, which is spread by animal bites, most commonly the bites of bats.

With the exception of rabies, these viruses all present with similar symptoms and signs, and cannot be differentiated clinically. The clinical manifestations of encephalitis differ from those of meningitis. The causative virus directly invades the cerebral cortex and produces abnormalities in upper cortical function. Patients may experience visual or auditory hallucinations. As described in case 6.3, patients may perform peculiar higher motor functions such as unbuttoning and buttoning a shirt or placing underwear over pants. Patients with encephalitis frequently develop seizures that are either grand mal or focal in character. They may also develop motor or sensory deficits such as ataxia. These symptoms and signs are usually accompanied by severe headache. As the disease progresses to cerebral edema, the patient may become comatose. Development of coma is associated with a poor prognosis. In herpes encephalitis, the typical vesicular herpetic lesions on the lip or face are not usually seen, because reactivated virus migrates up the Vth cranial nerve toward the central nervous system rather than toward the periphery.

Patients who contract rabies encephalitis often suffer the acute onset of hydrophobia. On attempting to drink water, they experience spasms of the pharynx. These spasms spread from the pharynx to the respiratory muscles, causing shallow, quick respirations. These abnormalities are thought to be the result of brain stem involvement and damage to the nucleus ambiguus in the upper medulla. Hyperactivity, seizures, and coma usually follow. Pituitary dysfunction is often evident and can result in diabetes insipidus (causing loss of free water) or inappropriate antidiuretic hormone secretion (causing hyponatremia). Cardiac arrhythmias and autonomic dysfunction are also common. Patients usually die within 1 to 2 weeks after the onset of coma. Less commonly, patients present with ascending paralysis resembling the Guillain–Barré syndrome and subsequently develop coma.

Diagnostic studies usually include CT or MRI scan with contrast. The MRI is more sensitive, detecting smaller lesions and early areas of edematous cerebral cortex. In herpes simplex encephalitis, involvement of the temporal lobes is the rule. In other forms of encephalitis, diffuse cerebral edema may be found in severe cases. As seen in case 6.3, however, these imaging studies are often normal. Electroencephalogram is particularly helpful in herpes simplex encephalitis, frequently demonstrating electrical spikes in the region of the infected temporal lobe. Lumbar puncture usually reveals a CSF WBC count below 500/mm^3, with a predominance of mononuclear cells. However, in early infection, PMNs may be noted, and this finding warrants a follow-up lumbar puncture to document a shift to lymphocytes. The CSF protein is usually normal or mildly elevated, and the CSF glucose is usually normal, although low glucose may be seen in herpes. In HSV-1 encephalitis increased numbers of red blood cells may also be found in the CSF.

With exception of rabies, a specific diagnosis is usually difficult to determine. Acute and convalescent serum should be sent for IgM and IgG titers to determine the viral causes of encephalitis. Samples of CSF should be cultured for virus in addition to bacteria and fungi. Throat swabs for viral culture are also recommended. The yield for viral cultures is highest early in the illness.

A CSF PCR for HSV is both sensitive and specific; where available, it is the diagnostic test of choice. In the absence of this test, brain biopsy of the affected temporal lobe remains the diagnostic procedure of choice. Herpes immunofluorescence stain of cortical tissue has an 80% yield. Viral culture of the brain should also be obtained (takes 1 to 5 days to grow). In herpes encephalitis, histopathology classically reveals Cowdry type A intranuclear inclusions. Other stains including smear for acid-fast bacilli and stains for fungi should also be performed.

With the exception of HSV-1, most of the common causes of viral encephalitis have no specific associated treatment. One possible approach is to initiate acyclovir therapy (10 mg/kg intravenously every 8 hours) while awaiting diagnostic tests, recognizing that a delay in therapy of herpes encephalitis worsens the prognosis.

KEY POINTS

About Viral Encephalitis

1. Three major categories:
   a) Mosquito-borne (arboviruses)
   b) Animal-to-human (rabies virus)
   c) Human-to-human [herpes simplex 1 (HSV-1), mumps, measles, Varicella, human herpesvirus 6; less commonly, Epstein–Barr virus, cytomegalovirus, and enteroviruses]

2. Symptoms of cortical dysfunction are evident:
   a) Hallucinations, repetitive higher motor activity such as dressing and undressing
   b) Seizures
   c) Severe headache
   d) Ataxia

3. Rabies causes distinct symptoms:
   a) Hydrophobia
   b) Rapid, short respirations
   c) Hyperactivity and autonomic dysfunction
   d) (Less commonly) ascending paralysis

4. Diagnosis is often presumptive, requiring acute and convalescent serum analysis.
   a) Cerebrospinal fluid (CSF) shows a white blood cell count below 500/mm^3, mild increase in protein, possibly red blood cells (in cases of HSV-1)
   b) Polymerase chain reaction of CSF diagnoses HSV, culture is seldom positive.
   c) A computed tomography or magnetic resonance imaging scan may show temporal lobe abnormalities in HSV-1 infection.
   d) An electroencephalogram may show localized temporal lobe abnormalities in HSV infection.
   e) Brain biopsy is likely necessary in the presence of temporal lobe abnormalities and no improvement on acyclovir.

5. Treat with acyclovir for possible HSV-1 infection.

6. Prevent disease: Avoid mosquito bites during epidemics. Wash wounds inflicted by rabies-infected animals; give immune globulin and rabies vaccine.

If temporal lobe abnormalities are found and if the patient fails to improve on acyclovir, a brain biopsy should be strongly considered. In other forms of encephalitis in which no focal cortical abnormalities are noted, the usefulness of brain biopsy remains to be determined. If HSV is confirmed by PCR, culture, or biopsy, intravenous acyclovir should be continued for 14 to 21 days.

The prognosis of viral encephalitis varies depending on the agent. A mortality of 50% to 60% is associated with HSV-1, and the frequency of neurologic sequelae is high. Early treatment reduces mortality. The mortality for rabies is nearly 100%, justifying vaccination of anyone who has potentially been exposed to the rabies virus. The prognoses for arboviruses depend on the patient's age, the extent of cortical involvement, and the specific agent. Eastern equine encephalitis tends to be the most virulent, having a 70% mortality; Western equine encephalitis is usually mild and often subclinical, infecting primarily young children. West Nile virus infection is also often subclinical or causes just mild disease; however, in elderly individuals, this virus can cause severe, life-threatening disease that can be accompanied by flaccid paralysis. Venezuelan equine encephalitis is also usually mild, and Japanese encephalitis varies in severity.

Management of rabies exposure is complex, and specific guidelines have been published by the Advisory Committee on Immunization Practices [Human rabies prevention—United States, 1999. Recommendations of the Advisory Committee on Immunization Practices (ACIP). *MMWR Recomm Rep.* 1999;48:1–21.f]. Bite wounds should be washed with a 20% soap solution and irrigated with a virucidal agent such as povidone iodine solution. Rabies immune globulin (20 IU/kg) should be injected around the wound and given intramuscularly. Several safe and effective anti-rabies vaccines are available. The vaccine should be given on days 0, 3, 7, 14, and 28.

■ CNS ABSCESS

BRAIN ABSCESS

POTENTIAL SEVERITY

Often subacute in onset, but may be life-threatening if improperly managed. Early neurosurgical consultation is of critical importance.

CASE 6.4

A 19-year-old white man noted the gradual onset of severe left frontal headache. The headache was sharp and constant, interfered with sleep, and was not relieved by asparin. Two weeks after the onset of the headache, the teen was noted to have a grand mal seizure associated with urinary incontinence that lasted 15 minutes. On admission to hospital, he was afebrile and alert, but somewhat confused. He was oriented to person, but not to time or place. Examination of the head, ears, nose, and throat showed teeth in poor repair, with evidence of several cavities and gingivitis. Fundoscopic exam revealed sharp disc margins. Mild left-sided weakness was noted on neurologic exam. A CT scan with contrast demonstrated a 3-cm, ring-enhancing lesion in the right frontal cortex. No evidence of sinusitis.

KEY POINTS

About the Clinical Manifestations of Brain Abscess

1. Symptoms are initially nonspecific, and a delay in diagnosis is common (2 weeks).
   a) Severe headache is often localized to the site where the abscess has formed.
   b) Neck stiffness noted in occipital brain abscess or after rupture into the ventricle.
   c) Alterations in mental status, inattentiveness, lethargy, coma (a bad prognostic sign) may be seen.
   d) Vomiting is associated with increased pressure in the cerebrospinal fluid (CSF).
2. Physical findings are often minimal: ·
   a) Fever not present in half of patients.
   b) Focal neurologic findings appear late.
   c) Papilledema, a late manifestation, seen in 25% of cases.
   d) Deficits in the VIth and IIIrd cranial nerves result from increased CSF pressure.
   e) Seizures most common in association with frontal brain abscess.

Prevalence and Pathogenesis

Brain abscess is an uncommon disease, found in about 1 in 10,000 general hospital admissions. Infection of the cerebral cortex can result from the direct spread of bacteria from another focus of infection (accounts for 20% to 60% of cases) or from hematogenous seeding.

DIRECT SPREAD

The direct spread of microorganisms from a contiguous site usually causes a single brain abscess. Primary infections that can spread directly to the cerebral cortex include:

1. Subacute and chronic otitis media and mastoiditis (spread to the inferior temporal lobe and cerebellum).
2. Frontal or ethmoid sinusitis (spread to the frontal lobes).
3. Dental infection (usually spreads to the frontal lobes).

The brain abscess in Case 6.4 likely originated from a dental focus. Brain abscess as a complication of ear infection has decreased in frequency, especially in developed countries. By contrast, brain abscess arising from a sinus infection remains an important consideration in adults and children alike. Bullet wounds to the brain devitalize tissue and may leave fragments of metal that can serve as a focus for infection. Other missiles that have been associated with brain abscesses are pencil-tip injury to the eye and a lawn dart. In such cases, brain abscess may develop many years after the injury. Brain abscess can occasionally result from facial trauma or as a complication of a neurosurgical procedure. The development of brain abscess

after neurosurgery may be delayed, with symptomatic infection occurring 3 to 15 months after the surgery.

HEMATOGENOUS SPREAD

Abscesses associated with bacteremia are usually multiple and are located in the distribution of the middle cerebral artery. Initially, they tend to be located at the junction of the gray and white matter, where brain capillary blood flow is slow and septic emboli are more likely to lodge. Microinfarction causes damage to the blood–brain barrier, allowing bacteria to invade the cerebral cortex.

Primary infections that lead to hematogenous seeding the brain include:

- Chronic pulmonary infections such as lung abscess and empyema, often in hosts with bronchiectasis or cystic fibrosis.
- Skin infections.
- Pelvic infections.
- Intra-abdominal infections.
- Esophageal dilation and endoscopic sclerosis of esophageal varices.
- Bacterial endocarditis (2% to 4% of cases).
- Cyanotic congenital heart diseases (most common in children).

No primary site or underlying condition can be identified in 20% to 40% of patients with brain abscess.

The location of a brain abscess reflects the site of the primary infection. In order of decreasing frequency, abscesses are most commonly found in the frontal or temporal, frontoparietal, parietal, cerebellar, and occipital lobes.

The histologic changes in the brain depend on the duration of infection. Early lesions (first 1 to 2 weeks) are poorly demarcated and are associated with localized edema. Acute inflammation is evident, but not tissue necrosis. This early stage is commonly called cerebritis. After 2 to 3 weeks, necrosis and liquefaction occur, and a fibrotic capsule surrounds the lesion.

Microbiology

The bacterial causes of brain abscess are highly variable. The pathogens involved vary depending on the site of the primary infection, the age of the patient (microorganisms often differ in children and adults), and the immune status of the host. The organism or organisms recovered from a brain abscess frequently provide clues about the primary site of infection and any potentially undiagnosed underlying conditions in the host.

Anaerobic bacteria are common constituents of brain abscesses, generally originating as part of the normal mouth flora. However, intra-abdominal or pelvic

---

KEY POINTS

About the Pathogenesis of Brain Abscess

1. Brain abscess has two major causes:
   a) Direct spread from middle ear, frontal sinus, or dental infection
   b) Hematogenous spread from chronic pulmonary, skin, pelvic, and intra-abdominal infection, also endocarditis, bacteremia after esophageal dilatation, cyanotic heart disease (multiple abscesses at the grey–white matter junction)
2. Abscess location can be frontal or temporal, frontoparietal, parietal, cerebellar, and occipital.
3. Cerebritis (acute inflammation and edema) progresses to necrosis, followed by fibrotic capsule formation.

infections can occasionally lead to bacteremia with an anaerobic organism that seeds the cerebral cortex. The anaerobes in such cases usually reflect colonic or female genital tract flora. The anaerobes most frequently cultured from brain abscesses include anaerobic streptococci, *Bacteroides* species (including *B. fragilis*), *Prevotella melaninogenica*, *Propionibacterium*, *Fusobacterium*, *Eubacterium*, *Veillonella*, and *Actinomyces*.

Aerobic gram-positive cocci are also frequently encountered, including *S. viridans*, *S. milleri*, microaerophilic streptococci, *S. pneumoniae* (rare), and *S. aureus*. *S. aureus* is a more frequent pathogen in brain abscess following trauma or a neurosurgical procedure. *S. milleri* is particularly common, and this organism possesses proteolytic enzymes that predispose to necrosis of tissue and formation of abscesses.

Aerobic gram-negative rods are not usually recovered in brain abscess except following neurosurgery or head trauma. When gram-negative rods are isolated, *E. coli*, *Pseudomonas*, *Klebsiella*, and *Proteus* species are most common. Rarer gram-negative rods include *H. aphrophilus*, *Actinobacillus actinomycetemcomitans*, *Salmonella*, and *Enterobacter* species.

IMMUNOCOMPROMISED HOST

In the immunocompromised patient, the range of organisms—particularly opportunistic pathogens—is considerably broader. *Toxoplasma gondii* can reactivate when the cell-mediated immune system becomes compromised. *Nocardia asteroides*, a common soil organism, can enter the bloodstream via the lungs and seed the cerebral cortex. *Aspergillus*, *Cryptococcus neoformans*, and *Coccidioides immitis* also can enter through the lungs and subsequently invade the cerebral cortex. Other pathogens causing brain abscess in the immunocompromised host include *Candida albicans*, mucormycosis (*Zygomyces*), *Cladosporium trichoides*, and *Curvularia* species.

Individuals infected with HIV frequently develop infections of the cerebral cortex. *Toxoplasma gondii* is the most common cause of brain abscess in these patients, but more than one CNS infection can occur simultaneously. Tuberculomas, cryptococcomas, early progressive multifocal leukoencephalopathy, and infection with *L. monocytogenes*, *Salmonella*, *Candida*, *Histoplasma*, and *Aspergillus* have all been reported to cause CNS lesions in association with HIV infection. In the patient with AIDS, CNS lymphoma also commonly mimics brain abscess (see Chapter 17).

IMMIGRANTS

Parasites are the most common cause of brain abscess in individuals who have previously lived outside the United States. Cysticercosis represents 85% of brain infections in Mexico City (see Chapter 12). Other parasites that can cause brain abscess include *Entamoeba histolytica*, *Schistosoma japonicum*, and *Paragonimus* species.

Clinical Symptoms and Signs

The symptoms of brain abscess tend come on gradually and are often nonspecific, delaying the diagnosis. The mean interval between the first symptom and diagnosis is 2 weeks.

As observed in case 6.4, headache is the most common symptom. It usually localizes to the side on which the abscess is located, but in some cases, the headache is generalized. As observed with bacterial meningitis, headache is usually severe, and it is not relieved by asparin or other over-the-counter pain medications. In patients with cyanotic heart disease and unexplained headache, the diagnosis of brain abscess must always be excluded.

About 15% of patients complain of neck stiffness mimicking meningitis. Meningismus is most commonly associated with occipital lobe brain abscess or with an abscess that has leaked into a lateral ventricle.

KEY POINTS

About the Causes of Brain Abscess

1. Anaerobes (from mouth flora, pelvis, and gastrointestinal tract):
   a) *Bacteroides* (may include *B. fragilis*)
   b) *Prevotella melaninogenica*
   c) *Propionibacterium, Fusobacterium, Eubacterium, Veillonella*
   d) *Actinomyces*
2. Aerobic gram-positive cocci:
   a) *Streptococcus milleri* (protease activity, predisposition to form abscesses)
   b) Microaerophilic streptococci
   c) *Staphylococcus aureus* (endocarditis, trauma, neurosurgery)
   d) *S. viridans*
3. Gram-negative rods (Escherichia coli, Pseudomonas, Klebsiella, Proteus) are rare. Haemophilus aphrophilus, Actinobacillus actinomycetemcomitans, Salmonella and Enterobacter are rarer.
4. Possibilities in the immunocompromised host:
   a) Toxoplasmosis
   b) *Nocardia*
   c) *Aspergillus, Cryptococcus neoformans*, and *Coccidioides immitis* (fungi)
5. Cysticercosis parasite a possibility in immigrants.

Table 6.6. Neurologic Manifestations of Brain Abscess

Location	Neurologic Deficits
Temporal	Wernicke's aphasia, homonymous superior quadranopsia, mild contralateral facial muscle weakness
Frontal	Drowsy, inattentive, disturbed judgment, mutism, seizures plus grasp, suck, and snout reflexes; contralateral hemiparesis when the abscess is large
Parietal	Impaired position sense, two-point discrimination, and stereognosis; focal sensory and motor seizures, homonymous hemianopsia; impaired opticokinetic nystagmus
Cerebellar	Ataxia, nystagmus (coarser on gaze toward the lesion); ipsilateral incoordination of arm and leg movements with intention tremor; rapid progression (usually not encapsulated)
Brain stem	Facial weakness and dysphagia, multiple other cranial nerve palsies, contralateral hemiparesis

Changes in mental status are common. In patients with frontal abscess, subtle disturbances in judgment and inattentiveness may be the primary symptom. Lethargy can progress to coma, and these changes are thought be primarily the consequence of cerebral edema and increased intracranial pressure. The development of coma is associated with a poor prognosis. Vomiting may also develop as a consequence of increased intracranial pressure.

The absence of fever does not exclude a diagnosis of brain abscess. A significant percentage of patients with the disease (45% to 50%) fail to mount a febrile response. Focal neurologic deficits usually develop days to weeks after the onset of headache and are observed in half of patients at the time of admission. The specific neurologic deficits depend on the location of the abscess (s Table 6.6). Palsies as a consequence of increased intracranial pressure on the VIth and IIIrd cranial nerve may be seen. Papilledema is a late manifestation of increased intracranial pressure and is found in 25% of patients. As observed in case 6.4, focal or grand mal seizures develop in 25% of patients and are most commonly associated with frontal lobe brain abscess.

Diagnosis

Focal symptoms (for example, unilateral headache) or signs (for example, unilateral cranial nerve deficits, hemiparesis) and papilledema suggest a space-occupying lesion in the cerebral cortex. In this circumstance, a lumbar puncture is contraindicated until this possibility is excluded. The asymmetric cerebral edema associated with brain abscess can cause brain stem herniation in 15% to 30% of patients if CSF pressure is reduced below the tentorium by lumbar puncture. A CT or MRI scan with contrast should be performed before lumbar puncture to exclude a focal cerebral lesion. Blood samples for culture should be drawn (positive in 15% of cases), and empiric parenteral antibiotic therapy initiated before the CT or MRI scan. If the study is negative, the lumbar puncture can then be performed.

COMPUTED TOMOGRAPHY SCAN

A CT scan is not as sensitive as MRI for diagnosing brain abscess, but it can frequently be obtained more easily on an emergent basis. When brain abscess is a serious consideration, the CT study must be performed with a contrast agent. The lesion has different appearances on scan depending on the duration of the infection, and these difference reflect the histopathology:

1. **Early cerebritis.** The lesion appears as an irregular area of low density that does not enhance following contrast injection.
2. **Later cerebritis.** The lesion enlarges and demonstrates a thick diffuse ring of enhancement following contrast injection. The ring of contrast enhancement represents breakdown of the blood–brain barrier and development of an inflammatory capsule (Figure 6.5).
3. **Late cerebritis.** Necrosis often develops with late cerebritis. Pre-contrast images reveal a ring of higher density than the surrounding edematous brain. Injection of contrast demonstrates a thin ring that is not of uniform in thickness.
4. **Healed abscess.** Once the abscess has healed, the resulting collagen capsule becomes isodense (same density as the surrounding tissue), and infusion of contrast no longer results in ring enhancement.

MAGNETIC RESONANCE IMAGING

An MRI scan is the diagnostic study of choice for evaluating brain abscess. The scan should be performed with gadolinium diethylenetriamine petaacetic acid, which crosses the damaged blood–brain barrier. This agent

and normal CSF protein (Table 6.3). On rare occasions, an abscess may rupture into the lateral ventricle, causing frank meningitis and a resulting CSF formula with a predominance of PMNs (up to 160,000/mm³), low glucose, and high protein.

Treatment

The goals of therapy are to sterilize the abscess or abscesses and reduce the mass effect caused by necrosis and cerebral edema. Because surgical drainage of the brain abscess is usually necessary, a neurosurgeon should be contacted as soon as the diagnosis is made.

ANTIBIOTICS

To cure brain abscess, prolonged intravenous antibiotic therapy (6 to 8 weeks) is required. A number of drugs can be chosen depending upon the probable pathogen or pathogens. Once the causative organisms have been isolated and susceptibility testing performed, the drug regimen can be modified.

High-dose penicillin remains the mainstay of therapy when a dental origin is suspected. Penicillin covers all mouth flora, including aerobic and anaerobic streptococci. Metronidazole is also recommended for most

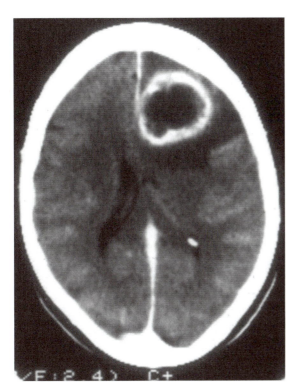

Figure 6–5. Computed tomography scan with contrast, showing a brain abscess. Note the large ring-enhancing lesion in the left frontal cortex, associated with marked edema and obliteration of the lateral ventricle.

increases the T1 intensity and causes more prominent enhancement of lesions than can be accomplished with CT scan. Compared with CT scan, MRI scan

- is more sensitive for detecting early cerebritis.
- is more sensitive for detecting satellite lesions and is capable of detecting smaller-diameter lesions (1-mm resolution).
- more accurately estimates the extent of central necrosis, ring enhancement, and cerebral edema.
- better visualizes the brainstem.

Lumbar puncture

As noted earlier in this chapter, lumbar puncture is contraindicated in patients with brain abscess because of the danger of herniation. When this test has been performed inadvertently, the cerebrospinal profile is indicative of a parameningeal infection—that is, moderate numbers of WBCs (fewer than 500), usually with a predominance of mononuclear cells; normal CSF glucose;

KEY POINTS

About the Diagnosis of Brain Abscess

1. Focal symptoms or neurologic signs plus papilledema suggest the possibilty of a space-occupying lesion; lumbar puncture is contraindicated.

2. After blood culture and empiric antibiotics, perform computed tomography (CT) or magnetic resonance imaging (MRI) scan with contrast.

3. An MRI is preferred over CT scan (detects early cerebritis and smaller lesions, and visualizes the brainstem).

4. Four stages detectable on imaging:
   a) Early cerebritis (edema, no ring enhancement).
   b) Later cerebritis (ring enhancement with early capsule, edema).
   c) Late cerebritis (necrosis, ring seen without contrast, thin, non-uniform contrast-enhancing ring).
   d) Healed abscess (no longer ring-enhancing, lesion becomes isodense).

5. Lumbar puncture is contraindicated.

patients, because this antibiotic readily penetrates brain abscesses; intralesional concentrations reach 40 μg/mL. This drug has excellent cidal activity against all anaerobes, but is not active against aerobic organisms. In most patients, a third-generation cephalosporin should also be included in the regimen to cover Enterobacteriaceae that may be present, particularly in patients with a brain abscess associated with a chronic ear infection. High-dose ceftriaxone or cefotaxime are equally effective and should be used unless *Pseudomonas aeruginosa* is strongly suspected. When *P. aeruginosa* is cultured, or when a brain abscess develops following a neurosurgical procedure, maximum doses of ceftazidime or cefepime should be used. In patients who develop brain abscess following a penetrating head trauma or craniotomy, and in the patient with *S. aureus* bacteremia, high-dose oxacillin or nafcillin needs to be included. Aminoglycosides, erythromycin, tetracyclines, and first-generation cephalosporins should not be used to treat brain abscess, because these drugs do not cross the blood–brain barrier.

SURGERY

Surgical drainage is generally required for both diagnosis and treatment. Needle aspiration is preferred in most cases, because this procedure reduces the extent of neurologic damage. In patients with a traumatic brain abscess, an open procedure is preferred to remove bone chips and foreign material. Surgical removal of the entire capsule greatly increases the likelihood of cure in fungal brain abscesses. In patients with early cerebritis without evidence of cerebral necrosis, and in patients with abscesses located in vital regions of the brain inaccessible to aspiration, surgery can be delayed or avoided. When a decision is made not to drain immediately, careful follow-up with sequential CT or MRI scans is critical. Following the initiation of empiric antibiotics for an established brain abscess, indications for surgical intervention include lack of clinical improvement within a week, depressed sensorium, signs of increased intracranial pressure, multiloculated abscess, abscess size exceeding 2.5 cm, and progressive increase in the ring diameter of the abscess. Contrast enhancement at the site of the abscess may persist for several months, and so that finding is not helpful for deciding on surgical intervention or continued antibiotic therapy.

GLUCOCORTICOIDS

Glucocorticoids should be given only to patients with evidence of mass effect and a depressed mental status. If used, intravenous dexamethasone should be administered at a loading dose of 10 mg, followed by 4 mg every 6 hours. The drug should be discontinued as soon as possible.

The addition of glucocorticoids has several disadvantages. These agents reduce contrast enhancement on CT

KEY POINTS

About the Treatment and Outcome of Brain Abscess

1. Antibiotic therapy must be prolonged (6 to 8 wks) and must use high doses of intravenous
   a) penicillin (covers mouth flora).
   b) metronidazole (concentrates in abscesses and kills all anaerobes).
   c) ceftriaxone or cefotaxime (covers gram-positive and gram-negative aerobes). If *Pseudomonas* is a possibility, substitute ceftazidime or cefepime.
   d) Nafcillin or oxacillin (for abscess following head trauma, neurosurgery, or *Staphylococcus aureus* bacteremia). Use vancomycin if methicillin-resistant *S. aureus* is suspected.

2. Neurosurgery usually required for culture and drainage. Always consult a neurosurgeon.
   a) Needle aspiration is usually preferred (less collateral damage).
   b) Open resection is recommended after head trauma and with fungal abscess.
   c) Use observation in cases of early cerebritis, with frequent follow-up imaging (computed tomography or magnetic resonance).

3. Use dexamethasone in the presence of mass effect and depressed mental status. Avoid when possible, because it
   a) reduces contrast enhancement during imaging.
   b) slows capsule formation and increases the risk of ventricular rupture.
   c) reduces antibiotic penetration into the abscess.

4. Mortality ranges from 0% to 30%. Poor prognosis is associated with
   a) rapid progression in hospital.
   b) coma on admission.
   c) rupture into the ventricle.

---

scan, making changes in abscess size more difficult to monitor. Glucocorticoids also slow capsule formation (increase the risk of ventricular rupture), and reduce antibiotic penetration into the abscess by improving the integrity of the blood–brain barrier.

Prognosis and Outcome

Mortality from brain abscess currently ranges from 0% to 30%. The use of CT and MRI has improved outcomes by allowing for earlier diagnosis and more accurate monitoring of response to therapy.

Poor prognostic factors for recovery include

- rapid progression of the infection before hospitalization,
- stupor or coma on admission (60% to 100% mortality), and
- rupture of the abscess into the ventricle (80% to 100% mortality).

Surviving patients experience a high incidence of neurologic sequelae (30% to 60%), recurrent seizures being the most common. This persistent problem most frequently follows frontal brain abscess.

INTRACRANIAL EPIDURAL AND SUBDURAL ABSCESS

POTENTIAL SEVERITY

Subdural abscess spreads rapidly. Emergency surgical drainage is life-saving.

Intracranial epidural and subdural abscesses are rare. They usually result from spread of infection from a nidus of osteomyelitis after neurosurgery, from an infected sinus (in particular the frontal sinus), or less commonly, from an infected middle ear or mastoid. In infants, subdural effusions may complicate bacterial meningitis; however, unlike the form seen in adults, they rarely require drainage. The bacteria causing these closed-space infections reflect the primary site of infection. *S. aureus* is most common, followed by aerobic streptococci. Other pathogens include *S. pneumoniae, H. influenzae*, and gram-negative organisms. Anaerobes such as anaerobic streptococci and *B. fragilis* can also be associated with this infection. Patients with sinusitis and chronic mastoiditis often have polymicrobial abscesses.

Epidural abscesses form between the skull and the dura (Figure 6.1). Because the dura is normally tightly adherent to the skull, this infection usually remains localized and spreads slowly, mimicking brain abscess in its clinical presentation. On exam, localized erythema, swelling, and tenderness of the subgaleal region may be seen. Subdural empyema in the cranial region progresses much faster than epidural abscess does, usually spreading rapidly throughout the cranium. Patients appear acutely ill and septic. They complain of severe headache that is localized to the site of infection, and nuchal rigidity commonly develops, suggesting the diagnosis of meningitis. Within 24 to 48 hours focal neurologic deficits are noted, and half of these patients develop seizures. Lumbar puncture is contraindicated because of the high risk of brain stem herniation. A CT scan with contrast should be performed, and in most instances, the images demonstrate the abscess and the overlying osteomyelitis, sinus infection, or mastoiditis. In early epidural or subdural abscess, MRI scan is capable of detecting early cortical edema and smaller collections of inflammatory fluid. In patients suspected of having early disease, whose CT scan is negative, an MRI scan should be performed.

Subdural empyema is a neurosurgical emergency. Immediate drainage is required to prevent death from cerebral herniation. Exploratory burr holes and blind drainage have been life-saving in rapidly progressing cases. Antibiotic therapy should be instituted immediately. The same regimens recommended for brain abscess are used. The mortality from subdural empyema remains high at 14% to 18%, the prognosis being especially poor in patients who are comatose. Epidural abscess is less dangerous, but also requires surgical drainage. Mortality is low; however, if left untreated, this infection can spread to the subdural space.

KEY POINTS

About Epidural and Subdural Intracranial Abscess

1. Associated with frontal sinusitis, mastoiditis, and neurosurgery.
2. *Staphylococcus aureus* are a common cause; otherwise, microbiology is similar to that in brain abscess.
3. Epidural abscess progresses slowly, requires surgical drainage.
4. Subdural abscess spreads quickly.
   a) Often mimics meningitis.
   b) Lumbar puncture is contraindicated; use computed tomography scan or magnetic resonance imaging emergently.
   c) Requires immediate drainage.
   d) Mortality ranges from 14% to 18%.

SPINAL EPIDURAL ABSCESS

> ## POTENTIAL SEVERITY
>
> *Often subacute in onset. Development of motor weakness indicates imminent spinal cord infarction and requires emergency surgical drainage.*

After the dura passes below the foramen magnum, it no longer adheres tightly to the bone surrounding the spinal cord. Both an anterior and a posterior space that contain fat and blood vessels are present. Infection can spread to the epidural space from vertebral osteomyelitis or disk-space infection. Infection of the epidural space following epidural catheter placement is increasingly common, as is postoperative infection following other surgical procedures in the area of the spinal cord. Skin and soft-tissue infections, urinary tract infections, and intravenous drug abuse can all lead to bacteremia and seeding of the epidural space. In approximately one third of patients, no primary cause is identified.

The inflammatory mass associated with infection can compress the nerve roots as they exit the spinal canal, causing radicular pain, and findings consistent with lower motor neuron dysfunction (decreased reflexes, loss of light touch and pain sensation in specific dermatomes). In addition to radicular pain, patients complain of localized back pain. These symptoms often are accompanied by malaise and fever. As the epidural mass expands, the spinal cord is compressed, resulting in upper motor neuron findings such as a positive Babinski's reflex, hyperreflexia, loss of motor function, and bladder dysfunction. Usually within 24 hours of the onset of paralysis, the spinal cord's vascular supply becomes irreversibly compromised, leading to infarction and permanent paraplegia. To prevent this devastating outcome, clinicians need to consider spinal epidural abscess in the differential diagnosis for back pain. In the patient with back pain and fever, spinal epidural abscess must be strongly considered.

A helpful clue can be derived from the physical examination. In posterior epidural abscesses, severe localized tenderness over the infected area is encountered. However, in anterior epidural abscesses (a rarer event) infection is deep-seated, and tenderness cannot be elicited. Epidural abscess formation can be readily visualized on MRI scan (Figure 6.6), which is the pre-

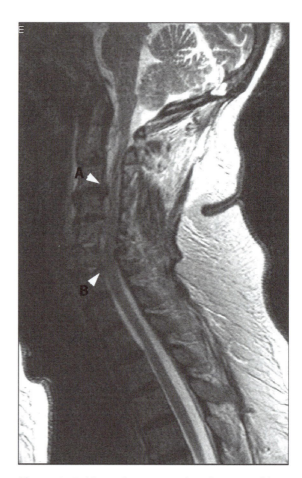

Figure 6–6. Magnetic resonance imaging scan with contrast, showing a *Staphylococcus aureus* epidural abscess. **A.** Sagittal view: Anterior mass can be seen compressing the spinal cord. Diffuse enhancement indicates extensive inflammation. The area of spinal canal narrowing is demarcated by the arrowheads. **B.** Axial view: An anterior epidural abscess is seen in the spinal canal (arrowheads) compressing the spinal cord (arrows) against the posterior wall of the canal. Pictures courtesy of Dr. Ron Quisling, University of Florida College of Medicine.

ferred test. A CT scan with gadolinium contrast is also an effective method of diagnosis, but is now seldom used.

The bacteriology of epidural abscess reflects the primary site of infection. *S. aureus*, including the methicillin-resistant form (MRSA), is cultured from more than half of cases. Gram-negative aerobes are the second most frequent cause, followed by aerobic streptococci, *S. epidermidis,* and anaerobes. *Mycobacterium tuberculosis* is

KEY POINTS

About Spinal Epidural Abscess

1. The spinal canal has both an anterior and a posterior epidural space containing fat and small vessels.

2. The spinal epidural space can become infected by
   a) spread of infection from osteomyelitis or disk space infection.
   b) spinal surgery or epidural catheter placement.
   c) hematogenous spread from skin or urinary tract infection or intravenous drug abuse.

3. Symptoms and signs include
   a) low back pain and fever.
   b) radicular pain accompanied by lower motor neuron deficits.
   c) signs of cord compression in later stages (Babinski's reflex, hyperreflexia, loss of motor function, bladder dysfunction). Within 24 hours of onset, irreversible paraplegia may occur.
   d) localized spinous process tenderness in posterior epidural abscesses.

4. In the patient with back pain and fever, always consider spinal epidural abscess.

5. Magnetic resonance imaging (MRI) scan with contrast is the diagnostic study of choice.

6. Treatment involves
   a) emergency surgical drainage if physical exam suggests neurologic compromise or MRI shows significant cord compression.
   b) Prolonged antibiotic therapy (4 to 6 weeks) with nafcillin or oxacillin, metronidazole, and ceftriaxone. If methicillin-resistant *Staphylococcus aureus* is suspected, vancomycin coverage is also required.

another important cause, most commonly associated with tuberculous infection of the thoracic vertebra.

Because of the unpredictability of neurologic complications, surgical decompression is recommended in all cases in which MRI scan suggests any neurologic compromise or evidence of significant cord compression. Drainage is combined with prolonged antibiotic treatment (4 to 6 weeks). High doses of nafcillin or oxacillin (or vancomycin if MRSA is suspected), ceftriaxone, and metronidazole are recommended as empiric therapy pending culture results.

FURTHER READING

Bacterial Meningitis

Choi C. Bacterial meningitis in aging adults. *Clin Infect Dis.* 2001;33:1380–1385.

de Gans J, van de Beek D. Dexamethasone in adults with bacterial meningitis. *N Engl J Med.* 2002;347:1549–1556.

Durand ML, Calderwood SB, Weber DJ, et al. Acute bacterial meningitis in adults: a review of 493 episodes. *N Engl J Med.* 1993;328:21–28.

Hussein AS, Shafran SD. Acute bacterial meningitis in adults. A 12-year review. *Medicine (Baltimore).* 2000;79:360–368.

Odio CM, Faingezicht I, Paris M, et al. The beneficial effects of early dexamethasone administration in infants and children with bacterial meningitis. *N Engl J Med.* 1991;324:1525–1531.

Swartz MN, Dodge PR. Bacterial meningitis—a review of selected aspects. *N Engl J Med.* 1965;272:725, 779, 842, 898, 954,1,003

Thomas KE, Hasbun R, Jekel J, Quagliarello VJ. The diagnostic accuracy of Kernig's sign, Brudzinski's sign, and nuchal rigidity in adults with suspected meningitis. *Clin Infect Dis.* 2002;35:46–52.

Tunkel AR, Hartman BJ, Kaplan SL, et al. Practice guidelines for the management of bacterial meningitis. *Clin Infect Dis.* 2004;39:1267–1284.

Uchihara T, Tsukagoshi H. Jolt accentuation of headache: the most sensitive sign of CSF pleocytosis. *Headache.* 1991;31:167–171.

Aseptic Meningitis

Isaacson E, Glaser CA, Forghani B, et al. Evidence of human herpesvirus 6 infection in 4 immunocompetent patients with encephalitis. *Clin Infect Dis.* 2005;40:890-893.

Kupila L, Vuorinen T, Vainionpaa R, Hukkanen V, Marttila RJ, Kotilainen P. Etiology of aseptic meningitis and encephalitis in an adult population. *Neurology.* 2006;66:75–80.

Encephalitis

Benson PC, Swadron SP. Empiric acyclovir is infrequently initiated in the emergency department to patients ultimately diagnosed with encephalitis. *Ann Emerg Med.* 2006;47:100–105.

Lury KM, Castillo M. Eastern equine encephalitis: CT and MRI findings in one case. *Emerg Radiol.* 2004;11:46–48.

Tuberculous Meningitis

Berger JR. Tuberculous meningitis. *Curr Opin Neurol.* 1994;7:191–200.

Offenbacher H, Fazekas F, Schmidt R, et al. MRI in tuberculous meningoencephalitis: report of four cases and review of the neuroimaging literature. *J Neurol.* 1991;238:340–344.

Patel VB, Padayatchi N, Bhigjee AI, et al. Multidrug-resistant tuberculous meningitis in KwaZulu–Natal, South Africa. *Clin Infect Dis.* 2004;38:851–856.

Thwaites GE, Nguyen DB, Nguyen HD, et al. Dexamethasone for the treatment of tuberculous meningitis in adolescents and adults. *N Engl J Med.* 2004;351:1741–1751.

Cryptococcal Meningitis

Ecevit IZ, Clancy CJ, Schmalfuss IM, Nguyen MH. The poor prognosis of central nervous system cryptococcosis among nonimmunosuppressed patients: a call for better disease recognition and evaluation of adjuncts to antifungal therapy. *Clin Infect Dis.* 2006;42:1443–1447.

Rex JH, Larsen RA, Dismukes WE, Cloud GA, Bennett JE. Catastrophic visual loss due to *Cryptococcus neoformans* meningitis. *Medicine (Baltimore).* 1993;72:207–224.

Brain Abscess

Corson MA, Postlethwaite KP, Seymour RA. Are dental infections a cause of brain abscess? Case report and review of the literature. *Oral Dis.* 2001;7:61–65.

Jansson AK, Enblad P, Sjolin J. Efficacy and safety of cefotaxime in combination with metronidazole for empirical treatment of brain abscess in clinical practice: a retrospective study of 66 consecutive cases. *Eur J Clin Microbiol Infect Dis.* 2004;23:7–14.

Seydoux C, Francioli P. Bacterial brain abscesses: factors influencing mortality and sequelae. *Clin Infect Dis.* 1992;15:394–401.

Su TM, Lan CM, Tsai YD, Lee TC, Lu CH, Chang WN. Multiloculated pyogenic brain abscess: experience in 25 patients. *Neurosurgery.* 2003;52:1075–1080.

Subdural and Epidural Abscess

Darouiche RO. Spinal epidural abscess. *N Engl J Med.* 2006;355:2012–20.

Dill SR, Cobbs CG, McDonald CK. Subdural empyema: analysis of 32 cases and review. *Clin Infect Dis.* 1995;20:372–386.

Mackenzie AR, Laing RB, Smith CC, Kaar GF, Smith FW. Spinal epidural abscess: the importance of early diagnosis and treatment. *J Neurol Neurosurg Psychiatry.* 1998;65:209–212.

Nussbaum ES, Rigamonti D, Standiford H, Numaguchi Y, Wolf AL, Robinson WL. Spinal epidural abscess: a report of 40 cases and review. *Surg Neurol.* 1992;30:225–231.

Rich PM, Deasy NP, Jarosz JM. Intracranial dural empyema. *Br J Radiol.* 2000;73:1329–1336.

Cardiovascular Infections

Time Recommended to Complete: 1 day

Frederick Southwick, M.D.

GUIDING QUESTIONS

1. Which cardiac lesions predispose to bacterial endocarditis?

2. If antibiotic prophylaxis is to be administered, when should the antibiotic be given?

3. What are the most common symptoms in subacute bacterial endocarditis?

4. When bacterial endocarditis is suspected, what are the skin lesions that should be searched for, and how often are they seen?

5. How should blood samples for culture be drawn if the clinician suspects bacterial endocarditis?

6. Are bacteriostatic antibiotics effective in the treatment of bacterial endocarditis?

7. In the patient with Staphylococcus aureus line-related bacteremia, how long should antibiotics be administered?

8. Which key physical finding is most helpful for detecting cardiac tamponade?

■ CARDIOVASCULAR INFECTIONS

INFECTIVE ENDOCARDITIS

POTENTIAL SEVERITY

Acute endocarditis is life-threatening and often requires surgical intervention. Subacute endocarditis is an indolent disease that can continue for months.

Epidemiology

Infective endocarditis remains a serious but relatively uncommon problem. The incidence varies from series to series, being estimated to be as high as 11 per 100,000 population, and as low as 0.6 per 100,000 population. The exact incidence is difficult to ascertain, because the definitions for endocarditis differ in many surveys. A reasonable estimate is probably 2 per 100,000 population. This means that a primary care physician will encounter only 1 to 2 cases over a working lifetime.

Endocarditis is more common in men than in women, and the disease is increasingly becoming a disease of elderly individuals. In recent series, more than half of the patients with endocarditis were over the age of 50 years. With available rapid treatment for group A streptococcal infections, the incidence of rheumatic heart disease has declined, eliminating this important risk factor for endocarditis in the young. With life expectancy increasing worldwide, the percentage of

KEY POINTS

About the Epidemiology of Infective Endocarditis

1. A rare disease; a primary care physician is likely to see just 1 to 2 cases in an entire career.
2. More common in men.
3. Increasingly a disease of elderly individuals.

elderly people will continue to rise, and the number of elderly patients with infective endocarditis can be expected to increase in the future.

Pathogenesis and Predisposing Risk Factors

HOST FACTORS

Infective endocarditis is usually preceded by formation of a predisposing cardiac lesion. Pre-existing endocardial damage leads to the accumulation of platelets and fibrin, producing nonbacterial thrombotic endocarditis (NBTE). This sterile lesion serves as an ideal site to trap bacteria as they pass through the bloodstream. Cardiac lesions that result in endocardial damage and predispose to the formation of NBTE include rheumatic heart disease, congenital heart disease (bicuspid aortic valve, ventricular septal defect, coarctation of the aorta, and Fallot's tetralogy), mitral valve prolapse, degenerative heart disease (calcific aortic valve disease), and prosthetic valve placement.

Risk factors for endocarditis reflect the pathogenesis of the disease. Patients with congenital heart disease and rheumatic heart disease, those with an audible murmur associated with mitral valve prolapse, and elderly patients with calcific aortic stenosis are all at increased risk. The higher the pressure gradient in aortic stenosis, the greater the risk of developing endocarditis. Intravenous drug abusers are at high risk of developing endocarditis as a consequence of injecting bacterially contaminated solutions intravenously.

Platelets and bacteria tend to accumulate in specific areas of the heart based on the Venturi effect. When a fluid or gas passes at high pressure through a narrow orifice, an area of low pressure is created directly downstream of the orifice. The Venturi effect is most easily appreciated by examining a rapidly flowing, rock-filled river. When the flow of water is confined to a narrower channel by large rocks, the velocity of water flow increases. As a consequence of the Venturi effect, twigs and other debris can be seen to accumulate on the downstream side of the obstructing rocks, in the area of lowest pressure.

Similarly, vegetations form on the downstream or low-pressure side of a valvular lesion. In aortic stenosis, vegetations tend to form in the aortic coronary cusps on the downstream side of the obstructing lesion. In mitral regurgitation, vegetations are most commonly seen in the atrium, the low-pressure side of regurgitant flow. Upon attaching to the endocardium, pathogenic bacteria induce platelet aggregation, and the resulting dense platelet–fibrin complex provides a protective environment. Phagocytes are incapable of entering this site, eliminating an important host defense. Colony counts in vegetations usually reach

---

> ### KEY POINTS
>
> ### About Host Factors in the Pathogenesis of Infective Endocarditis
>
> 1. Nonbacterial thrombotic endocarditis (NBTE) results from valve damage that is followed by platelet and fibrin deposition.
> 2. NBTE results from
>   a) rheumatic heart disease,
>   b) congenital heart disease (bicuspid valve, ventricular septal defect),
>   c) mitral valve prolapse,
>   d) degenerative valve disease (calcific aortic valve disease), or
>   e) prosthetic valve.
> 3. Venturi effect results in vegetation formation on the low-pressure side of high-flow valvular lesions.
> 4. Disease of the mitral or aortic valve is most common; disease of tricuspid valve is rarer (usually seen in intravenous drug abusers).

10^9 to 10^{11} bacteria per gram of tissue, and these bacteria within vegetations periodically lapse into a metabolically inactive, dormant phase.

The frequency with which the four valves become infected reflects the likelihood of endocardial damage. Shear stress would be expected to be highest in the valves exposed to high pressure, and most cases of bacterial endocarditis involve the valves of the left side of the heart. The mitral and aortic valves are subjected to the highest pressures and are the most commonly infected. Right-sided endocarditis is uncommon (except in the case of intravenous drug abusers), and when right-sided disease does occur, it most commonly involves the tricuspid valve. The closed pulmonic valve is subject to the lowest pressure, and infection of this valve is rare.

Patients with prosthetic valves must be particularly alert to the symptoms and signs of endocarditis, because the artificial material serves as an excellent site for bacterial adherence. Patients who have recovered from an episode of infective endocarditis are at increased risk of developing a second episode.

BACTERIAL FACTORS

The organisms responsible for infective endocarditis are sticky. They adhere more readily to inert surfaces and to the endocardium. Streptococci that express

<table>
<tr><td colspan="2">

KEY POINTS

About Bacterial Factors in the Pathogenesis of Infective Endocarditis

1. Bacteria with high dextran content stick to non-bacterial thrombotic endocarditis (NBTE) more readily; they also cause dental caries.
   a) *Streptococcus viridans* is the leading cause of subacute bacterial endocarditis.
   b) *S. bovis* also has high dextran content; associated with colonic carcinoma.
2. *Candida albicans* adheres well to NBTE; *C. krusei* adheres poorly.

</td></tr>
</table>

Table 7.1. Causes of Bacteremia Potentially Leading to Endocarditis

Procedure or manipulation	Positive blood culture (%)
Dental	
Dental extraction	18–85
Periodontal surgery	32–88
Gum chewing	15–51
Tooth brushing	0–26
Oral irrigation device	27–50
Upper airway	
Bronchoscopy (rigid scope)	15
Intubation or nasotracheal suction	16
Gastrointestinal	
Upper gastrointestinal endoscopy	8–12
Sigmoidoscopy or colonoscopy	0–9.5
Barium enema	11
Liver biopsy (percutaneous)	3–13
Urologic	
Urethral dilatation	18–33
Urethral catheter	8
Cystoscopy	0–17
Transurethral prostatectomy	12–46

from Everett ED, Hirschmann JV. Transient bacteremia and endocarditis prophylaxis. A review. *Medicine (Baltimore).* 1977; 56:61–77

dextran on the cell wall surface adhere more tightly to dental enamel and to other inert surfaces. Streptococci that produce higher levels of dextran demonstrate an increased ability to cause dental caries and to cause bacterial endocarditis. *Streptococcus viridans*, named for their ability to cause green ("alpha") hemolysis on blood agar plates, often have a high dextran content and are a leading cause of dental caries and bacterial endocarditis. *S. mutans*, and *S. sanguis* are the species in this group that most commonly cause endocarditis.

One group D streptococcus, *S. bovis*, produces high levels of dextran and demonstrates an increased propensity to cause endocarditis. This bacterium often enters the bloodstream via the gastrointestinal tract as a consequence of a colonic carcinoma. *S. viridans* also express the surface adhesin FimA, and this protein is expressed in strains that cause endocarditis. *Candida albicans* readily adheres to NBTE in vitro and causes endocarditis, particularly in intravenous drug abusers and in patients with prosthetic valves. *C. krusei* is non-adherent and seldom causes infective endocarditis.

Adherence to specific constituents in the NBTE also may be important virulence characteristics. For example, pathogenic strains of *S. sanguis* are able to bind to platelet receptors, and endocarditis-causing strains of *Staphylococcus aureus* demonstrate increased binding to fibrinogen and fibronectin.

CAUSES OF BACTEREMIA LEADING TO ENDOCARDITIS

Before bacteria can adhere to NBTE, they must gain entry to the bloodstream. Whenever a mucosal surface heavily colonized with bacterial flora is traumatized, a small number of bacteria enter the bloodstream, where they are quickly cleared by the spleen and liver. As outlined in Table 7.1, dental manipulations frequently

<table>
<tr><td>

KEY POINTS

About Causes of Bacteremia Potentially Leading to Infective Endocarditis

1. Causes of bacteremia that can lead to infective endocarditis.
   a) Dental manipulations (extraction, periodontal surgery), oral irrigators (Waterpik)
   b) Tonsillectomy
   c) Urology procedures (urethral dilatation, cystoscopy, prostatectomy
   d) Pulmonary procedures (rigid bronchoscopy, intubation)
   e) Gastrointestinal (GI) procedures (upper GI endoscopy, sigmoidoscopy, colonoscopy)

</td></tr>
</table>

precipitate transient bacteremia. Patients undergoing dental extraction or periodontal surgery are at particularly high risk, but gum chewing and tooth brushing can also lead to bacteremia. Oral irrigation devices such as the Waterpik should be avoided in patients with known valvular heart disease or prosthetic valves, because these devices precipitate bacteremia more frequently than simple tooth brushing does. Other manipulations that can cause significant transient bacteremia include tonsillectomy, urethral dilatation, transurethral prostatic resection, and cystoscopy. Pulmonary and gastrointestinal procedures cause bacteremia in a low percentage of patients.

Causes of Infective Endocarditis

The organisms most frequently associated with infective endocarditis are able to colonize the mucosa, enter the bloodstream, and adhere to NBTE or native endocardium (see Table 7.2). In native valve endocarditis, *Streptococcus* species are the most common cause, representing more than half of all cases. *S. viridans* species are most frequent, followed by *S. bovis*. *Staphylococcus* species are the second most common cause, and in

some recent series, they have exceeded the streptococci in frequency. *Staphylococcus aureus* predominates, with coagulase-negative staphylococci playing a minor role. Enterococci (*S. faecalis* and *S. faecium*) are now classified separately from the streptococci, and in most series, these organisms are the third most common cause of infective endocarditis. Other rarer organisms include gram-negative aerobic bacteria, and the HACEK (*Haemophilus aphrophilus, Actinobacillus - actinomycetemcomitans, Cardiobacterium hominis, Eikenella corrodens*, and *Kingella kingae*) group. These slow-growing organisms are found in the mouth and require CO_2 for optimal growth. They may not be detected on routine blood cultures that are discarded after 7 days. Anaerobes, *Coxiella burnetii* ("Q fever endocarditis"), and *Chlamydia* species are exceedingly rare causes. In about 3% to 5% of cases, cultures are repeatedly negative.

In intravenous drug abusers, the microbiology differs, with *S. aureus* and gram-negative organisms predominating (Table 7.2). In certain areas of the country—for example, Detroit, Michigan—methicillin-resistant *S. aureus* (MRSA) is the predominant pathogen. *Pseudomonas aeruginosa*, found in tap water, is

Table 7.2. Microorganisms That Cause Infective Endocarditis

Organism	Native valve (%)	IV drug abuser (%)	Prosthetic valve	
			Early (%)	Late (%)
Streptococcus spp.	60–80	15	<10	35
S. viridans	30–40	5	<5	25
S. bovis	10	<5	<5	<5
Other	<5	<5	<5	<5
Staphylococcus spp.	20–35	50	50	30
Coagulase-positive	10–27	50	20	10
Coagulase-negative	1–3	<5	30	20
Enterococcus spp.	5–18	8	<5	<5
Gram-negative bacilli	<5	15	20	20
Miscellaneous bacteria	<5	5	5	5
HACEK group	<5	<1	<1	<5
Corynebacterium and *Propionibacterium*	<1	<5	<5	<5
Anaerobes	<1	<1	<1	<1
Fungi	<5	5	5	5
Coxiella burnetii	<1	<1	<1	<1
Polymicrobial	<1	<5	<5	<5
Culture-negative	3–5	3–5	<5	<5

Adapted from Schlant RC, Alexander RW, O'Rourke RA, Soonneblick EH, eds. Hurst's The Heart. 8th ed. New York, NY: McGraw–Hill; 1994: pp. 1681–1709.

KEY POINTS

About the Causes of Infective Endocarditis

1. Native valve endocarditis:
   a) Most common cause is streptococci: *S. viridans* is number one, then *S. faecalis* (*Enterococcus*) and *S. bovis* (associated with colonic cancer)
   b) *Staphylococcus aureus* is the second most common cause.
   c) HACEK group is an uncommon cause, but consider in culture-negative cases (hold blood cultures for more than 7 days).
2. Intravenous drug abusers:
   a) Most common cause is *S. aureus*.
   b) Gram-negative aerobic bacilli are the second most common cause; *Pseudomonas aeruginosa*
   c) Fungi
   d) Multiple organisms
3. Prosthetic valve:
   a) "Early" is the result of nosocomial pathogens: *S. aureus*, coagulase-negative staphylococci, gram-negative bacilli, fungi
   b) "Late" (more than 2 months post-op) is the result of mouth and skin flora: *S. viridans*, coagulase-negative staphylococci, *S. aureus*, gram-negative bacilli, fungi

the most common gram-negative organism. Streptococci also are common, particularly *Enterococcus* and *S. viridans* species. Fungi, primarily *C. albicans*, is another important cause of endocarditis in this population. Polymicrobial disease is also more frequent.

The causes of prosthetic valve endocarditis depend on the timing of the infection (Table 7.2). The development of endocarditis within the first 2 months after surgery ("early prosthetic valve endocarditis") is primarily caused by nosocomial pathogens. Staphylococcal species (coagulase-positive and -negative strains alike), gram-negative aerobic bacilli, and fungi predominate. In disease that develops more than 2 months after surgery ("late prosthetic valve endocarditis"), organisms originating from the mouth and skin flora predominate: *S. viridans* species, *S. aureus*, and coagulase-negative staphylococci being most common. Gram-negative aerobic bacilli and fungi are less common, but still important pathogens.

Clinical Manifestations

CASE 7.1

A 78-year-old retired advertising executive was admitted to the hospital with a chief complaint of increasing shortness of breath and ankle swelling. About 15 weeks before admission, he had had some dental work done. About 2 weeks after that work was completed, he began to experience shortness of breath following any physical exertion. He also noted increasing fatigue, night sweats, and intermittent low-grade fever. At that time, a diastolic murmur, II/VI was noted along the left sternal border, maximal at the third intercostal space. He was treated as an outpatient with diuretics for left-sided congestive heart failure (CHF).

The day before admission, he began experiencing increasingly severe shortness of breath. He also began coughing frothy pink phlegm, and he arrived in the emergency room gasping for air.

Physical examination showed a temperature of 39°C, blood pressure of 106/66 mm Hg, a pulse of 85 per minute regular, and a respiratory rate of 36 per minute. The patient appeared lethargic and had rapid shallow respirations. His teeth were in good repair. No hemorrhages or exudates were seen in the fundi. With the patients sitting at a 30-degree angle, the jugular veins were distended to the level of his jaw; diffuse wheezes and rales were heard in lower two thirds of both lung fields. The heart demonstrated a loud S3 gallop, II/VI nearly holosystolic murmur heard loudest in the left third intercostal space radiating to the apex, and a II/VI diastolic murmur heard best along left sternal border. Liver and spleen were not palpable. Pitting edema of the ankles(2+) extending midway up the thighs was noted. Nail beds had no splinter hemorrhages. Pulses were 2+ bilaterally.

The laboratory workup found a white blood cell (WBC) count of 11,700/mm³, with 69% polymorphonuclear leukocytes, 4% band forms, 22% lymphocytes, and 3% mononuclear cells, and a hematocrit of 30%, normochromic, normocytic. Urinalysis showed 1+ protein with 10 to 20 red blood cells and 5 to 10 white blood cells per high-power field. The patient's erythrocyte sedimentation rate was 67 mm/h. An electrocardiogram showed normal sinus rhythm, with left bundle branch block. A chest radiograph revealed extensive diffuse perihilar infiltration bilaterally. Four of four blood cultures were positive for S. viridans.

HISTORY

When the event leading to bacteremia can be identified, the incubation period usually required before symptoms develop is less than 2 weeks. In case 7.1, the onset of symptoms occurred 15 days after dental work. Because symptoms of endocarditis are usually nonspecific, a delay of 5 weeks occurs, on average, between the onset of symptoms and diagnosis. In case 7.1, the delay was 3 months.

As observed in this patient, the most common symptom is a low-grade fever. Body temperature is usually only mildly elevated in the 38°C range, and with the exception of acute endocarditis, it seldom rises above 40°C. Fever is frequently accompanied by chills and less commonly by night sweats. Fatigue, anorexia, weakness, and malaise are common complaints, and the patient often experiences weight loss. Myalgias and arthralgias are also common complaints. Patients are often mistakenly suspected of having a malignancy, connective tissue disease, or other chronic infection such as tuberculosis.

Another prominent complaint in a smaller percentage of patients is low back pain. Debilitating back pain that limits movement can be the presenting complaint, and health care personnel should always consider infective endocarditis as one possible cause of low back pain and fever. Systemic emboli can result in sudden hemiparesis or sudden limb pain as a consequence of tissue ischemia. In all patients who suffer a sudden accident consistent with an embolic stoke, infective endocarditis should be excluded.

In addition to a subacute onset, some patients can present with rapid onset (hours to days) of symptoms and signs. Acute infective endocarditis is most commonly associated with *S. aureus* or enterococci, and occasionally with *S. pneumoniae*. Fever is often high, 40°C, accompanied by rigors. These patients are usually brought to the emergency room acutely ill. The likelihood of serious cardiac and extravascular complications is higher in these patients, particularly those with acute *S. aureus* endocarditis. Rapid diagnosis and treatment are mandatory to reduce valvular destruction and embolic complications.

PHYSICAL FINDINGS

The classical physical findings of infective endocarditis should be carefully searched for. Fever is the rule and is detected in 95% of patients. A heart murmur is almost

---

KEY POINTS

About the History in Infective Endocarditis

1. Nonspecific symptoms usually begin 2 weeks after initial bacteremia.
2. On average, diagnosis takes 5 weeks from onset of symptoms.
3. Low-grade fever is most common, may be accompanied by night sweats.
4. Fatigue, malaise, generalized weakness, anorexia, and weight loss are common; mimics cancer.
5. Myalgias and arthralgias may suggest a connective tissue disease.
6. Low back pain can be the initial primary complaint. Consider endocarditis, epidural abscess, and osteomyelitis when back pain is accompanied by fever.
7. Infective endocarditis must be excluded in all cases of embolic cerebrovascular accident, particularly in younger patients.
8. In acute endocarditis, fever is high (40°C range), and the patient appears acutely ill.

KEY POINTS

About the Physical Findings in Infective Endocarditis

1. A cardiac murmur is heard in nearly all patients.
   a) Absence of a murmur should call into question the diagnosis of infective endocarditis.
   b) Classic changing murmur is rare, but it may occur with rupture of chordae tendinae.
   c) New aortic regurgitation is the result of infective endocarditis until proven otherwise.
2. Embolic phenomenon are found in up to 50% of cases.
   a) are most common in the conjunctiva; clusters can be found anywhere.
   b) Splinter hemorrhages, linear streaks, are found under nails.
   c) Osler nodes, painful raised lesion in the pads of the fingers or toes, are evanescent.
   d) Janeway lesions, red macules, are more persistent and most common in acute endocarditis attributable to *Staphylococcus aureus*.
   e) Roth spots are retinal hemorrhages with a clear center.
3. Splenomegaly can be found; left upper quadrant tenderness can occur with embolic infarction.
4. Check all pulses as a baseline because of the risk of obstructive emboli.
5. Perform a thorough neurologic exam; a sudden embolic stroke can develop.

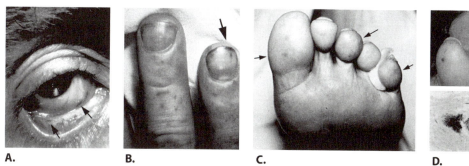

A.   **B.**   **C.**   **D.**

Figure 7–1. Embolic phenomena in infective endocarditis. **A.** Conjunctival petechiae: Arrows point to two discrete linear hemorrhages. **B.** Nail-bed splinter hemorrhage: Multiple petechiae are seen on both fingers. Arrow points to a splinter hemorrhage underlying the nail bed. **C.** Osler nodes: Arrows point to subtle discolorations of the pads of the toes. These sites were raised and tender to palpation. **D.** Janeway lesions: Painless hemorrhagic lesions (left). Biopsy of a typical lesion shows thrombosis and intravascular gram-positive cocci (right). Culture was positive for *Staphylococcus aureus.* *See color image on color plate 1 & 2*

always seen. The absence of an audible murmur should call into question the diagnosis of endocarditis, except in cases of right-sided endocarditis or infection of a mural thrombus (rare). Although classically described as a changing murmur, the character of the murmur usually does not change significantly over time unless a valve leaflet is destroyed (occurs most commonly with *S. aureus*) or a chordae tendinae ruptures. Detection of a new aortic regurgitant murmur is a bad prognostic sign and is commonly associated with the development of CHF, as described in case 7.1. The most common cause of acute aortic regurgitation is infective endocarditis; therefore, if a high-pitched diastolic murmur radiating along the left sternal border is heard, the initial workup should always include blood cultures. In case 7.1, the diagnosis was delayed because this man's outpatient physician did not exclude infective endocarditis as the cause of the new diastolic murmur.

Careful attention must be paid to the fundi, skin, nail beds, and peripheral pulses, because manifestations attributable to emboli are noted in more than half of infective endocarditis cases. Fundoscopic exam may reveal classic Roth spots, retinal hemorrhages with pale centers, or, more commonly, flame-shaped hemorrhages. One of the most common locations to detect petechial - hemorrhages is the conjunctiva [Figure 7.1(A)]. This finding is not specific for endocarditis, however; it is also seen in patients after cardiac surgery and in patients with thrombocytopenia.

Clusters of petechiae can be seen on any part of the body. Other common locations are the buccal mucosa, palate, and extremities. Presence of petechiae alone should be considered a nonspecific finding. The splinter hemorrhages (linear red or brownish streaks) that develop under the nail beds of the hands and feet are caused by emboli lodging in distal capillaries [Figure 7.1(B)]. These lesions can also be caused by trauma to the fingers or toes. Osler nodes are small pea-sized subcutaneous, painful erythematous nodules that arise in the pads of the fingers and toes and in the thenar eminence [Figure 7.1(C)]. They are usually present only for a brief period, disappearing within hours to days. Janeway lesions are most commonly seen in association with *S. aureus* infection [Figure 7.1(D)]. These hemorrhagic plaques usually develop on the palms and soles. Bacteria can sometimes be visualized on a skin biopsy of the lesion [Figure 7.1(D)]. It must be kept in mind that, as observed in case 7.1, about half of all patients with infective endocarditis will demonstrate no physical evidence of peripheral emboli. The absence of embolic phenomena therefore does not exclude the diagnosis.

Other findings can include clubbing of the fingers and toes. As a consequence of earlier diagnosis and treatment, this manifestation is less common than in the past, but it may be found in patients with prolonged symptoms. Another commonly reported finding is splenomegaly. Some patients experience left upper quadrant pain and tenderness as result of splenic infarction caused by septic emboli. Joint effusions are uncommon; however, diffuse arthralgias and joint stiffness are frequently encountered.

Finally, all pulses should be checked periodically. A sudden loss of a peripheral pulse, accompanied by limb pain, warrants immediate arteriography to identify and extract occluding emboli. A thorough neurologic exam must also be performed. Confusion, severe headache, or focal neurologic deficits should be further investigated by computed tomography (CT) or magnetic resonance imaging (MRI) scan with contrast of the head looking for embolic infarction, intracerebral hemorrhage, or brain abscess.

LABORATORY FINDINGS

Laboratory abnormalities are nonspecific in nature. Case 7.1 had many of the typical laboratory findings of infective endocarditis. Anemia of chronic disease is noted in 70% to 90% of subacute cases. A normocytic, normochromic red cell morphology, low serum iron, and low iron binding capacity characterize this form of anemia. Peripheral leukocyte count is usually normal. The finding of an elevated peripheral WBC count should raise the possibility of a myocardial abscess or another extravascular focus of infection. Leukocytosis is also often found in patients with acute bacterial endocarditis. The erythrocyte sedimentation rate, a measure of chronic inflammation, is almost always elevated. With the exception of patients with hemoglobinopathies that falsely lower the rate of red blood cell sedimentation, the finding of a normal sedimentation rate virtually excludes the diagnosis of infective endocarditis. In nearly all cases, C-reactive protein, another inflammatory marker, is also elevated. A positive rheumatoid factor is detected in half of these patients, and elevated serum globulins are found in 20% to 30% of cases. Cryoglobulins, depressed complement levels, positive tests for immune complexes, and a false positive serology for syphilis are other nonspecific findings that may accompany infective endocarditis. Urinalysis is frequently abnormal, with proteinuria being found in 50% to 65% of cases, and hematuria in 30% to 50%. These abnormalities are the consequence of embolic injury or deposition of immune complexes causing glomerulonephritis.

A chest X-ray should be performed in all patients with suspected endocarditis. In patients with right-sided disease, distinct round cannonball-like infiltrates may be detected; these represent pulmonary emboli. In cases of acute mitral regurgitation or decompensated left-sided failure because of aortic regurgitation, diffuse alveolar fluid may be detected, indicating pulmonary edema. Finally the patient's electrocardiogram should be closely monitored. The finding of a conduction defect raises concern that infection has spread to the conduction system; in some cases, this spread may progress to complete heart block. In case 7.1, the PR interval was prolonged, and this patient subsequently developed complete heart block. Findings consistent with myocardial infarct may be detected when emboli are released from vegetations in the coronary cusps into the coronary arteries.

Diagnosis

BLOOD CULTURES

Blood cultures are the critical test for making a diagnosis of infective endocarditis. As compared with most tissue infections—such as pneumonia and pyelonephritis—that result in the intermittent release of large numbers of bacteria into the blood, infective endocarditis is associated with a constant low-level bacteremia (Figure 7.2). The vegetation is like a time-release capsule, with bacteria

---

KEY POINTS

About the Laboratory Findings in Infective Endocarditis

1. Anemia of chronic disease is found in most patients.
2. The peripheral white blood cell count is normal, unless myocardial abscess or acute disease is present.
3. Manifestations of chronic antigenemia mimic a connective tissue disorder:
   a) Elevated sedimentation rate and C-reactive protein
   b) Positive rheumatoid factor
   c) Elevated immunoglobulins, cryoglobulins, and immune complexes
   d) Decreased complement
   e) Hematuria and proteinuria
4. A chest radiograph may be abnormal:
   a) Circular, cannonball-like lesions in embolic right-sided endocarditis
   b) Pulmonary edema pattern secondary to left-sided congestive heart failure
5. Monitor the electrocardiogram closely; conduction defects can progress to complete heart block.

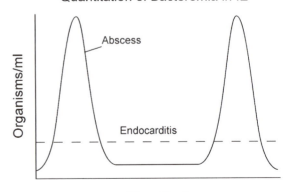

Figure 7–2. Concentration of bacteria in the bloodstream over time in infective endocarditis versus bacteremia caused by other infections.

being constantly released in small numbers into the bloodstream. It is this constant antigenic stimulus that accounts for the rheumatic complaints and multiple abnormal serum markers associated with infective endocarditis.

To document the presence of a constant bacteremia, blood samples for culture should be drawn at least 15 minutes apart. In patients with suspected subacute infective endocarditis, three blood cultures are recommended over the first 24 hours. In these patients, antibiotics should be withheld until the blood cultures are confirmed to be positive because administration of even a single dose of antibiotics can lower the number of bacteria in the bloodstream to undetectable levels and prevent identification of the pathogen. However, if the patient is acutely ill, three samples for culture should be drawn over 45 minutes, with empiric therapy begun immediately thereafter.

Because the number of bacteria in the blood is usually low (approximately 100/mL), a minimum of 10 mL of blood should be inoculated into each blood culture flask. Lower volumes reduce the yield and may account for many culture-negative cases. Routinely, blood cultures are held in the microbiology laboratory for 7 days and are discarded if negative. However, if a member of the slow-growing HACEK group is suspected, the laboratory must be alerted to hold the blood cultures for 4 weeks and to subculture the samples on chocolate agar in 5% CO_2. If nutritionally deficient streptococci are suspected, specific nutrients need to be added to the blood culture medium.

The sensitivity of blood cultures is excellent, yields being estimated to be 85% to 95% on the first blood culture and improving to 95% to 100% with a second blood culture. The third blood culture is drawn primarily to document the constancy of the bacteremia; it does not significantly improve overall sensitivity. The administration of antibiotics within 2 weeks of blood cultures lowers the sensitivity, and patients who have received antibiotics often require multiple blood cultures spaced over days to weeks to identify the cause of the disease.

ECHOCARDIOGRAPHY

Echocardiography is the other essential test that all patients with suspected infective endocarditis must receive. Transthoracic echocardiography (TTE) is relatively insensitive (44% to 63%) for detecting vegetations as compared with transesophageal echocardiography (TEE: 94% to 100% sensitivity), which can detect vegetations smaller than 3 mm. As compared with TTE, TEE more readily detects extravalvular extension of infection (87% vs. 28% sensitivity); and more accurately visualizes valve perforations (95% vs. 45% sensitivity). A TEE is also preferred for investigating prosthetic valve endocarditis. When accompanied

---

KEY POINTS

About the Diagnosis of Infective Endocarditis

1. Blood cultures document constant bacteremia with an endocarditis-associated pathogen:
   a) Blood cultures spaced at least 15 minutes apart, three over 24 hours for subacute bacterial endocarditis.
   b) Large volumes of blood (at least 10 mL) need to be added to blood culture flasks.
   c) Blood cultures are usually negative for at least 7 days after an antibiotic is given.
2. Documentation of endocardial involvement [transesophageal echocardiography (TEE) is more sensitive than transthoracic echocardiography]; TEE always preferred in prosthetic valve endocarditis.
3. Duke criteria are helpful in making the clinical diagnosis of infective endocarditis in the absence of pathologic tissue.

---

by Doppler-color flow analysis, echocardiography can assess valve function, myocardial contractility, and chamber volume—vital information for deciding on surgical intervention.

THE MODIFIED DUKE CRITERIA

A definitive diagnosis of infective endocarditis in the absence of valve tissue histopathology or culture is often difficult, and many investigations of this disease have been plagued by differences in the clinical definition of infective endocarditis. Clinical criteria have been established that allow cases to be classified as definite and possible (Table 7.3). Using the modified Duke criteria, a finding of 2 major criteria, or 1 major criterion and 3 minor criteria, or 5 minor criteria classifies a case as definite infective endocarditis. A finding of 1 major and 1 minor criterion, or 3 minor criteria, classifies a case as possible infective endocarditis.

Complications

In the modern antibiotic era, complications associated with infective endocarditis remain common, with approximately 60% of patients experiencing one complication; 25%, two; and 8%, three or more complications.

CARDIAC COMPLICATIONS

Complications involving the heart are most frequent, occuring in one third to one half of patients. Congestive

Tabel 7.3. Modified Duke Criteria for the Diagnosis of Bacterial Endocarditis

Major criteria	Minor criteria	Definite infective endocarditis	Possible infective endocarditis
1. Two separate blood cultures, both positive for typical endocarditis-associated organisms, including *Staphylococcus aureus* OR Persistent positive blood cultures—two more than 12 hours apart, or three, or a majority from among more than four, during 1 hour. 2. Evidence of endocardial involvement by positive echocardiogram (for patients with possible infective endocarditis, TEE is recommended) OR New regurgitant murmur 3. Positive Q fever serology (antiphase I IgG > 1:800), or single blood culture positive for *Coxiella burnetii*	1. Predisposing heart condition 2. Fever of 38°C or more 3. Vascular phenomena 4. Immunologic phenomena 5. Single positive blood culture with typical organisms 6. Previous minor criterion of suspicious lesion on TTE now eliminated	2 major criteria, or 1 major criterion and 3 minor criteria, or 5 minor criteria	1 major and 1 minor criterion, or 3 minor criteria

TEE = transesophageal echocardiography; TTE = transthoracic echocardiography; IgG = immunoglobulin G.

Li JS, Sexton DJ, Mick N, et al. Proposed modifications to the Duke criteria for the diagnosis of infective endocarditis. *Clin Infect Dis.* 2000;30:633–638.

heart failure is the most common complication that leads to surgical intervention. Destruction of the valve leaflets results in regurgitation. Less commonly, vegetations become large enough to obstruct the outflow tract and cause stenosis. Perivalvular extension of infection also requires surgical intervention. This complication is more common with aortic valve disease, and spread from the aortic valvular ring to the adjacent conduction system can lead to heart block. This complication should be suspected in the infective endocarditis patient with peripheral leukocytosis, persistent fever while on appropriate antibiotics, or an abnormal conduction time on electrocardiogram. Transesophageal echo detects most cases, and this test should be performed in all patients with aortic valve endocarditis. Less common complications include pericarditis and myocardial infarction.

SYSTEMIC EMBOLI

Pieces of the vegetation—consisting of a friable collection of platelets, fibrin, and bacteria—frequently break off and become lodged in arteries and arterioles throughout the body. Small emboli are likely released in all cases of endocarditis, but they are symptomatic in only one sixth to one third of patients. Patients with large vegetations (exceeding 10 mm) and vegetations on the anterior leaflet of the mitral valve are at higher risk for systemic emboli. Because the right brachiocephalic trunk (innominate artery) is the first vessel to branch from the ascending aortic arch, emboli have a higher likelihood of passing through that vessel and into the right internal carotid artery.

The second branch coming off the aortic arch is the left common carotid artery, and the likelihood of emboli entering this vessel is also higher. These anatomic considerations probably account for the observation that two thirds of left-sided systemic emboli from the heart lodge in the central nervous system. In addition to sudden neurologic deficits, patients can experience ischemic limbs and splenic and renal infarction.

Patients with right-sided endocarditis frequently develop recurrent pulmonary emboli. Symptomatic emboli more commonly occur in patients with *S. aureus* and fungal endocarditis and in patients infected with slow-growing organisms such as those in the HACEK group. Antibiotic therapy is associated with fibrotic changes in the vegetation, and after 2 weeks of therapy, the risk of emboli is markedly reduced.

MYCOTIC ANEURYSMS

Infectious emboli can become lodged at arterial bifurcations, where they occlude the vasa vasorum or the entire vessel lumen, damaging the muscular layer of the vessel. The systemic arterial pressure causes ballooning of the weakened vessel wall and formation of an aneurysm. Aneurysms are most commonly encountered in the middle cerebral artery, abdominal aorta, and mesenteric arteries. On occasion, these aneurysms can burst, resulting in intracerebral or intra-abdominal hemorrhage. Because of the increased risk of hemorrhage, anticoagulation should be avoided in patients with infective endocarditis. Mycotic aneurysms are most commonly encountered in *S. aureus* endocarditis.

NEUROLOGIC COMPLICATIONS

Complications arising in the central nervous system are second only to cardiac complications in frequency, being seen in 25% to 35% of patients. In addition to embolic stokes and intracerebral hemorrhage, patients can develop encephalopathy, meningitis, meningoencephalitis, and brain abscess. In the past, development of a neurologic deficit was considered a contraindication to cardiac surgery. More recent experience indicates that surgery within 1 week of the neurologic event is not accompanied by worsening neurologic deficits.

RENAL COMPLICATIONS

Significant renal failure (serum creatinine above 2 mg/dL) can develop in up to one third of patients, with the likelihood of this complication being higher in elderly patients and in those with thrombocytopenia. Renal dysfunction can be caused by immune-complex glomerulonephritis, renal emboli, and drug-induced interstitial nephritis. Glomerulonephritis results from deposition of immune complex in the basement membranes of the glomeruli, resulting in the microscopic changes of membranoproliferative disease. Urinalysis reveals hematuria and mild proteinuria. Red cell casts are observed in glomerulonephritis, but not in interstitial nephritis. Glomerulonephritis usually improves rapidly with antibiotic therapy.

Treatment

ANTIBIOTICS

Whenever possible, the antibiotic therapy of subacute infective endocarditis should be based on the antibiotic sensitivities of the offending organism or organisms (Table 7.4 lists doses). Because bacteria are protected

---

KEY POINTS

About Complications Associated with Infective Endocarditis

1. Cardiac complications occur in up to half of patients:
   a) Congestive heart failure
   b) Myocardial abscess (aortic disease associated with conduction defects)
   c) Myocardial infarction (rare complication of aortic disease)
2. Two thirds of systemic emboli go to the cerebral cortex.
3. Neurologic complications can arise from emboli:
   a) Embolic stroke (most commonly with *Staphylococcus aureus*, fungi, and HACEK group organisms)
   b) Mycotic aneurysms (most common with *S. aureus* infection)
   c) Encephalopathy, meningitis, and brain abscess
4. Renal complications are possible:
   a) Membranoproliferative glomerulonephritis resulting from deposition of immune complex
   b) Interstitial nephritis
   c) Embolic damage

---

from neutrophil ingestion by the dense coating of fibrin found in the vegetation, bactericidal antibiotics are required to cure this infection. To design the most effective regimen, minimal bactericidal levels should be determined for multiple antibiotics, and combinations of these antibiotics tested for synergy (see Chapter 1). The goal is to achieve serum cidal levels of 1:8 to 1:32, these levels of cidal activity being associated with cure.

A second important principle of antibiotic therapy is the requirement for prolonged treatment. The concentrations of bacteria in the vegetation are high, and a significant percentage of the bacteria slow their metabolism and stop actively dividing for significant periods. These conditions prevent immediate sterilization by cidal antibiotics that require active bacterial growth for their action (penicillins, cephalosporins, and glycopeptide antibiotics). To prevent relapse, most curative regimens are continued for 4 to 6 weeks. One exception is uncomplicated subacute bacterial endocarditis caused by *S. viridans* species. The combination of penicillin G and gentamicin is synergistic and is associated with more rapid killing of bacteria in vegetations.

Table 7.4. Antibiotic Therapy for Infective Endocarditis

Drug	Dose	Relative efficacy	Comments (duration 4–6 weeks unless otherwise noted)
Acute—empiric			
Vancomycin, plus	30 mg/kg IV q24h, divided q12h		Vancomycin more slowly cidal; whenever possible use an alternative
ampicillin, plus	12 g IV q24h, divided q4h		
gentamicin	1 mg/kg IV q8h		
Culture-negative			
Ampicillin, plus	12 g IV q24h, divided q4h		
gentamicin	1 mg/kg IV q8h		
Prosthetic—empiric			
Vancomycin, plus	1 g IV q12h		Duration 6–8 weeks
gentamicin, plus	1 mg/kg IV q8h		Duration 2 weeks
rifampin	600 mg PO q24h		Duration 6–8 weeks
Streptococcus viridans			
Penicillin G OR	24×10^6 U IV q24h[a] or divided q4h	First line	Short course if uncomplicated. Use sensitivity testing to determine best regimen
Ampicillin, plus gentamicin	12 g IV q24h, divided q4h		Duration 2 weeks
	1 mg/kg IV q8h or 3 mg/kg q24h		Duration 2 weeks
Ceftriaxone, plus	2 g IV q24h	Alternative	Short course if uncomplicated; duration 2 weeks for both
gentamicin	1 mg/kg IV q8h		
Vancomycin	30 mg/kg IV q12h	Alternative	For the penicillinallergic patient; duration 4 weeks
Enterococcus			
Ampicillin OR	12 g IV q24h, divided q4h	First line	Relapse is common in the absence of gentamicin; use sensitivity to determine best regimen
Penicillin G, plus	24×10^6 U IV q24h or divided q4h		Duration 2–6 weeks
gentamicin	1 mg/kg IV q8h		
Methicillin-sensitive Staphylococcus aureus (MSSA)			
Nafcillin or	12 g q24h[a] or	First line	Addition of gentamicin may shorten bacteremia, but has no effect on final outcome; duration 6 weeks (either one)
Oxacillin, with or without	divided q4h		
gentamicin	3 mg/kg IV q24h	Duration 3–5 days	For non-anaphylactic
Cefazolin, with or without	2 g IV q8h duration 6 weeks	Second line	reactions to penicillin
gentamicin	3 mg/kg IV q24h	Duration 3–5 days	

(Continued)

Table 7.4. *(Continued)*

Drug	Dose	Relative efficacy	Comments (duration 4–6 weeks unless otherwise noted)
Methicillin-resistant Staphylococcus aureus (MRSA)			
Vancomycin	30 mg/kg IV q24h, divided q12h	First line	Slow response; duration 6 weeks
Daptomycin	6 mg/kg IV q24h	First line	Comparable outcome to vancomycin. Staphylococcus aureus *(tricuspid)*
Nafcillin or	12 g IV q24h[a] or	First line	Short course effective if no metastatic lesions
Oxacillin, plus gentamicin	divided q4h 1 mg/kg IV q8h		and MSSA; duration 2 weeks Duration 6 weeks
Ciprofloxacin, plus	750 mg PO q12h	Second line	May be effective in MSSA; duration 4 weeks
rifampin	300 mg PO q12h		Duration 4 weeks

Based on the American Heart Association guidelines 2005.

Combination therapy for 2 weeks results in cure rates similar to those with penicillin alone for 4 weeks. A 2-week course of ceftriaxone and gentamicin achieves comparable results. The gentamicin dose should be adjusted to maintain peak serum levels of 3 μg/mL, the concentration required to achieve synergy.

In acute bacterial endocarditis, intravenous empiric antibiotic therapy should be initiated immediately after three blood samples for culture have been drawn. The combination of vancomycin, ampicillin, and gentamicin is recommended to cover the most likely pathogens (*S. aureus*, including MRSA; *S. pneumoniae*, and enterococci), pending culture results. Empiric therapy for culture-negative subacute bacterial endocarditis should include ampicillin and gentamicin to cover for enterococci, the HACEK group, and nutritionally deficient streptococci.

Table 7.4 outlines the regimens for each specific bacterial cause of endocarditis. Whenever possible, a synergistic regimen consisting of a β-lactam antibiotic and an aminoglycoside is preferred. One exception to this rule is *S. aureus*. Combination therapy with nafcillin or oxacillin and gentamicin may shorten the duration of positive blood cultures, but has not been shown to improve mortality or overall cure rates, and therefore dual antibiotic therapy is not recommended. With the exception of ceftazidime, minimum inhibitory concentrations (MICs) for cephalosporins correlate well with therapeutic response, and these agents are often therapeutically equivalent to the semisynthetic penicillins. The β-lactam antibiotics are preferred over vancomycin because vancomycin is less rapidly cidal, and failure rates of up to 40% have been reported when *S. aureus* endocarditis is treated with vancomycin. Daptomycin has been shown to be non-inferior to vancomycin in MRSA bacteremia and endocarditis. In the penicillin-allergic patient with methicillin-sensitive *S. aureus* endocarditis, β-lactam desensitization should be strongly considered. In patients with enterococcal endocarditis, cephalosporins are ineffective and should not be used. Maximal doses of intravenous penicillin or ampicillin combined with gentamicin are preferred, and this combination is recommended for the full course of therapy. However, one series noted comparable cure rates when gentamicin was administered for the first 2 weeks of therapy. Vancomycin combined with gentamicin is a suitable alternative in the penicillin-allergic patient. With the exception of uncomplicated infection with *S. viridans* species, antibiotic treatment should be continued for 4 to 6 weeks.

Antibiotic therapy for prosthetic valve endocarditis presents a particularly difficult challenge. The deposition of biofilm on the prosthetic material makes cure with antibiotics alone difficult, and the valve often has to be replaced. Some patients with late-onset prosthetic valve endocarditis caused by very antibiotic-sensitive organisms can be cured by antibiotic treatment alone. In patients with coagulase-negative staphylococci, a combination of intravenous vancomycin (1 g twice daily), and rifampin (300 mg three times daily) for more than 6 weeks, plus gentamicin (1 mg/kg three times daily) for 2 weeks, is the preferred treatment for methicillin-resistant strains. For methicillin-sensitive strains, nafcillin or oxacillin (2 g every four hours) should be substituted for vancomycin.

Intravenous drug abusers with uncomplicated tricuspid valve *S. aureus* endocarditis can be treated with 2 weeks of intravenous nafcillin or oxacillin (2 g every four hours) combined with tobramycin (1 mg/kg three times daily). This abbreviated regimen is not recommended in HIV-antibody-positive patients. An oral regimen of ciprofloxacin (750 mg twice daily) and rifampin (300 mg twice daily) for 4 weeks has also proved effective, provided that the *S. aureus* strain is sensitive to ciprofloxacin.

SURGERY

Medical therapy alone is often not curative, particularly in prosthetic valve endocarditis. In a significant percentage of patients, surgical removal of the infected valve or debridement of vegetations greatly increases the likelihood of survival. As a consequence, in recent years, the threshold for surgery has been lowered.

In almost all cases of infective endocarditis, the cardiologist and cardiac surgeon should be consulted early in the course of the illness. The decision to operate is often complex, and appropriate timing of surgery must balance the risk of progressive complications with the risk of intraoperative and postoperative morbidity and mortality. Indications for surgery include these:

1. **Moderate-to-severe CHF.** Congestive hear failure is the most frequent indication for surgery. A delay in surgery often results in a fatal outcome because of irreversible left ventricular dysfunction. In patients with CHF, death can be very sudden.

2. **More than one systemic embolus.** The ability to predict the likelihood of recurrent emboli by echocardiography is questionable. In some studies, large vegetations (exceeding 10 mm in diameter) and vegetations on the anterior leaflet of the mitral valve were found to have a higher probability of embolizing.

3. **Uncontrolled infection.** *S. aureus* is one of the most common pathogens to cause persistently positive blood cultures. Extravascular foci of infection should always be excluded before surgical intervention is considered.

4. **Resistant organisms or fungal infection.** The mortality in fungal endocarditis approaches 90%, and with the exception of a rare case of *Candida albicans*, cures have not been achieved by medical therapy alone.

5. **Perivalvular/myocardial abscess.** With the exception of very small abscesses, these lesions usually enlarge on medical therapy and require surgical debridement and repair.

As discussed earlier in "Neurologic complications", a focal neurologic deficit is not an absolute contraindication to surgery. Whenever possible, surgery should be delayed until blood cultures are negative to reduce the risk of septic intraoperative complications. However, even in the setting of ongoing positive blood cultures, infection of the new valve is uncommon, particularly if the surgeon thoroughly debrides the infected site. Relapse following surgery is rare (0.8%) and has not been shown to be related to positive blood cultures at the time of surgery or to positive valve cultures. Identification by PCR of the bacterial cause of valve tissue infection is a promising experimental method that should make diagnosis and treatment of culture-negative bacterial endocarditis more accurate.

Prognosis

Cure rates depend on the organism involved and the valve infected. *S. aureus* remains a particularly virulent pathogen and continues to be associated with a 50% mortality in patients over the age of 50 years. Patients with an infected aortic valve accompanied by regurgitation also have a 50% mortality. Fungal infections and infections with gram-negative aerobic bacilli are associated with poor outcomes. Development of CHF or onset of neurologic deficits is associated with a worse prognosis. Patients with early prosthetic valve endocarditis often do poorly despite valve replacement, with cure rates ranging from 30% to 50%. Late prosthetic valve endocarditis has a better outcome. In patients with late prosthetic valve infection with *S. viridans* species, cure rates of 90% have been achieved when antibiotic therapy is accompanied by surgery and 80% with antibiotic treatment alone. Patients with *S. epidermidis* late prosthetic valve endocarditis have been cured 60% of the time medically, and they have a 70% cure rate when medical treatment is combined with valve replacement.

Prevention

The efficacy of prophylaxis for native-valve endocarditis has never been proved. As documented in Table 7.1, individuals probably experience multiple episodes of transient bacteremia each day, and this cumulative exposure is hundreds of times greater than a single procedure. As a consequence of these concerns, the American Heart Association now recommends antibiotic prophylaxis only for high-risk patients. High-risk patients are defined as patients with prosthetic valves (including bioprosthetic and homograft valves), a past history of endocarditis, complex cyanotic

---

KEY POINTS

About Prophylaxis in Infective Endocarditis

1. The efficacy of prophylaxis has not been proved; however, it is considered the standard of care.
2. Give to high-risk (prosthetic valve, previous endocarditis, cyanotic heart disease, surgical shunt) and moderate-risk (rheumatic and other acquired valvular dysfunction, hypertrophic cardiomyopathy, mitral valve prolapse with regurgitation) patients.
3. Give in time to achieve peak antibiotic levels at the time of the invasive procedure.

---

congenital heart disease, or surgically constructed systemic pulmonary shunts.

Invasive procedures that warrant prophylaxis include these:

• Dental procedures (dental extractions and gingival surgery carry the highest risk)
• Tonsillectomy and adenoidectomy
• Surgical procedures that involve intestinal or respiratory mucosa

The timing of antibiotic prophylaxis is important. The antibiotic should be administered before the procedure and timed so that peak serum levels are achieved at the time of the procedure. Table 7.5 outlines the suggested agents and schedules.

INTRAVASCULAR CATHETER-RELATED INFECTIONS

POTENTIAL SEVERITY

Can be life-threatening. Often prolong hospital stay, and can be complicated by metastatic lesions and bacterial endocarditis.

CASE 7.2

A 53-year-old white woman was admitted to the hospital with complaints of severe shaking during infusion of her hyperalimentation solution. She had been

Table 7.5. Doses and Schedules of Prophylactic Antibiotics in Native-Valve Endocarditis

Patients	Agent	Schedule
Dental, oral, and upper respiratory procedures—all patients, oral administration		
Non-penicillin-allergic	Amoxicillin	2 g PO 1 hour pre-procedure
Penicillin-allergic	Clindamycin OR Cephalexin or cefadroxil OR Azithromycin OR clarithromycin	600 mg PO 1 hour pre-procedure 2 g PO 1 hour pre-procedure 500 mg PO 1 hour pre-procedure
Dental, oral, and upper respiratory procedures-all patients, parenteral administration		
Non-penicillin-allergic	Ampicillin	2 g IM or IV 30 minutes pre-procedure
Penicillin-allergic	Clindamycin OR Cefazolin	600 mg IV 30 minutes pre-procedure 1 g IM or IV 30 minutes pre-procedure Cephalosporins should not be given to a patient with a history of an immediate hypersensitivity reaction to penicillin.

receiving intravenous hyperalimentation for 16 years for a severe dumping syndrome that prevented eating by mouth. She had had multiple complications from her intravenous lines, including venous occlusions and line-associated bacteremia, requiring 24 line replacements. She had last been admitted 6 months earlier with Enterobacter cloacae infection of her intravascular catheter requiring line removal and intravenous cefepime. At that time, a tunneled catheter had been placed in her left subclavian vein, and she had been doing well until the evening before admission. As she was infusing her solution, she developed rigors, and her temperature rose to 39.2°C. She continued to experience chills and developed a headache.

On physical examination, her temperature was found to be 38°C and her blood pressure, 136/50 mm Hg. She was nontoxic appearing. A II/VI systolic ejection murmur was noted along the left sternal border (present for years). The site of the catheter was not erythematous or tender. Two blood cultures were positive for Escherichia coli. The sample from the catheter became culture-positive 6 hours after being drawn, and a simultaneous peripheral blood sample became culture-positive 5 hours after that (11 hours after being drawn).

Epidemiology and Pathogenesis

More than 200,000 nosocomial bloodstream infections occur annually in the United States. A large proportion of these infections are related to intravascular devices. Bacteria most commonly infect catheters by tracking subcutaneously along outside of the catheter into the fibrin sheath that surrounds the intravascular segment of the catheter. Bacteria can also be inadvertently introduced into the hub and lumen of the catheter from the skin of a caregiver or as a consequence of a contaminated infusate. Less commonly, catheters can be infected by hematogenous spread caused by a primary infection at another site.

Once bacteria invade the fibrin sheath surrounding the catheter, they generate a biofilm that protects them from attack by neutrophils. This condition makes sterilization by antibiotics alone difficult. The risk of infection is greater for some devices than others:

1. Catheters
   a) Internal jugular > vein femoral vein > subclavian
   b) Non-tunneled > tunneled
   c) Centrally inserted central venous > peripherally inserted central
   d) Conventional tips > silver-impregnated tips
   e) Hemodialysis > others

2. Ports and other devices
   a) Tunneled > totally implanted
   b) Hyperalimentation > standard infusion

Regular exchange of central venous catheters over guidewires does not reduce the incidence of infection. In fact, reinsertion of a catheter through an infected soft-tissue site can precipitate bacteremia.

The organisms most commonly associated with intravascular device infection are skin flora. Gram-positive cocci predominate, with coagulase-negative staphylococci being most common, followed by *S. aureus*. Coagulase-negative staphylococci produce a glycocalyx that enhances its adherence to synthetic

Clinical Manifestations and Diagnosis

The clinical presentation of intravascular device–related infection is nonspecific, generally involving fever, chills, and malaise. The finding of purulence around the intravascular device is helpful, but this sign is not always present. The absence of an alternative source for bacteremia should always raise the possibility of intravascular device infection. As observed in case 7.2, the abrupt onset of chills or hypotension during infusion of a solution through a device strongly suggests catheter-associated infection or contamination of the infusate. The rapid resolution of symptoms following removal of the device, plus positive blood cultures for coagulase-negative staphylococci, corynebacteria, or a fungus are other findings that suggest an infected intravascular device. However, the absence of these findings does not exclude the diagnosis.

Rapid diagnosis can be achieved by drawing 100 µL blood from the catheter while still in place, subjecting the sample to cytospin, and performing Gram and acridine

---

KEY POINTS

About the Epidemiology and Pathogenesis of Intravascular Catheter-Related Infections

1. Bacteria infect catheters in three ways:
   a) Skin flora migrate along the catheter track
   b) Bacteria are injected into the port
   c) Hematogenous spread occurs
2. Catheter location and type affect the risk of infection.
3. Regular exchange of central venous catheters over guidewires does not reduce the incidence of infection; the technique is not recommended, because it can precipitate bacteremia.
4. Gram-positive cocci predominate:
   a) Coagulase-negative staphylococci are the most common, adhere to catheters using a glycocalyx
   b) *S. aureus*
   c) Enterococci
   d) Corynebacteria
5. Gram-negative organisms account for one third of infections:
   a) *Enterobacter* species, *Escherichia coli*, *Acinetobacter* species, *Pseudomonas* species, and *Serratia* species.
   b) *Klebsiella* species, *Citrobacter*, or non-aeruginosa strains of *Pseudomonas* are associated with contaminated infusate.
6. *Candida albicans* also forms an adherent glycocalyx; associated with high glucose solutions.

KEY POINTS

About the Clinical Manifestations and Diagnosis of Intravascular Catheter–Related Infections

1. Symptoms are nonspecific. These historical facts are suggestive:
   a) Rigors or chills associated with infusion
   b) Resolution of symptoms on removal of the intravenous catheter
   c) Blood cultures positive for *Staphylococcus epidermidis*, corynebacteria, or *Candida albicans*
2. Purulence around the catheter site provides strong evidence, but this sign is absent in many cases.
3. Cytospin Gram or acridine orange staining of catheter sample provides rapid diagnosis.
4. Roll and sonication methods can be used for quantitating bacteria on the catheter tip. Surveillance cultures are not recommended.
5. Blood samples for culture should be drawn simultaneously from the catheter and the peripheral veins.
   a) Bacterial growth from the catheter sample that is 5 to 10 times that from the peripheral sample is quantitative for catheter infection.
   b) Positive bacterial growth from a catheter more than 2 hours earlier than positive growth in a peripheral sample indicates catheter infection.

---

materials such as catheter tips. Enterococci and corynebacteria are other common gram-positive pathogens. Gram-negative bacilli account for up to one third of infections, with *Klebsiella pneumoniae*, *Enterobacter* species, *E. coli*, *Pseudomonas* species, *Acinetobacter* species, and *Serratia* species being most common. Positive blood cultures for *Klebsiella*, *Citrobacter*, and non-aeruginosa strains of *Pseudomonas* suggest a contaminated infusate.

Fungi now account for 20% of central venous catheter infections, *Candida albicans* predominating. Like coagulase-negative staphylococci, *C. albicans* is able to form a glycocalyx that enhances adherence to catheters. Patients receiving high glucose solutions for hyperalimentation are at particularly high risk for this infection.

orange staining. However, this method is less sensitive than culture of the removed catheter tip. Two methods for testing the catheter are recommended. The roll method (catheter is rolled across the culture plate) is semiquantitative (positive with 15 cfu or more); the vortex or sonication method (releases bacteria into liquid media) is quantitative (positive with 100 cfu or more). The roll method detects bacteria on the outer surface of the catheter; the vortex or sonication method also detects bacteria from the lumen. The sonication method is more sensitive, but more difficult to perform than the roll method is. The use of antibiotic- and silver-impregnated catheters may lead to false negative results with these methods. Cultures of removed catheter tips should be performed only when a catheter-related bloodstream infection is suspected. Routine surveillance culturing of removed catheter tips is not recommended.

When an intravascular device infection is suspected, at least two and preferably three blood samples for culture should be drawn: one set from the intravenous catheter and one to two sets from the peripheral veins. A negative blood culture from a sample drawn from the intravenous line is very helpful in excluding the diagnosis of catheter-related bloodstream infection. A positive culture requires clinical interpretation. As in case 7.2, when catheter removal is not desirable, quantitative blood culturing has been recommended. A finding of colony counts from the catheter sample that are 5 to 10 times those found from the peripheral samples suggests catheter-related infection.

A more practical approach (used in case 7.2) takes advantage of the automated colorimetric continuous monitoring of blood cultures now available in most clinical microbiology laboratories. The time required to detect bacteria in the catheter sample is compared to the time required in the peripheral sample. Detection of bacteria in the catheter sample more than 2 hours earlier than in the peripheral sample suggests a catheter-associated infection. In case 7.2, the history of rigors during intravenous infusion combined with the earlier detection of bacteria in the catheter culture than in the peripheral culture provided strong evidence that the infection originated in the intravascular device.

Treatment

Empiric antibiotic therapy should be initiated after appropriate cultures have been obtained. Vancomycin is usually recommended to cover for MRSA and for methicillin-resistant coagulase-negative staphylococci. In the severely ill or immunocompromised patient, additional coverage for gram-negative bacilli is recommended with an anti-pseudomonal third- (ceftazidime) or fourth-generation (cefepime) cephalosporin. In the severely ill patient, the catheter should be removed immediately. The catheter should also be removed if fever persists and blood cultures continue to be positive beyond 48 hours, and if the patient is infected with virulent, difficult-to-treat pathogens (*S. aureus*; gram-negative bacilli, particularly *Pseudomonas aeruginosa*; and fungi). Polymicrobial bacteremia suggests heavy contamination of the line and usually warrants catheter removal. Other indications for removal include neutropenia, tunnel or pocket infection, valvular heart disease or endocarditis, septic thrombophlebitis, or the presence of metastatic abscesses.

The duration of therapy has not been examined in carefully controlled trials. Therapy is usually continued for 2 weeks in uncomplicated infection. For patients with coagulase-negative staphylococci, treatment for 5 to 7 days is sufficient if the catheter is removed, but treatment should be continued for a minimum of 2 weeks if the catheter is left in place. In complicated infections in which bacteremia continues despite removal of the catheter, treatment must be continued for 4 to 6 weeks. On average, most catheter-associated infections are treated for 3 weeks. Because of the high incidence of relapse, follow-up blood cultures are important if the line was kept in place.

The salvage rate for tunnel catheters can be improved by filling the catheter lumen with pharmacologic concentrations of antibiotic—termed "antibiotic lock therapy." For gram-positive infections, vancomycin (25 mg in 5 mL of solution) is usually recommended, and for gram-negative bacilli, gentamicin (5 mg in 5 mL) is the agent of choice. This treatment exposes the bacteria to very high concentrations of antibiotic that are more likely to penetrate the biofilm. Antibiotic lock therapy is particularly helpful in tunnel catheters, because the associated infections usually develop within the catheter lumen. Cure rates from 60% to 80% have been achieved.

Because of the ability of *S. aureus* to attach to and destroy normal heart valves (70% of *S. aureus* endocarditis cases occur on previously normal heart valves), infection with this pathogen poses a unique challenge. The duration of therapy after prompt catheter removal is best guided by TEE. The presence of valvular vegetations on TEE warrants 4 weeks of therapy; the absence of vegetations by this test allows treatment to end after 2 weeks without significant risk of relapse. Short-course therapy should be considered only in patients who promptly defervesce on antibiotic therapy and who do not have valvular heart disease or an extravascular focus of infection.

In patients infected with *Candida* species, the intravenous catheter must be removed. Because of the high risk of *Candida* endophthalmitis (10% to 15%), catheter removal must be accompanied by antifungal therapy in untreated patients. In uncomplicated *C. albicans* infection, fluconazole (400 mg daily for more than 14 days) is as effective as amphotericin B and is accompanied by minimal toxicity. Therapy with systemic amphotericin B (0.3 to 1 mg/kg daily) is warranted in the presence of fungemia resulting from other, more resistant strains such

KEY POINTS

About the Treatment of Intravascular Catheter–Related Infections

1. The catheter should be removed if
   a) the patient is severely ill.
   b) fever and positive blood cultures persist for more than 48 hours.
   c) a virulent organism is the infecting agent.
   d) bacteremia is polymicrobial.
   e) tunnel infection, neutropenia, endocarditis, metastatic infection, or septic thrombophlebitis is present.
2. Empiric therapy is vancomycin and an antipseudomonal third- or fourth-generation cephalosporin.
3. Duration of therapy has not been studied.
   a) Average duration is 3 weeks.
   b) For coagulase-negative staphylococci, continue treatment for 7 to 10 days if the line has been removed, and 2 weeks if line has been kept in place.
   c) For complicated infections, continue treatment for 4 to 6 weeks.
4. Antibiotic lock therapy improves cure rate for tunneled catheters (vancomycin, gentamicin).
5. Infection with *S. aureus* has a high risk for endocarditis; transesophageal echocardiography helpful in determining the duration of therapy.
6. For *Candida albicans* infection, always remove the line, and treat for 2 weeks to prevent endophthalmitis.
   a) Fluconazole for uncomplicated catheter-related infection.
   b) Amphotericin B for severely ill, neutropenic, or resistant fungus– infected patients.

as *C. krusei*, prolonged positive blood cultures, severe systemic complaints, or neutropenia.

MYOCARDITIS

POTENTIAL SEVERITY

Fulminant myocarditis can be fatal or lead to chronic CHF. Most cases are self-limiting and are followed by full recovery.

The true incidence of myocarditis (inflammation of the heart) is unknown, because most cases are asymptomatic. It has been estimated that 1% to 5% of systemic viral illnesses have myocardial involvement. Young males are at higher risk for serious myocarditis, as are pregnant women, neonates, and immunocompromised patients.

Causes and Pathogenesis

Viruses are a major cause of myocarditis, and specific causation has been identified by PCR in nearly 40% of patients with myocarditis. Adenoviruses and enteroviruses (*Coxsackievirus* B and echoviruses) are most commonly detected, but many other viruses have been implicated, including cytomegalovirus and Epstein–Barr virus, varicella virus, mumps, influenza, and *Vaccinia* (following smallpox vaccination) viruses. Patients with asymptomatic HIV infection have a high incidence of myocarditis (1.6% annually).

Many bacteria have also been implicated as causes of myocarditis, including *Legionella* and *Chlamydia* species. Spirochetes can invade the heart, and patients with Lyme disease may present with cardiac arrhythmias (see Chapter 13). Severe disseminated fungal infections can result in myocarditis. Parasites are also implicated: *Trypanosoma cruzi* attack the heart in 30% of patients with Chagas' disease, and heavy infestation with *Trichinella* can cause fatal myocarditis (see Chapter 12).

Viruses directly invade myocytes and can cause direct damage to the infected cells. The immune response to infection also causes cytotoxicity. T cells predominate the myocyte infiltration, accompanied by macrophages and B cells. Circulating auto-antibodies directed against mitochondria and contractile proteins are frequently detected. Cytokines and oxygen-free radicals have also been implicated as contributors to myocyte damage. Forced exercise, pregnancy, use of steroids or nonsteroidal anti-inflammatory agents, consumption of ethanol, and nutritional deficiencies have all been implicated as factors that predispose to symptomatic myocarditis.

Clinical Manifestations, Diagnosis, and Treatment

The pace of illness and the symptoms vary greatly from patient to patient. Some patients experience a flu-like illness that can be accompanied by chest pain when the pericardium is involved. Other patients present with arrhythmias or symptoms and signs of right- and left-sided CHF. Left ventricular dilatation can lead to expansion of the mitral valve ring and a mitral regurgitant murmur.

Cardiac enzymes are elevated in a few cases. Levels of creatinine kinase antibodies are elevated in only 5% of cases and cardiac troponin I in 34%. Elevations are most commonly detected within the first month of symptoms and suggest ongoing myocyte necrosis. Acute and convalescent viral titers may be drawn and will detect recent viral infections, but this test should not be considered proof of a viral cause. Echocardiography is very helpful for assessing cardiac contractility, chamber size, valve function, and wall thickness. Contrast-enhanced MRI allows for detection of the extent and degree of inflammation, parameters that correlate with left ventricular function and clinical status. Definitive diagnosis requires endomyocardial biopsy. Timing of the biopsy and interpretation by an experienced pathologist are critical. Analysis by PCR of biopsy tissue remains experimental, and the specificity and sensitivity of the assay remains to be determined.

Treatment for viral myocarditis is evolving. In patients with persistent virus in the myocardium, β-interferon administration has been associated with clearance of the virus and improvement in myocardial function. Immunosuppressive agents have failed to improve outcome, and administration of immunoglobulins has not been proved to be of benefit. Exercise restriction limits the work required by the inflamed heart and has been shown to be beneficial in a mouse model of viral myocarditis. In-hospital cardiac monitoring may be required during the acute phase of myocarditis to prevent potentially life-threatening arrhythmias. Anti-arrhythmic drugs must be used cautiously because of their negative inotropic effects. To reduce the risk of mural thrombi and systemic emboli, warfarin anticoagulation should be considered in patients with an ejection fraction below 20%. In most cases of viral myocarditis, patients recover completely; however those with fulminant disease may die. Severe cardiac damage can lead to refractory CHF that can be corrected only with cardiac transplantation.

PERICARDITIS

POTENTIAL SEVERITY

Viral pericarditis usually has a self-limiting benign course. However, patients with purulent pericarditis have a high mortality and require emergent care.

KEY POINTS

About Myocarditis

1. Primarily caused by adenoviruses and enteroviruses (*Coxsackievirus* B and echoviruses).

2. In asymptomatic HIV, incidence of myocarditis is 1.6% annually.

3. Risk factors for symptomatic disease include forced exercise, pregnancy, steroids or nonsteroidal anti-inflammatory agents, consumption of ethanol, and nutritional deficiencies.

4. Many patients are asymptomatic. Some develop
   a) flu-like illness, sometimes with chest pain;
   b) arrhythmias, and
   c) congestive heart failure (CHF).

5. A physical exam reveals S3 gallop (indicating left-sided CHF), mitral regurgitation resulting from ring dilatation.

6. In a few cases, cardiac enzymes are elevated.

7. Echocardiography is very helpful; magnetic resonance imaging allows for assessment of the extent of inflammation.

8. Endomyocardial biopsy combined with analysis by polymerase chain reaction is experimental.

9. Treatment includes β-interferon, bed rest, drugs for congestive heart failure and arrhythmias, anticoagulation.

10. Full recovery is usual; however, fulminant cases may require heart transplant.

Pathogenesis

Inflammation of the pericardium has multiple infectious and noninfectious causes. Of cases in which a cause can be determined, a virus is most common. The same viruses that invade the myocardium also attack the pericardium. Bacteria can also cause pericarditis, resulting in purulent disease. In the antibiotic era, pericarditis has become rare. *S. aureus*, *S. pneumoniae*, and other streptococci are the leading causative organisms, although virtually any bacterium can cause purulent pericarditis. The pericardium can become infected as a result of hematogenous spread (the most common route today) or by spread from a pulmonary, myocardial, or subdiaphragmatic focus. Purulent pericarditis can also be a delayed complication of a penetrating injury or cardiac surgery. Postoperative infections are most commonly caused by *S. aureus*, gram-negative aerobic rods, and *Candida* species.

Tuberculous pericarditis results from hematogenous spread during primary disease, from lymphatics draining the respiratory tract, or from direct spread originating in the lung or pleura. Initially, infection causes fibrin deposition and development of granulomas containing viable mycobacteria; gradual accumulation of pericardial fluid—initially containing polymorphonu-clear leukocytes, and then eventually lymphocytes, monocytes, and plasma cells—follows. Finally, the effusion is absorbed, and the pericardium thickens, becomes fibrotic, and calcifies. Over time, the pericardial space shrinks, causing constrictive pericarditis.

Clinical Manifestations

Clinical manifestations of pericarditis vary depending on the cause. Viral and idiopathic pericarditis usually present with substernal chest pain, which is usually sharp and made worse by inspiration. Pain is also worsened by lying supine, the patient preferring to sit up and lean forward. In acute bacterial pericarditis, the patient suddenly develops fever and dyspnea, and only one third of patients complain of chest pain. Because of the lack of specific symptoms, a diagnosis of purulent pericarditis is often not considered, and the diagnosis is made only at autopsy. Tuberculous pericarditis is more insidious in clinical onset. Vague, dull chest pain, weight loss, night sweats, cough, and dyspnea are most commonly reported.

The classic physical findings of pericarditis include a scratchy three-component friction rub (as result of the moving heart rubbing against the abnormal pericardium during atrial systole), early ventricular filling, and ventricular systole. When the pericardial effusion increases in volume, the friction rub usually disappears. The hemodynamic consequences of the pericardial effusion can be assessed by checking for pulsus paradoxicus; a value exceeding 10 mm Hg indicates significant tamponade. A second hemodynamic consequence of pericardial tamponade is a rise in right ventricular filling pressure. High right-sided pressure causes an increase in jugular venous distension and abnormal jugular venous pulsations with a loss of Y descent. The patient often has a rapid respiratory rate and complains of dyspnea. However, because of the equalization of right- and left-sided cardiac pressures, pulmonary edema does not develop, and the lung fields are clear on auscultation.

KEY POINTS

About the Causes, Pathogenesis, and Clinical Manifestations of Pericarditis

1. Pericarditis has three forms:
   a) Viral, with enteroviruses most common (*Coxsackievirus* and *Echovirus*)
   b) Purulent, which is usually hematogenous (multiple organisms, including *Staphylococcus aureus*)
   c) Tuberculous, which is usually seeded during primary disease, but can spread from a pulmonary focus
2. Main symptom is substernal chest pain, which is relieved by sitting forward. Pain is less common in purulent pericarditis and has a gradual onset in tuberculous disease.
3. Physical exam shows
   a) three-component friction rub early; rub later disappears with increased pericardial fluid.
   b) pulsus paradoxicus (exceeding 10 mm Hg is abnormal).
   c) jugular venous distension with depressed Y descent.

KEY POINTS

About the Diagnosis and Treatment of Pericarditis

1. Echocardiography should be performed immediately:
   a) Allows for assessment of pericardial thickness, pericardial fluid, and tamponade.
   b) Can be used to guide emergency pericardiocentesis.
2. Electrocardiogram shows diffuse ST and T changes, depressed PR interval, decreased QRS voltage, electrical alternans.
3. Pericardiocentesis only for those with tamponade or suspected of having purulent pericarditis. Pericardial biopsy improves the diagnostic yield.
4. Viral or idiopathic pericarditis is self-limiting.
   a) Use nonsteroidal agents only if no myocarditis.
   b) Colchicine can be used.
5. Purulent pericarditis requires emergency surgical drainage and systemic antibiotics. Mortality is 30%.
6. Tuberculous pericarditis is treated with
   a) a four-drug antituberculous regimen, and
   b) prednisone to prevent constriction (20% to 50% incidence during treatment).
   c) Calcific form requires pericardiectomy.

Diagnosis and Treatment

Electrocardiogram is abnormal in 90% of patients and may show diffuse ST segment elevation, depression of the PR segment, and (when the effusion is large) decreased QRS voltage and electrical alternans. The electrocardiography findings are usually not specific, and when pericarditis is being considered, echocardiography is the critical test that needs to be ordered. The echocardiogram readily detects pericardial thickening and pericardial fluid accumulation. In life-threatening tamponade, echocardiography can be used to guide pericardiocentesis. In the absence of hemodynamic compromise, pericardiocentesis is not recommended because of the low diagnostic yield and moderate risk of the procedure. However, in patients with significant pericardial tamponade, pericardial fluid yields a diagnosis in one quarter of cases, and pericardial biopsy in half of patients. Pericardial fluid and tissue biopsy can be performed surgically. In an emergency, echocardiography-guided catheter pericardiocentesis can be performed. In patients with a thickened pericardium, a percutaneous pericardial biopsy can safely be performed.

Viral and idiopathic pericarditis are usually benign self-limiting disorders that can be treated with bed rest. Nonsteroidal anti-inflammatory agents are helpful for reducing chest pain, but they should probably be avoided in patients with accompanying myocarditis. Colchicine (1 mg daily) may also be helpful for reducing symptoms in cases of idiopathic disease.

In patients with purulent pericarditis, surgical drainage of the pericardium should be performed emergently, accompanied by systemic antibiotic therapy. This disease continues to generate a 30% mortality.

Tuberculous pericarditis should receive four-drug antituberculous therapy. However, during treatment, 20% ro 50% of patients progress to constrictive pericarditis. This complication can be prevented by simultaneous administration of oral prednisone (60 mg for 4 weeks, 30 mg for 4 weeks, 15 mg for 2 weeks, and 5 mg for 1 week). Patients who have developed calcific tuberculous pericarditis at the time of diagnosis require pericardiectomy for relief of symptoms.

FURTHER READING

Bacterial Endocarditis

Baddour LM, Wilson WR, Bayer AS, et al. Infective endocarditis: diagnosis, antimicrobial therapy, and management of complications: a statement for healthcare professionals from the Committee on Rheumatic Fever, Endocarditis, and Kawasaki Disease, Council on Cardiovascular Disease in the Young, and the Councils on Clinical Cardiology, Stroke, and Cardiovascular Surgery and Anesthesia, American Heart Association: endorsed by the Infectious Diseases Society of America. *Circulation.* 2005;111:e394–e434.

Breitkopf C, Hammel D, Scheld HH, Peters G, Becker K. Impact of a molecular approach to improve the microbiological diagnosis of infective heart valve endocarditis. *Circulation.* 2005;111:1415–1421.

Dhawan VK. Infective endocarditis in elderly patients. *Clin Infect Dis.* 2002;34:806–812.

Fowler VG Jr, Miro JM, Hoen B, et al. *Staphylococcus aureus* endocarditis: a consequence of medical progress. *JAMA.* 2005;293:3012–3021.

Hoen B, Alla F, Selton-Suty C, et al. Changing profile of infective endocarditis: results of a 1-year survey in France. *JAMA.* 2002;288:75–81.

McDonald JR, Olaison L, Anderson DJ, et al. Enterococcal endocarditis: 107 cases from the international collaboration on endocarditis merged database. *Am J Med.* 2005;118:759–766.

Morris AJ, Drinkovic D, Pottumarthy S, MacCulloch D, Kerr AR, West T. Bacteriological outcome after valve surgery for active infective endocarditis: implications for duration of treatment after surgery. *Clin Infect Dis.* 2005;41:187–194.

Mylonakis E, Calderwood SB. Infective endocarditis in adults. *N Engl J Med.* 2001;345:1318–1330.

Piper C, Korfer R, Horstkotte D. Prosthetic valve endocarditis. *Heart.* 2001;85:590–593.

Ramsdale DR, Turner-Stokes L. Prophylaxis and treatment of infective endocarditis in adults: a concise guide. *Clin Med.* 2004;4:545–550.

Intravascular Device Infection

Bouza E, Burillo A, Munoz P. Catheter-related infections: diagnosis and intravascular treatment. *Clin Microbiol Infect.* 2002;8:265–274.

Mermel LA, Farr BM, Sherertz RJ, et al. Guidelines for the management of intravascular catheter-related infections. *Clin Infect Dis.* 2001;32:1249–1272.

Raad I, Hanna HA, Alakech B, Chatzinikolaou I, Johnson MM, Tarrand J. Differential time to positivity: a useful method for diagnosing catheter-related bloodstream infections. *Ann Intern Med.* 2004;140:18–25.

Safdar N, Fine JP, Maki DG. Meta-analysis: methods for diagnosing intravascular device-related bloodstream infection. *Ann Intern Med.* 2005;142:451–466.

Myocarditis

Bowles NE, Ni J, Kearney DL, et al. Detection of viruses in myocardial tissues by polymerase chain reaction. evidence of adenovirus as a common cause of myocarditis in children and adults. *J Am Coll Cardiol.* 2003;42:466–472.

Kuhl U, Pauschinger M, Schwimmbeck PL, et al. Interferon-beta treatment eliminates cardiotropic viruses and improves left ventricular function in patients with myocardial persistence of viral genomes and left ventricular dysfunction. *Circulation.* 2003;107:2793–2798.

Kuhl U, Pauschinger M, Seeberg B, et al. Viral persistence in the myocardium is associated with progressive cardiac dysfunction. *Circulation.* 2005;112:1965–1970.

Lewis W. Cardiomyopathy in AIDS: a pathophysiological perspective. *Prog Cardiovasc Dis.* 2000;43:151–170.

Pericarditis

Aikat S, Ghaffari S. A review of pericardial diseases: clinical, ECG and hemodynamic features and management. *Cleve Clin J Med.* 2000;67:903–914.

Adler Y, Finkelstein Y, Guindo J, et al. Colchicine treatment for recurrent pericarditis. A decade of experience. *Circulation.* 1998;97:2183–2185.

Levy PY, Corey R, Berger P, et al. Etiologic diagnosis of 204 pericardial effusions. *Medicine (Baltimore).* 2003;82:385–391.

Trautner BW, Darouiche RO. Tuberculous pericarditis: optimal diagnosis and management. *Clin Infect Dis.* 2001;33:954–961.

Gastrointestinal and Hepatobiliary Infections

8

Time Recommended to complete: 3 days

Frederick Southwick M.D.

GUIDING QUESTIONS

1. What are the three most common bacterial causes of infectious diarrhea, and how are these infections contracted?

2. Which test is useful for differentiating viral from bacterial diarrhea?

3. How does Clostridium difficile *cause diarrhea, and how is pseudomembranous colitis diagnosed?*

4. What are the findings that suggest the development of spontaneous peritonitis?

5. How do abdominal abscesses usually form, and how are they best managed?

6. Which pathogen most commonly causes peptic ulcer disease?

7. How do hepatic abscesses usually develop, and which bacteria are most commonly cultured?

8. What are the three most common forms of viral hepatitis, and how are they contracted?

9. What are the major complications of viral hepatitis?

■ INFECTIOUS DIARRHEA

POTENTIAL SEVERITY

Can be life-threatening in infants, young children, and elderly people. Most individuals with this illness can be managed as outpatients.

Diarrheal illness is one of the leading causes of death worldwide, accounting for nearly 2.5 million deaths annually. It is most commonly encountered in developing countries and is a less serious problem in the United States. Still, the incidence of diarrhea in the United States has been estimated to be 1 episode per person per year.

With appropriate medical care, these infections are rarely fatal. The pathogens that cause diarrhea can be transmitted through food, through water, or through person-to-person spread. Differences in these modes of transmission reflect differences in the ability of each pathogen to survive in the environment. They also reflect the inoculum size required for a given pathogen to cause disease.

ACUTE DIARRHEA
Bacterial Diarrhea

POTENTIAL SEVERITY

These disorders are usually self-limiting, but can be fatal in infants, elderly people, and people who develop enteric fever.

The three most common bacterial causes of acute infectious diarrhea are *Salmonella*, *Shigella*, and *Campylobacter*. Other important bacterial pathogens include *Escherichia coli*, *Vibrio parahaemolyticus*, and *Yersinia enterocolitica*. Each of these pathogens has unique life-cycle and virulence characteristics. The various causes of acute bacterial diarrhea are usually not distinguishable clinically, and diagnosis requires isolation of the organism on stool culture.

CASE 8.1

A 52-year-old black woman with rheumatoid arthritis for 24 years was admitted to the hospital with complaints of fever and diarrhea for the preceding 24 hours.

One month earlier she had been hospitalized for neck surgery and received a 10-day course of a broad-spectrum antibiotic (ceftazidime). Antibiotic treatment was completed the day of discharge (18 days before her second admission). She was doing well in a rehabilitation hospital until 3 days prior to admission, when she developed a fever to 38.9°C associated with shaking chills and persistent severe watery diarrhea (25 to 30 bowel movements daily). One day before admission, she noted abdominal cramps, nausea, vomiting, and anorexia. The rehabilitation nurse found the woman's blood pressure to be 70/50 mm Hg, and referred her to the emergency room. Medications: asparin and large quantities of antacids.

Epidemioly: Her son had brought her an egg salad sandwich from Famous Deli, which they shared 16 hours before onset of the illness. Her son also has severe diarrhea.

Physical examination: Temperature 39°C, blood pressure 70/50 mm Hg, pulse rate of 120 per minute, and respiratory rate 20 per minute. She was moderately ill-appearing, with dry mucous membranes and a dry, fissured tongue. Abdomenal exam revealed hyperactive bowel sounds and mild diffuse tenderness No skin lesions were seen.

Laboratory findings: White blood cell (WBC) count of 7100/mm³, with 10% polymorphonuclear leukocytes (PMNs), 63% bands, 19% lymphocytes; blood urea nitrogen of 63 mg/dL; and serum creatinine of 2.1 mg/dL. Methylene blue smear of the stool: few PMNs and few mononuclear cells. Gram stain: mixed flora. Stool culture: Salmonella enteritidis.

MICROBIOLOGY, PATHOGENESIS, AND EPIDEMIOLOGY

Table 8.1 summarizes the characteristics of the most common bacterial uses of diarrhea.

Salmonella

Salmonella is an aerobic gram-negative bacillus that can grow readily on simple culture media. It is motile, and most strains do not ferment lactose. As a consequence of DNA sequencing, the speciation of *Salmonella* has recently been revised, and the related nomenclature has become complex.

From a clinical standpoint, the simplest approach is to differentiate typhoidal salmonella (primarily *S. typhi* and *S. paratyphi*) from the many nontyphoidal serotypes that primarily cause gastroenteritis (*S. enteritidis*, *S. typhimurium* most common). One nontyphoidal strain of note is *S. choleraesuis*. This serotype has a higher likelihood of causing bacteremia.

S. typhi is adapted to humans and rarely infects other animals; however, the other *Salmonella* species readily infect both wild and domestic animals. These organisms attach to epithelial cells in the small intestine and colon.

KEY POINTS

About Salmonella Gastroenteritis

1. Gram-negative bacillus, does not ferment lactose, motile.
2. Attaches to intestinal and colonic cells, and injects proteins that stimulate internalization.
3. Spreads to mesenteric nodes; *Salmonella choleraesuis* and *S. typhi* often enter the bloodstream.
4. The organism is acid-sensitive, with 10-4 to 10-8 organisms required for infection. Risk factors for disease include
   a) antacid use,
   b) prior antibiotics (reduces competition by normal flora), and
   c) depressed immune function (AIDS and transplant patients, sickle cell disease).
5. Contracted from contaminated foods (more commonly in the summer months):
   a) Chicken products (eggs, undercooked meat)
   b) Contaminated processed foods (ice cream, unpasteurized goat cheese, whitefish, contaminated fruits and vegetables)
   c) Infected pet turtles, rodents, iguanas, birds
   d) Contaminated water supply (*S. typhi*)

Table 8.1. Bacterial Diarrhea: Causative Pathogens, Epidemiology, Stool Findings

Causative organism	Epidemiology	Stool[a] PMNs	RBCs	Comments
Salmonella	Foodborne, *S. typhi* waterborne	2+	Rare	May have monocytes in stool; contaminated meat and milk products
Shigella	Person-to-person	4+	3+	Mucous, tenesmus; daycare centers in the United States
Campylobacter	Foodborne	4+	3+	Gram-stain positive (seagull-like gram-negative bacilli), chicken
Escherichia coli				
Enterotoxigenic	Waterborne	0	0	Cholera-like illness with watery diarrhea; developing countries, travelers' diarrhea
Enteroaggregative	Foodborne and waterborne			Watery diarrhea; developing countries, travelers' diarrhea
Enteropathogenic	Foodborne, waterborne, person to person	0	0	Children under 3 years of age; developing countries
Enterohemorrhagic	Foodborne	±	4+ visible	O157:H7, contaminated beef, vegetables, mayonnaise, cider
Enteroinvasive	Foodborne	4+	3+	Rare, developing countries
Vibrio parahaemolyticus	Foodborne	0	0	Raw seafood (sushi); common in Japan
Vibrio cholera	Waterborne	0	0	Developing countries
Yersinia	Foodborne	4+	3+	Common in Europe, rare in the United States; can mimic appendicitis
Clostridium difficile	Antibiotic-associated	2–4+	0–3+	Early disease, watery diarrhea; later, extensive colitis

[a] PMNs = polymorphonuclear leukocytes; RBCs = red blood cells, 4+ = many PMN per hpf, 3+ moderate numbers per hpf, 2 + few PMN per hpf.

Once attached they inject into host cells specific proteins that cause the formation large ruffles that surround the bacteria, internalizing them into large vacuoles. There, *Salmonella* are able to replicate and eventually lyse the infected cell, escaping into the extracellular environment and in some cases gaining entry to the bloodstream to cause bacteremia. *S. typhi* is particularly adept at surviving within cells. It often causes little intestinal epithelial damage and little diarrhea, primarily entering mesenteric lymph nodes and the bloodstream to cause classic enteric fever. *S. choleraesuis* is also adept at invading the bloodstream. It is the most common cause of nontyphoidal *Salmonella* bacteremia.

Studies in normal volunteers have revealed that large numbers of bacteria (10-4 to 10-8 organisms) are required to produce symptomatic disease. However, epidemiologic studies suggest that infection can result from ingestion of 200 organisms. Stomach acidity kills many *Salmonella* before they enter the more hospitable intestinal tract, but in gastrectomy patients or those who use antacids (as in case 8.1), the number of organisms required to cause disease is markedly reduced. The critical inoculum size is also affected by the normal bowel flora. Reduction in the flora as a result of prior antibiotic treatment reduces competition for nutrients (as in case 8.1) and allows *Salmonella* to more readily multiply within the bowel lumen. Depressed immune function increases the risk of salmonellosis, patients with AIDS and lymphoma and other neoplasms being at higher risk. Patients with sickle cell disease have an increased incidence of *Salmonella* bacteremia that is often complicated by osteomyelitis.

Because large numbers of *Salmonella* organisms are required to cause disease, gastroenteritis is almost always associated with ingestion of heavily contaminated food. In case 8.1, the sandwich from the delicatessen likely had become contaminated. Because chickens often excrete *Salmonella* in their stools, eggs, egg products, and undercooked chicken are the foods most commonly associated with disease. Contamination of processed foods—examples include ice cream, unpasteurized goat cheese, paprika-powdered potato chips, and whitefish—has resulted in large outbreaks of salmonellosis. *Salmonella*-infected human or animal feces can contaminate fruits and vegetables. Pet turtles, iguanas, rodents, and birds can carry large numbers of organisms, and can infect humans, particularly young children. Contamination of the water supply with sewage also can lead to gastrointestinal infection. *S. typhi* is frequently contracted from contaminated water, and typhoid fever is most commonly found in developing countries where sanitation is poor. Salmonella infections are more common in the summer months, when the warmer temperatures allow the organism to multiply more rapidly on contaminated foods.

Shigella

The gram-negative *Shigella* bacillus is nonmotile and does not ferment lactose. It grows readily on standard media. The four major serologic groups, A through D, are common to different areas of the world. Group A *Shigella dysenteriae* and group D *S. boydii* are seldom found in the United States, where the species most commonly encountered are group B *S. flexneri* and group D *S. sonnei*.

Shigella contains a series of surface proteins that induce intestinal epithelial cells and M cells to ingest it. Like *Salmonella*, this organism injects proteins into host cells, stimulating ruffling. Unlike *Salmonella*, the phagocytosed *Shigella* uses a surface hemolysin to lyse the phagosome membrane and escape into the cytoplasm. There, the bacterium induces the assembly of actin rocket tails that propel it through the cytoplasm. When the bacterium reaches the cell periphery, it pushes outward to form membrane projections that can be ingested by adjacent cells, efficiently spreading directly from cell to cell. *Shigella* produces a cytotoxic Shiga toxin and induces premature cell death. This combination of efficient cell-to-cell spread and host-cell destruction produces superficial ulcers in the bowel mucosa and induces an extensive acute inflammatory response that usually prevents entry of *Shigella* into the bloodstream.

Shigella is relatively resistant to acid, and can survive in the gastric juices of the stomach for several hours. This characteristic explains why ingestion of as few as 200 bacteria can cause disease. The organism first takes up residence in the small intestine. After several days, it is cleared by the small intestine, but then invades the colon, where it causes an intense inflammatory response, forming microabscesses and mucosal ulcerations.

Because such a low inoculum is required to cause disease, the epidemiology of *Shigella* is different from that of *Salmonella*. *Shigella* has no intermediate animal hosts; the bacteria reside only in the intestinal tract of humans. The primary mode of spread is person-to-person by

KEY POINTS

About *Shigella* Dysentery

1. Gram-negative rod, does not ferment lactose, nonmotile.
2. Induces ruffling of host cells; once internalized, escapes to the cytoplasm.
   a) Moves through the cytoplasm and spreads from cell to cell by polymerizing actin.
   b) Accelerates cell death, forming plaques of necrotic cells.
   c) Induces marked inflammation and rarely invades the bloodstream.
3. Resistance to gastric acid means that a small numbers of organisms (200 bacteria) can cause disease.
4. Initially grows in the small intestine, and then spreads to the colon.
5. Spreads from person to person. Daycare centers, toilet seats, contaminated water are vectors. Can be spread by flies. Less commonly foodborne.

anal–oral transmission. Foodborne and waterborne outbreaks may also occur as a consequence of fecal contamination—incidents that are most commonly reported in developing countries, where public health standards are poor. Toilet seats can become heavily contaminated by *Shigella*, which may account for some cases in the United States. Children in daycare centers have a high incidence of infection, as do institutionalized individuals, particularly mentally challenged children. On U.S. Indian reservations, high numbers of *Shigella* dysentery cases have been reported. In tropical areas, spread of *Shigella* has been attributed to flies, and epidemics of shigellosis have been reported to correlate with heavy fly infestations.

Campylobacter

Campylobacter are comma-shaped gram-negative rods that, on microscopic examination, are often paired in a distinctive seagull shape. *Campylobacter* are microaerophilic, and with the exception of *Campylobacter fetus*, are unable to grow at 25°C. Ideal growth conditions for *C. jejuni*, the strain that most commonly causes diarrhea, are 42°C, 6% oxygen, and 5% to 10% carbon dioxide. Other bowel flora often overgrow on routine Mac-Conkey's medium, and so selective Campy–BAP medium (10% sheep blood in *Brucella* agar containing amphotericin B, cephalothin, vancomycin, polymyxin B, and trimethoprim) is recommended.

KEY POINTS

About *Campylobacter* Gastroenteritis

- -

1. *Campylobacter* is a coma-shaped gram-negative rod, micro-aerophilic.

2. Grows best at 42°C, requires Campy-BAP selective medium or other bowel flora overgrow. Only *C. fetus* can grow at 25°C.

3. Internalized by and lives in monocytes and intestinal epithelial cells; induces cell death, bowel ulceration, and intense inflammation.

4. *C. fetus* is carried by monocytes to the bloodstream; it resists serum bactericidal activity and causes persistent bacteremia.

5. Like *Salmonella*, *Campylobacter* is sensitive to gastric acid and requires a high inoculum (more than 10^4 bacteria).

6. Epidemiology is similar to that of *Salmonella*. *C. jejuni* is primarily responsible for diarrhea.
   a. Survives well in chickens because of their high body temperature (30% of carcasses test positive).
   b. Carried in water, raw milk, sheep, cattle, swine, and reptiles.

The life cycle of *Campylobacter* is not as well defined as that of *Salmonella* and *Shigella*. It can be ingested by monocytes, where it can survive within the cells for 6 to 7 days. Endocytosis by intestinal epithelial cells and M cells is also likely to occur. Once intracellular, *Campylobacter* induces cell death and tissue necrosis leading to ulceration of the bowel wall and intense acute inflammation. Possibly as a consequence transport by monocytes, *Campylobacter* can gain entry into the bloodstream. *C. fetus*, subspecies *fetus*, is particularly adept at causing bacteremia, often causing little or no diarrhea. This strain's resistance to the bactericidal activity of serum may explain its ability to produce persistent bacteremia leading to vascular infections, soft-tissue abscesses, and meningitis.

Like *Salmonella*, *Campylobacter* is sensitive to acid, and large numbers of organisms (more than 10^4) are therefore required to cause disease. The epidemiology of *Campylobacter* is similar to that of *Salmonella*. *C. jejuni* is the species that primarily causes diarrhea. This species frequently contaminates poultry, and its high carriage rate may be partly explained by the high body temperature in birds, a condition that would be expected to enhance growth of *C. jejuni*. This organism is 10 times more frequently cultured from commercial chicken carcasses than *Salmonella* is (approximately 30% vs. 3%). *C. jejuni* can also be carried in water, raw milk, sheep, cattle, swine, and reptiles. As observed with *Salmonella*, infections are more common in the summer months.

Escherichia coli

Multiple strains of *E. coli* can cause diarrheal illness. These strains cannot easily be distinguished from the nonpathogenic strains of *E. coli* that normally colonize the bowel. Experimental serotyping methods are available that can identify specific lipopolysaccharide antigens (O antigens) and flagellar antigens (H antigens) associated with specific pathogenic characteristics. The diarrhea-causing *E. coli* strains are generally divided into five major classes based on their mechanisms of virulence:

1. **Enterotoxigenic (ETEC) strains.** Colonize the small bowel and produce a cholera-like or heat-stable toxin that stimulates secretion of chloride, causing watery diarrhea. These organisms are most commonly encountered in developing countries and are contracted from water contaminated with human sewage. These strains are a major cause of travelers' diarrhea.

2. **Enteroaggregative (EaggEC) strains.** Adhere in large aggregates to human colonic mucosa and produce a low-molecular-weight enterotoxin that causes watery diarrhea. The diarrhea is often prolonged. These strains are contracted by ingesting contaminated water or food. Enteroaggregative *Esch. coli* are reported in developing countries and are an important cause of travelers' diarrhea.

3. **Enteropathogenic (EPEC) strains.** Adhere to the small bowel and induce the polymerization of actin filaments to form a pedestal directly beneath the site of bacterial attachment. This process is associated with mild inflammation and usually causes watery diarrhea. These strains are transmitted by contaminated food or water and by person-to-person spread in nurseries. This disease primarily affects children under the age of 3 years, and it is more common in developing countries.

4. **Enterohemorrhagic (EHEC) strains.** Produce verotoxins or Shiga-like cytotoxins that inhibit protein synthesis and cause cell death. In certain strains, the toxin damages vascular endothelium in the bowel and glomeruli, causing hemorrhagic inflammatory colitis and hemolytic uremic syndrome. The strain most commonly associated with this syndrome is O157:H7; however, other toxin-producing serotypes are being identified with increasing frequency. Cattle appear to be the primary reservoir, and the disease is most commonly associated with ingestion of undercooked contaminated ground beef. Less commonly, cases have developed after

KEY POINTS

About *Escherichia coli* Gastroenteritis

1. Serotyping identifies specific O (lipopolysaccharide) and H antigens (flagellar proteins).
2. Five pathogenic classes have been defined:
   a) Enterotoxigenic (ETEC): Produce a cholera-like toxin. Spread by water contaminated with human sewage in developing countries. Cause of travelers' diarrhea.
   b) Enteroaggregative (EaggEC): Adhere as large aggregates. Enterotoxin produces watery diarrhea. Cause of travelers' diarrhea.
   c) Enteropathogenic (EPEC): Induce pedestals that cause mild inflammation. Produce watery diarrhea primarily in children under 3 years of age. Person-to-person spread in developing countries.
   d) Enterohemorrhagic (EHEC): Produce verotoxins or Shiga-like cytotoxin. Damage vessels. The O157:H7 strain causes hemolytic–uremic syndrome. Cattle are the primary reservoir. Spread by undercooked hamburger, unpasteurized milk, contaminated apple cider, and mayonnaise.
   e) Enteroinvasive (EIEC): Similar to *Shigella*. Require large inoculum. Seen in developing countries.

consumption of unpasteurized milk or contaminated apple cider, spinach, lettuce, or commercial mayonnaise. Person-to-person spread can occur in daycare centers and nursing homes. This infection is found primarily in industrialized nations and usually occurs during the summer months.

5. **Enteroinvasive (EIEC) strains.** Invade colonic epithelial cells by the same mechanisms that *Shigella* uses. The EIEC strains do not produce toxins, but rather cause an inflammatory colitis that is indistinguishable from that caused by *Shigella*. These strains require ingestion of a large inoculum (10^8 organisms) to cause disease. Outbreaks are rare and are usually associated with contaminated foods in developing countries.

Vibrio

The two primary strains of *Vibrio* associated with diarrhea are *V. cholera* and *V. parahaemolyticus*. This small, slightly curved gram-negative rod has a single flagellum at one end that causes the bacterium to move erratically under the microscope. The organism can be isolated from the stool using thiosulfate, citrate, bile salt, sucrose agar, or tellurite taurocholate gelatin agar.

V. cholera

The *V. cholera* strain gains entry to the small bowel when the host ingests contaminated water (requires 10^3 to 10^6 organisms to cause disease) or food (requires 10^2 to 10^4 organisms). Neutralization of stomach acid lowers the inoculum required to cause disease. The organisms attaches to the small intestine, where it produces cholera toxin. This exotoxin binds to a specific receptor in the bowel mucosa that activates adenylate cyclase, causing an increase in cyclic adenosine monophosphate (cAMP). Elevated cAMP in turn promotes secretion of chloride and water, causing voluminous watery diarrhea.

V. cholera is able to grow and survive in aquatic environments—particularly in estuaries, where it attaches to algae, plankton, and shellfish. During periods when the environment is unfavorable for growth, the organism can convert to a dormant state that can no longer be cultured. The bacteria can also form a "rugose"—an aggregate of bacteria surrounded by a protective biofilm that blocks killing by chlorine and other disinfectants. These

KEY POINTS

About *Vibrio cholera* Diarrhea

1. *Vibrio* is a slightly curved gram-negative bacillus with a single flagellum. It requires a special culture medium (tellurite taurocholate gelatin).
2. Spread by contaminated water (10^3 to 10^6 organisms) or food (10^2 to 10^4 organisms).
3. Attaches to the small intestine, and produces cholera toxin. Binds to a receptor that increases cyclic adenosine monophosphate, and thereby promotes chloride and water secretion.
4. Survives in algae, plankton, and shellfish. Can convert to dormant state or form aggregates surrounded by biofilm (rugose).
5. Non-cholera toxin strains are seen in the Gulf of Mexico.
6. Cholera toxin strains are spread by contaminated water in India, Bangladesh, Asia, Africa, Europe, South America (Peru), and Central America. Outbreaks occur in the hot seasons of the year.

characteristics allow *V. cholera* to persist in water and shellfish. Oysters harvested during the summer months off the Gulf Coast of the United States are frequently positive for *V. cholera*. Fortunately, these strains do not produce cholera toxin, and they cause only occasional cases of gastroenteritis. Cholera toxin–producing strains are usually found in areas of poor sanitation, where fecal contamination of food and water are common.

This organism is capable of producing large epidemics or pandemics, with major outbreaks frequently taking place in India and Bangladesh. Epidemics have also been reported in Asia, Africa, and Europe. In 1991, a large outbreak occurred in Peru, and cholera has been reported in other regions of South America and in Central America. Epidemics usually begin during the hot seasons of the year.

V. parahaemolyticus

The *V. parahaemolyticus* strain is halophilic ("salt loving") and grows in estuaries and marine environments, attaching to plankton and shellfish. Little is known about its pathogenesis, except for the close correlation between hemolysis and ability to cause disease. Nonhemolytic strains are almost always avirulent.

V. parahaemolyticus produces an enterotoxin and causes moderate bowel inflammation, resulting in mild to moderately severe diarrhea. Clams and oysters that filter large volumes of water become heavily contaminated with *V. parahaemolyticus*, and the ingestion of raw or undercooked shellfish is the primary cause of human disease. Other forms of inadequately cooked seafood can harbor small numbers of *Vibrio*, and the tradition of eating uncooked seafood (sushi) explains the high incidence of *V. parahaemolyticus* diarrhea in Japan. The increasing popularity of sushi in the United States is likely to be accompanied by an increasing incidence of that illness.

KEY POINTS

About *Vibrio parahaemolyticus* Diarrhea

1. Thrives in salt water and concentrates in shellfish.
2. Nonhemolytic strains are nonpathogenic.
3. Produces an enterotoxin that causes moderate inflammation and watery diarrhea.
4. Very common in Japan, being contracted from sushi.
5. Incidence may increase in the United States as sushi becomes more popular.

KEY POINTS

About *Yersinia* Gastroenteritis

1. Aerobic gram-negative bacillus; requires a large inoculum (10^9).
2. Infects terminal ileum, and resulting mesenteric node inflammation mimics appendicitis.
3. Common in northern Europe, South America, Africa, and Asia; rare in the United States.
4. Acquired from contaminated meat products and milk; grows at 4°C.
5. Most common in children; more frequent during winter months.

Yersinia

Y. enterocolitica is a gram-negative bacillus that grows aerobically on standard media. Large numbers of organisms must be ingested to cause disease (10^9 organisms). The organism primarily invades the mucosa of the terminal ileum, causing painful enlargement of the mesenteric nodes. As a consequence of right-sided abdominal pain, *Yersinia* enterocolitis can be mistaken for appendicitis.

Yersinia infection is rare in the United States, being more commonly reported in northern Europe, South America, Africa, and Asia. The disease usually occurs in children. *Y. enterocolitica* is generally contracted from contaminated meat products, and because this bacterium can grow at 4°C, refrigerated meats are a particular concern. Contamination of pasteurized milk has been associated with several outbreaks in the United States. In contrast with other forms of bacterial diarrhea that peak during the summer months, most cases of *Y. enterocolitica* occur during the winter months.

CLINICAL MANIFESTATIONS

Gastroenteritis

Acute diarrhea is defined as diarrhea lasting less than 14 days, emphasizing the self-limiting nature of the infections. With the exception of certain strains of *E. coli* and *Vibrio*, most cases of bacterial diarrhea present with enterocolitis. As illustrated in case 8.1, the incubation period after ingestion of *Salmonella*-contaminated food is usually 8 to 24 hours (*Shigella*: 36 to 72 hours; EHEC: 4 days).

Enterocolitis is characterized by diarrhea and abdominal pain. Stools may be frequent but small, or (as in Case 8.1) the diarrhea may voluminous. In some patients, stool may be watery as a consequence of increased secretion of fluids into the bowel. Watery diarrhea is most commonly encountered in ETEC, EPEC, EaggEC, and *Vibrio* infections. Other patients have purulent, mucousy stools. This latter form of diarrhea is most commonly encountered in *Shigella* dysentery, reflecting the exuberant acute inflammatory response of the bowel. Stools may be bloody as a result of bowel ulceration and tissue necrosis. Bloody stools are most commonly encountered in *Shigella*, *Campylobacter*, EHEC, and EIEC. Visible blood in the stool is particularly prominent with EHEC, often causing the patient to seek medical attention. In patients with significant colonic involvement, tenesmus and marked pain on attempting to defecate are common complaints.

On physical exam, a significant percentage of patients have fever, usually in the 38°C to 39°C range. However patients with EHEC are often afebrile. Abdominal exam reveals hyperactive bowel sounds, reflecting increased peristalsis. Diffuse tenderness is typical, usually not accompanied by guarding or rebound. In some cases, however, severe tenderness with rebound may be present, suggesting the diagnosis of acute appendicitis or cholecystitis. The peripheral leukocyte count is often normal, but some patients develop moderate leukocytosis. Fluid loss can be profound, leading to hypotension and electrolyte abnormalities. Positive

---

KEY POINTS

About Enteric Fever

1. Caused by Salmonella typhi, S. paratyphi, Campylobacter fetus, and Yersinia enterocolitica.
2. Incubation period is 8 to 14 days, longer with lower inocula.
3. Influenza-like syndrome: headache, muscle aches, malaise, lethargy, nonproductive cough.
4. Mild abdominal discomfort that worsens, with constipation or minimal bloody diarrhea.
5. Progresses to high fever (40°C) and slow pulse, septic shock, and bowel perforation.
6. Skin shows small rose-colored macules ("rose spots").
7. Normochromic, normocytic anemia; leukopenia.
8. Positive blood cultures in 90% of patients in the first week.

KEY POINTS

About the Clinical Presentation of Bacterial Diarrhea

1. Incubation periods are 8 to 24 hours for *Salmonella*, 36 to 72 hours for *Shigella*, and 4 days for EHEC.
2. Diarrhea varies in volume and consistency:
   a. Watery with enteropathogenic, enterotoxigenic, enteroaggregative, and *Vibrio*
   b. Mucousy with *Shigella*
   c. Bloody with *Shigella*, *Campylobacter*, enterohemorrhagic, and enteroinvasive
3. Abdominal pain is associated with hyperactive bowel sounds and diffuse tenderness; in some cases, severe pain may mimicking appendicitis or cholecystitis.
4. When the colon is involved, tenesmus and pain on defecating are seen, most commonly with *Shigella*

---

blood cultures can accompany *Salmonella* enterocolitis, but are rare in *Shigella* or *C. jejuni* infections.

Enteric fever—Typhoid fever is most commonly associated with *S. typhi* and *S. paratyphi*. The incubation is usually 8 to 14 days, being longer with a lower inoculum. Fever is the first manifestation, and the disease usually mimics an influenza-like illness, characterized by continuous frontal headache, generalized aches, malaise, anorexia, and lethargy. A large percentage of patients also have a nonproductive cough. Most patients complain of mild abdominal discomfort and constipation that is often followed by bloody diarrhea during the second week of the illness. Also during the second week, fever increases to 40°C, and the patient often becomes severely ill. Abdominal pain and distension worsen, and mental status dulls. By the third week, in the absence of antibiotic treatment, a significant percentage of patients recover, but 10% die of septic shock or bowel perforation.

On physical examination, the pulse may inappropriately slow despite the high fever (temperature–pulse dissociation). The abdomen is often markedly distended and tender during the later phases of the disease, and splenomegaly is noted in a significant percentage of patients. By the second to third week, small (2 mm to 5 mm) rose-colored maculopapular lesions that blanch on pressure develop on the upper abdomen and chest regions in 80% of patients. Rose spots usually persist for 2 to 4 days. Normochromic normocytic anemia and moderate peripheral leukopenia (WBC count in the range of 2500/mm^3) are common. Some patients may have a mild elevation in peripheral leukocyte count.

Blood cultures are positive in 90% of patients during the first week and in 50% during the second week. Stool cultures remain positive for many weeks. *C. fetus* and *Y. enterocolitica* can produce a syndrome that is clinically indistinguishable from typhoid fever.

DIAGNOSIS

Direct examination of the stool using a methylene blue stain should be performed in all severely ill patients to assess the cellular response. The presence of PMNs on stool smear strongly suggests acute bacterial enterocolitis, but the same result may also be seen in amoebic dysentery and in antibiotic-associated pseudomembranous colitis. An abundant PMN response is seen in *Shigella, Campylobacter*, and EIEC infections (Table 8.1). Cases of *Salmonella* enterocolitis tend to have a less vigorous PMN response in the stool, and patients with *S. typhi* may demonstrate increased numbers of fecal monocytes.

The sensitivity of leukocyte stool smear varies depending on the clinical laboratory. Fecal lactoferrin (a iron-binding protein found in PMNs) is a more sensitive and specific (90% to 100%) test for differentiating acute bacterial enterocolitis from viral gastroenteritis, but it is not widely available. Gram stain can also be performed, and the finding of seagull-shaped gram-negative forms is highly suggestive of *Campylobacter*. The bacterial culture is positive in approximately 5% of cases of acute diarrhea. There-

fore cultures should be obtained only in patients with severe disease in which hospitalization is being considered, in patients with bloody diarrhea, or in cases in which an outbreak is suspected. The stool sample should be planted immediately on the appropriate media to maximize sensitivity. In the case of *Campylobacter*, special selective media and microaerophilic conditions must be used (see the earlier discussion of this specific pathogen). Pathogenic strains of *E. coli* cannot be readily identified by culture; immunologic and molecular biologic methods are required. Slide agglutination using specific antiserum against O antigens has been performed in several epidemics. For investigative purposes, primers for polymerase chain reaction (PCR) and probes for DNA hybridization are also available.

TREATMENT AND OUTCOME

Moat cases of bacterial enterocolitis are self-limiting, usually lasting 3 to 7 days. They may not require antibiotic therapy (Table 8.2). Fluid and electrolyte replacement is generally the most important supportive measure. Agents that slow peristalsis are contraindicated in patients with bacterial enterocolitis who have fever or bloody stools. These drugs may prolong fever, increase the risk of bacteremia, lead to toxic megacolon, and prolong fecal excretion of the pathogen. Bowel splints can also exacerbate the hemolytic uremic syndrome. Antibiotic therapy for *Salmonella* enterocolitis prolongs carriage in the stool and has not been shown to shorten the duration of gastroenteritis. Antibiotics are specifically contraindicated in patients with EHEC, because they may exacerbate the hemolytic uremic syndrome.

Patients with typhoid fever should receive immediate antibiotic treatment. Chloramphenicol was the treatment of choice until recently, but relapses occurred with that regimen, and increasing numbers of *S. typhi* have become resistant to chloramphenicol. A fluoroquinolone (ciprofloxacin, levofloxacin) or a third-generation cephalosporin (ceftriaxone) are the recommended first-line regimens.

To prevent potential complications associated with bacteremia, nontyphoidal salmonella should also be treated with antibiotics when this disease develops in neonates, people over age of 50 years, immunocompromised patients, and patients with prosthetic valves or vascular grafts. Antibiotic therapy should be continued only for 48 to 72 hours, or until the patient no longer has a fever. An oral fluoroquinolone, amoxicillin, or trimethoprim–sulfamethoxazole are generally recommended.

To prevent person-to-person spread and shorten the course of shigellosis, trimethoprim–sulfamethoxazole or ciprofloxacin are usually administered.

KEY POINTS

About the Diagnosis of Bacterial Diarrhea

1. Direct examination of the stool using methylene blue stain assesses polymorphonuclear leukocyte (PMN) response.

   a) Abundant PMNs are seen in *Shigella, Campylobacter*, and enteroinvasive *Escherichia coli* infection.

   b) *Salmonella* infections produces moderate PMNs; with *S. typhi,* monocytes may be seen,

   c) PMNs are also seen with amoebic dysentery and *Clostridium difficile* toxin–associated diarrhea.

2. A Gram stain showing seagull-shaped gram-negative forms indicates *Campylobacter* infection.

3. Culture stools using both standard media and *Campylobacter*-selective media.

4. *E. coli* strains can be identified by slide agglutination tests using specific O antisera.

Table 8.2. Antibiotic Treatment of Acute Bacterial Diarrhea

Cause	Treatment	Duration	Comments
Salmonella			
Nontyphoidal	Ciprofloxacin 500 mg PO q12h OR levofloxacin 400 mg PO q24h	5–7 days	Treatment prolongs the carrier state, avoid in most cases; for exceptions see text
Typhoid fever	Ciprofloxacin 500 mg PO q12h OR ceftriaxone 2 gm IV q24h Children: azithromycin 1 g, then 500 mg PO × 6 days	10–14 days	Delay in therapy increases risk of death; chloramphenicol no longer used in the United States
Shigella			
	Ciprofloxacin 500 mg PO q12h, OR levofloxacin 400 mg PO q24h OR TMX-sulfa 1 double-strength tablet q12h	3 days	Sterilizes the stool and reduces secondary cases
Campylobacter jejuni			
	Azithromycin 500 g PO q24h OR ciprofloxacin 500 mg PO q12h	3 days	Treatment within 4 days shortens the course; fluoroquinolone resistance increasing
Escherichia coli			
Enterotoxigenic Enteroaggregative Enteropathogenic Enteroinvasive	Ciprofloxacin 500 mg PO q12h OR levofloxacin 400 mg PO q24h	3 days	Shortens the course of illness
Enterohemorrhagic	No treatment		Also avoid anti-motility drugs; both increase toxin release and worsen hemolytic uremic syndrome; supportive care only
Vibrio parahemolyticus			
	No treatment		Antibiotics do not shorten the course of illness
Vibrio cholera			
	Ciprofloxacin 1 g PO Alternative (adults): doxycycline 300 mg PO	1 dose 1 dose	Reduces diarrhea volume; hydration most important;
Yersinia enterocolitica			
	Doxycycline 100 mg IV q12h PLUS gentamicin 5 mg/kg IV q24h Alternative: ciprofloxacin 500–750 mg PO q12h	3–7 days	Treat only very severe disease; efficacy of antibiotics not proven
Clostridium difficile			
	Metronidazole 500 mg PO q8h Alternative: Nitazoxanide 500 mg PO Q12H Preferred for severe colitis: vancomycin 125–500 mg PO q6h	10 days	Discontinue all other antibiotics if possible, nitazoxinide may be helpful in cases refractory to metronidazole

---

KEY POINTS

About the Treatment of Bacterial Diarrhea

1. These diseases are self-limiting, and seldom require antibiotic treatment.
2. Fluid and electrolyte replacement are most important.
3. Avoid agents that slow peristalsis, which increases the risk of bacteremia, and prolongs fever and the carrier state.
4. Antibiotic treatment of *Salmonella* gastroenteritis prolongs the carrier state. However, to prevent complications associated with bacteremia, use ciprofloxacin, amoxicillin, or trimethoprim–sulfamethoxazole to treat
   a) neonates,
   b) people over the age of 50 years, and
   c) immunocompromised patients or those with prosthetic valves or synthetic vascular grafts.
5. Treat enteric fever emergently with ciprofloxacin or ceftriaxone.
6. Trimethoprim–sulfamethoxazole or ciprofloxacin reduces person-to-person spread of *Shigella*.
7. Erythromycin, azithromycin, or ciprofloxacin shortens the carrier state in *Campylobacter jejuni* infection.
8. *Yersinia* is not usually treated; in severe cases, use trimethoprim–sulfamethoxazole, ciprofloxacin, ceftriaxone.
9. *Vibrio parahaemolyticus* usually not treated.
10. Ciprofloxacin for 3 to 5 days shortens the course of travelers' diarrhea.

KEY POINTS

About Prevention of Bacterial Diarrhea

1. Investigation of sources of contamination is a cost-effective preventive measure.
2. Fecal carriage after *Salmonella* infection may continue for an extended period.
   a) The carrier state can often be eradicated by prolonged therapy (4 to 6 weeks) with amoxicillin or ciprofloxacin.
   b) Carrier state often cannot be eliminated in patients with gallstones.

PREVENTION

Public health measures are the most efficient and cost-effective way of reducing these diseases. By understanding the epidemiology of each pathogen, the public health investigator can track down the source of bacterial contamination and prevent additional cases.

After symptomatic disease, *Salmonella* fecal carriage may continue for an extended period, particularly if the patient received antibiotics. This carriage represents a potential health hazard for food handlers. The carrier state can usually be eradicated by prolonged therapy with amoxicillin (standard dose for 4 to 6 weeks) or a fluoroquinolone (ciprofloxacin: standard dose for 4 to 6 weeks). In patients with gallstones, the carrier state often cannot be eliminated.

For individuals visiting areas endemic for travelers' diarrhea, a nonabsorbable rifamycin derivative, rifaximin, 200 mg orally, once or twice daily is protective.

Antibiotic-Associated Diarrhea

POTENTIAL SEVERITY

Undiagnosed C. difficile can progress to severe colitis that may require colectomy or result in bowel perforation and death.

Antibiotic-associated diarrhea develops in up to 30% of hospitalized patients. Systemic antibiotics reduce the normal flora and interfere with bacterial breakdown of carbohydrates. The increased concentrations of undigested carbohydrate increase the intraluminal osmotic

---

Although antibiotic treatment of *C. jejuni* diarrhea has not been proven to shorten the course of the illness, it has been shown to shorten the carrier state. Useful antibiotics include erythromycin, azithromycin, or ciprofloxacin. Recently, ciprofloxacin-resistant strains have been reported.

Y. enterocolitica is not usually treated; however, in severe cases, trimethoprim–sulfamethoxazole, a fluoroquinolone, or a third-generation cephalosporin may be administered.

V. parahaemolyticus usually does not require treatment. The course of travelers' diarrhea can be shortened to 1.5 days from 3 to 5 days by a brief course of ciprofloxacin.

load, preventing water resorption and causing watery diarrhea. Antibiotic-induced reductions in the normal bowel flora also permit overgrowth by resistant bacteria. *Staphylococcus aureus* and *Candida* species were suggested as possible causes of this diarrhea, but subsequent studies failed to reveal a clear association. Overgrowth of *Klebsiella oxytoca* has been shown to accompany hemorrhagic colitis, and a cytotoxin has been identified in the stool indicating that this organism can account for some cases of antibiotic-associated diarrhea; however, the most frequent causative agent is *C. difficile*. This pathogen has been implicated in 20% to 30% of patients with antibiotic-associated diarrhea and 50% to 75% of those who develop antibiotic-associated colitis.

MICROBIOLOGY, PATHOGENESIS, AND EPIDEMIOLOGY

C. difficile is an obligate anaerobe, spore-forming, gram-positive rod. The organism's name reflects the difficulty of isolated the pathogen on routine media. A cycloserine, cefoxitin, fructose agar with an egg-yolk base is capable of selecting this organism from total fecal flora.

When the bowel flora is exposed to broad-spectrum antibiotics, *C. difficile* overgrows and releases two high-molecular-weight exotoxins, toxin A and toxin B, which bind to and kill cells in the bowel wall.

KEY POINTS

About the Microbiology, Pathogenesis, and Epidemiology of *Clostridium difficile*

1. Obligate anaerobic, spore-forming, gram-positive rod.
2. Produces two cytotoxins, toxin A and toxin B, that bind to and kill host cells.
3. Bowel wall necrosis leads to acute inflammation.
4. A disease of hospitalized patients. Risk factors include
   a) broad-spectrum antibiotic administration (reduces competing normal flora; clindamycin is associated with the highest incidence, followed by ampicillin/amoxicillin and cephalosporins).
   b) cancer chemotherapy.
   c) bowel enemas or stimulants, enteral feedings.
   d) underlying disease in elderly patients or recent gastrointestinal surgery.
5. Spread from patient to patient by hospital personnel through spores carried on hands, clothes, or equipment.

A third toxin, binary toxin, an actin-specific adenosine diphosphate ribosyl transferase, has been detected in up to two thirds of recent *C. difficile* isolates and may be associated with more severe disease. Exposure of tissue-cultured cells to filtrate from *C. difficile*–infected feces resulted in dramatic cytopathic changes, including rounding up and detachment of cells. Death of colonic cells results in the formation of shallow ulcers, an exuberant acute inflammatory response, and the formation of pseudomembranes that are readily seen by colonoscopy. Early lesions are superficial, but as the disease progresses and the toxin levels increase, inflammation can extend through the full thickness of the bowel.

This disease develops in 10% of patients hospitalized for more than 2 days. *C. difficile* diarrhea is rarely encountered in outpatients. The incidence of disease is higher in elderly patients and in those who have severe underlying diseases or have undergone gastrointestinal surgery. An increased incidence is also associated with broad-spectrum antibiotics (clindamycin, ampicillin, amoxicillin, and cephalosporins are associated with the highest incidence), anticancer chemotherapy (methotrexate, 5-fluorouracil, doxorubicin, cyclophosphamide), bowel enemas or stimulants, enteral feedings, and close proximity to another patient with *C. difficile* diarrhea. This infection is spread from patient to patient by hospital personnel. Spores can be readily carried on hands, clothes, and stethoscopes. Numerous hospital outbreaks have been reported, and these outbreaks occur more commonly on wards where clindamycin is frequently administered.

CLINICAL MANIFESTATIONS

C. difficile causes a spectrum of disease manifestations, from an asymptomatic carrier state to fulminant colitis. The severity of symptoms does not appear to relate to amount of toxin released into the stool, but may relate to the number of toxin receptors in the host's bowel. High titers of immunoglobulin G (IgG) directed against toxin A appear to be protective and are often high in the asymptomatic carrier. The most common form of symptomatic disease is diarrhea without colitis.

Diarrhea usually begins 5 to 10 days after the initiation of antibiotics. However, diarrhea can develop up to 10 weeks after completion of antibiotic therapy. The diarrhea is usually watery, consisting of 5 to 15 bowel movements daily. Crampy, bilateral lower quadrant pain that decreases after a bowel movement, low-grade fever, and mild peripheral blood leukocytosis are common characteristics. Pseudomembranous colitis presents with the same symptoms and findings, except that pseudomembranes are seen on colonoscopy and marked thickened of the colonic bowel wall is seen on computed tomography (CT) scan.

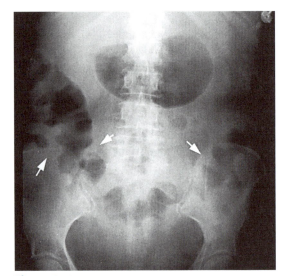

Figure 8–1. Abdominal radiograph demonstrating prominent thumbprinting seen in *Clostridium difficile* colitis. Arrows point to thickened folds of the large intestine, indicative of marked bowel edema. Picture courtesy of Pat Abbitt, University of Florida College of Medicine

These forms of *C. difficile*–induced diarrhea can be difficult to differentiate clinically from the most common form of antibiotic-associated diarrhea, osmotic diarrhea. Lack of fever or leukocytosis, absence of PMNs in the stool, and improvement when oral intake is reduced favor osmotic diarrhea.

Fulminant colitis develops in 2% to 3% of patients infected with *C. difficile*. This disease is associated with severe morbidity and a high mortality. Diarrhea is usually present; however, some patients develop constipation. Abdominal pain is usually diffuse and severe and can be associated with hypoactive bowel sounds, abdominal distension, and guarding. Findings of peritonitis can develop and usually indicate bowel perforation. Toxic megacolon (bowel loops dilated to more than 7 cm) is a feared complication. Full-thickness involvement of the bowel wall leads to bowel distension and air–fluid levels visible on abdominal CT scan or X-ray. Thumbprinting is often seen, reflecting submucosal edema, which can mimic bowel ischemia (Figure 8.1). Sigmoidoscopy must be performed cautiously under these conditions because of the high risk of perforation. Marked elevation in the peripheral WBC count (25,000 to 35,000 /mm^3) is common. The development of lactic acidosis usually indicates impending bowel perforation and irreversible bowel damage that requires immediate surgical intervention.

DIAGNOSIS

Stool smear demonstrates PMNs in half of cases and may be heme-positive. Stool culture for *C. difficile* is not recommended because this organism is difficult and expensive to isolate, and because culture yields many false positive results. Diagnostic laboratories have therefore focused on toxin detection.

The original cytotoxicity assay remains the definitive test. Stool filtrate is overlaid onto fibroblasts. If the toxin is present, the cells round up and eventually detach from the monolayer. Specificity is confirmed if these effects are blocked by incubating the filtrate in advance with toxin-neutralizing antibody. The assay is sensitive (94% to 100%) and specific (99%) when performed by experienced personnel, but it is expensive and requires 2 to 3 days to perform.

Enzyme-linked immunoabsorbent assay (ELISA) kits that detect toxins A and B are now preferred as the initial screening test. They are rapid and less expensive, and they have a comparable specificity, but a lower sensitivity (70% to 90%). Many assays detect only toxin A and fail to detect a small percentage of *C. difficile* strains that exclusively produce toxin B. In cases in which the diagnosis is strongly suspected, a negative ELISA assay should be confirmed by the cytotoxic assay.

Sigmoidoscopy is usually not required, because patients with positive findings almost always have a positive toxin test. With caution, endoscopy can be performed in the patient who requires immediate diagnosis, who is unable to produce stool, or in whom other colonic disorders are also being considered. A significant percentage of patients will have negative findings; however, the presence of pseudomembranes is considered diagnostic.

TREATMENT, OUTCOME, AND PREVENTION

Whenever possible, the first step should be to discontinue the offending antibiotic or antibiotics. In many cases, patients will fully recover without further intervention. This approach is preferred when symptoms are mild, because it allows the bowel to recolonize with competing normal flora and prevents relapse. In contrast, administration of metronidazole or vancomycin is associated with a 10% to 25% relapse rate.

As in other forms of diarrhea, fluids and electrolytes need to be replaced. Diarrhea serves to protect the mucosa by flushing away *C. difficile* toxins; antiperistaltic agents must therefore be avoided. Use of such agents increases the risk of full-blown colitis and toxic megacolon. If these measurers are not effective or practical, specific therapy with oral metronidazole (250 mg four times pwe dy for 10 days) should be initiated. Asymptomatic patients colonized with *C. difficile* should not be treated. Recurrent disease is common as a consequence of residual spores in the stool that are not killed by the antibiotic. First-time recurrences should be treated with the same regimen used to treat the initial episode. Oral vancomycin should be avoided whenever possible because of the increased risk of selecting for vancomycin-resistant enterococci. Nearly all strains of *C. difficile* are killed by metronidazole, and bactericidal levels are readily achieved in the bowel of symptomatic patients. Cure rates of 95% have been reported with the use of this agent. Recent observational studies suggest a trend toward poorer cure rates and higher relapse rates.

Oral vancomycin (125 mg four times daily for 10 days) should be reserved for patients with severe disease. The bowel does not absorb vancomycin, and stool levels of vancomycin reach concentrations that are 1000 to 3000 times the minimum inhibitory concentration for *C. difficile*. Unlike metronidazole levels, which decrease in stool as the integrity of the bowel mucosa improves, vancomycin levels remain high throughout the course of the disease. Response rates and relapse rates for oral vancomycin are comparable to those for oral metronidazole. In the patient who is unable to take oral medications, intravenous metronidazole (500 mg every 8 hours) should be administered. Intravenous metronidazole is excreted in the biliary tract, and therapeutic levels of the

---

KEY POINTS

About the Diagnosis, Treatment, and Prevention of *Clostridium difficile* Diarrhea

1. Diagnosis:
   a) In 50% of cases, PMNs are found in a stool smear.
   b) Enzyme-linked immunoabsorbent assay for toxins A and B is the preferred assay. Many assays detect only toxin A and can miss *C. difficile* that produces only toxin B.
   c) The cytotoxicity assay remains the definitive test, but it is expensive and takes several days.
   d) Endoscopy is usually not required, and risks perforation.

2. Treatment:
   a) Drugs must be orally administered (except for metronidazole).
   b) Metronidazole is the treatment of choice; intravenous metronidazole is also effective, being excreted in bile.
   c) Use vancomycin only for severe illness because of the risk of superinfection with vancomycin-resistant enterococci.
   d) Nitazoxanide comparable to metronidazole in initial trials.
   e) Tolevamer binds toxins A and B, but doesn't change bowel flora.
   f) Severe disease may require bowel resection; mortality is 30% to 50%.
   g) Relapse is common because of residual spores. Re-treat with metronidazole.

3. Prevention:
   a) Spread by hospital personnel; hand washing is critical.
   b) Limiting clindamycin use may reduce the attack rate.

---

antibiotic are achieved in the stool. Intravenous vancomycin fails to achieve significant intraluminal bowel concentrations and is not recommended.

Two new medications recently became available. Oral nitazoxanide 500 mg twice daily for 7 to 10 days demonstrated response rates comparable to those with metronidazole. Tolevamer, a soluble high-molecular-weight anionic polymer, binds *C. difficile* toxins A and B without altering the other gastrointestinal flora. In mild-to-moderate disease 2 g in an oral dose every

8 hours demonstrated response rates comparable to those with oral vancomycin and with a trend toward reduced relapse rates. Tolevamer also binds potassium and can cause hypokalemia.

The most feared complications of pseudomembranous colitis are toxic megacolon and bowel perforation. These complications arise in a small proportion of patients (0.4% to 4%), but are associated with a high mortality (30% to 50%). Persistent fever, marked elevation of the peripheral WBC count, lack of response to antibiotics, and marked bowel thickening on CT scan are worrisome findings. They warrant consultation with a general surgeon. When these complications arise, bowel resection and ileostomy are recommended.

Standard infection control measures must be scrupulously followed to prevent hospital personnel from spreading *C. difficile* spores from patient to patient. Thorough hand washing can never be overemphasized. Prolonged broad-spectrum antibiotics should be avoided whenever possible. Limiting the use of clindamycin has proved effective in reducing the attack rate in several hospital outbreaks.

Viral Diarrhea

POTENTIAL SEVERITY

A self-limiting disease that can cause dehydration.

Viral diarrhea is the most common form of the disease, usually causing mild self-limiting watery diarrhea. The viruses most common associated with viral diarrhea are noroviruses, rotaviruses, enteric adenoviruses, and astroviruses.

VIROLOGY, PATHOGENESIS, AND EPIDEMIOLOGY

Norovirus

The single-stranded RNA *Norovirus* belongs to the calicivirus family, a group that derives its name from the distinct cup- or chalice-like indentations of the viral capsid seen on electron microscopy. Because no convenient method is known for propagating the virus, and no animal model of *Norovirus* gastroenteritis exists, little is known about its pathogenesis. Histopathology from infected human volunteers has revealed that the virus causes blunting of villi and PMN infiltration of the lamina propria in the jejunum. Patients present with the acute onset of nausea, vomiting, and watery diarrhea. The virus is shed in the stool for 24 to 48 hours

after the onset of illness, and it also is present in high concentrations in vomitus. Ingestion of 100 viral particles can cause disease.

Infection is transmitted by contaminated water and food and by person-to-person spread. In addition to contaminated drinking water, swimming pools and lakes can transmit the disease. Norovirus is relatively resistant to chlorine. Shellfish are a leading food source, and because the virus is relatively heat-resistant, cooking contaminated shellfish does not completely eliminate the risk of infection. Infected food handlers can contaminate food, resulting in large outbreaks. Large outbreaks have also been reported in closed environments such as ships, military installations, hospitals, and nursing homes. Norovirus is more commonly associated with outbreaks in adults, but infants and children may also be infected by this virus or another member of the calicivirus group.

Rotavirus

The name *Rotavirus* (from the Latin *rota*, meaning wheel) for this double-stranded RNA virus is derived from the wheel-like appearance of the viral capsid on

KEY POINTS

About Viral Diarrhea

1. Viral diarrhea is the most common form of infectious diarrhea.
2. The disease is caused primarily by four viral groups:
   a) *Norovirus* ("Norwalk"): This calicivirus blunts intestinal villi, causes mild malabsorption, is resistant to chlorine, is spread by contaminated water (including swimming pools), and primarily infects adults.
   b) *Rotavirus*: Causes lactase deficiency, and primarily infects infants. Resists hand washing. Peaks in winter.
   c) Enteric adenovirus 40, 41: Infects infants and young children; peaks in the summer months.
   d) *Astrovirus*: Infects children in pediatric wards and elderly people in nursing homes.
3. Clinical spectrum varies from mild, watery diarrhea to severe nausea, vomiting, and fever. No polymorphonuclear leukocytes are found in the stool. Commercial Enzyme-linked immunoabsorbent assays for *Rotavirus* are available.
4. Self-limiting diseases; use supportive care with hydration.

electron micrographs. It is a member of the reovirus family. Rotaviruses are able to replicate in mature villous epithelial cells in the small intestine. The viral capsid attaches to and penetrates the peripheral membrane of the host cell and enters the cytoplasm. Diarrhea is thought to be caused by loss of absorption by epithelial villi, lactase deficiency, and a decrease in the intestinal concentrations of other dissacharidases. The virus may also increase chloride secretion.

Rotavirus is the most common cause of infant diarrhea, and by age 3 years, more than 90% of children have acquired antibodies. Repeated infections may occur, indicating minimal cross-protection between strains. Adults may also contract the infection, most commonly from infected children as a consequence of fecal–oral transmission. The virus is resistant to hand washing and to many commonly used disinfectants, but it is inactivated by chlorine. It is able to survive on surfaces, in water, and on the hands for prolonged periods. In developed countries, infections most commonly occur during the winter months.

Enteric Adenoviruses

Two serotypes (adenovirus 40 and 41) of this double-stranded DNA virus have been associated with diarrhea. They are the second most frequent cause of nonbacterial gastroenteritis in infants and young children. Infections occur most commonly during the summer months.

Astrovirus

The single-stranded RNA astroviruses have the appearance of a five- or six-pointed star on electron micrographs. Astroviruses have been associated with outbreaks of gastroenteritis in children on pediatric wards and in elderly patients in nursing homes. The prevalence of this virus is lower than those for the other known causes of viral gastroenteritis.

CLINICAL MANIFESTATIONS, DIAGNOSIS, AND TREATMENT

CASE 8.2

A young physician arrived in Tuba City, Arizona, to work in an Indian health service clinic. Three days later, he became ill with mild mid-abdominal cramps and watery diarrhea, but denied fever. He continued working, added additional salt and fluid to his diet, and was inconvenienced, but not incapacitated by his illness. On the third day of symptoms, a stool smear revealed no PMNs, and a bacterial culture grew no pathogens.

The clinical manifestations of viral diarrhea vary. At one end of the clinical spectrum, the patient may experience mild watery diarrhea with minimal symptoms as described in Case 8.2; at the other extreme, the patient may develop severe nausea, vomiting, abdominal cramps, headache, myalgias, and fevers to 39°C. Stool smear reveals no leukocytes, and cultures are negative for bacterial pathogens.

Identification of the specific viral agent is usually not possible. The infecting agents are most readily identified by their appearance on electron microscopy. The PCR technique shows promise for identifying Norovirus in stool and in the environment. Commercial ELISA assays for Rotavirus are available and provide satisfactory results. These diseases are self-limiting and last 2 to 6 days depending on the agent. Maintaining hydration is the primary goal of therapy.

CHRONIC DIARRHEA

As compared with acute diarrhea, which lasts less than 14 days, chronic diarrhea is defined as diarrhea lasting more than 30 days. Persistent diarrhea defines a diarrheal illness that lasts for more than 14 days.

Parasitic Diarrhea

Amoebiasis can mimic bacterial enterocolitis; other parasites, such as *Giardia lamblia*, *Cryptosporidium*, *Isospora belli*, and *Microsporidium* often present with complaints that mimic viral gastroenteritis. However, in most instances, these parasitic infections are not self-limiting; they persist for prolonged periods.

AMOEBIASIS

Life Cycle and Epidemiology

Amoebiasis is caused by *Entamoeba histolytica*. Other amoebic species found in the feces of humans, including *Entamoeba coli*, *Entamoeba dispar*, *Entamoeba moshkovskii*, *Entamoeba hartmanni*, *Entamoeba polecki*, *Endolimax nana*, and *Iodamoeba buetschlii* do not cause disease in humans. *Entamoeba histolytica* trophozoites are large (10 to 60 μm in diameter) and contain lucent cytoplasm, a single nucleus, and multiple intracellular granules (Figure 8.2). They crawl by chemotaxis, using an actin-based mechanism that is similar to that used by human macrophages and neutrophils.

Trophozoites attach to specific galactose receptors on host cells, and after contact, rapidly kill the host cells by a calcium-dependent mechanism. The amoeba also releases numerous proteolytic enzymes that break down the cell matrix of the anchoring host. Flask-shaped mucosal ulcers may be found in the colon at sites of trophozoite invasion. Ulcers can extend into the submucosa and result in invasion of the bloodstream.

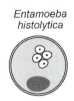 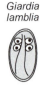

Entamoeba histolytica   *Giardia lamblia*   *Cryptosporidium parvum*   *Isospora belli*   microsporidia

├─ 10µm ─┤

Figure 8–2. Parasites that cause diarrhea. Each pathogen is schematically drawn to scale and represents the form most commonly detected on stool smear.

Amoebae can also travel up the portal vein and form abscesses in the liver. Because *Entamoeba histolytica* can lyse host neutrophils, acute inflammatory cells are rarely seen in regions of active infection. Immunity against amoebae is mediated primarily by generation of immunoglobulin A antibodies and by cell-mediated immune response. Patients with depressed cell-mediated immunity are at greater risk for disseminated disease.

In addition to its trophozoite form, *Entamoeba histolytica* forms dormant cysts under unfavorable environmental conditions. The cyst has a distinctive morphology, consisting of a rounded structure with three or four distinct nuclei (Figure 8.2). These hardy cysts can remain viable for months outside the host in moist, warm environments. Trophozoites are very sensitive to the acid pH

of the stomach; however, cysts readily survive the gastric environment, and ingestion of single cyst can cause active infection. Cysts can be spread from person to person by the fecal–oral route and by contaminated food and water. In developing countries, a large proportion of the population becomes infected with *Entamoeba histolytica*, and the infected individuals usually carry the parasite in their stool for 12 months. In the United States, institutionalized patients, particularly the mentally challenged, have a high incidence of stool carriage and disease. An increased incidence has also been observed in sexually promiscuous homosexual males. The risk of amoebiasis is increased by travel to a developing country and is particularly high in individuals who reside in the endemic area for more than 1 month.

Clinical Manifestations

Symptoms depend on the degree of bowel invasion. Superficial bowel infection is associated with watery diarrhea and nonspecific gastrointestinal complaints. Invasive intestinal disease presents with the gradual onset, over 1 to 3 weeks, of abdominal pain and bloody diarrhea associated with tenesmus and abdominal tenderness. Fever is noted in some patients. Amoebiasis can be mistaken for ulcerative colitis, and administration of corticosteroids can dramatically worsen the disease and lead to toxic megacolon. Amoebic liver abscess can develop in conjunction with colitis. Patients complain of right upper quadrant pain and can also experience pain referred to the right shoulder. Hepatomegaly is noted in half of all cases.

Diagnosis and Treatment

Stool smears usually demonstrate PMNs. However, because the amoebic trophozoites destroy human PMNs, the numbers are often lower than are seen in patients with shigellosis. In amoebiasis, stools are always heme-positive, reflecting trophozoite invasion and destruction of bowel mucosa. In acute hepatic disease, alkaline phosphatase may not be elevated, but it rises in chronic hepatic infection.

Previously, the diagnosis was made by identifying trophozoites or cysts in the stool. However, two non-

---

KEY POINTS

About Life Cycle and Epidemiology of Amoebiasis

1. Caused by *Entamoeba histolytica*, a parasite that contains ingested red blood cells and that is 10 to 60 µm in diameter.
2. Parasite binds to galactose receptors on host cells and kill them, causes flask-like ulcers.
3. Able to invade the portal vein and form abscesses in the liver.
4. Able to lyse host polymorphonuclear leukocytes. Acute inflammatory cells are rarely seen in areas of infection. Specific anti-IgA antibodies and cell-mediated immunity provide protection.
5. Dormant cysts can survive for month in moist, warm environments.
6. Cysts can contaminate food and water.
7. Very common in developing countries.
8. In the United States, the paraxiate is found in institutionalized patients, sexually promiscuous homosexuals, and tourists.

<table>
</table>

KEY POINTS

About the Clinical Manifestations, Diagnosis, and Treatment of Amoebiasis

1. Clinical presentation depends on the degree of invasion:
   a) Watery diarrhea is associated with superficial infection.
   b) Bloody diarrhea, tenesmus, abdominal pain, and tenderness with more invasive disease.
   c) Can be misdiagnosed as ulcerative colitis; corticosteroids can lead to toxic megacolon.
   d) Right upper quadrant, right shoulder pain, hepatomegaly seen with liver abscess.

2. Diagnosis:
   a) Stool smears show fewer polymorphonuclear leukocytes (PMNs) than are seen with shigellosis (trophozoites destroy PMNs).
   b) Stools are always heme-positive.
   c) Alkaline phosphatase elevated in chronic, but not acute hepatic abscess.
   d) Stool examination is insensitive; fecal antigen or polymerase chain reaction is recommended.
   e) Serum is anti-amoebic antibody positive in most patients after 1 week of symptoms.
   f) Aspirate from liver abscess shows brownish, sterile liquid without PMNs; parasite not usually seen, and antigen may not be detected.

3. Treatment: Metronidazole for active disease; iodoquinol or paromomycin for carrier state.

pathogenic species *Entamoeba dispar* and *Entamoeba moshkovskii* cannot be morphologically distinguished from *Entamoeba histolytica*. Fecal *Entamoeba histolytica* antigen tests have proven to be more sensitive and specific than stool smears, and they are now the diagnostic test of choice. Identification in stool by the PCR method is also sensitive and specific, but is not widely available. These tests should be ordered in conjunction with a serum anti-amoebic antibody. The latter test is positive in most patients who have had symptomatic disease for more than 1 week. However, antibodies persist for life and therefore are not helpful in detecting reinfection.

Abdominal CT scan should be performed in patients with symptoms consistent with hepatic disease. This test readily identifies abscesses. Serum anti-amoebic antibodies are elevated in 99% of patients with hepatic amoebic abscess. Aspiration of the abscess

yields sterile, odorless, brownish liquid without PMNs. Amoebae are not generally seen, and are only rarely cultured because the parasite concentrates in the walls of the abscess. Antigen is detected in hepatic fluid in only 40% of cases.

Invasive enterocolitis and hepatic abscess should be treated with oral metronidazole (750 mg every 8 hours for 10 days) or tinidazole [2 g daily, divided into three doses, for 3 to 5 days (not available in the United States.)]. For asymptomatic cyst excretors, oral iodoquinol (650 mg every 8 hours for 20 days) or paromomycin (25 to 35 mg/kg daily, divided into three doses, for 7 days) is recommended. Diloxanide furoate (500 mg orally every 8 hours for 10 days) can be used as an alternative therapy.

GIARDIA LAMBLIA

Life Cycle and Epidemiology

Like amoebae, *Giardia lamblia*, an enteric flagellated protozoan, has two stages: the free-living trophozoite, and the dormant cyst. The trophozoite consists of a dorsal convex surface and a flat disk-shaped ventral surface composed of microtubules and micro-ribbons, two nuclei, and four pairs of flagella. On stained preparations, it has the appearance of a bearded human face (Figure 8.2). Trophozoites adhere to gastrointestinal endothelial cells, disrupt the brush border, cause dissacharidase deficiency, and induce inflammation. All of these mechanisms are thought to account for watery diarrhea and malabsorption. Cell-mediated and

KEY POINTS

About the Pathogenesis and Epidemiology of Giardiasis

1. *Giardia* exists as trophozoites and dormant cysts.
2. Trophozoites attach to gastrointestinal endothelial cells, causing malabsorption and inflammation.
3. *Giardia* cysts are spread by contaminated water (and sometimes food) and person-to-person contact.
4. Infection occurs worldwide. Common in mountainous regions of the United States.
5. A disease of campers (sterilization of water critical for prevention), daycare centers, and sexually active homosexuals.

humoral immunity both play a role in host defense. Patients with X-linked agammaglobulinemia have an increased risk of contracting severe prolonged disease, emphasizing the contribution of humoral immunity. Under unfavorable environmental conditions *Giardia* can form dormant cysts that are excreted in the stool, and account for spread of disease.

Giardiasis is found throughout the world; it is a common infection in the United States. Giardia cysts are most commonly spread by contaminated water, and multiple waterborne outbreaks have occurred in mountainous regions of the Northeast, Northwest, and Rocky Mountain States, and in British Columbia. Campers must aggressively sterilize drinking water from mountain streams to prevent this common infection. Foodborne outbreaks are increasingly being recognized. *Giardia* can also be transmitted from person to person in daycare centers and other confining institutions. This pathogen also has been spread from person to person by sexually active homosexuals.

Clinical Manifestations, Diagnosis, and Treatment

A patient with this parasite usually has only mild symptoms or is asymptomatic. Adults may complain of abdominal cramps, bloating, diarrhea, anorexia, nausea,

---

KEY POINTS

About the Clinical Manifestations, Diagnosis, and Treatment of Giardiasis

1. Clinical manifestations are usually mild The disease is self-limiting, 4 to 6 weeks.
   a) Adult have mild symptoms: abdominal cramps, anorexia, watery diarrhea, nausea, and belching.
   b) Children have more severe watery diarrhea.
   c) A chronic malabsorption syndrome can develop, primarily with immunoglobulin deficiency.
2. Diagnosis:
   a) Stool smear shows no polymorphonuclear leukocytes; cysts are seen in 90% of cses after three stool exams.
   b) Enzyme-linked immunoabsorbent assay or immunofluorescence antigen are the tests of choice.
   c) Endoscopy no longer necessary.
3. Treat with metronidazole.

---

and malaise. Belching is also a common complaint. Children most often develop watery diarrhea. Symptoms usually resolve spontaneously in 4 to 6 weeks. Chronic disease is less common and results in malabsorption, chronic diarrhea, and weight loss.

A diagnosis of giardiasis should be considered in all patients with prolonged diarrhea. Stool smears reveal no PMNs. Examination for cysts using concentration techniques have a 90% yield after three stool samples. Today, ELISA or immunofluorescence antigen tests with high sensitivity (up to 98%) and specificity (90% to 100%) are available, and they are now the test of choice. Endoscopy and duodenal biopsy, or duodenal aspiration, are no longer necessary in most cases. Oral metronidazole (250 mg every 8 hours for 5 to 7 days) is the treatment of choice.

CHRONIC DIARRHEAL ILLNESSES PRIMARILY ASSOCIATED WITH IMMUNOCOMPROMISED HOSTS

The *Cryptosporidium* intestinal protozoan survives and replicates within the intestinal microvilli, eventually generating oocysts that are excreted in the stool and are responsible for the spread of infection (Figure 8.2). Autoinfection can also occur, explaining how ingestion of small numbers of oocysts can cause severe, persistent infection in the immunocompromised host. Loss of cell-mediated immunity increases the risk of infection and explains the higher incidence of *Cryptosporidium* intestinal disease in AIDS patients.

Cryptosporidium is classified as an intestinal coccidian; it is related to malarial organisms. The mechanisms by which *Cryptosporidium* causes diarrhea are not completely understood. The pathogen affects intestinal ion transport and causes inflammatory damage to the intestinal microvilli, resulting in malabsorption. This parasite is carried in the intestinal tract of many animals and is also found in water. The oocyst is resistant to chlorination, and large outbreaks resulting from contaminated drinking water supplies have been reported. Infection can also be transmitted in contaminated swimming pools, and an outbreak in a water park has been described. Ingestion of 130 oocysts causes diarrheal disease in 50% of volunteers. Person-to-person spread has also been reported and can occur in households or in institutional settings such as daycare centers and hospitals. Animal-to-person spread can take place after exposure to infected farm animals.

The intestinal coccidian *Isospora belli* is found more frequently in tropical environments, but has been identified as a cause of watery diarrhea in AIDS patients in the United States. A characteristic oocyst is excreted in the stool (Figure 8.2).

The obligate intracellular parasite known as *Microsporidium* is very small in comparison with the other parasites that cause diarrhea (Figure 8.2). It was known to be a common pathogen in insects and fish; however, in 1985, intestinal microsporidiosis was first described in an patient with AIDS. This parasite causes significant diarrhea only in immunocompromised hosts. It infects mucosal epithelial cells, causing villous atrophy, and may ascend into the biliary tract to cause cholangitis. The diagnosis is made by demonstrating the organisms in stool or after intestinal biopsy. Giemsa, Ziehl–Nielsen, or Gram stain may be used to identify the organism.

Clinical Manifestations, Diagnosis, and Treatment

Cryptosporidium, *Isospora belli*, and *Microsporidium* all present with chronic watery diarrhea, often associated with abdominal cramps. Most cases occur in immunocompromised hosts, most frequently patients with AIDS. Children and immunocompetent adults can develop symptomatic cryptosporidiosis, and acute disease may be followed by chronic intestinal symptoms associated with fatigue, headaches, eye, and joint pains. Minimal findings are noted on physical examination. Patients may appear malnourished and be dehydrated.

Diagnosis can be made by stool smear. Stool samples should be stained not only with iodine, but also with modified Kinyoun's acid-fast stain, and concentrated. *Cryptosporidium* cysts are acid-fast; however, fecal smears have proved less specific and sensitive than fecal antigen tests that are now commercially available. *Isospora belli* sporocysts are transparent and can easily be overlooked. In addition to being acid-fast, they demonstrate blue autofluorescence when observed under a fluorescence microscope with a 330 to 380 nm ultraviolet filter. A modified trichrome stain is recommended for the diagnosis of *Microsporidium*, which stains the cysts reddish-pink. A number of fluorescence stains that are sensitive and specific for *Microsporidium* are commercially available (for example, Calcofluor white stain from Sigma–Aldritch).

Children and immunocompetent adults with persistent *Cryptosporidium* should be treated with oral nitazoxanide for 3 days (adults: 500 mg twice daily; children 1 to 3 years: 100 mg twice daily; children 4 to 11 years: 200 mg twice daily). For treatment of patients with HIV, HAART (highly active antiretroviral therapy) should be combined with 14 days of nitazoxanide treatment. This agent is not effective when the patient's CD4 count falls below 50 cells/μL.

Isospora belli can be effectively treated with trimethoprim–sulfamethoxazole (1 double-strength tablet every 6 hours for 10 day, then twice daily for 3 weeks). In

---

KEY POINTS

About *Cryptosporidium*, *Isospora belli*, and *Microsporidium*

1. Survive and multiply on or in the mucosal epithelial cells of the intestine.
2. *Cryptosporidium* can spread by contamination of the water supply (oocysts resist chlorination). Small numbers of oocysts—as few as 130—can cause disease.
3. Primarily infect AIDS patients with severely depressed cell-mediated immunity.
4. Cause watery diarrhea and abdominal cramps, dehydration, and malnutrition.
5. Diagnosis is made by stool smear:
   a) *Cryptosporidium* cysts are confirmed by modified Kinyoun acid–fast stain
   b) *Isospora belli* sporocysts are transparent and acid-fast positive; they fluoresce under ultraviolet light
   c) Modified trichrome and fluorescence stains are sensitive and specific for *Microsporidium*.
6. Treatment:
   a) Nitazoxanide for *Cryptosporidium* in children and chronically symptomatic adults.
   b) Trimethoprim–sulfamethoxazole for *Isospora belli*.
   c) Fumagillin effective for *Microsporidium*.

---

sulfa-allergic patients, pyrimethamine (75 mg/kg daily for 3 to 4 weeks), combined with folinic acid (10 to 25 mg daily) has proved to be a successful alternative. Treatment of *Microsporidium* with oral albendizole (400 mg twice daily for 3 weeks) leads to clinical improvement; however, most patients relapse when the medication is discontinued. Fumagillin (20 mg every 8 hours for 2 weeks), an antibiotic derived from *Aspergillus fumigatus*, results in clearance of spores, but relapse occurs in a few patients. Fumagillin is toxic to bone marrow and may result in reversible neutropenia or thrombocytopenia, or both.

■ INTRA-ABDOMINAL INFECTIONS

The overall incidence of intra-abdominal infections is difficult to ascertain, but certainly this group of diseases accounts for a significant number of admissions through the emergency room. Intra-abdominal infections often fall at the interface of internal medicine and surgery. In many cases, the infectious disease specialist, gastroenterologist, radiologist, and general surgeon need to coordinate their care to assure the most favorable outcome.

PRIMARY OR SPONTANEOUS PERITONITIS

POTENTIAL SEVERITY

A frequently fatal infection that requires immediate paracentesis and empiric antibiotic therapy.

Microbiology and Pathogenesis

In adults, spontaneous (primary) peritonitis develops in patients with severe cirrhosis and ascites. Ascites caused by congestive heart failure, malignancy, and lymphedema can also be complicated by this infection. Bacteria may enter the peritoneal space by hematogenous spread, lymphatic spread, or migration through the bowel wall. In patients with severe cirrhosis, the reticuloendothelial system of the liver is often bypassed secondary to shunting, increasing the risk of prolonged bacteremia. Bowel motility is also slowed in these patients, resulting in bacterial overgrowth. The most common pathogens are enteric bowel flora, *E. coli* being most common, followed by *K. pneumoniae. Streptococcus pneumoniae* and other streptococci, including enterococci, may also be cultured. *S. aureus* and anaerobes are infrequently encountered.

Clinical Manifestations

The initial symptoms and signs may be subtle, and physicians need to maintain a low threshold for diagnostic and therapeutic intervention. Fever is the most common manifestation, and initially, it is often low grade (38°C range). Abdominal pain is usually diffuse and constant, and differs from the usual sensation of tightness experienced with tense ascites. A third common manifestation is a deterioration of mental status. Infection is well known to exacerbate hepatic encephalopathy. Diarrhea may precede other symptoms and signs, and is usually precipitated by overgrowth of the bowel flora. Abdominal tenderness is diffuse and not associated with guarding, because the

---

KEY POINTS

About the Microbiology, Pathogenesis, and Clinical Presentation of Primary Peritonitis

1. Most commonly associated with end-stage liver disease and portal hypertension.
2. Organisms infect the ascitic fluid by hematogenous spread, lymphatic spread, and bowel leakage.
3. Infecting organisms:
   a) Enteric gram-negative pathogens are most common (*Escherichia coli* and *Klebsiella pneumoniae*).
   b) *Streptococcus pneumoniae* and enterococci are also possibilities.
   c) Anaerobes and *Staphylococcus aureus* are uncommon.
4. Clinical presentation may be subtle:
   a) Low-grade fever (38°C)
   b) Constant, diffuse abdominal pain without guarding
   c) Worsening mental status

---

ascites separates the visceral and parietal peritoneum, preventing severe inflammatory irritation of the abdominal wall muscles. In the late stages of infection, rebound tenderness may be elicited. If hypotension and hypothermia develop before antibiotics are initiated, the prognosis is grave.

Diagnosis

The diagnosis of spontaneous peritonitis is made by sampling the ascitic fluid. Needle aspiration of peritoneal fluid is a simple and safe procedure. Significant bleeding requiring transfusion occurs in less than 1% of patients, despite abnormally elevated prothrombin times in a high percentage of cases. Paracentesis is a minimally traumatic procedure and does not require prophylactic plasma transfusions.

Proper handling of the samples is critical for making an accurate diagnosis. A minimum of 10 mL of ascitic fluid should be inoculated into a blood culture flask. Care must be taken to exchange the needle used to penetrate the skin for a new sterile needle that is used to puncture the blood culture flask. A second sample should be inoculated into a tube containing anticoagulant for cell counts. If this precaution is not taken, the ascites fluid may clot, preventing accurate cytologic analysis. A third tube should be sent to measure total protein, albumin, lactic dehydrogenase (LDH), glucose, and amylase levels. A separate syringe or tube should also be sent for Gram stain.

The leukocyte count in the ascitic fluid of patients with spontaneous peritonitis almost always exceeds 300 cells/mm^3 with predominance of PMNs. The diagnosis is strongly suggested by an absolute PMN count exceeding 250/mm^3. Urinalysis leukocyte esterase strips can be used to rapidly assess acute inflammation, a reading of 2+ or higher indicating probable infection. Gram stain is positive in 20% to 40% of cases. Other ascites fluid values help to differentiate primary from secondary peritonitis. High total protein, LDH, and amylase, accompanied by low glucose in the ascitic fluid are more commonly found in secondary peritonitis and should raise the possibility of bowel perforation.

Treatment and Outcome

Empiric therapy should be initiated emergently. Delays in therapy can result in sepsis, hypotension, lactic acidosis, and death. In the patient with cirrhosis and ascites who has fever, abdominal pain, or tenderness, changes in mental status, or more than 250 PMNs/mm^3 in their ascitic fluid, antibiotics should be initiated as soon as blood, urine, and ascites fluid cultures have been obtained. A third-generation cephalosporin (cefotaxime or ceftriaxone) covers most of the potential pathogens. If secondary peritonitis is suspected, anaerobic coverage with metronidazole should be added. Treatment should be continued for 5 to 10 days, depending on the response to therapy.

Mortality remains high in this disease (60% to 70%), reflecting the severe underlying liver disease in these patients and the serious nature of the infection. Early diagnosis may reduce mortality to the 40% range. Death is often the result of end-stage cirrhosis, spontaneous peritonitis being a manifestation of this terminal disease. Patients who have had a first bout of spontaneous peritonitis should strongly be considered for liver transplant.

Intermittent prophylaxis may be considered in patients at risk for recurrent spontaneous peritonitis. Prophylactic regimens have included trimethoprim–sulfamethoxazole (1 double-strength tablet orally for 5 of 7 days) or oral ciprofloxacin (750 mg once weekly).

SECONDARY PERITONITIS

POTENTIAL SEVERITY

A life-threatening illness that usually requires acute surgical intervention.

Microbiology and Pathogenesis

Spillage of bowel flora into the peritoneal cavity has multiple causes. Perforation of a gastric ulcer, appendicitis with rupture, diverticulitis, bowel neoplasm, gangrenous bowel resulting from strangulation or mesenteric artery insufficiency, and pancreatitis are some of the diseases that commonly lead to secondary peritonitis.

The types of organisms associated with peritonitis depend on the site of mucosal breakdown. Gastric perforation most commonly results in infection with mouth flora, including streptococci, *Candida*, lactobacilli, and anaerobes. Perforation in the lower regions of the bowel result in infections with mixed enteric flora. In the colon, bacterial concentrations in feces average 10^{11} colony-forming units per milliliter. Anaerobes constitute a major component, *Bacteroides fragilis* being one of the most common

---

KEY POINTS

About the Diagnosis, Treatment, and Outcome of Spontaneous Peritonitis

1. Paracentesis needs to be performed when this diagnosis is considered:
   a) New sterile needle to inoculate 10 mL fluid into a blood culture flask
   b) Cell count from an anticoagulated sample showing more than 250 leukocytes per cubic millimeter, with predominance of polymorphonuclear leukocytes (PMNs, is a positive result).
   c) Gram stain positive in 20% to 30% of patients.
   d) Elevated protein, lactate dehydrogenase, and amylase, with low glucose suggests secondary peritonitis.
2. Start empiric antibiotics emergently, as soon as cultures are obtained:
   a) Use Ceftriaxone or cefotaxime.
   b) Add metronidazole if secondary peritonitis is suspected
   c) Mortality is 60% to 70%, reduced to 40% with early treatment.
3. Marker of severe end-stage liver disease. Patients should be considered for liver transplant.
4. Trimethoprim–sulfamethoxazole or ciprofloxacin prophylaxis is recommended for patients at risk.

KEY POINTS

About the Microbiology and Pathogenesis of Secondary Peritonitis

1. Bacteriology depends on the site of perforation.
   a) Gastric perforation: Mouth flora, including *Candida* and anaerobes are common.
   b) Lower bowel contains 10^{11} bacteria/mL, and perforation causes massive soilage: Anaerobes are a major component, *Bacteroides fragilis* being common; among aerobic gram-negative bacteria, *Escherichia coli* predominates; *Klebsiella, Proteus*, and *Enterobacter* species are also common; gram-positive *Streptococcus viridans*, enterococci, and *Clostridia perfringens* are also seen.
2. Peritoneum exudes 300 mL to 500 mL of proteinaceous material hourly, with masses of polymorphonuclear lymphocutes; cleared by the lymphatics, but then reach the bloodstream. Fibrinous material can wall off abscesses.
3. Metabolic acidosis, hypoxia, multi-organ failure, and death may follow.

KEY POINTS

About the Clinical Presentation of Secondary Peritonitis

1. Abdominal pain is usually sharp and begins at the site of spillage.
2. Any movement or deep breathing worsens the pain.
3. Peritoneal inflammation causes abdominal spasm (guarding) and rebound.
4. Rectal tenderness may be found.
5. Elderly patients often lack the typical findings of peritonitis.

---

species. Aerobic gram-negative bacteria are abundant, *E. coli* predominating. *Klebsiella, Proteus*, and *Enterobacter* species are also common. Gram-positive bacteria also are found in the bowel flora, with *S. viridans*, enterococci, and *C. perfringens* predominating.

The peritoneal response to infection is usually rapid and exuberant. Large quantities of proteinaceous exudate are released into the peritoneum, and a massive influx of PMNs and macrophages occurs. The influx of fluid can result in intravascular fluid losses of 300 mL to 500 mL hourly. Mechanically, the diaphragmatic lymphatic system can clear large numbers of bacteria quickly, but once in the lymphatic system, the bacteria usually invade the bloodstream. Phagocytic cells ingest large numbers of bacteria and kill them. Deposition of fibrinous exudate can wall off the infection to form discrete abscesses. When the peritoneal host defense is overwhelmed, the patient develops metabolic acidosis, tissue hypoxia, irreversible shock, and multi-organ failure. Death follows.

Clinical Manifestations

The anterior peritoneum is richly enervated, and the first manifestation of inflammation is abdominal pain that is usually sharp, localized to the initial site of spillage, and aggravated by motion. Pain is almost always accompanied by loss of appetite and nausea. Fever, chills, constipation, and abdominal distension are common. Patients usually lie still in bed, breathing with shallow respirations. Fever, tachycardia, and hypotension develop in the later stages.

On abdominal exam, the bowel sounds are decreased or absent, and the abdomen is tender to palpation. Guarding and involuntary spasm of the abdominal muscles can result in a board-like abdomen. If slow compression of the abdomen followed by rapid release of pressure causes severe pain, the patient has rebound tenderness, indicating peritoneal irritation. On rectal exam, tenderness can often be elicited. Elderly patients often fail to present with the classic findings of peritonitis. They often have only mild to moderate tenderness, and do not exhibit guarding or rebound. A high index of suspicion must be maintained when an elderly patient presents with abdominal pain. These patients are at increased risk for diverticulitis, perforated colonic carcinoma, and bowel ischemia.

Diagnosis and Treatment

Serial abdominal examinations, careful monitoring of vital signs, and peripheral WBC count are helpful in deciding whether an exploratory laparotomy is necessary. A high peripheral WBC count in the range 17,000 to 25,000 WBCs per cubic millimeter with an increased percentage of PMNs and band forms is usually noted. A normal peripheral leukocyte count without a predominance of PMNs should call into question the diagnosis of secondary peritonitis. Supine and upright abdominal X-rays should be performed to exclude free air under the diaphragm (indicative of bowel or gastric perforation), to assess the bowel gas pattern, and to search for areas of thickened edematous bowel wall. A chest X-ray must always be performed to exclude lower lobe pneumonia, which can cause ileus and upper quadrant tenderness mimicking peritonitis. A CT scan of the abdomen and pelvis following oral and intravenous contrast is now considered the initial diagnostic test of choice for patients with suspected intra-abdominal infection. This diagnostic procedure often obviates the need for exploratory laparotomy and can assist in the accurate diagnosis of appendicitis, localization and needle aspiration of abscesses, and identification of areas of bowel obstruction.

Antibiotic treatment should be initiated emergently in patients suspected of secondary peritonitis.

Broad-spectrum antibiotic coverage is necessary to cover the multiple organisms infecting the peritoneum. A number of regimens have been recommended. Single agents are available that are effective for community-acquired infections of mild to moderate severity; these include high doses of cefoxitin, cefotetan, and ticarcillin–clavulanate. Imipenem–cilastatin or meropenem can be used as a single agent in severe peritonitis or in hospital-acquired or resistant infections. Combination therapy is often used in severe cases:

1. Cefoxitin or cefotetan plus gentamicin

2. Metronidazole and a third-generation cephalosporin (ceftriaxone, cefotaxime, ceftizoxime)

3. Metronidazole plus a fluoroquinolone (ciprofloxacin, levofloxacin, gatifloxacin)

4. Clindamycin plus aztreonam

When secondary peritonitis is being considered, a general surgeon should be consulted emergently. Repeated abdominal exam allows the surgeon to follow the progression of findings and if tenderness becomes more diffuse and guarding and rebound increase, exploratory laparotomy is often required for diagnosis, drainage, and bowel repair. Peritoneal irrigation is performed intraoperatively, and drains are placed at sites where purulent collections are noted. Multiple operations are often required for the surgical treatment of patients with diffuse purulent peritonitis. Antibiotic coverage should be adjusted based on the cultures and sensitivities of the intraoperative cultures.

SECONDARY PERITONITIS ASSOCIATED WITH PERITONEAL DIALYSIS

Bacterial peritonitis is a frequent complication of chronic ambulatory peritoneal dialysis and is the most frequent reason for discontinuation of that therapy. *S. aureus*, including methicillin-resistant strains (MRSA), or a single gram-negative bacteria are most commonly associated with this infection. The incidence of *S. epidermidis* infection has decreased over the past decade. *Pseudomonas aeruginosa* grows readily in water and is the causative agent in up to 5% of cases. Fungal peritonitis has become increasingly common. Atypical mycobacteria and, less commonly, *Mycobacterium tuberculosis* have also caused peritonitis in this setting.

As observed in spontaneous peritonitis, fever and diffuse abdominal pain are the most common complaints. The peritoneal dialysis fluid usually becomes cloudy as a consequence of inflammatory cells. Peritoneal fluid WBC counts usually exceed 100 /mm^3, with a predominance of PMNs. A predominance of lymphocytes should raise the possibility of fungal or tuberculous infection. Cultures of the peritoneal fluid (two cultures,

10 mL in each blood culture flask) and Gram stain should be obtained. Yield from a Gram stain is low, but properly obtained peritoneal cultures are positive in more than 90% of cases. Blood cultures should be obtained if systemic symptoms are present, but such cultures are rarely positive.

After samples for culture have been obtained, antibiotic should be added to the dialysate. Initial empiric therapy should include a first-generation cephalosporin (cefazolin 500 mg/L loading dose, followed by 125 mg/L in each dialysate bag), or vancomycin if MRSA is suspected (1000 mg loading dose, followed by 25 mg in each bag), and an aminoglycoside (gentamicin or tobramycin 0.6 mg/kg or amikacin 2 mg/kg per exchange, once daily). Once-daily aminoglycoside therapy rather than constant treatment is recommended to reduce the risk of ototoxicity. If the patient fails to improve within 48 hours, removal of the dialysis catheter should be considered.

HEPATIC ABSCESS

POTENTIAL SEVERITY

Usually presents subacutely. With appropriate drainage and antibiotics, prognosis is excellent.

Pathogenesis and Microbiology

Spread of pyogenic infection to the liver can occur in multiple ways. Biliary tract infection is most common, followed by portal vein bacteremia associated with intra-abdominal infection, primarily appendicitis, diverticulitis, or inflammatory bowel disease. Direct extension into the liver from a contiguous infection can occur after perforation of the gallbladder or duodenal ulcer, or in association with a perinephric, pancreatic, or subphrenic abscess. Penetrating wounds and postoperative complications may result in liver abscess. Bacteremia from any source can seed the liver via the hepatic artery and result in the formation of multiple abscesses. In approximately one quarter of cases, a cause cannot be determined.

The bacteriology of this infection reflects the primary site of infection. As in secondary peritonitis, this infection is usually polymicrobial. Anaerobes are commonly cultured, including *Bacteroides* species. *Fusobacterium*, *Peptostreptococcus*, and *Actinomyces* species, and microaerophilic streptococci (*S. milleri* being most common) are frequently found. Enteric gram-negative rods are also important pathogens, *K. pneumoniae* (particularly the K1 serotype) being most common. *Candida* can also invade the liver, candidal abscesses usually occurring in leukemia patients following chemotherapy-induced neutropenia. Amoebic liver abscess is rare, but complicates 3% to 9% of patients with amoebic colitis.

Clinical Manifestations

Fever with or without chills is the most common presenting complaint. It may also be the only complaint, hepatic abscess being one of the more common infectious causes of fever of undetermined origin (See Case 3.1). Abdominal pain develops in about half of these patients, often confined to the right upper quadrant. Pain is usually dull and constant. Weight loss (more than 10 pounds in less than 3 months) is another frequent complaint. Physical exam often reveals tenderness over the liver. Jaundice is rare. In patients with abscess in the upper regions of the right hepatic lobe, pulmonary exam may reveal decreased breath sounds on that side because of atelectasis or pleural effusion.

Diagnosis, Treatment, and Outcome

With the exception of amoebic liver abscess, the peripheral WBC count is usually elevated (above 20,000/mm^3), with increased numbers of immature neutrophils. Serum alkaline phosphatase is also elevated in most cases. Blood cultures are positive in up to half of patients. Abdominal CT scan is the most sensitive test for identifying liver abscesses; it demonstrates a discrete area of attenuation at the abscess site. Ultrasound is somewhat less sensitive, but also useful. Abscesses are found most commonly in the right lobe of the liver. If a single large abscess is noted, amoeba serology should be ordered. That test is positive in more than 90% of patients with amoebic hepatic abscess. Ultrasound and CT can both be used to guide needle aspiration for culture and drainage. A finding of brownish fluid without a foul odor suggests the possibility of amoebic abscess.

Initial empiric antibiotic therapy should be identical to that for secondary peritonitis. The antibiotic regimen can subsequently be tailored to the abscess culture results. Percutaneous drainage in combination with antibiotics is now the treatment of choice. Open surgical drainage should be considered in patients who continue to have fever after 2 weeks of antibiotic treatment and percutaneous drainage. Open surgery may also be required in patients with biliary obstruction, multiloculated abscesses (other than *Echinococcus*—see Chapter 12), and highly viscous abscesses. Mortality was high in early series (approaching 100%) when abscesses were not drained; however, with modern antibiotics and drainage techniques, nearly 100% of patients are now cured.

PANCREATIC ABSCESS

> ### POTENTIAL SEVERITY
>
> *A serious, but usually not fatal, complication of pancreatitis that presents subacutely.*

Pancreatic abscesses usually arise as complication of pancreatitis. Release of pancreatic enzymes leads to tissue necrosis. Subsequently, necrotic tissue can become

---

KEY POINTS

About the Clinical Manifestations, Diagnosis, and Treatment of Liver Abscess

1. May present as fever of unknown origin.
   a) Dull right upper quadrant pain is associated with right upper quadrant tenderness.
   b) Leukocytosis and elevated alkaline phosphatase are seen.
2. Computed tomography scan is the diagnostic study of choice.
3. With a single abscess, use serology to rule out amoebiasis.
4. Treat with percutaneous drainage and broad-spectrum antibiotic coverage (same regimens as for secondary peritonitis).
5. Use open drainage for the patient with
   a) biliary obstruction,
   b) multiloculated abscess (other than *Echinococcus*), or
   c) viscous exudate.

KEY POINTS

About Pancreatic Abscess

1. Necrotic tissue can become infected by contaminated bile or hematogenous spread.
2. Abscesses are polymicrobial
3. Use computed tomography scan and ultrasound to guide drainage.
4. Open surgical drainage and debridement of necrotic tissue is usually required.
5. The same broad-spectrum coverage used for secondary peritonitis is recommended.
6. Fatal outcome is more likely in elderly patients.

infected by reflux of contaminated bile or by hematogenous spread. Like other intra-abdominal abscesses, pancreatic abscesses are usually polymicrobial. Ultrasound and CT scan are employed for culture and drainage. Because of the significant quantity of necrotic tissue, open drainage and debridement are usually required in combination with broad-spectrum antibiotics. The same antibiotic regimens recommended for secondary peritonitis offer excellent empiric coverage pending cultures and sensitivities. Survival is improved by early surgical drainage. A fatal outcome is more likely in elderly patients, who more often have accompanying biliary tract disease.

CHOLECYSTITIS AND CHOLANGITIS

POTENTIAL SEVERITY

An acute, potentially life-threatening infection that can be complicated by sepsis. Rapid treatment reduces morbidity and mortality.

Pathogenesis and Microbiology

Biliary obstruction is most frequently caused by gallstones and results in increased pressure in and distension of the gallbladder. These changes compromise blood flow and interfere with lymphatic drainage, leading to tissue necrosis and inflammation, which lead to cholecystitis. Although infection is not the primary cause of acute cholecystitis, obstruction prevents flushing of bacteria from the gallbladder and is associated with infection in more than half of all cases. If treatment is delayed, infection can spread from the gallbladder to the hepatic biliary ducts and common bile duct, causing cholangitis.

The organisms associated with cholecystitis and cholangitis reflect the bowel flora and are similar to the organisms encountered in secondary peritonitis. *E. coli*, *Klebsiella* species, enterococci, and anaerobes are most frequently cultured from biliary drainage.

Clinical Manifestations

The acute onset of right upper quadrant pain, high fever, and chills are most common. Jaundice may also be noted, fulfilling Charcot's triad (fever, right upper quadrant pain, and jaundice). On physical exam, marked tenderness over the liver is commonly elicited. Hypotension may be present, indicating early gram-negative sepsis. Elderly patients may not complain of pain, presenting solely with hypotension. Marked peripheral leukocytosis with increased numbers of PMNs and band forms is the rule.

KEY POINTS

About Cholecystitis and Cholangitis

1. Caused by obstruction of the biliary tree, leading to necrosis and inflammation.
2. Polymicrobial infection occurs in more than half of cases. *Escherichia coli*, *Klebsiella* species, enterococci, and anaerobes.
3. Charcot's triad—fever, right upper quadrant pain, and jaundice—may be noted. Elderly patients may present with hypotension and no abdominal pain.
4. Diagnosis:
   a) Elevated alkaline phosphatase, gamma-glutamyl transpeptidase, and bilirubin. Transaminases can occasionally reach 1000 IU.
   b) Abdominal ultrasound is the preferred diagnostic screening tool.
   c) Endoscopic retrograde cholangiopancreatography (ERCP) confirms the diagnosis and for treatment.
5. Treatment:
   a) Broad-spectrum antibiotics (ampicillin plus gentamicin, imipenem, metronidazole plus levofloxacin).
   b) Biliary drainage and stone removal by ERCP is now the treatment of choice. Also used to dilate the sphinter of Oddi and to place stents to maintain flow.
   c) Percutaneous drainage an option for urgent decompression.
   d) Surgery is required for perforated or gangrenous gallbladder.
6. Mortality in severe cholangitis approaches 50%.

Liver function tests are usually consistent with obstruction, demonstrating an elevated serum alkaline phosphatase, gamma-glutamyl transpeptidase, and bilirubin. On rare occasions, serum aminotransferase enzymes, reflecting hepatocellular damage, may also be elevated (up to 1000 IU) as a result of microabscess formation in the liver. Blood cultures are frequently positive.

Diagnosis and Treatment

Ultrasonography is the preferred diagnostic study, and it can usually detect gallstones, dilatation of the gallbladder, and dilatation of the biliary ducts, including the common bile duct. Other adjunctive tests may include CT scan or magnetic resonance imaging; however, these tests are generally not recommended for initial screening. Endoscopic retrograde cholangiopancreatography (ERCP) is helpful for confirming the diagnosis, dilating the sphinter of Oddi, removing stones, and placing stents to maintain biliary flow in constricted, fibrotic biliary channels. This procedure should be performed under antibiotic coverage and should be avoided in cases of cholangitis because of the risk of precipitating high-level bacteremia.

Broad-spectrum antibiotics should be initiated immediately. Regimens similar to those for secondary peritonitis may used. Many experts prefer ampicillin and gentamicin because this regimen covers enterococci in addition to the enteric gram-negative pathogens. Imipenem also covers enterococci, plus the enteric gram-negative rods and anaerobes. Despite its poor activity against enterococci, levofloxacin has also proved effective. Metronidazole may be added to the levofloxacin to improve anaerobic coverage.

Prompt surgical intervention is required for patients with a gangrenous gallbladder and gallbladder perforation. In cases of acute cholecystitis, decompression of the gallbladder and stone removal is now most commonly accomplished by ERCP. Percutaneous drainage is another option for decompression. Urgent decompression should be performed in patients with persistent abdominal pain, hypotension, fever above 39°C, and mental confusion. Outcome is usually favorable for mild-to-moderate disease, but mortality approaches 50% in those with severe cholangitis.

HELICOBACTER PYLORI–ASSOCIATED PEPTIC ULCER DISEASE

POTENTIAL SEVERITY

A chronic disease that causes discomfort, but is not life-threatening.

Microbiology and Pathogenesis

Helicobacter pylori is a small, curved, microaerophilic gram-negative rod that is closely related to *Campylobacter*. This organism is able to survive and multiply within the gastric mucosa. Most *H. pylori* live freely in this environment; however, a small number adhere exclusively to gastric epithelial cells, forming adherence pedestals similar to those observed with enteropathogenic *E. coli*. This organism demonstrates corkscrew-like motility, allowing it to migrate within the gastric and duodenal mucosa. All pathogenic strains express high concentrations of urease, allowing them to generate ammonium ions that buffer

the gastric acid. Colonization with *H. pylori* may be associated with accumulation of increased numbers of inflammatory cells in the lamina propria of gastric epithelial cells. Production of inflammatory cytokines reduces somatostatin levels and causes an increase in gastrin levels. Chronic inflammation caused by *H. pylori* is thought to produce aplastic changes in the gastric mucosa that may lead to gastric carcinomas.

Clinical Manifestations, Diagnosis, and Treatment

Patients with *H. pylori* peptic ulcer disease usually have the classic symptom of dyspepsia: burning pain several hours after meals that is relieved by food and antacids. Belching, indigestion, and heartburn are also frequent

---

KEY POINTS

About *Helicobacter pylori*–Associated Peptic Ulcer Disease

1. This small, curved, microaerophilic gram-negative rod
   a) survives on the mucosal surface of the stomach, and
   b) synthesizes high concentrations of urease, which produces ammonium ions to neutralize acid.
2. Dyspepsia, belching, and heartburn are the most common symptoms.
3. Diagnosis:
   a) Test only symptomatic patients.
   b) Endoscopic biopsy with CLOtest for urease is preferred.
   c) Culture only for refractory cases.
   d) Urease breath test is expensive, but accurate.
   e) Enzyme-linked immunoabsorbent antibody test produces false positives in patients over 50 years of age; titer decreases with treatment.
4. Treatment:
   a) Proton pump inhibitor, plus amoxicillin, plus clarithromycin (for the penicillin-allergic, replace amoxicillin with metronidazole)
   b) Proton pump inhibitor, plus bismuth, plus amoxicillin, plus clarithromycin (or metronidazole or tetracycline)
   c) For relapse, use a proton pump inhibitor, plus levofloxacin, plus amoxicillin

complaints. Other than mild mid-epigastric tenderness, the physical examination is usually normal.

Testing for *H. pylori* is recommended only in symptomatic patients. Noninvasive tests include the urease breath test, in which the patient ingests ^{13}C- or ^{14}C-labeled urea, and their breath is analyzed for ^{13}C or ^{14}C over the next hour. This test requires expensive equipment, but it is specific and sensitive. Measurement of IgG antibody levels by ELISA assay is now commercially available, and this test is inexpensive and sensitive. False negatives may occur in elderly individuals. A stool antigen test is also available, and in the absence of proton pump inhibitor (PPI) administration or gastrointestinal bleeding, it is also sensitive and specific. All three tests may become negative with treatment and can be used to monitor response to therapy. The urea breath test remains the most accurate method for documenting cure.

Diagnosis is most commonly made by endoscopic biopsy. A biopsy specimen should be first tested for urease (CLO test) which has high sensitivity and specificity in patients not taking bismuth, H_2 blockers, or PPIs. Biopsy is the most cost-effective diagnostic method. Specimens can also be cultured using selective media and microaerophilic conditions. Culture to obtain antibiotic sensitivities should be performed in patients who have proved refractory to therapy. *H. pylori* can also be visualized using silver, Gram, or Giemsa stain, and by immunofluorescence.

Multiple regimens have been used to treat *H. pylori*, and the ideal regimen has not been determined. Triple therapy with a PPI (lansoprazole 30 mg or omeprazole 20 mg twice daily), oral amoxicillin (1 g twice daily), and oral clarithromycin (500 mg twice daily) for 2 weeks is associated with a 90% cure rate. In the patient who is penicillin-allergic, oral metronidazole (500 mg twice daily) can be substituted for amoxicillin. A PPI can also be combined with bismuth (525 mg every 6 hours) and two other oral antibiotics (amoxicillin, clarithromycin, metronidazole, tetracycline). For patients who relapse, triple therapy with oral levofloxacin (500 mg) combined with amoxicillin and a PPI has been found to be superior to quadruple therapy with bismuth, tetracycline (500 mg every 6 hours), metronidazole, and a PPI.

VIRAL HEPATITIS

POTENTIAL SEVERITY

Fulminant hepatitis is rare, but usually fatal. Chronic active hepatitis can lead to liver failure and require liver transplantation.

Acute viral hepatitis is a common disease that affects approximately 700,000 people in the United States annually. Three viral agents, hepatitis A, hepatitis B, and hepatitis C virus are primarily responsible for acute hepatitis. Less common causes include hepatitis D ("delta agent") and hepatitis E. A number of other viral agents affect multiple organs in addition to the liver. Epstein–Barr virus and cytomegalovirus are the most common viruses in this category. Less commonly, herpes simplex viruses, Varicella virus, coxsackievirus B, measles, rubella, rubeola, and adenovirus can infect the liver. Fulminant hepatitis is rare, but serious, occurring in approximately 1% of cases with icteric hepatitis. Fulminant disease is most commonly reported with hepatitis B or D, but it is also reported in pregnant woman with hepatitis E.

Clinical Manifestations of Acute Hepatitis

No clinical feature definitively differentiates one form of viral hepatitis from another.

Acute viral hepatitis has four stages of illness:

1. **Incubation period.** This period varies from a few weeks to 6 months, depending on the viral agent (Table 8.3). During this period, the patient has no symptoms.

2. **Preicteric stage.** The symptoms during this stage are nonspecific. The most common initial complaint is malaise, with patients reporting a general sense of not feeling well. Fatigue may also be a prominent complaint, accompanied by generalized weakness. Anorexia, nausea, and vomiting are other common symptoms. Loss of taste for cigarettes is reported among smokers. Dull right upper quadrant pain is also a frequent complaint. Some patients experience a flu-like illness consisting of myalgias, headache, chills, and fever. A few develop a serum-sickness syndrome consisting of fever, rash, and arthritis or arthralgias. These symptoms are the result of immune-complex (virus plus antibody) deposition. Most of the symptoms associated with viral hepatitis dramatically resolve with the onset of jaundice.

3. **Icteric stage.** This stage begins 4 to 10 days after the onset of the preicteric stage. Jaundice and dark urine are the classic symptoms. Scleral icterus may go unnoticed; it is best visualized in natural rather than artificial light. Pale-colored stools can develop as a consequence of reduced excretion of bile pigments. Immune-complex formation at this stage can result in vasculitis (primarily with hepatitis B), and glomerulonephritis can develop in association with hepatitis B or C infection.

4. **Convalescent stage.** The duration of this phase depends on the severity of the attack and the viral etiology.

Table 8.3. Clinical Characteristics of the Various Forms of Viral Hepatitis

Virus type	Incubation period	Epidemiology	Sequelae
Hepatitis A	4 Weeks	Fecal–oral Foodborne Waterborne Sexually transmitted	Self-limiting disease; can relapse up 6 months post primary attack; fulminant hepatitis rare
Hepatitis B	12 Weeks	Person to person Blood and blood products Other body fluids IV drug abuse Sexually transmitted	Chronic infection common (90% neonates, 20% to 50% children, 5% to 10% adults); hepatocellular carcinoma
Hepatitis C	6–10 Weeks	Person to person Blood and blood products IV drug abuse Sexually transmitted (rare) Higher risk with HIV infection	Usually a chronic infection; cirrhosis in 25%; requires liver transplant; hepatocellular carcinoma
Hepatitis D + B	12 Weeks	Person to person Blood and blood products Other body fluids IV drug abuse Sexually transmitted Household contacts	Same as hepatitis B; Hepatic failure more common among IV drug abusers
Hepatitis E	4 Weeks	Fecal–oral route Only in developing countries	Self-limiting disease; fulminant hepatitis in pregnancy

The most prominent physical finding is icterus that can be detected in the sclera or under the tongue when bilirubin levels reach 2.5 to 3.0 mg/dL. Slight hepatic enlargement with mild-to-moderate tenderness is common. Tenderness can be elicited by placing one hand over the liver and pounding this site gently with the fist of the other hand (termed "punch tenderness"). The skin may exhibit scratch marks as result of severe pruritus. Fulminant hepatitis may be accompanied by hepatic encephalopathy, causing depression in mental status and asterixis (irregular flapping of the outstretched hands after forcible dorsiflexion).

Laboratory findings are distinctive in viral hepatitis. Aminotransferase levels—aspartate aminotransferase (AST) and alanine aminotransferase (ALT)— often increase to between 1000 and 2000 IU, and the ratio of AST/ALT is usually less than 1. In alcoholic hepatitis, the latter ratio is usually more than 1.5. Alkaline phosphatase, a reflection of biliary obstruction or cholestasis, is only mildly elevated. Similarly, LDH is only mildly elevated. Transaminase values usually peak in the early icteric stage. Direct and indirect bilirubin fractions are usually equally elevated. High levels of direct or conjugated bilirubin suggest cholestasis, and high levels of indirect or unconjugated bilirubin usually indicate red blood cell hemolysis that can develop in patients with viral hepatitis who also have glucose-6-dehydrogenase deficiency or sickle cell anemia. Significant elevation of the prothrombin time is a bad prognostic sign. A prothrombin time above 100 s indicates irreversible hepatic damage, and these patients should be promptly considered for liver transplant.

In fulminant hepatitis, disseminated intravascular coagulation can develop, leading to thrombocytopenia. Liver biopsy is generally not required to diagnose acute viral hepatitis. This test should be performed when several causes of hepatitis are possible or when therapy is being considered. Histopathologic examination classically reveals ballooning and hepatocyte necrosis, disarray of liver lobules, mononuclear cell infiltration, and cholestasis.

Chronic hepatitis can follow acute hepatitis B and C infections. Particularly in patients with hepatitis C, chronic infection can follow asymptomatic acute infection. Most patients experience no symptoms until they progress to liver failure. In most instances of hepatitis C, hepatic failure takes more than 20 years; in hepatitis B virus infection, hepatic failure usually occurs more rapidly. Elevations of transaminase values are often detected during routine screening. Levels are usually mildly to moderately elevated and do not exceed 7 to 10 times normal values. Mild fatigue may develop, causing the patient to seek medical attention. Other patients may present with symptoms and signs of cirrhosis. Chronic generation of high antibody levels directed against the virus can result in the production of immune complexes that deposit in the glomeruli and the small- to medium-sized blood vessels, causing membranous glomerulonephritis and vasculitis in some patients with chronic disease. Polyarteritis nodosa is frequently associated with persistent hepatitis B infection.

Hepatitis A

VIROLOGY, PATHOGENESIS, AND EPIDEMIOLOGY

Hepatitis A is a small, non-enveloped single-stranded RNA virus. This picornavirus is highly resistant to

heating and drying. It is inactivated by chlorine and does not survive well in buffered saline, but in protein solutions such as milk, the virus is able to withstand high temperatures for brief periods. In tissue culture, the virus is not cytopathic, and replication has to be detected by immunofluorescence staining of antibodies. Isolation of the wild-type virus is often unsuccessful, making tissue culture an ineffective diagnostic tool.

The virus enters the host via the gastrointestinal tract, traversing the intestine and infecting the hepatocyte, where it survives and multiplies within the cell cytoplasm.. The virus infects primarily hepatocytes, and it is then released into the bloodstream and excreted into the bile, resulting in high levels of virus in the stool. Hepatocyte damage is caused by the host's cell-mediated immune response. Peak titers of virus in the blood and stool occur just before or when liver function tests become abnormal. Virus continues to be excreted in the feces for several weeks.

Hepatitis A causes an estimated 1.4 million cases of acute hepatitis worldwide. This virus is spread by the fecal–oral route and is highly infectious. Spread occurs readily in households. Preschool daycare centers are an important source of infection, because children under the age of 2 years develop asymptomatic disease and excrete high concentrations of the virus in their stool. The virus can then readily spread to nonimmune parents and caretakers. Sexual transmission of the virus occurs in male homosexuals, and intravenous drug abusers readily spread the virus to each other. Spread by blood transfusions is rare, however. Common-source outbreaks occur as consequence of contaminated water, milk, and food. Raw and or undercooked clams, oysters, and mussels are major sources of foodborne disease. These bivalve shellfish filter large volumes of contaminated water, concentrating the virus. Two large foodborne outbreaks were recently described in the United States, one caused by contaminated frozen strawberries and the second by contaminated green onions from Mexico. Infected food handlers have caused several outbreaks, and hand-washing is an important measure for preventing spread of this disease. Breakdowns in sanitary conditions that occur during natural disasters and war increase the risk of hepatitis A. Inactivation of the virus can readily be accomplished by treating potentially contaminated surfaces with a 1:100 dilution of household bleach.

CLINICAL COURSE AND DIAGNOSIS

After a 4-week incubation period, patients infected with hepatitis A usually experience the acute onset of a flu-like illness. The disease is usually self-limiting, resolving within 2 to 3 months (Figure 8.3). However, 10% of hospitalized patients follow a relapsing course characterized by improvement followed by a second episode of jaundice that usually develops 6 to 12 weeks later, but that can occur up to 6 months after the first symptomatic attack. Prolonged, but benign, cholestasis has also been reported. Patients with hepatitis A do not develop chronic hepatitis. Young children who have a less robust immune response to the virus often have few symptoms and do not develop jaundice. Fulminant hepatitis is a rare complication and occurs more frequently in patients who are coinfected with hepatitis C or hepatitis B.

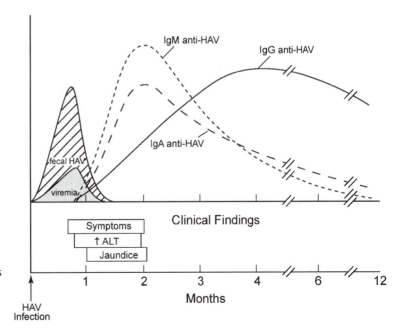

Figure 8–3. Clinical course of hepatitis A virus (HAV). IgM, A, G = immunoglobulins M, A, G; ALT = alanine aminotransferase. Vertical axis = relative concentration (Schematic adapted from Hoeprich Infectious Diseases, 1994)

The diagnosis is made by measuring serum anti-hepatitis A immunoglobulin M (IgM) antibody titers. levels are observed at the time of symptomatic disease and usually persist for 6 months. Anti-hepatitis A IgG antibodies progressively increase. Low titers are observed during early symptomatic disease, but they continue to rise, peaking at about 4 months. The heightened IgG titers persist for decades (Figure 8.3).

TREATMENT AND PREVENTION

Most people can be managed as outpatients. No therapy is available to alter the course of infection. Strict bed rest is not warranted, and moderate activity as tolerated is now recommended. In patients with fulminant hepatitis, exchange transfusions and glucocorticoids fail to

---

KEY POINTS

About the Treatment and Prevention of Hepatitis A

1. No therapy is available.
2. Pooled immunoglobulin is protective if given within 2 weeks of exposure.
3. Immunoglobulin prophylaxis is recommended for
   a) household and sexual contacts,
   b) daycare center staff and attendees,
   c) classroom contacts in school-centered outbreaks,
   d) persons residing or working in institutions with crowded living conditions,
   e) hospital personnel with direct contact with feces or body fluids from an infected patient, and
   f) travelers to endemic areas.
4. Prophylaxis is not recommended for casual contacts or in common-source outbreaks.
5. Vaccine indications are evolving. Vaccine should be give to
   a) children over the age of 2 years,
   b) homosexual men,
   c) intravenous drug abusers,
   d) heterosexuals with multiple sexual partners,
   e) people requiring repeated administration of concentrated coagulation factors.
   f) people with occupational risk of exposure, and
   g) Patients with preexisting chronic liver disease.

---

alter the clinical course, and liver transplantation may be required for survival.

Administration of pooled human immunoglobulin has been shown to prevent or reduce the symptoms of hepatitis A. Prophylaxis should be given within 2 weeks of exposure. The duration of protection is dose-dependent, with intramuscular administration of 0.02 mL/kg affording 2 months of protection, and 0.06 mL/kg usually providing protection for 5 months. Administration of immunoglobulin should be considered in U.S. residents who plan to travel in endemic areas outside of the usual tourist routes. Postexposure prophylaxis is recommended after recognition of the index case for household and sexual contacts; daycare center staff and attendees; classroom contacts in school-centered outbreaks; people residing or working in institutions with crowded living conditions such as prisons, military barracks, and facilities housing disabled people; and for hospital personnel who have come in direct contact with feces or body fluids from an infected patient. Prophylaxis is not recommended for casual contacts and is not effective for common-source outbreaks, because the outbreak will not become apparent until after the 2-week window of immunoglobulin efficacy.

A safe and effective formalin-killed vaccine is available and is now being given to children over the age of 2 years in many areas of the country. As a consequence, the incidence of Hepatitis A in these regions has decreased by two thirds. The vaccine should also be considered for individuals at high risk of hepatitis A: homosexual men, intravenous drug abusers, heterosexuals with multiple sexual partners, individuals requiring repeated administration of concentrated coagulation factors, and people with an occupational risk of exposure. The vaccine is also recommended for patients with pre-existing chronic liver disease. The duration of protection has been estimated to be 20 to 30 years.

Hepatitis E

This small, single-stranded RNA virus is related to the caliciviruses. Its pathogenesis, epidemiology, and clinical manifestations are similar to those of hepatitis A (Table 8.3). The virus is secreted in the stool and spread by the fecal–oral route. Outbreaks have been associated with contaminated water in India, Nepal, Southeast Asia, Africa, China, and Mexico. Infection occurs in areas where sanitation is poor and fecal contamination of water is likely. Indigenous cases have not been reported in the United States, Canada, or the developed countries of Europe and Asia. In those countries, infection is reported in tourists who have traveled to endemic areas. As observed with hepatitis A, the disease is self-limiting and does not result in chronic hepatitis. The hepatitis E virus can cause fulminant hepatitis in pregnant women in their third trimester, with resulting mortality rates of 15% to 25%. The diagnosis can be made by PCR of serum and by a rise in IgM antibody against hepatitis E. Injections of immunoglobulin have not been proven to protect against hepatitis E, and no vaccine is currently available.

Hepatitis B

VIROLOGY AND PATHOGENESIS

Hepatitis B is a small, enveloped, spherical, partially double-stranded DNA virus classified as a hepadnavirus. The outer core contains lipid and the hepatitis B surface antigen (HBsAg—Figure 8.4). The host directs viral-neutralizing antibody (anti-HBV) against the HBsAg. The bloodstream of infected patients contains not only fully competent viral particles, but an even higher abundance of defective viral particles that form small spheres and filaments. These latter forms are noninfectious and are composed of HbsAg and host membrane lipid.

The virus has a unique tropism for hepatocytes and a narrow host range that includes humans, chimpanzees, and a few other higher primates. Hepatitis B virus cannot be reliably maintained in tissue-culture cells. It survives in serum for months at 4°C and for years frozen at –20°C, but it is killed within 2 minutes when heated to 98°C and when treated with many detergents. Hepatitis B viral DNA can integrate into host cell DNA, and that integration may account for the increased incidence of hepatocellular carcinoma in patients who are chronic carriers of hepatitis B virus. These inserts may alter the expression of critical regulatory genes and upregulate host oncogenes.

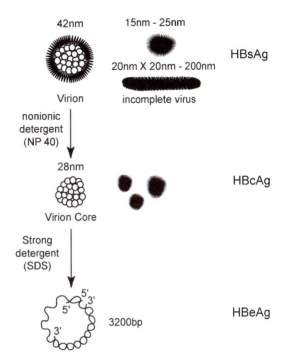

Figure 8–4. Schematic of the various forms of hepatitis B virus antigen: surface antigen (HBsAg), intracellular core antigen (HBcAg), and secreted core antigen (HBeAg). (Schematic adapted from Hoeprich Infectious Diseases, 1994)

EPIDEMIOLOGY

Hepatitis B virus is spread from person to person primarily by blood and blood products. Blood transfusion remains a major mode of transmission in the United States; however, screening of donors has reduced the risk to 1 in 63,000 transfusions. Screening tests fail to exclude a small percentage of donors who have infectious viral particles in their blood despite being negative for HBsAg. Hepatitis B virus is also found in other body fluids, including urine, bile, saliva, semen, breast milk, and vaginal secretions. It is not found in feces, however. Membrane contact with any of these body fluids can result in transmission. The virus can be spread to sexual partners, and it is prevalent in homosexual men and heterosexuals with multiple partners. It can be readily spread from mother to neonate at the time of vaginal delivery—a common mode of transmission in developing countries. Intravenous drug abusers have a high incidence of hepatitis B. Reuse of needles has also led to transmission of the virus during placement of tattoos and ear-piercing. Crowded environments, such as institutions for the mentally handicapped, favor spread. The virus has also been spread to transplant organ recipients when the donated organ originates from

---

KEY POINTS

About Hepatitis E

1. This single-stranded RNA virus is related to the caliciviruses.
2. Incubation period is 1 month.
3. Transmitted by the fecal–oral route.
4. Reported in developing countries with poor sanitation, but not in the United States, except in travelers.
5. The disease is self-limiting.
6. Causes fulminant hepatitis in women in their third trimester of pregnancy.
7. No blood test is available.
8. Pooled immunoglobulins are not helpful for prevention.

a hepatitis B–infected donor. Hepatitis B virus infection is very common; 280,000 primary infections occur annually in the United States, and the virus is estimated to have infected approximately 5% of the world's population.

CLINICAL COURSE AND DIAGNOSIS

The clinical picture of hepatitis B is similar to that of hepatitis A, with two major differences: the average incubation period (12 weeks) is longer than with hepatitis A, and hepatitis B is not always self-limiting. Symptoms usually resolve over 1 to 3 months, and transaminase values usually return to normal within 1 to 4 months. Afterward, the full virus remains in the liver for a decade, and in a significant percentage of patients, elevations in transaminase values persist for more than 6 months. This latter finding indicates progression to chronic active hepatitis. The percentage that progress to chronic disease is age dependent, being 90% in neonates, 20% to 50% in children 1 to 5 years of age, and 5% to 10% in adults.

A number of serum tests are available to assist in the diagnosis of hepatitis B. These tests are based on the general understanding of the structure and life cycle of the virus (Figures 8.4 and 8.5):

1. **Viral capsid surface antigen and the antibody directed against the surface antigen (anti-HBs).** The HBsAg test was the first available for detecting hepatitis B. HBsAg appears in serum within 1 to 10 weeks after exposure; its disappearance within 4 to 6 months indicates recovery (Figure 8.5). The persistence of HBsAg beyond 6 months indicates chronic disease. The disappearance of HBsAg may be preceded by the appearance of anti-HBs, and during this period, patients may develop a serum-sickness-like illness. In a large percentage of patients, anti-HBs does not rise to detectable levels for several weeks to months after the disappearance of HBsAg. During this window HBsAg and anti-HBs are both negative (Figure 8.5), and if these two tests alone are used for screening blood donors, a small percentage of infected donors may be missed. To prevent this occurrence, blood banks also test for IgM antibody directed against HBcAg (see point 2). Anti-HBs rises slowly over 6 to 12 months and usually persists for life, providing protection against reinfection.

2. **Antibody directed against the core antigen (anti-HBc).** HBcAg is detected in infected hepatocytes, but is not released into serum; however, IgM antibody directed against HBcAg (anti-HBc) is usually the earliest anti-hepatitis B antibody detected in the infected patient (Figure 8.5). The IgM anti-HBc is usually interpreted as a marker for early acute disease; however, in some patients, anti-HBc IgM levels can persist for up to 2 years after acute infection, and in patients

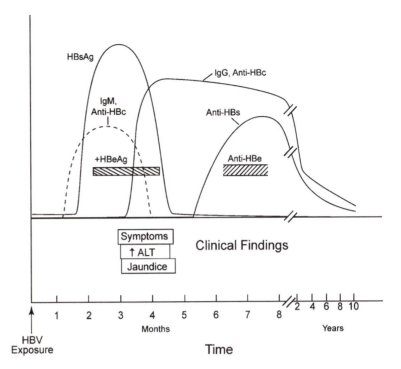

Figure 8–5. Clinical course of hepatitis B. HBsAg = hepatitis surface antigen; HBeAg = secreted core antigen; IgM = immunoglobulin M; ALT = alanine aminotransferase. Vertical axis = relative concentration (Schematic adapted from Hoeprich Infectious Diseases, 1994)

with chronic active hepatitis, IgM antibody levels can rise during periods of exacerbation. An anti-HBc IgM titer is particularly helpful for screening blood donors, because this antibody is usually present during the window between HBsAg disappearance and anti-HBs appearance. The IgG antibodies directed against the core antigen develop in the later phases of acute disease and usually persist for life.

3. **Secreted core antigen (HBeAg) and its antibody (anti-HBe).** Naked DNA strands and associated proteins make up HBeAg (Figure 8.4). The presence of HBeAg in serum indicates active viral replication, and it persists in patients with chronic disease, its presence correlating with infectivity. As the patient with acute hepatitis B recovers, HBeAg disappears, and anti-HBe appears. Seroconversion from HBeAg to anti-HBe usually corresponds with the disappearance of hepatitis B virus DNA from the serum.

4. **Hepatitis B viral DNA (HBV-DNA).** Quantitation of viral DNA in serum is most commonly used in the assessment of patients with chronic active hepatitis. In the patient with acute hepatitis, this test provides no significant advantages over that for HBeAg. Both tests indicate active viral replication. In patients with fulminant hepatitis, assays for HBV-DNA has been positive in the absence of other positive markers for hepatitis B.

TREATMENT AND PREVENTION

The approach to the treatment of acute hepatitis B is identical to that of hepatitis A, being that no therapeutic intervention can alter the course of acute disease. Prevention requires education of those who engage in high-risk behaviors, screening of the blood supply, and universal precautions by hospital personnel. High-titer hepatitis B immunoglobulin reduces the incidence of clinical hepatitis B. Immunoglobulin is prepared from the serum of patients with high titers of anti-HBs, and ameliorates the severity of infection if given within 7 days of exposure (0.05 to 0.07 mL/kg intramuscularly).

A safe and effective recombinant hepatitis B vaccine is available, and vaccination should be initiated in most individuals at the time of exposure. This vaccine is now recommended for all neonates. In the United States, vaccination is also recommended for all children who did not receive the vaccine as a neonate. Among adults, vaccination is recommended for health care workers, laboratory workers who handle blood and blood products, patients who require repeated blood transfusions or clotting factors, hemodialysis patients, morticians, people with multiple sexual partners, intravenous drug users, residents and staff of closed institutions such as prisons and institutions for the mentally handicapped, and household and sexual contacts of carriers. The vaccine should be given intramuscularly in three doses at months 0, 1 to 2, and 6 to 12. In neonates born to mothers with

<table>
<tr><td>

KEY POINTS

About the Clinical Manifestations and Diagnosis of Hepatitis B

1. Incubation period is 12 weeks.
2. Acute disease is clinically similar to Hepatitis A; however, persistent infection can develop in
   a. 90% of infants,
   b. 20% to 50% of children 1 to 5 years of age, and
   c. 5% to 10% of adults.
3. Diagnosis is made by serologic testing:
   a) Hepatitis B surface antigen (HBsAg) appears within 10 weeks of exposure and persists for 4 to 6 months; persistence beyond 6 months indicates chronic disease.
   b) Antibody to hepatitis B surface antigen (anti-HBs) often develops after HBsAg disappears; anti-HBs usually persists for life. Anti-HBs and HBsAg may be negative during this "window" transition period.
   c) Immunoglobulin M (IgM) antibody against hepatitis B intracellular core antigen (anti-HBc) is an early marker for acute disease, but it can persist for 2 years and can increase during exacerbations of chronic active hepatitis. Used for blood screening.
   d) Hepatitis B secreted core antigen (HBeAg) indicates active viral replication. Disappearance HBeAg and appearance of antibody against it (anti-HBe) indicates clearance of the virus.
   e) Quantitation of hepatitis B DNA is used to assess response to therapy of chronic disease.

</td><td>

KEY POINTS

About the Treatment and Prevention of Acute Hepatitis B

1. Treatment is the same as that for Hepatitis A: supportive measures.
2. Hepatitis B immunoglobulin should be given within 7 days of exposure.
3. Recombinant vaccine is safe and efficacious and should be given to
   a) health care workers,
   b) laboratory workers who handle blood and blood products,
   c) patients requiring repeated blood transfusions or clotting factors,
   d) hemodialysis patients,
   e) morticians,
   f) people with multiple sexual partners,
   g) intravenous drug abusers,
   h) residents and staff of closed institutions, and
   i) household and sexual contacts of carriers.

</td></tr>
</table>

unknown or positive HBsAg, status, the first dose of vaccine should be given within 12 hours of delivery, with the booster doses given at 1 and 6 months. The vaccine is highly effective, and has markedly reduced the incidence of hepatitis B in health care workers.

Treatment and Prognosis of Chronic Hepatitis B

Patients with a positive HBsAg for more than 20 weeks are defined as chronic HBsAg carriers. The carrier state develops in 5% to 10% of adults. The course of chronic disease depends on the balance between viral replication and the host's immune response. This chronic illness has several stages:

1. **Replicative phase, immune tolerance.** During this phase, the host's immune system demonstrates

tolerance to the virus, allowing active replication. Hepatic inflammation is minimal. This stage can persist for 20 to 30 years in neonates.

2. **Replicative phase, immune clearance.** The immune system recognizes the virus as a foreign antigen, and active inflammation ensues. Symptoms of hepatitis may develop, although most patients remain asymptomatic. Liver function tests become abnormal, indicating active hepatitis. During this phase, the virus may clear from the serum. In some patients, however, viral replication may continue, and those patients are said to have had an episode of abortive immune clearance.

3. **Nonreplicative phase.** In this phase, HBeAg is negative, and anti-HBe appears. In some of these patients, HBsAg may persist and may be associated with progression of liver disease.

Patients with persistent HbsAg and ongoing hepatic inflammation can progress to cirrhosis and liver failure. Chronic carriage of hepatitis B is also associated with an increased risk of hepatocellular carcinoma, and HBsAg-positive individuals who develop cirrhosis have an annual 1.6% incidence of hepatocellular carcinoma. To prevent these complications, treatment is recommended in chronic carriers of hepatitis B virus with positive HBeAg. The goal of therapy is to achieve HBeAg seroconversion

---

KEY POINTS

About Chronic Hepatitis B

1. Chronic disease is defined as positive HBsAg for more than 20 weeks.
2. Three stages:
   a) Replicative stage with immune tolerance, laboratory findings within normal limits, viral load high.
   b) Replicative stage with immune clearance, laboratory findings are abnormal.
   c) Non-replicative stage, HBeAg disappears, HBsAg may persist.
3. Chronic carriers can progress to cirrhosis and hepatic failure. Risk of hepatocellular carcinoma is increased.
4. Treatment:
   a) Multiple antiviral agents are being tested.
   b) Interferon α reserved for patients with persistent HBeAg and elevated transaminase values.

---

from positive to negative. Patients with normal transaminase values at the time of therapy have a poorer response rate, and many experts do not recommend treatment under those conditions.

The treatment of chronic hepatitis B is rapidly evolving, and the efficacy of a number of antiviral agents—including emtricitabine, entecavir, clevudine, telbivudine, valtorcitabine, tenofovir, alamifovir, pradefovir, and remofovir—is being explored. Treatment with lamivudine alone selects for lamivudine-resistant virus within 1 year. Experience with antiretroviral treatment suggests that combination therapy will prove more efficacious, and combination trials are also under way. Interferon α has potent antiviral effects and is also undergoing therapeutic trials; however, this agent is expensive and is associated with a high incidence of unpleasant side effects (see Chapter 1). Treatment is usually reserved for patients who have persistent HBeAg and elevated transaminase values. Co-infection with HIV and hepatitis virus adds further complexity to patient management. When possible, antiretroviral therapy should include tenofovir and emtricitabine (combination pill: Truvada) in combination with a non-nucleoside reverse transcriptase inhibitor or a protease inhibitor (see Chapter 17).

Hepatitis D

The hepatitis D virion is a small, single-stranded RNA virus that is surrounded by a single hepatitis D antigen and a lipoprotein envelope provided by hepatitis B. The hepatitis D virus, also called delta agent, can replicate only in a human host who is co-infected with hepatitis B. When the D virus is present, hepatitis B replication is suppressed. Hepatitis D virus replicates at very high levels in the nuclei of hepatocytes. During acute disease, it is thought to be directly responsible for cytotoxic damage in those cells. Clinically, hepatitis D+B is indistinguishable from hepatitis B. A higher incidence of hepatic failure has been noted with combined infection in intravenous drug abusers. The rate of progression to chronic active hepatitis is the same.

Hepatitis D virus is endemic in the Mediterranean basin, having been first discovered in Italy. A high prevalence is also seen in the eastern Asia (Pacific Islands, Taiwan, Japan). Person-to-person spread may be the result of mucosal contact with infected body fluids or injection of blood or blood products. Spread among household contacts is common and is associated with poor hygiene and low socioeconomic status. The virus can be spread by sexual contact and is common among intravenous drug abusers. In the Western hemisphere, infection with hepatitis D virus is uncommon, being found primarily in individuals requiring multiple blood transfusions or coagulation products, and in abusers of intravenous drugs. The diagnosis is made by measuring anti-hepatitis D IgM and IgG serum titers. No specific treatment is available for hepatitis D. Measures designed to prevent hepatitis B also eliminate the risk of this virus.

KEY POINTS

About Hepatitis D ("Delta Agent")

1. This single-stranded RNA virus surrounded by a hepatitis B envelope.
2. Replicates only in the presence of hepatitis B virus.
3. Replicates rapidly in the host cell nucleus.
4. Clinically indistinguishable from other forms of acute hepatitis.
5. Person-to-person spread by body fluids and blood or blood products:
   a) Sexual contact
   b) Intravenous drug abuse
   c) Multiple blood transfusions (U.S. patients)
6. Diagnosis by anti-hepatitis D immunoglobulin M and G serum titers.

Hepatitis C

VIROLOGY, PATHOGENESIS, AND EPIDEMIOLOGY

Hepatitis C is a single-stranded RNA virus that is thought to be enveloped. As the virus replicates, it demonstrates ineffective proofreading, generating multiple mutations and virions (called "quasi-species") in the blood. These constant mutations allow the virus to evade the host's immune system and cause chronic disease. The virus cannot be propagated by routine methods, explaining the great difficulty encountered in originally identifying the cause of non-A, non-B transfusion-associated hepatitis.

Hepatitis C has a very narrow host range, infecting only humans and chimpanzees. Within the liver, the virus infects only hepatocytes, leaving biliary epithelium and stromal cells uninfected. The mechanism of hepatocyte damage has not been clarified, but probably involves both cytopathic and immune-mediated mechanisms. In addition to acute hepatitis, the virus can cause chronic persistent hepatitis and chronic active hepatitis. The latter disease is characterized by periportal infiltration with lymphocytes and piecemeal necrosis. It is often followed by fibrosis, leading to cirrhosis.

This virus has a worldwide distribution, and in the United States, seroprevalence ranges from 0.25% in low-risk blood donors to 2% among those who exhibit

---

KEY POINTS

About the Pathogenesis and Epidemiology of Hepatitis C

1. Single-stranded RNA virus.
2. Viral replication is associated with inaccurate proofreading and multiple mutations, yielding multiple quasi-species (a mechanism for evading the immune system).
3. Infects only hepatocytes in the liver; infects only humans and chimpanzees.
4. In the United States, 2.4 million are chronically infected.
5. Spread by
   a) blood and blood products,
   b) intravenous drug abuse,
   c) mother-to-neonate contact (less common than in hepatitis B), and
   d) sexual contact (rare).
6. Higher risk of infection in HIV-infected individuals.

KEY POINTS

About the Clinical Manifestations and Diagnosis of Hepatitis C

1. Incubation period is 6 to 10 weeks.
2. Only 25% of patients will develop symptoms of acute hepatitis.
3. Between 50% and 75% of patients progress to chronic infection.
4. Diagnosis:
   a) An enzyme-link immunoabsorbent assay detects antibodies directed against specific hepatitis C antigens with 95% sensitivity.
   b) In low-risk populations, confirmation by recombinant immunoblot assay is suggested,
   c) Polymerase chain reaction methods are able to detect viral load.

---

high-risk behaviors such as intravenous drug abuse. A similar range of seroprevalence is encountered internationally. Approximately 150,000 new cases develop annually in the United States, and 2 to 4 million people are estimated to have chronic disease. The infection is spread primarily by the parenteral administration of blood or blood products and by needle sharing among intravenous drug abusers. Spread from an infected mother to her neonate is reported, but this form of transmission is less common than is observed with hepatitis B. The risk is higher in mothers who are co-infected with HIV. Sexual transmission may occur, but it is less efficient than in the case of hepatitis B virus or HIV. Co-infection with hepatitis C and HIV is common in the United States and has created new therapeutic challenges (see Chapter 17).

CLINICAL MANIFESTATIONS AND DIAGNOSIS

The incubation period for hepatitis C is 6 to 10 weeks. A high proportion of acute attacks remain asymptomatic, with only one quarter of infected patients experiencing the typical symptoms of acute hepatitis. Hepatitis C alone does not cause fulminant hepatitis, but 50% to 70% of acutely infected patients are estimated to progress to chronic hepatitis C infection. Serum transaminase values fluctuate during chronic illness. During some periods, they may be normal; at other times, they increase to 7 to 10 times normal values.

Disease is detected by an ELISA assay designed to measure antibodies directed against specific hepatitis C antigens. The most recent generation of this test (E12)

---

has a greater than 95% sensitivity and a high positive predictive value. In low-risk populations, the ELISA assay should be confirmed by recombinant immunoblot assay. This latter test has a higher specificity and, when positive, indicates true infection. Detection of serum viral RNA by the PCR method allows for quantitation of the serum viral load, and some assays claim to detect levels as low as 100 copies per milliliter.

TREATMENT AND PROGNOSIS

Unlike hepatitis B (which may spontaneously clear over time), hepatitis C seldom clears spontaneously. Approximately 20% to 25% of patients progress to cirrhosis over a period of 20 to 30 years. Hepatitis C is one of the leading causes of hepatic failure requiring liver transplant (20% to 50% of liver transplants in the United States). Like chronic hepatitis B, chronic hepatitis C is associated with an increased incidence of primary hepatocellular carcinoma.

Treatment with pegylated interferon α-2a once weekly, combined with oral ribavirin (1 to 1.2 g daily) results in the best response rates, and is now recommended as initial therapy for hepatitis C. After 12 weeks of therapy, a quantitative test for haepatitis C RNA should be performed. If a greater than 2 log decline is observed, treatment should be continued for 48 weeks. Duration of therapy and rates of response vary with the virus genotype.

FURTHER READING

Infectious Diarrhea

Chen XM, Keithly JS, Paya CV, LaRusso NF. Cryptosporidiosis. *N Engl J Med.* 2002;346:1723–1731.

DuPont HL. Travelers' diarrhea: antimicrobial therapy and chemoprevention. *Nat Clin Pract Gastroenterol Hepatol.* 2005;2:191–198.

Glass RI, Noel J, Ando T, et al. The epidemiology of enteric caliciviruses from humans: a reassessment using new diagnostics. *J Infect Dis.* 2000;181(Suppl 2):S254–S261.

Guerrant RL, Van Gilder T, Steiner TS, et al. Practice guidelines for the management of infectious diarrhea. *Clin Infect Dis.* 2001;32:331–351.

Haque R, Huston CD, Hughes M, Houpt E, Petri WA Jr. Amebiasis. *N Engl J Med.* 2003;348:1565–1573.

Johnson KE, Thorpe CM, Sears CL. The emerging clinical importance of non-O157 Shiga toxin-producing *Escherichia coli. Clin Infect Dis.* 2006;43:1587–1595.

Musher DM, Musher BL. Contagious acute gastrointestinal infections. *N Engl J Med.* 2004;351:2417–2427.

Okeke IN, Nataro JP. Enteroaggregative *Escherichia coli. Lancet Infect Dis.* 2001;1:304–313.

Sirinavin S, Garner P. Antibiotics for treating salmonella gut infections. *Cochrane Database Syst Rev.* 2000;:CD001167.

Tarr PI, Gordon CA, Chandler WL. Shiga-toxin-producing *Escherichia coli* and haemolytic uraemic syndrome. *Lancet.* 2005;365:1073–1086.

Thielman NM, Guerrant RL. Clinical practice. Acute infectious diarrhea. *N Engl J Med.* 2004;350:38–47.

Antibiotic-Associated Diarrhea

Bartlett JG. Clinical practice. Antibiotic-associated diarrhea. *N Engl J Med.* 2002;346:334–339.

Högenauer C, Langner C, Beubler E, et al. *Klebsiella oxytoca* as a causative organism of antibiotic-associated hemorrhagic colitis. *N Engl J Med.* 2006;355:2418–2426.

Loo VG, Poirier L, Miller MA, et al. A predominantly clonal multi-institutional outbreak of *Clostridium difficile*–associated diarrhea with high morbidity and mortality. *N Engl J Med.* 2005;353:2442–2449.

Louie TJ, Peppe J, Watt CK, et al. Tolevamer, a novel nonantibiotic polymer, compared with vancomycin in the treatment of mild to moderately severe *Clostridium difficile*–associated diarrhea. *Clin Infect Dis.* 2006;43:411–420.

Musher DM, Logan N, Hamill RJ, et al. Nitazoxanide for the treatment of *Clostridium difficile* colitis. *Clin Infect Dis.* 2006;43:421–427.

Sougioultzis S, Kyne L, Drudy D, et al. *Clostridium difficile* toxoid vaccine in recurrent *C. difficile*–associated diarrhea. *Gastroenterology.* 2005;128:764–270.

Primary and Secondary Peritonitis

Alapati SV, Mihas AA. When to suspect ischemic colitis. Why is this condition so often missed or misdiagnosed? *Postgrad Med.* 1999;105:177–180,183–184,187.

Castellote J, Lopez C, Gornals J, et al. Rapid diagnosis of spontaneous bacterial peritonitis by use of reagent strips. *Hepatology.* 2003;37:893–896.

Gupta H, Dupuy DE. Advances in imaging of the acute abdomen. *Surg Clin North Am.* 1997;77:1245–1263.

Kim DK, Yoo TH, Ryu DR, et al. Changes in causative organisms and their antimicrobial susceptibilities in CAPD peritonitis: a single center's experience over one decade. *Perit Dial Int.* 2004;24:424–432.

Navasa M, Rodes J. Management of ascites in the patient with portal hypertension with emphasis on spontaneous bacterial peritonitis. *Semin Gastrointest Dis.* 1997;8:200–209.

Piraino B, Bailie GR, Bernardini J, et al. Peritoneal dialysis–related infections recommendations: 2005 update. *Perit Dial Int.* 2005;25:107–131.

Liver Abscess

Kaplan GG, Gregson DB, Laupland KB. Population-based study of the epidemiology of and the risk factors for pyogenic liver abscess. *Clin Gastroenterol Hepatol.* 2004;2:1032–1038.

Rahimian J, Wilson T, Oram V, Holzman RS. Pyogenic liver abscess: recent trends in etiology and mortality. *Clin Infect Dis.* 2004;39:1654–1659.

Yu WL, Ko WC, Cheng KC, et al. Association between *rmpA* and *magA* genes and clinical syndromes caused by *Klebsiella pneumoniae* in Taiwan. *Clin Infect Dis.* 2006;42:1351–1358.

Helicobacter Pylori

Ernst PB, Peura DA, Crowe SE. The translation of *Helicobacter pylori* basic research to patient care. *Gastroenterology.* 2006;130:188–206, quiz 212–213.

Saad RJ, Schoenfeld P, Kim HM, Chey WD. Levofloxacin-based triple therapy versus bismuth-based quadruple therapy for persistent *Helicobacter pylori* infection: a meta-analysis. *Am J Gastroenterol.* 2006;101:488–496.

Hepatitis A

Levy MJ, Herrera JL, DiPalma JA. Immune globulin and vaccine therapy to prevent hepatitis A infection. *Am J Med.* 1998;105:416–423.

Wasley A, Samandari T, Bell BP. Incidence of hepatitis A in the United States in the era of vaccination. *JAMA.* 2005;294:194–201.

Wheeler C, Vogt TM, Armstrong GL, et al. An outbreak of hepatitis A associated with green onions. *N Engl J Med.* 2005;353:890–897.

Hepatitis B

Lee WM. Hepatitis B virus infection. *N Engl J Med.* 1997;337:1733–1745.

Nakhoul F, Gelman R, Green J, Khankin E, Baruch Y. Lamivudine therapy for severe acute hepatitis B virus infection after renal transplantation: case report and literature review. *Transplant Proc.* 2001;33:2948–2949.

Saag MS. Emtricitabine, a new antiretroviral agent with activity against HIV and hepatitis B virus. *Clin Infect Dis.* 2006;42:126–131.

Yuki N, Nagaoka T, Yamashiro M, et al. Long-term histologic and virologic outcomes of acute self-limited hepatitis B. *Hepatology.* 2003;37:1172–1179.

Hepatitis C

Iwasaki Y, Ikeda H, Araki Y, et al. Limitation of combination therapy of interferon and ribavirin for older patients with chronic hepatitis C. *Hepatology.* 2006;43:54–63.

Moradpour D, Wolk B, Cerny A, Heim MH, Blum HE. Hepatitis C: a concise review. *Minerva Med.* 2001;92:329–339.

Strader DB, Wright T, Thomas DL, Seeff LB. Diagnosis, management, and treatment of hepatitis C. *Hepatology.* 2004;39:1147–1171.

Genitourinary Tract Infections and Sexually Transmitted Diseases

9

Time Recommended to Complete: 2 days

Frederick Southwick, M.D.

GUIDING QUESTIONS

1. What are the virulence factors that allow bacteria to infect the urinary tract, and where do the bacteria come from?

2. What are the host factors that help to prevent infection of the urinary tract?

3. Which symptoms and signs help the clinician to differentiate upper tract (pyelonephritis) from lower tract disease (cystitis)?

4. How useful is the urinary sediment in diagnosing urinary tract infection?

5. When should a urine culture be ordered, and what represents a true positive culture? What does 10^5 CFU/mL mean?

6. How is prostatitis contracted, and which organisms are most likely to cause this infection?

7. How do the treatments of acute and chronic prostatitis differ?

8. How is urethritis differentiated from cystitis?

9. Does delay in treating urethritis lead to any serious complications in women?

10. What are the physical findings that accompany pelvic inflammatory disease (PID)?

11. Why should physicians have a low threshold for diagnosing and treating PID?

12. What are the most common causes of genital ulcers, and how can they be differentiated on clinical exam?

13. What are the three stages of syphilis, and how are they treated?

14. How do the VDRL (Venereal Disease Research Laboratory) and RPR (rapid plasma reagin) tests differ from the FTA-ABS (fluorescent treponemal antigen–antibody absorption) test, and how should these tests be utilized?

15. What is the leading cause of venereal warts, and what are the potential long-term consequences of having this infection?

POTENTIAL SEVERITY

Often outpatient infections; however, the development of pyelonephritis or pelvic inflammatory disease can lead to sepsis and death. These infections need to be promptly treated.

■ GENITOURINARY TRACT INFECTIONS

URINARY TRACT INFECTION

Urinary tract infections (UTIs) are the most common infections seen in outpatient practice. Clinicians must understand the different types of UTIs and know how to diagnose and treat them.

Pathogenesis

Any discussion of UTI must take into account bacterial virulence factors and host factors. The balance between the ability of a specific bacterium to invade the urinary tract and the ability of the host to fend off the pathogen determines whether the human host will develop a symptomatic UTI.

BACTERIAL FACTORS

Bacteria generally gain entry into the urinary system by ascending the urethra into the bladder and then, in some cases, ascending the ureters to the renal parenchyma. The organism that most commonly infects the urinary tract is *Escherichia coli*, and certain strains of *E. coli* are more likely to cause a UTI. These strains possess advantageous virulence characteristics, including increased ability to adhere to the epithelial cells of the urethra and increased resistance to serum cidal activity and hemolysin production. *E. coli* adhere by their fimbria or pili, distinct protein hairlike structures on the bacterial surface. Pyelonephritis strains are the most adherent; cystitis strains tend to be intermediately adherent.

Two types of fimbriae are important for determining whether *E. coli* causes lower or upper tract infection. Type I fimbriae specifically adhere to mannosylated proteins on the surface of bladder epithelial cells. Bacteria that adhere by type I fimbriae can be readily detached from epithelial cells by exposing them to mannose ("mannose–sensitive"). Some strains of *E. coli* have a second type of fimbriae called P fimbriae that adhere to glycophospholipids embedded in the outer surface of the plasma membrane of uroepithelial cells. The adherence of P fimbriae is not weakened by mannose exposure (mannose-resistant receptors). Patients with cystitis tend to be infected with *E. coli* that express type I fimbriae, while the *E. coli* that cause upper-tract disease are more likely to express P fimbriae. These differences represent a classic example of bacterial tropism. Trimethoprim–sulfamethoxazole (TMP-SMX), an agent used to prevent UTI, reduces the synthesis and expression of the fimbria adhesion molecules.

A number of other virulence factors contribute to the ability of urinary pathogens to survive and grow in the urinary tract. Because urine is an incomplete growth media, bacteria must be capable of synthesizing several essential nutritional factors before they can grow in urine. Bacterial synthesis of guanine, arginine, and glutamine are required for optimal growth. Pathogenic *Proteus mirabilis* produces ureases that appear to play an important role in the development of pyelonephritis. Motile bacteria can ascend the ureter against the flow of urine. Endotoxins can decrease ureteral peristalsis, slowing the downward flow of urine and enhancing the ability of gram-negative bacteria to ascend into the kidneys.

HOST FACTORS

Urine contains high concentrations of urea and generally has a low pH. These conditions inhibit bacterial growth. The urine of pregnant women tends to be more suitable for bacterial growth, and patients with diabetes often have glucose in their urine, making that urine a better culture medium. These factors help to explain why pregnant women and diabetic patients have an increased incidence of UTI.

Mechanical factors probably are the most important determinants for the development of UTI. Mechanical factors can be grouped into three risk categories:

1. **Obstruction.** The flushing mechanism of the bladder protects the host against infection of the urinary tract. When bacteria are introduced into the bladder, the organisms generally are cleared from the urine. Obstruction of urinary flow is one of the most important predisposing factors for the development of a UTI. Prostatic hypertrophy and urethral strictures can lead to bladder outlet obstruction. Defective bladder contraction associated with spinal cord injury also results in poor bladder emptying. These conditions result in a significant volume of urine remaining in the bladder after voiding ("increased post-void residual"), which markedly increases the likelihood of infection. Intrarenal obstruction caused by renal calculi, polycystic kidney disease, and sickle cell disease also increase the risk of renal infection. *Proteus* and other urea-splitting organisms can cause stone formation and can become entrapped within the stones. Another mechanical problem that increases the risk of upper tract disease is vesicoureteral reflux (defective bladder–ureteral valves).

2. **Urethra Length.** Women have a short urethra, which increases the risk of bacteria entering the bladder. The incidence of UTI in women (1% to 3% of women) is much higher than that in men (0.1% or less until later years). At least 10% to 20% of all women develop a symptomatic UTI at some point during their lifetime. Trauma to the urethra by sexual intercourse and the use of a diaphragm both increase the risk of UTI. Colonization of the vaginal area near the urethra is an important risk factor for UTI in women. This event is thought to proceed the development of UTI. Immunoglobulin A (IgA) and G (IgG) antibodies against cell wall antigens have been described. The exact role of immunoglobulins in protecting against colonization and invasion of the urinary tract remains to be determined.

3. **Urethra Bypass.** Bladder catheterization bypasses the urethra. Within 3 to 4 days of catheterization,

cystitis generally develops unless a sterile closed drainage system is used. Unfortunately, even the most sterile handling of the bladder catheter only delays the onset of infection. All patients with a bladder catheter in place will eventually develop a UTI.

Once bacteria begin to actively grow in the bladder, they stimulate an acute inflammatory response. Polymorphonuclear leukocytes (PMNs) are attracted by chemoattractants released by epithelial cells and bacteria. Over time, bacteria are capable of migrating up the ureters and reaching the kidney. The renal medulla is particularly susceptible to invasion by bacteria. The high concentrations of ammonia in the medulla inactivate complement, and the high osmolality in this region inhibits migration of PMNs. Once bacteria enter the

Table 9.1. Common Urinary Tract Pathogens

	Outpatient	Inpatient
Escherichia coli	75%	Common
Klebsiella	15%	Common
Proteus	5%	Common
Enterococci	2%	Common
Staphylococcus epidermidis	<2%	Common
Group B streptococci	<2%	Common
Pseudomonas	Rare	Common

renal parenchyma, they are able to enter the bloodstream and cause septic shock.

Causes

Most organisms that cause UTIs come from the fecal and vaginal flora (Table 9.1):

E. coli is by far the most common pathogen in uncomplicated outpatient UTI. *Klebsiella* and *Proteus* are less common. In young, sexually active women *Staphylococcus saprophyticus* accounts for 5% to 15% of cases of cystitis. In patients who experience recurrent infections, have been instrumented, or have anatomic defects or renal stones, *Enterobacter*, *Pseudomonas*, and enterococci are more commonly cultured. *Candida* species are frequently encountered in hospitalized patients who are receiving broad-spectrum antibiotics and have a bladder catheter. Two other important nosocomial pathogens are *S. epidermidis* and *Corynebacterium* group D2. In 95% of cases, UTIs are caused by a single organism. Patients with structural abnormalities are more likely to have polymicrobial infections.

KEY POINTS

About the Pathogenesis of Urinary Tract Infections

1. Certain bacterial characteristics predispose to urinary tract infection (UTI):
   a) Type I and P fimbriae (adhere to mannose-sensitive and -insensitive host cell receptors)
   b) Hemolysin production
   c) Resistance to serum cidal activity
   d) Ability to synthesize essential amino acids arginine and glutamine
   e) Urease production (*Proteus mirabilis*)
2. Certain host characteristics predispose to UTI:
   a) Urine usually inhibits bacterial growth [exceptions occur in pregnant women and patients with diabetes (glucose)].
   b) Mechanical properties can make bacterial growth more likely:
      i) Obstruction (flushing can be inhibited by prostatic hypertrophy, urethral stricture, defective bladder contraction, renal stones, vesicoureteral reflux).
      ii) Short urethra length and colonization of the vaginal area lead to higher risk in women (1% to 3% annual incidence compared with less than 0.1% in men).
      iii) Bladder catheterization bypasses the urethra.
   c) High ammonia in the renal medulla blocks complement, and high osmolality inhibits polymorphonuclear leukocytes.

KEY POINTS

About the Causes of Urinary Tract Infection

1. *Escherichia coli* is the most frequent pathogen, followed by *Klebsiella* and *Proteus*.
2. *Staphylococcus saprophyticus* causes 5% to 15% of cystitis cases in young, sexually active women.
3. Nosocomial infections usually involve *Enterobacter*, *Pseudomonas*, enterococci, *Candida*, *S. epidermidis*, and *Corynebacterium*.

CASE 9.1

A 23-year-old white woman was admitted to the hospital with complaints of left flank pain for 4 days and fever for 2 days. One week before admission (4 weeks after her honeymoon), she noted mild burning on urination. Four days before admission, she noted left flank pain. Two days before admission, she experienced fever associated with rigors and increasingly severe flank pain. She gave a past medical history of recurrent UTI over the past 5 years, requiring antibiotic treatment once annually. She denied vaginal discharge and was completing her menstrual cycle.

The physical examination showed a blood pressure of 80/50 mm Hg, a pulse of 125 per minute, and a temperature of 37.8°C. She appeared very ill and in pain. The remainder of her physical exam was normal, except for mild left costovertebral angle tenderness. No suprapubic tenderness was elicited. Her pelvic exam was within normal limits.

Laboratory workup revealed a white blood cell (WBC) count of 10,200/mm³, with 81% PMNs and 2% bands; a hematocrit of 36%, a blood urea nitrogen of 3mg/dL, and a serum creatinine of 0.4mg/dL. A urinalysis showed a specific gravity of 1010 g/mL, a pH of 5, 100 WBCs per high-power field (normal: 0–5), and 0–2 red blood cells per high-power field (normal). No protein or glucose was detected. A urine culture showed more than 10^5 E. coli, and 2 of 2 blood cultures grew E. coli.

Clinical Manifestations

Patients with cystitis usually experience acute-onset dysuria (pain, tingling, or burning in the perineal area during or just after urination). Dysuria results from inflammation of the urethra. In addition, patients need to urinate frequently, because inflammation of the bladder results in increasing suprapubic discomfort when the bladder is distended and may cause bladder spasms that interfere with bladder distension. Some patients note blood in the urine caused by inflammatory damage to the bladder wall.

As illustrated by case 9.1, the clinical manifestations of upper-tract disease usually overlap with those of lower-tract disease (Table 9.2). However, in addition to symptoms of cystitis, patients with pyelonephritis are more likely to experience fever and chills, costovertebral angle pain, nausea and vomiting, and hypotension. Certain risk factors increase the likelihood of

Table 9.2. Symptoms in Lower and Upper Urinary Tract Disease

Cystitis	Pyelonephritis
	All cystitis symptoms, plus
Burning	Fever
Frequency	Chills
Urgency	Costovertebral angle pain
Suprapubic pain	Nausea and vomiting
Dysuria	Hypotension

upper-tract disease. Patients with diabetes mellitus often experience subacute pyelonephritis that clinically mimics cystitis. Elderly patients have a higher probability of

---

KEY POINTS

About the Clinical Manifestations of Urinary Tract Infection

1. Symptoms of cystitis and pyelonephritis overlap.
2. Cystitis symptoms include dysuria, urinary frequency, hematuria, suprapubic discomfort.
3. Pyelonephritis symptoms include fever and chills, nausea and vomiting, tachycardia, hypotension, and costovertebral angle pain and tenderness. The disease is more likely to occur in
   a) diabetic patients (who often have only symptoms of cystitis),
   b) elderly patients (who may present with confusion or somnolence), or
   c) patients who have had cystitis symptoms for more than 7 days.
4. Asymptomatic bacteriuria is defined as a positive culture with no symptoms, and usually without pyuria.
   a) Treat pregnant women to prevent low birthweight neonates.
   b) Treat adolescent children to prevent renal scarring.
5. Urethritis can be mistaken for cystitis; usual indicators are fewer than 10^5 bacteria on culture and a lack of suprapubic tenderness.
6. Vaginitis can mimic cystitis; pelvic exam is a must if symptoms are associated with vaginal discharge.

having upper-tract disease and a higher risk for developing bacteremia. Patients who have had symptoms for more than 7 days are also at increased risk for pyelonephritis. When antibiotic treatment for cystitis is delayed for this period, bacteria have time to migrate up the ureters and infect the kidneys.

Another clinical condition (most commonly encountered in elderly women) is called asymptomatic bacteriuria. This condition is defined as a positive urine culture without symptoms. Urinalysis usually shows no WBCs or an insignificant number. This form of bacteriuria does not need to be treated unless the patient is pregnant or a child is of preschool age. Treatment is recommended in pregnant women because these patients are at increased risk of developing pyelonephritis. In preschool children, asymptomatic bacteriuria can result in renal scarring and interfere with normal growth of the kidneys.

Urethritis—inflammation of urethra—can be confused with cystitis. The primary symptom is burning on urination. Colony counts resulting from urine culture are less than 10^5 organisms per milliliter (see "Diagnosis," next), and the patient usually does not experience suprapubic pain or urinary frequency. Women with vaginitis can also experience burning on urination. Therefore, in a woman with symptoms suggestive of cystitis or urethritis accompanied by a vaginal discharge, a pelvic exam is warranted to exclude a pelvic infection.

The physical findings associated with UTI are usually minimal. Patients with cystitis may have suprapubic tenderness. Patients with pyelonephritis often are febrile and may be hypotensive and have an elevated heart rate. They often are acutely ill, appearing toxic. Costovertebral angle or flank tenderness resulting from inflammation and swelling of the infected kidney may be noted. In elderly patients, pyelonephritis and gram-negative sepsis may lead to confusion and somnolence. Urinalysis and urine culture should therefore always be included in the workup for acute changes in the mental status of an elderly patient.

Diagnosis

A microscopic examination of urinary sediment should be performed for all patients (Figure 9.1).

Following a careful cleaning of the perineal area, a midstream sample should be obtained and centrifuged for 5 minutes at 2000 rpm. On examination under a high-power lens (100 × oil immersion objective), each leukocyte represents 5 to 10 cells per milliliter of urine. More than 10 WBCs per high-power field is considered abnormal and represents pyuria. The dipstick leukocyte esterase test is rapid, sensitive, and specific for detecting pyuria. However, false negative tests may occur, and in patients with a negative leukocyte esterase test and symptoms suggestive of a UTI, a microscopic urinalysis

is recommended. The finding of WBC casts is strong evidence for pyelonephritis (a rare finding).

Increased protein in the urine also commonly accompanies UTI. Unspun urinary Gram stain is very helpful and should be performed in all patients with suspected pyelonephritis. The presence of one or more bacteria per oil immersion field indicates more than 10^5 organisms per milliliter. This bacterial concentration is unlikely to represent contamination, and in combination with pyuria and appropriate symptoms, it indicates active infection.

Urine culture is not required as part of the initial evaluation in young sexually active women with suspected cystitis. However in all other patients, a urine

---

KEY POINTS

About the Diagnosis of Urinary Tract Infection

1. Urinalysis should be performed in all patients with a possible urinary tract infection (UTI):
   a) More than 10 white blood cells per high-power field indicates pyuria.
   b) Leukocyte esterase dip stick is usually sensitive.

2. Unspun urine Gram stain can be helpful; 1 bacterium per high-power field indicates 10^5 organisms per milliliter.

3. Urine culture requires quantitation to differentiate contamination from true infection.
   a) Not required in sexually active adult women with early symptoms of cystitis.
   b) More than 10^5 organisms per milliliter indicates infection. Symptomatic women can have as few as 10^3 organisms.
   c) IDSA guidelines recommend using more than 10^3 organisms per milliliter as an indication of infection in symptomatic patients.
   d) Cultures must be processed immediately.
   e) Follow-up culture is warranted in the patient who experiences relapse of symptoms after completion of antibiotics.

4. Ultrasound is the imaging study of choice. Use in
   a) patients with upper-tract disease and persistent fever on antibiotics.
   b) preschool girls with a second UTI, or in boys or men with a UTI.

5. Intravenous pyelogram may be required to further delineate anatomic defects, but avoid in multiple myeloma or renal failure.

6. In patients not responding to antibiotics, use computed tomography scan with contrast to exclude perinephric abscess.

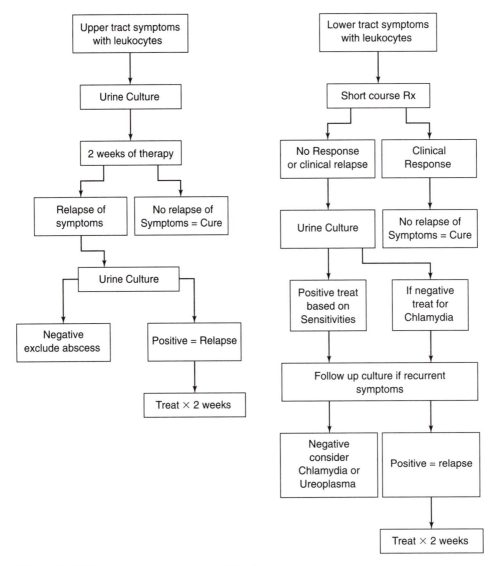

Figure 9–1. How to manage urinary tract infection.

sample for culture should be obtained. Urine in the bladder is normally sterile. Because the urethra and periurethral areas are very difficult to sterilize, even carefully collected specimens are contaminated. By quantitating bacteria in midstream, clean-voided urine, it is possible to statistically differentiate contamination from true infection. In women, infection is generally associated with more than 10^5 organisms per milliliter, and in men, in whom the number of contaminating bacteria tends to be lower, true infection has been found to be associated with bacterial counts of exceeding 10^3 per milliliter. These statistical values are helpful guidelines;

however, in one third of young women with symptomatic lower-tract infection, sample can contain fewer than 10^5 organisms. The Infectious Disease Society of America (IDSA) recommends that, in women with symptoms suggestive of a UTI, a colony count of 10^3 or greater should be considered significant.

It is important that urine cultures be processed immediately or stored at 4°C for no longer than 24 hours before the sample is plated on growth media. Improper handling of urine samples renders colony counts unreliable, and under these conditions, quantitative urine cultures cannot be used to differentiate true infection from contamination. Routine follow-up urine cultures after completion of therapy is not cost-effective, but a urine culture is indicated if the patient experiences recurrent symptoms of a UTI upon completion of therapy. Patients with presumed cystitis who experience recurrent symptoms and have a positive urine culture following short-course therapy (see "Treatment," next) are likely to be infected with an antibiotic-resistant organism or to have upper-tract disease (see Figure 9.1).

Which patients should undergo imaging studies to exclude an anatomic defect of the urinary tract?

Because anatomic defects are unlikely in young sexually active women with cystitis, imaging studies are not recommended in this population. However relapse after therapy in women (indicative of upper-tract disease) warrants investigation, as does probable upper-tract disease in any patients. Other situations that warrant investigation of the urinary tract anatomy include a second UTI in a preschool girl and a UTI in a boy and man at any age. Any patient with upper-tract disease on antibiotic therapy who fails to defervesce within 48 to 72 hours should be studied to exclude anatomic obstruction.

Ultrasonography is recommended as the imaging study of choice. Urinary tract ultrasonography is sensitive, specific, inexpensive, and safe. Ultrasound can detect congenital anatomic abnormalities, renal stones, ureteral obstruction, hydronephrosis, kidney swelling, and bladder distension. Intravenous pyelogram may be required in some patients to further delineate the anatomic abnormalities demonstrated by sonogram. To exclude the diagnosis of perinephric abscess, contrast-enhanced computed tomography (CT) scan should be considered in patients who fail to respond to antibiotics. In the setting of renal failure or multiple myeloma, intravenous contrast often exacerbates renal dysfunction and should be avoided.

Treatment

LOWER TRACT DISEASE

Short-course therapy is generally recommended (Table 9.3) for lower-tract disease. Although single-dose therapy may be effective, the preferred regimen is 3 days of antibiotics. Trimethoprim–sulfamethoxazole, cephalexin, cefpodoxime proxetil, norfloxacin, or ciprofloxacin are all generally effective treatment. Short-course therapy has also proved efficacious in elderly women with cystitis. In regions with a high incidence of TMP-SMX–resistant *E. coli*, 7 days of nitrofurantoin has been recommended as a fluoroquinolone-sparing regimen for uncomplicated cystitis. Short-course therapy should not be used in men, in patients with upper-tract symptoms, and in women whose symptoms span more than 7 days, or in diabetic patients (who often have chronic pyelonephritis with lower-tract symptoms).

UPPER TRACT DISEASE

Patients with upper-tract disease should receive a longer course of therapy. Two weeks of antibiotics are required. If the patient is not toxic and has not been vomiting, oral antibiotics can be used. A fluoroquinolone is recommended for empiric therapy. If a specific agent is identified and sensitivities are known, then TMP-SMX, cefpodoxime axetel, or amoxicillin–clavulanate may be used.

Patients with suspected bacteremia (high fever, shaking chills, hypotension) and patients with nausea and vomiting should be hospitalized for intravenous antibiotic therapy. The Gram stain usually reveals gram-negative rods. Multiple antibiotic regimens are effective. Intravenous ciprofloxacin has been found to be superior to intravenous TMP-SMX. Other effective regimens include gentamicin or tobramycin, a third-generation cephalosporin (ceftriaxone), or aztreonam. In patients who demonstrate more severe, life-threatening septic shock, an aminoglycoside should be combined with a

---

KEY POINTS

About the Treatment of Urinary Tract Infection

1. Cystitis: short course, 3 days (exceptions: boys and men, diabetic patients, women with symptoms for more than 7 days, and elderly people)
   a) Trimethoprim–sulfamethoxazole (TMP-SMX)
   b) Ciprofloxacin or levofloxacin
   c) Cefpodoxime proxetil
   d) Ciprofloxacin
2. Uncomplicated pyelonephritis: 2 weeks (not septic, not vomiting can use oral antibiotics)
   a) Fluoroquinolone preferred for empiric therapy
   b) If sensitivities known: TMP-SMX, cefpodoxime proxetil, or amoxicillin–clavulanate
3. Suspected bacteremia (chills, septic, hypotensive, vomiting): hospitalize, use intravenous antibiotics
   a) Third-generation cephalosporin (ceftriaxone)
   b) Ciprofloxacin
   c) Gentamicin
   d) Aztreonam
4. Extremely ill patient: usually treated with an aminoglycoside and a second antibiotic
   a) Cefepime
   b) Ciprofloxacin or levofloxacin
   c) An anti-pseudomonal penicillin
   d) A carbapenem

Table 9.3. Empiric Therapy for Urinary Tract Infection

Drug	Dose	Duration (days)
Uncomplicated cystitis—oral regimens		
Levofloxacin	250 mg q24h	3
Ciprofloxacin	100–250 mg q12h or 500 mg q24h	3
Trimethoprim–sulfamethoxazole	160/800 mg q12h	3
Trimethoprim	100 mg q12h	3
Cefpodoxime proxetil	100 mg q12h	3–7
Nitrofurantoin macrocrystals	50 mg q6h	7
Nitrofurantoin monohydrate macrocrystals (Macrobid)	100 mg q12h	7
Amoxicillin–clavulanate	500 mg q12h	7
Uncomplicated pyelonephritis—oral regimens		
Ciprofloxacin	500 mg q12h	14
Ciprofloxacin XR	1000 mg q24h	
Levofloxacin	250–500 mg q24h	
Ofloxacin	200–300 mg q12h	
Norfloxacin	400 mg q12h	
Lomefloxacin	400 mg q12h	
Enoxacin	400 mg q12h	
Uncomplicated pyelonephritis—oral regimens (sensitivities known)		
Trimethoprim–sulfamethoxazole	160/800 mg q12h	14
Cefpodoxime proxetil	100 mg q12h	
Amoxicillin–clavulanate	500 mg q12h	
Ceftriaxone	1 g q24h	
Uncomplicated pyelonephritis—intravenous regimens		
Ciprofloxacin	200–400 mg q12h	14
Levofloxacin	250–500 mg q24h	
Ofloxacin	200–400 mg q12h	
Gentamicin (± ampicillin)[a]	3–5 mg/kg q24h	
Ampicillin (+ gentamicin)[a]	1–2 g q6h	
Aztreonam	1 g q8–12h	
Complicated pyelonephritis—intravenous regimens (if extremely ill, use combination therapy; see text)		
Cefepime	1 g q12h	14
Ciprofloxacin	400 mg q12h	
Levofloxacin	500 mg q24h	
Ofloxacin	400 mg q12h	
Gentamicin (+ ampicillin)[a]	3–5 mg/kg q24h	
Ampicillin (+ gentamicin)[a]	1–2 g q6h	
Ticarcillin–clavulanate	3.2 g q8h	
Piperacillin–tazobactam	3.375 g[a] q6–8h	
Imipenem–cilastatin	250–500 mg q6–8h	

[a] Use if *Enterococcus* is suspected.

KEY POINTS

About Prevention of Urinary Tract Infections

1. Voiding or single-dose trimethoprim–sulfamethoxazole after intercourse reduces urinary tract infections (UTIs) in women,

2. In patients with anatomic defects that predispose to UTI, use daily low-dose trimethoprim–sulfamethoxazole or nitrofurantoin.

3. Antibiotic prophylaxis for bladder catheters is not recommended.

fourth-generation cephalosporin, an anti-pseudomonal penicillin (ticarcillin–clavulanate or piperacillin–tazobactam) or a carbapenem (see Chapter 2). If the patient relapses, a 2-week course of therapy should be repeated. If relapse follows the second treatment, a 4- to 6-week course should then be given. All patients with relapse should be studied for anatomic defects or stones.

Prevention

Patients with frequent symptomatic recurrences should receive preventive therapy. In sexually active women, voiding immediately after intercourse is often helpful. Administration of a single dose of TMP-SMX immediately after intercourse is even more effective. In children and other patients with anatomic defects, low dose (½ tablet) TMP-SMX daily or 50 mg of nitrofurantoin daily usually eliminates recurrent infection. Antibiotic prophylaxis for patients with indwelling bladder catheters is not effective and simply selects for antibiotic-resistant pathogens.

PROSTATITIS

POTENTIAL SEVERITY

Acute prostatitis can lead to sepsis and requires acute empiric antibiotic therapy.

Causes and Pathogenesis

Gram-negative bacteria are the most common cause of prostatitis. *E. coli* is most frequent, followed by *Klebsiella*, *Proteus*, and (less commonly) *Pseudomonas*, *Enterobacter* species, and *Serratia marcescens*. Prostate infection is com-

monly associated with a UTI and may serve as a reservoir for recurrent UTIs. With the exception of enterococci, gram-positive pathogens are uncommon. Cases of *Staphylococcus* species prostatitis have also been reported. The cause of culture-negative prostatitis has not been clarified. *Chlamydia* is a possible cause in these cases.

The mechanism by which bacteria usually reaches the prostate is reflux of infected urine. The prostate contains a potent antibacterial substance called prostatic antibacterial factor. The production of this zinc-containing compound is markedly reduced during prostatitis, allowing active growth of bacteria. Infection results in an influx of PMNs, edema, intraductal desquamation, and cell necrosis.

Symptoms and Clinical Findings

Patients with acute bacterial prostatitis experience fever, chills, dysuria, and urinary frequency. If the prostate becomes extremely swollen, bladder outlet

KEY POINTS

About Prostatitis

1. Primarily caused by gram-negative enteric organisms:
   a) *Escherichia coli* is most frequent.
   b) *Klebsiella* and *Proteus* are also cultured; *Pseudomonas*, *Enterobacter* species, and *Serratia* are less common.
   c) Gram-positive pathogens are rare, except for enterococci.

2. Pathogenesis is unclear:
   a) Reflux from urethra [often associated with a urinary tract infection (UTI)]
   b) Depletion of prostatic antibacterial factor

3. Clinical manifestations:
   a) Acute prostatitis—fever, chills, dysuria, and urinary frequency; bladder outlet obstruction. Prostate tender (do not massage, can precipitate bacteremia).
   b) Chronic prostatitis—low-grade fever, myalgias, and arthralgias, recurrent UTIs

4. Diagnosis: By urine or blood culture, or both

5. Treatment:
   a) Acute disease—trimethoprim–sulfamethoxazole (TMP-STX) or ciprofloxacin
   b) Chronic disease—prolonged therapy with TMP-STX or ciprofloxacin (6 to 12 weeks); may require prostatectomy

obstruction may develop. On physical examination, the patient often appears septic and has a high fever. Moderate tenderness of the suprapubic region is often seen. On rectal exam, the prostate is exquisitely tender and diffusely enlarged.

In chronic prostatitis, symptoms may be subtle. Back pain, low-grade fever, myalgias, and arthralgias are the most common complaints. These patients often present with recurrent UTIs.

Diagnosis

In acute bacterial prostatitis, massage of the inflamed prostate is contraindicated because of a high risk of precipitating bacteremia. The causative agent can usually be identified by urine culture. Blood cultures may also prove to be positive. Diagnosis and treatment of chronic prostatitis is difficult, and is best managed by an experienced urologist. Quantitative culturing of the first void urine, midstream urine, and prostatic massage sample or post

prostatic massage urine sample are recommended to differentiate cystitis and urethritis from chronic prostatitis.

Treatment

Initial empiric therapy for acute bacterial prostatitis should include coverage for Enterobacteriaceae. Ciprofloxacin or TMP-SMX in the doses recommended in Table 9.3 are useful. Once the culture result is available, treatment can be modified. Therapy should be prolonged: 4 to 6 weeks. It should be kept in mind that most antibiotics do not penetrate the lipophilic, acidic environment of the prostate; however, just as is observed in meningitis, the marked inflammation in acute prostatitis allows for antibiotic penetration. Patients usually respond quickly to intravenous therapy, allowing the switch to an oral regimen.

In chronic prostatitis, antibiotic penetration is critical for effective treatment. Trimethoprim is lipid-soluble and readily penetrates the prostate. The fluoroquinolones have also proved effective for treatment of chronic prostatitis. Treatment must be very prolonged. Therapy with oral TMP-SMX (1 double-strength tablet twice daily) or fluoroquinolone (ciprofloxacin 500 mg twice daily) should be continued for 6 to 12 weeks. Relapses are frequent, and prostatectomy may be required for cure.

KEY POINTS

About Urethritis

1. Causes:
   a) *Chlamydia trachomatis* and *Neisseria gonorrhoeae* are associated with a purulent discharge.
   b) *Ureaplasma urealyticum* and noninfectious causes are non-purulent.
2. Symptoms and signs:
   a) Burning on urination, worse with concentrated urine after alcohol consumption
   b) Staining of underwear, mucous in the urine.
   c) Meatus erythematous, milky discharge from penis
3. Diagnosis:
   a) Primarily by DNA probes
   b) Gram stain—In gonorrhea, intracellular gram-negative diplococci almost always found; negative Gram stain indicates nongonococcal disease (NGU)
   c) Culture of *N. gonorrhoeae* using 5% CO_2 has to be planted immediately
4. Treatment:
   a) Third-generation cephalosporin or a fluoroquinolone for gonorrhea
   b) Macrolide, tetracycline, fluoroquinolone, or sparfloxacin for NGU

■ SEXUALLY TRANSMITTED DISEASES

POTENTIAL SEVERITY

These (usually outpatient) infections can cause significant discomfort, but are rarely life-threatening.

Sexually transmitted diseases (STDs) are a common outpatient problem and warrant continued public health measures, including education and tracking of secondary cases. The incidence of these infections rises in association with reductions in public health funding. The importance of aggressive case-finding and early treatment cannot be overemphasized.

URETHRITIS

Causes

Urethritis can be caused by *Chlamydia trachomatis* and *Neisseria gonorrhoeae*. These infections are associated with a purulent or mucousy penile discharge in men and pyuria in women. *Ureaplasma urealyticum* and noninfectious causes (trauma, allergic, and chemical) also result in symptoms of urethritis, but are not associated with pyuria.

Symptoms

Patients with urethritis usually experience burning on urination, but have no other symptoms. The severity of dysuria varies greatly. Burning may be worse when passing concentrated urine or after drinking alcohol. This symptom is usually accompanied by a urethral discharge that often stains the undergarments. The urethral discharge may vary greatly in quantity and color, and can be primarily purulent or can also contain significant mucous. Some patients note mucous strands in their urine.

Clinical Findings

Examination reveals erythema of the urethral meatus, and milking of the urethra often yields a purulent material that can be cultured, used for DNA probe analysis, and applied to a slide for Gram stain. If a discharge cannot be expressed, a small calcium alginate urethral swab can be gently inserted at least 2 cm into the urethra. Because patients with urethritis often have multiple STDs, the perineal area, inguinal nodes, and vagina or penis need to be carefully examined for skin and mucous membrane lesions (see the subsection on syphilis later in this chapter).

Diagnosis

Gram stain of the urethral discharge is very helpful. A finding of more than 4 PMNs per oil-immersion field is always abnormal and is seen in most cases of acute symptomatic urethritis. In nearly all cases of gonococcal urethritis, gram-negative diplococci will be observed within the PMNs. The absence of intracellular bacteria strongly suggests non-gonococcal urethritis (NGU), which is caused primarily by *C. trachomatis*.

Urinalysis of the first 10 mL of urine, followed by a midstream sample, is useful for differentiating cystitis from urethritis. The finding of a higher number of PMNs in the first void sample as compared with the midstream sample strongly suggests the diagnosis of urethritis. In patients with cystitis, equal numbers of PMNs should be found in both samples. In many STD clinics, DNA probes of urethral samples or urine are used to diagnose *N. gonorrhoeae* and *C. trachomatis*. Urethral culture is now seldom used to diagnose *N. gonorrhoeae*. *Neisseria* requires 5% CO_2, and because the organism does not tolerate drying, samples must be immediately planted on selective Thayer–Martin agar plates. Culture for *U. urealyticum* is problematic and is not recommended. At the present time, diagnosis of this pathogen is usually presumptive and is based on clinical findings. It must be kept in mind that many patients with gonococcal urethritis also have NGU.

Treatment

When *N. gonorrhoeae* is identified, treatment with a third-generation cephalosporin or a fluoroquinolone is recommended (see Table 9.4). Because of the high likelihood of a concomitant NGU, this regimen should in most cases be accompanied by azithromycin or doxycycline (for doses, see Table 9.4). About 10% of *U. urealyticum* are resistant to doxycycline. If urethritis is refractory to doxycycline, then a macrolide, a fluoroquinolone, or sparfloxacin are effective treatment.

PELVIC INFLAMMATORY DISEASE

Causes and Pathogenesis

Pelvic inflammatory disease (PID) is primarily a disease of young, sexually active women. It is the most common gynecologic disease managed in emergency rooms, with an estimated 1 million cases being diagnosed annually in the United States. The disease is caused by spread of

---

KEY POINTS

About the Causes and Pathogenesis of Pelvic Inflamatory Disease

1. Primarily caused by *Neisseria gonorrhoeae* and *Chlamydia trachomatis*. Other, less common, pathogens include
   a) *Streptococcus pyogenes* and *Haemophilus influenzae* (most frequently accompany gonorrhea and chlamydia).
   b) group B streptococci, *Escherichia coli*, *Klebsiella* species, *Proteus mirabilis*, and anaerobes (least frequent).
2. Cervical canal usually prevents vaginal flora from invading the endometrium.
   a) Menstruation allows bacteria to bypass the cervix, with pelvic inflammatory disease (PID) usually begining 7 days after menstruation.
   b) Delayed treatment of urethritis leads to PID (15% of cases progress to PID).
3. Risk factors for PID:
   a) Young age (sexually active teenagers at highest risk)
   b) Multiple sexual partners
   c) Past history of PID

Table 9.4. Treatment Regimens for Sexually Transmitted Diseases CDC Guidelines 2006

Drug	Dose	Relative Efficacy	Comments
Gonococcal urethritis			
Cefixime	400 mg PO once	First line	
Ceftriaxone	125 mg IM once	First line	Some discomfort with the IM injection
Ciprofloxacin	500 mg PO once	First line	Increased resistance to fluoroquinolones in Honolulu, Hawaii
Ofloxacin	400 mg PO once		
Levofloxacin	250 mg PO once (500 mg q24h for disseminated disease)		
Combine with azithromycin or doxycycline	2 g PO once 100 mg PO q12h for 7 days		
Spectinomycin	2 g IM once	Alternative	
Ceftizoxime	500 mg IM once	Alternative	
Cefoxitin with probenecid	2 g IM 1 g PO once	Alternative	
Disseminated gonococcal disease			
Ceftriaxone	1 g IV or IM q24h	First line	Continue for 24–48 hours; after clinical improvement, switch to an oral regimen to complete 7 days minimum
Cefotaxime, or ceftizoxime	1 g IV q8h 1 g IV q8h	Alternative	Same duration and PO regimen as for ceftriaxone
Ciprofloxacin, or ofloxacin, or levofloxacin	400 mg IV q12h 400 mg IV q12h 250 mg IV q24h	Alternatives	Same duration and PO regimen as for ceftriaxone
Spectinomycin	2 g IM q24h	Alternative	Same duration and PO regimen as for ceftriaxone
Non-gonococcal urethritis			
Azithromycin	1 g PO once	First line	
Doxycycline	100 mg PO q12h for 7 days	First line	
Erythromycin base	500 mg PO q6h for 7 days	Alternative	
Ofloxacin	300 mg PO q12h for 7 days	Alternative	
Levofloxacin	500 mg PO q24h for 7 days	Alternative	
Amoxicillin	500 mg PO q8h for 7 days	Alternative	In pregnancy only
Metronidazole, plus azithromycin	2 g PO once 1 g PO once		Use if recurrent urethritis to treat *Trichomonas vaginalis*
Pelvic inflammatory disease—IV regimens			
(A) Cefotetan, or cefoxitin, plus doxycycline	2 g IV q12h 2 g IV q6h 100 mg PO q12h for 14 days	First line	Continue for 24 hours after improvement

(Continued)

Table 9.4. (Continued)

Drug	Dose	Relative Efficacy	Comments
Pelvic inflammatory disease—IV regimens			
(B) Clindamycin, plus gentamicin	900 mg IV q8h 1.5 mg/kg IV q8h, or 7 mg/kg IV q24h	First line	Continue IV for 24 hours after improvement, then switch to clindamycin 450 mg PO q6h to complete 14 days
Ofloxacin, or levofloxacin, with or without metronidazole	400 mg IV q12h 500 mg IV q24h 500 mg IV q8h	Alternative	Metronidazole adds anaerobic coverage
Ampicillin/sulbactam, plus doxycycline	3 g IV q6h 100 mg IV or PO q12h	Alternative	
Pelvic inflammatory disease—"Oral" regimens			
(A) Ofloxacin, or levofloxacin, with or without metronidazole	400 mg PO q12h 500 mg PO q24h 500 mg PO q12h for 14 days	First line	
(B) Ceftriaxone, or cefoxitin, plus doxycycline, with or without metronidazole	250 mg IM once 2 g IM + probenecid 1 g 100 mg PO q12h for 14 days 500 mg PO q12h for 14 days	First line	Metronidazole adds anaerobic coverage
Genital ulcers: Herpes simplex—first episode			
Acyclovir	400 mg PO q8h for 7–10 days	First line	Less expensive
Acyclovir	200 mg PO 5 times daily, 7–10 days	First line	Less expensive
Famciclovir	250 mg PO q8h for 7–10 days	First line	
Valacyclovir	1 g PO q12h for 7–10 days	First line	
Genital ulcers: Herpes simplex—episodic therapy, HIV-negative			
Acyclovir	Same as first episode, for 5 days	First line	Less expensive
Acyclovir	800 mg q12h for 5 days	First line	Less expensive
Acyclovir	800 mg q8h for 2 days	First line	
Famciclovir	125 mg q12h for 5 days	First line	
Famciclovir	1000 mg q12h for 1 day	First line	
Valacyclovir	500 mg PO q12h for 3 days	First line	
Valacyclovir	1 g q24h for 5 days	First line	
Genital ulcers: Herpes simplex—episodic therapy, HIV-positive			
Acyclovir	Same as first episode, for 5–10 days	First line	Less expensive
Famciclovir	500 mg PO q12h for 5–10 days	First line	
Valacyclovir	1 g PO q12h for 5–10 days	First line	
Genital ulcers: Herpes simplex—daily suppressive therapy, HIV-negative			
Acyclovir	400 mg PO q12h	First line	Less expensive
Famciclovir	250 mg PO q12h	First line	
Valacyclovir	500 mg PO q24h	First line	
Valacyclovir	1 g PO q24h	First line	

(Continued)

Table 9.4. *(Continued)*

Drug	Dose	Relative Efficacy	Comments

Drug	Dose	Relative Efficacy	Comments
Genital ulcers: Herpes simplex—daily suppressive therapy, HIV-positive			
Acyclovir	400–800 mg q12h or q8h	First line	Less expensive
Famciclovir	500 mg q12h	First line	
Valacyclovir	500 mg q12h	First line	
Genital ulcers: Chancroid			
Azithromycin	1 g PO once	First line	Most convenient
Ceftriaxone	250 mg IM once	First line	IM injection painful
Ciprofloxacin	500 mg PO q12h for 3 days	First line	
Erythromycin base	500 mg PO q6h for 7 days	First line	Least convenient
Genital ulcers: Lymphogranuloma venerium			
Doxycycline	100 mg PO q12h × 21 days	First line	
Erythromycin base	500 mg PO q6h for 21 days	First line	No data on azithromycin
Donovanosis			
Doxycycline	100 mg PO q12h for 21 days	First line	
Ciprofloxacin	750 mg q12h for 21 days	Alternative	
Erythromycin base	500 mg q6h for 21 days	Alternative	
Azithromycin	1 g PO weekly × 3	Alternative	
Trimethoprim–sulfamethoxazole	1 double-strength tablet PO q12h for 21 days	Alternative	
Syphilis—primary and secondary			
Benzathine penicillin	2.4×10^6 U IM once	First line	Weekly re-treatmenr for 3 doses
Doxycycline	100 mg PO q12h for 14 days	Alternative	For penicillin-allergic patients
Tetracycline	500 mg PO q6h for 14 days	Alternative	For penicillin-allergic patients
Azithromycin	2 g PO once	Alternative	For penicillin-allergic patients; less effective, requires close follow-up
Latent syphilis—Early (less than 1 year)			
Benzathine penicillin	2.4×10^6 U IM once	First line	
Latent syphilis—Late or tertiary (except neurosyphilis)			
Benzathine penicillin	2.4×10^6 U IM weekly ×3	First line	
Latent syphilis—Neurosyphilis			
Aqueous penicillin G	$3–4 \times 10^6$ U IV q4h for 10–14 days	First line	
Procaine penicillin, plus probenecid	2.4×10^6 U IM q24h 500 mg PO q6h for 10–14 days	First line	A painful regimen
Ceftriaxone	2 g IV q24h for 10–14 days	Alternative	
Bacterial vaginosis			
Metronidazole	500 mg PO q12h for 7 days	First line	
Metronidazole gel 0.75%	One full applicator (5 g)	First line	
Trichomoniasis			
Metronidazole	2 g PO once	First line	
Tinidazole	2 g PO once	First line	
Metronidazole	500 mg q12h for 7 days	Alternative	

cervical microbes to the endometrium, fallopian tubes, ovaries, and surrounding pelvic structures.

The vagina contains multiple organisms, with *Lactobacillus* being the predominant organism. The endocervical canal serves as a protective barrier, preventing the vaginal flora from entering the upper genital tract and maintaining a sterile environment. Menstruation allows the vaginal flora to bypass this barrier, and as a consequence, most cases of PID begin within 7 days of menstruation. Nearly all cases of community-acquired PID are now believed to be sexually transmitted.

The organisms that most commonly cause pelvic inflammatory disease are *N. gonorrhoeae* and *C. trachomatis*. If treatment of urethritis is delayed, infection of the vaginal area can spread to the uterus and cause PID. Approximately 15% of both gonococcal and chlamydial urethritis cases progress to PID. These two pathogens may be accompanied by growth of other pathogenic organisms, most commonly *Streptococcus pyogenes* and *Haemophilus influenzae*. Other pathogens include group B streptococci, *E. coli*, *Klebsiella* species, *Proteus mirabilis*, and anaerobes (primarily *Bacteroides*, *Prevotella*, *Peptococcus*, and *Peptostreptococcus* species).

Factors that increase the risk of PID include younger age (sexually active teenagers have the highest disease incidence), multiple sexual partners, and a past history of PID. The use of condoms and spermicidal agents protect against this infection. The placement of an IUD does not increase the risk for PID in women with a stable monogamous relationship.

Symptoms and Clinical Findings

Lower abdominal pain is the most common complaint of women with PID. Onset of pain often occurs during or immediately after menses. Pain may be worsened by jarring movements or sexual intercourse. Approximately one third of women experience uterine bleeding. Other complaints include fever and vaginal discharge.

On physical examination only about half of patients are febrile. Abdominal exam usually reveals bilateral lower quadrant tenderness. Rebound and hypoactive bowel sounds may also be present. The finding of right upper quadrant tenderness suggests the development of perihepatitis (Fitz–Hugh–Curtis syndrome), noted in about 10% of cases. On pelvic exam, cervical motion tenderness and a purulent endocervical discharge provide strong evidence for PID. Adnexal and uterine tenderness should also be present or the diagnosis of PID should be questioned. Tenderness is usually symmetric in uncomplicated PID. The finding of increased tenderness in one adnexa or palpation of an adnexal mass suggests a tubo-ovarian abscess. Others diseases that may present with similar clinical findings—appendicitis, ectopic

---

KEY POINTS

About the Clinical Manifestations of Pelvic Infalmmatory Disease

1. Lower abdominal pain during or immediately following menses,
   a) made worse by jarring motions,
   b) accompanied by vaginal bleeding (one third of cases), and
   c) commonly presenting with vaginal discharge.
2. On physical exam,
   a) only half of patients have fever.
   b) bilateral lower quadrant tenderness and cervical, uterine, and bilateral adnexal tenderness are present.
   c) right upper quadrant tenderness indicates Fitz–Hugh–Curtis syndrome.
   d) localized tenderness to one adnexa suggests tubo-ovarian abscess.

---

pregnancy, diverticulitis, adnexal torsion, rupture or hemorrhage of an ovarian cyst, nephrolithiasis, pancreatitis, and perforated bowel—should also be considered.

Diagnosis

During the initial evaluation, a pregnancy test should be performed to exclude the possibility of tubo-ovarian pregnancy. A complete blood count should also be performed, although an elevated peripheral WBC count is observed in only half of PID cases. The erythrocyte sedimentation rate and level of C-reactive protein are more reliable indicators of inflammation, and normal values make the diagnosis of PID unlikely. Urinalysis to exclude cystitis or pyelonephritis is recommended in all cases. Pyuria may also be present in patients with urethritis and PID; therefore, if urethritis is suspected, a first void should be compared to a midstream urine sample as described for urethritis. Microscopic examination of the vaginal discharge usually reveals more than 3 WBCs per high-power field and has proved to be the most sensitive test (approximately 80%) for PID. Nevertheless, a number of other disorders can also cause a purulent discharge, giving the test a low specificity (approximately 40%). Tests for chlamydia and gonococcus also need to be performed for all patients with suspected PID. Ultrasound should be performed in patients with suspected tubo-ovarian abscess. Laparoscopy has high specificity

---

KEY POINTS

**About the Diagnosis and Treatment
of Pelvic Inflammatory Disease**

1. No specific test is available for pelvic inflammatory disease (PID); diagnosis is usually clinical:
   a) Erythrocyte sedimentation rate and C-reactive protein are elevated. Normal values make thes diagnosis unlikely.
   b) On examination of vaginal exudate, more than 3 white blood cells per high-power field is 80% sensitive and 40% specific.
2. Definitive diagnosis can be made by
   a) Laparoscopy (low sensitivity; should be reserved for the seriously ill patient).
   b) Histologic evidence of endometritis on biopsy.
   c) Imaging revealing thickened, fluid-filled oviducts with or without free pelvic fluid or tubo-ovarian swelling.
3. To prevent infertility and chronic pain, the threshold for treatment should be low:
   a) Outpatient treatment—ofloxacin or levofloxacin, plus metronidazole for 14 days or 1 dose of ceftriaxone, plus doxycycline with or without metronidazole for 14 days.
   b) Inpatient treatment—cefoxitin or cefotetan, plus doxycycline, or clindamycin plus gentamicin.
   c) Laparoscopy to rule out tubo-ovarian abscess; laparotomy to rule out ruptured abscess.

---

for PID, but low sensitivity, failing to reveal significant abnormalities in half of all cases. Laparoscopy should be reserved for patients who are seriously ill, and in whom another competing diagnosis such as appendicitis is suspected. It should also be performed in patients who remain acutely ill despite outpatient treatment or 72 hours of inpatient therapy.

There is no definitive test for the diagnosis of PID. Guidelines from the U.S. Centers for Disease Control and Prevention (CDC) state that a definitive diagnosis of PID requires one of three findings:

1. Histologic evidence of endometritis in a biopsy.
2. An imaging technique revealing thickened fluid-filled oviducts with or without free pelvic fluid or tubo-ovarian swelling.
3. Laparoscopic abnormalities consistent with PID.

Because of the difficulty of achieving a definitive diagnosis and the potential harm to a woman's reproductive health from delayed treatment, the CDC also recommends that "health care providers should maintain a low threshold for the diagnosis of PID." Young, sexually active women with the appropriate risk factors and clinical findings should be presumptively managed as having PID.

Treatment

To prevent potential complications and minimize the sequelae of PID, prompt empiric antibiotic therapy is recommended. For outpatient therapy, treat with ofloxacin or levofloxacin plus metronidazole for 14 days. Alternatively, a single dose of ceftriaxone combined with a 14-day course of doxycycline with or without metronidazole is recommended by the CDC (see Table 9.4).

For inpatient therapy, cefotetan or cefoxitin should combined with doxycycline. This regimen should be continued until 24 hours after significant clinical improvement, and should then be followed by oral doxycycline to complete 14 days of therapy. An alternative inpatient regimen consists of clindamycin and gentamicin, followed by oral clindamycin or doxycycline to complete 14 days of therapy (see Table 9.4). If tubo-ovarian abscess is suspected, or the patient fails to respond within 72 hours, laparoscopy should be performed and areas of loculated pus drained percutaneously or transvaginally. If a leaking or ruptured abscess is suspected, laparotomy should be performed immediately. The sequelae following PID can include infertility, chronic pelvic pain, and an increased risk of ectopic pregnancy.

GENITAL ULCERS

The most commonly diagnosed and treated venereal diseases of the skin and mucous membranes are genital ulcers.

Causes

The most common cause of genital ulcers in the United States is herpes genitalis (usually attributable to herpes simplex type II), followed by syphilis (*Treponema pallidum*) and chancroid (*Haemophilus ducreyi*). Lymphogranuloma venerium (LGV: *C. trachomatis*) and Behcet's syndrome (unknown cause) are rarer. In India, Papua New Guinea, the West Indies, and parts of Africa and South America, donovanosis or granuloma inguinale (*Calymmatobacterium granulomatosis*) is a major cause of genital ulcers. Trauma can also lead to ulceration. With the exception of Behcet's syndrome, these diseases are sexually transmitted. A complete sexual history and a past history of sexually transmitted diseases must therefore be obtained.

Clinical Findings

Certain clinical features tend to favor one causative agent over another. However, these rules should be applied with caution, because the "classic" findings are seen in only one third of cases. Thus, the following physical findings, although specific, are insensitive (see Table 9.5):

1. **Ulcer number and location.** The number of ulcers has been purported to be helpful; however, because of the wide variability in ulcer number in each disease, recent studies indicate that this characteristic is not helpful. The one exception is herpes simplex virus (HSV), which frequently presents as a cluster of vesicles and ulcers. The location of the ulcers is helpful in differentiating Behcet's syndrome from other causes. This idiopathic inflammatory disease involves the mouth, conjunctiva, and joints in addition to the genitalia. In Behcet's syndrome, ulcers usually form on the scrotum or vulva rather than on the penis, anus, or vagina as observed with the venereal diseases.

2. **Ulcer size.** The size of the ulcers may be helpful in differentiating potential causes. The multiple ulcers of HSV tend to be the same size; the ulcers associated with chancroid tend to vary in size and may coalesce to form a giant lesion.

3. **Ulcer tenderness.** Tenderness on palpation is most commonly noted in HSV and chancroid, but is present in about one third of syphilitic ulcers.

4. **Appearance of ulcer base and edges.** The appearance of the base of the ulcer helps to differentiate chancroid and Behcet's syndrome from syphilis and herpes. In chancroid, the base is ragged and necrotic; in Behcet's, it is yellow and necrotic. Syphilitic and HSV ulcers have clean-appearing bases. The characteristics of the ulcer edge can also be helpful. In chancroid, the edge tends to be undermined, and induration is minimal. In cases of syphilis, the edge is usually markedly indurated. In HSV and chancroid, an erythematous border is usually seen. In donovanosis, the edge has a unique, stark white appearance.

5. **Inguinal adenopathy.** Inguinal lymphadenopathy is commonly encountered with genital ulcers. In chancroid and herpes genitalis, the inguinal nodes are often exquisitely tender; in primary and secondary syphilis, nodes tend to be rubbery and only minimally tender. In chancroid, these nodes commonly become fluctuant and contain significant quantities of pus. Fluctuant nodes are also often encountered in LGV. In that disease, the genital ulcer usually heals

Table 9.5. Clinical Characteristics of Genital Ulcers

Disease	Ulcer characteristics				Adenopathy
	Number	Location	Tenderness	Appearance	
Herpes simplex virus	Clusters	Labia, penis	Tender	Uniform size, clean base, erythematous border	Very tender inguinal nodes
Syphilis	1–2	Vagina, penis	One third tender	Clean base, indurated border	Rubbery, mildly tender
Chancroid	—	Labia, penis	Tender	Can be large; ragged and necrotic base, undermined edge	Very tender fluctuant inguinal nodes
Lymphogranuloma venerium	—	Labia, penis	Painless	Ulcer lasts 2–3 weeks, spontaneously heals at time of fluctuant adenopathy	Fluctuant inguinal nodes, "groove sign"
Donovanosis	Kissing lesions	Labia, penis	Painless	Clean, beefy red base; stark white heaped-up edges	Nodes usually firm, can mimic lymphogranuloma venerium
Behcet's syndrome	—	Mouth, scrotum or vulva	Painful	Yellow necrotic base	Adenopathy minimal

spontaneously, and 3 to 6 weeks later, the patient develops markedly enlarged and tender inguinal nodes that become fluctuant (called "secondary LGV"). Infection also commonly spreads to the femoral nodes. The inguinal ligament that separates the inguinal from the femoral nodes forms a groove or indentation resulting in the "groove sign," a classic sign associated with this disease.

Diagnosis

The CDC recommends that the diagnosis be made clinically and that patients be treated empirically. It is important to keep in mind that clinical diagnosis is accurate less than 50% of the time. However, the commercially available diagnostic tests either have a low sensitivity, are impractical because of the time required to obtain results, or are too costly. In many instances, follow-up is not possible, and therefore diagnosis and treatment must occur during a single clinic visit.

At a minimum, patients with genital ulcers should have blood drawn for a VDRL (Venereal Disease Research Laboratory) or RPR (rapid plasma reagin) test, and when possible, that test should be repeated in 1 month if the first is negative. Recognizing the increased risk of HIV among patients with genital ulcers, all patients should receive HIV counseling and HIV antibody testing. In areas in which chancroid is prevalent and the ulcer appearance is suggestive, a Gram stain of scrapings from the ulcer edge should be performed looking for gram-negative rods arranged in parallel arrays having the appearance of a "school of fish" (while keeping in mind that this test is not very sensitive). When available, culturing of samples using selective media should be performed. Also when available, these additional tests should be performed: darkfield microscopy of an ulcer scraping, looking for corkscrew-appearing spirochetes (syphilis); a Tzanck preparation, looking for multinucleated giant cells; and a viral culture looking for HSV. In areas in which LGV is prevalent or in cases in which the classic findings are observed, LGV serology should be ordered. A potentially highly sensitive and specific test that is currently available only for investigational purposes is called the multiplex polymerase chain reaction (M-PCR). The M-PCR uses primers that are capable of identifying the three most common causes of genital ulcers: HSV, *H. ducreyi*, and *T. pallidum*.

Treatment

Empiric therapy depends on the clinical findings, the prevalence of STDs in the area, and the likelihood of follow-up. In most cases, empiric therapy for HSV and syphilis are recommended. For the first episode of HSV, treatment should consist of 7 to 10 days of acyclovir, valacyclovir, or famciclovir (see Table 9.4). For primary

---

KEY POINTS

About Genital Ulcers

1. Genital ulcers have five major causes: herpes simplex virus (HSV), syphilis, chancroid, lymphogranuloma venerium (LGV), donovanosis, and Behcet's syndrome
2. Diagnosis is usually made by the clinical characteristics of the ulcer (not always reliable):
   a) Size and location
   b) Pain and tenderness
   c) Appearance of base and edges
   d) Lymphadenopathy
3. Laboratory studies include VDRL (Venereal Disease Research Laboratory), HIV antibody, Gram stain (for suspected chancroid), viral culture for HSV, LGV serum titers, dark-field exam for syphilis
4. Treatment:
   a) HSV—acyclovir, valacyclovir, or famciclovir
   b) Syphilis—penicillin
   c) Chancroid—azithromycin or ceftriaxone
   d) Donovanosis—trimethoprim–sulfamethoxazole or doxycycline
   e) LGV—doxycycline or erythromycin

---

syphilis, penicillin is the drug of choice. Recommendations for treatment and follow-up are outlined in the subsection on syphilis (next). In areas in which chancroid is prevalent, coverage of *Haem. ducreyi* should also be included. Chancroid is effectively treated with single oral dose of azithromycin or intramuscular ceftriaxone. Other effective regimens include erythromycin base and ciprofloxacin. If LGV is strongly suspected, doxycycline is the preferred treatment. Alternatively, erythromycin can be used. Donovanosis is treated with TMP-SMX or doxycycline.

SYPHILIS

POTENTIAL SEVERITY

Not life-threatening, but untreated primary infection can lead to debilitating complications 20 to 30 years later.

Epidemiology

The syphilis spirochete, *T. pallidum*, is spread from person to person primarily by sexual intercourse or passage through the placenta, causing congenital disease. Less commonly, close contact with an active lesion (such as kissing) or transfusion of fresh blood from a patient with early-disseminated disease can result in transmission.

The incidence of syphilis has waxed and waned over the past 50 years as a consequence of changing sexual practices and changing government commitments to public health departments. The history of syphilis is a rich one, and the spirochete is purported to have infected many famous political figures and artists, including Henry VIII, Frederick the Great, Pope Alexander VI, Oscar Wilde, Ludwig von Beethoven, and Franz Schubert.

Syphilis abruptly appeared in Europe during the 15th century, and severe epidemics of secondary syphilis, then called "the great pox," were reported in the 16th century. It is estimated that, by the late 19th century, 10% of the population was infected with syphilis. In 1942, just prior to the widespread use of penicillin, 575,000 new cases of syphilis (approximately 4 per 1000 population) were reported in the United States. With testing and antibiotic treatment, the number of new cases dropped to 6500 annually in the 1950s, but it then increased in the 1960s with the advent of the sexual revolution. With the rise of homosexual promiscuity in the late 1970s and early 1980s, 50% of new cases in the United States were reported in homosexual men. Many of these patients were also co-infected with HIV. Educational programs encouraging "safe sex" with condoms reduced the incidence in the homosexual community during late 1980s and early 1990s. However, at the same time, the incidence of syphilis increased dramatically in the heterosexual African American and Hispanic populations. By 1992, as a consequence of aggressive public health measures, the annual incidence of syphilis in the United States was reduced to 28,000 from 50,000. Most recently, with the improved success of antiretroviral therapy, the fear of AIDS has decreased, and many individuals have falsely concluded that HIV is now easily treatable. With this reduced fear, "safe sex" practices have been ignored, and the incidence of syphilis has again begun to climb.

Pathogenesis and Clinical Manifestations

Syphilis is caused by *T. pallidum*, a fragile bacterium that is long (5 to 20 μm) and very thin (0.1 to 0.2 μm). This member of the spirochete family is so thin that it cannot be visualized by standard light microscopy; however, it can be seen by darkfield or phase microscopy. These two techniques use condensers that shine light at an oblique angle, accentuating the long, corkscrew morphology of the organism. The live spirochete moves gracefully by a characteristic flexing motion. This bacterium cannot be grown in vitro; it requires cultivation in animals, rabbits being the most commonly used for live cultures. *T. pallidum* divides slowly, by binary fission, with a doubling time of 30 hours. (Most conventional bacteria double every 60 minutes.)

The natural history of syphilis can be broken down into three stages:

1. Primary syphilis
2. Secondary syphilis
3. Latent syphilis

PRIMARY SYPHILIS

Following sexual intercourse, the organism is able to penetrate the skin, and it begins multiplying subcutaneously at the site of entry. The presence of the organism stimulates infiltration by PMNs, followed by T lymphocytes and specific antibodies that are generated in response to the infection. The development of this inflammatory response leads to skin ulceration and the formation of a painless chancre (described in the preceding subsection on genital ulcers) approximately 3 weeks after exposure. Spirochetes can be readily identified by darkfield microscopy of skin scrapings from the ulcer.

SECONDARY SYPHILIS

Once the treponemes penetrate the skin, they quickly migrate to the lymphatics and gain entry to the bloodstream, disseminating widely throughout the body. Symptomatic secondary disease occurs in approximately 30% of patients. A skin rash is noted in 90% of patients

---

KEY POINTS

About the Epidemiology of Syphilis

1. Transmitted by sexual intercourse.
2. Can cross the placenta and cause congenital disease.
3. Direct contact with an infected lesion can occasionally spread the disease, as can a blood transfusion drawn from a patient with early disseminated disease.
4. Annual incidence in the United States is 28,000 cases.
5. Incidence waxes and wanes depending on changes in sexual practices and public health funding.

and usually consists of pink to red macular, maculopapular, papular, or pustular lesions. The lesions usually begin on the trunk and spread to the extremities, often involving the palms and soles. In areas of increased moisture such as the groin, the lesions may coalesce, producing painless, gray-white, erythematous, highly infectious plaques called condyloma lata. Patches of alopecia may result in a moth-eaten appearance to the

eyebrows or beard. Rash is often accompanied by diffuse lymphadenitis. Enlargement of the epitrochlear nodes is particularly suggestive of secondary syphilis.

The manifestations of secondary disease usually begin 2 to 8 weeks after exposure. At this stage, organisms can be found in the blood, skin, central nervous system, and aqueous humor of the eye. In addition to the skin and lymph nodes, almost any organ in the body can be affected. Basilar meningitis may develop that can result in deficits of cranial nerves III, VI, VII, and VIII. These deficits are manifested as pupillary abnormalities, diplopia, facial weakness, hearing loss, and tinnitus. Anterior uveitis, immune-complex glomerulonephritis, syphilitic hepatitis, synovitis, and periostitis are other disease manifestations. Secondary syphilis has been called "The Great Imitator," and serology for syphilis should always be ordered in a patient with unexplained skin rash, lymphadenopathy, lymphocytic meningitis, neurologic deficit, bone and joint abnormalities, glomerulonephritis, or hepatitis.

LATENT SYPHILIS

After dissemination is controlled by the immune system, the organisms can persist in the body without causing symptoms. During the latent period, the spirochetes slow their metabolism and doubling time. "Latent syphilis" is defined as the asymptomatic period more than 1 year after primary infection—a period that often lasts 20 to 30 years. Before that year ends, patients are at risk of symptomatic relapse and are therefore considered infectious. During the latent period, specific antibodies directed against *T. pallidum* can be detected by the fluorescent treponemal antibody absorption assay (FTA-ABS) or by various hemagglutinin tests (see the subsection on diagnosis and treatment).

TERTIARY OR LATE SYPHILIS

Patients with syphilis who remain untreated have a 40% risk of developing late syphilis. This disease causes three major syndromes:

1. Late neurosyphilis
2. Cardiovascular syphilis
3. Late benign gummas

Late Neurosyphilis

Arteritis can develop in the small vessels of the meninges, brain, and spinal cord, resulting in multiple small infarcts that can cause hemiparesis, generalized or focal seizures, and aphasia. This neurologic disease is called meningovascular syphilis, and usually occurs 5 to 10 years after primary infection. Meningovascular syphilis should always be considered in the younger patient who suffers a cerebrovascular accident.

KEY POINTS

About Late Neurosyphilis

1. Meningovascular syphilis causes arteritis and cerebral infarction. Can be a rare cause of stroke in younger patients. Occurs within 5 to 10 years of primary disease

2. General paresis arises from direct damage to the cerebral cortex by spirochetes, 15 to 20 years after primary disease. Includes
   a) emotional lability, paranoia, delusions, hallucinations, megalomania; and
   b) tremors, hyperreflexia, seizures, slurred speech, Argyll Robertson pupils, optic atrophy.

3. Tabes dorsalis is caused by demyelination of the posterior column, 15 to 20 years after primary disease. Includes
   a) ataxic gait, loss of position sense, lightening pains, absence of deep tendon reflexes, loss of bladder function; and
   b) Charcot's joints, skin ulcers.

4. Argyll Robertson pupils
5. Loss of deep tendon reflexes
6. Impotence, loss of bladder function, fecal incontinence
7. Neuropathy leading to Charcot's joints (caused by persistent trauma) and traumatic skin ulcers

Cardiovascular Syphilis

Arteritis involves the feeding vessels of the aorta (the vasa vasorum), resulting in necrosis of the media of the vessels and progressive dilatation of the aorta that can lead to aortic regurgitation, congestive heart failure, and coronary artery stenosis, causing angina. Less commonly, asymptomatic saccular aneurysms of the ascending aortic, transverse, and (rarely) descending aorta may develop. Chest X-ray may demonstrate streaks of calcification in the aorta, suggesting the diagnosis. Cardiovascular manifestations arise 15 to 30 years after primary infection in 10% of untreated patients.

Later benign Gummas

A gumma is a nonspecific granulomatous-like lesion that can develop in skin, bone, mucous membranes, or, less commonly, in other organs. In the antibiotic era,

The spirochetes can also cause direct damage to the neural cells within the cerebral cortex and spinal cord. Cortical damage results in a constellation of clinical manifestations called "general paresis" that usually develops 15 to 20 years after the primary infection:

1. **Personality disorder.** Includes emotional lability, paranoia, loss of judgment and insight, and carelessness in appearance.
2. **Psychiatric disturbances.** May include delusions, hallucinations, and megalomania.
3. **Distinct neurologic abnormalities.** Include abnormal pupillary response (small pupils that fail to react to light, but that accommodate to near vision by dilating), termed Argyll Robertson pupils; hyperreactive reflexes; tremors of the face, hands, and legs; seizures; speech disturbances, particularly slurred speech; and optic atrophy.

Demyelination of the posterior column, dorsal roots, and dorsal root ganglia gives rise to the constellation of symptoms and signs called tabes dorsalis:

1. Ataxic, wide-based gait with foot slap
2. Loss of position sense and vibratory, deep pain, and temperature sensation
3. Lightning-like pains of sudden onset and rapid radiation

KEY POINTS

About Cardiovascular Syphilis and Late Benign Gummas

1. Arteritis of the vasa vasorum causes damage to the aortic vessel wall, 15 to 30 years after primary disease. Includes
   a) dilatation of the proximal aorta, leading to aortic regurgitation and congestive heart failure; and
   b) saccular aneurysms, primarily of the ascending and transverse aorta.
   c) Chest radiographs may demonstrate linear calcifications of the aorta.

2. Gummas are granulomatous-like lesions, rare today, except in patients with AIDS.
   a) Skin gummas can break down, forming a chronic ulcer.
   b) Lytic bone lesions can cause tenderness and draining sinuses.
   c) Mass lesions of cerebral cortex, liver, and gastric antrum.

these lesions are rare, except in patients with AIDS. In the skin, the gumma can break down and form a chronic non-healing ulcer. Bone gummas usually develop in the long bones and are associated with localized tenderness, bony destruction, and chronic draining sinuses. Visceral gummas can be found in any organ, most commonly presenting as mass lesions in the cerebral cortex, liver, and gastric antrum.

Diagnosis and Treatment

The diagnosis of syphilis is complicated by the fact that *T. pallidum* cannot be cultured in vitro. Primary and secondary disease can be diagnosed by using darkfield microscopy to examine skin scrapings. This test is not readily available in many laboratories, and it requires a skilled technician. More recently, fluorescently conjugated antitreponemal antibodies have proved to be more sensitive than darkfield microscopy, but the test is more technically demanding. The antibody can also be used to identify the spirochete in biopsy specimens. Identification of treponemal DNA by PCR is under development, but no test is currently commercially available. Serologic testing remains the primary method of diagnosis in most cases. The CDC has published extensive guidelines for the serodiagnosis and treatment of syphilis (see "Further Reading" at the end of this chapter).

Two classes of serologic tests are available:

Non-treponemal Tests. measure levels of the antibody to cardiolipin–cholesterol–lecithin antigen (previously called reagin). The most commonly used tests in this class are the VDRL and the RPR, both of which measure the highest dilution of serum that causes the antigen to flocculate on a slide. In 2% of cases, a prozone phenomenon is observed. That is, when the antibody titer is high, a flocculate is not observed in the undiluted sample, probably as a consequence of an imbalance between antigen and antibody. When the same sample is diluted antibody:antigen ratios are more balanced and a flocculate develops.

The VDRL or RPR titer is usually highest in secondary or early latent disease. After appropriate treatment, the titer usually decreases to less than 1:4, and in one quarter of patients, the VDRL or RPR becomes negative. In patients with primary or secondary syphilis, the titer usually declines to a quarter of its former value within 6 months of treatment and to one eighth by 12 months. In patients with late syphilis, the decline is usually slower, reaching one quarter of former values over a period of 12 months. A titer change to one quarter of former values or lower is considered significant. The rate of titer decline is slower in patients with prolonged infection, a history of recurrent infection, and a high initial titer. In a small number of patients, the test remains persistently positive. These patients are called chronic persisters. A persistent elevation represents a false positive, persistent active infection, or re-infection, particularly when the titer remains elevated above 1:4. False positive tests are rarely encountered with the modern, more highly purified antigen, being most commonly observed in patients with connective tissue disease or HIV infection. The non-treponemal test is recommended for screening and to monitor the response to antibiotic therapy.

Specific Treponemal Tests. measure specific antibodies directed against the T. pallidum spirochete. The FTA-ABS is the standard indirect immunofluorescence antibody test. Serum is absorbed with nonpathogenic treponemes to remove nonspecific cross-reactive antibodies. A 1:5 dilution of the serum is then mixed with pathogenic T. pallidum harvested from infected rabbits, and antibody binding is measured by subsequently incubating the spirochetes with a fluorescence-conjugated antihuman IgG antibody. This test is very specific, but it is difficult to quantify and does not

---

KEY POINTS

About Testing for Syphilis

1. Non-treponemal tests: The VDRL (Venereal Disease Research Laboratory) and RPR (rapid plasma reagin) test the ability of serum to flocculate a cardiolipin–cholesterol–lecithin antigen.
   a) Modern tests produce only occasional false positive results, usually connective tissue disease.
   b) Prozone phenomenon observed in 2% of cases.
   c) Can be used as a marker of response to therapy.
2. Treponemal tests measure antibody directed against the treponeme.
   a) Specific and sensitive, but antibody titers may persist for life.
   b) Not useful for assessing disease activity, used to verify a positive VDRL or RPR.
3. Tests of cerebrospinal fluid (CSF):
   a) A VDRL of the CSF is positive in one half of neurosyphilis cases.
   b) A peripheral VDRL is positive in three quarters of cases.
   c) Specific treponemal test is positive in all cases, should be ordered when considering neurosyphilis.

predict active disease. A positive treponemal antibody test indicates only that the patient has been exposed to syphilis in the past.

Other tests with similar specificity are the TPHA (*T. pallidum* hemagglutination assay) and MHATP (micro-hemagglutination *T. pallidum*) test. Specific treponeme tests are used to verify a positive VDRL or RPR, but cannot be used to follow response to therapy. One of these tests should also be ordered in patients with suspected neurosyphilis who have a negative VDRL.

In patients with latent disease, the cerebrospinal fluid should be examined if ophthalmic signs or symptoms are noted, if evidence suggests tertiary syphilis, if the patient's VDRL or RPR titer fails to decline following appropriate therapy, or if the patient develops HIV infection in association with late latent syphilis or syphilis of unknown duration. Neurosyphilis is accompanied by WBC counts in the cerebrospinal fluid of 10 to 400/mm^3, with a predominance of lymphocytes and elevated protein (45 to 200 mg/dL). A cerebrospinal fluid VDRL is positive in about half of active cases. The peripheral VDRL or RPR is negative in about one quarter of cases of neurosyphilis; however, the peripheral FTA-ABS is usually reactive. Therefore, when neurosyphilis is suspected, a specific antitreponemal test needs to be ordered to exclude the diagnosis.

Treatment

Penicillin remains the treatment of choice for all forms of syphilis, and the efficacy of penicillin is well documented. However the optimal dose and duration of therapy have never been proved by well-designed studies. Because of the slow rate of growth of *T. pallidum*, therapy for a minimum of 2 weeks and therapeutic concentrations of 0.03 μg/mL or higher are thought to be important to insure killing. Intramuscular benzathine penicillin maintains constant serum concentrations of antibiotic, but may not maintain cidal serum levels. It is therefore important that patients receiving conventional intramuscular benzathine penicillin receive appropriate follow-up testing to document cure.

The Jarisch–Herxheimer reaction is a well-described systemic reaction that follows initiation of antibiotic treatment in patients with syphilis. Patients experience the abrupt onset of fever, chills, muscle aches, and headache. These symptoms are often accompanied by hyperventilation, tachycardia, flushing, and mild hypotension. These symptoms usually begin 1 to 2 hours after the first dose of antibiotic is given, and they most commonly follow penicillin treatment. A Jarisch–Herxheimer reaction is reported in most secondary syphilis cases (70% to 90%), but can occur with antibiotic treatment at any stage of syphilis (10% to 25%). Patients should be warned of the high likelihood

of this reaction and informed that the symptoms are self-limiting, lasting approximately 12 to 24 hours. The Jarisch–Herxheimer reaction can be aborted by simultaneously administering a single dose of oral prednisone (60 mg) with the first dose of antibiotic. Prednisone pretreatment is recommended for pregnant women and patients with symptomatic cardiovascular syphilis or neurosyphilis. Asparin every 4 hours for 24 to 48 hours will also ameliorate the symptoms.

Current recommendations for the treatment of the various stages of syphilis are listed below and summarized in Table 9.4:

Primary and Secondary Syphilis. A single intramuscular dose of benzathine penicillin G 2.4 million units remains the recommended treatment regimen. Patients should be reexamined at 6 months and 1 year. Treatment failure or reinfection is diagnosed if symptoms persist or recur, or if the VDRL or RPR titer increases by a factor of 4. Under these circumstances, the patient should be evaluated for HIV infection, a lumbar puncture should be performed, and the patient re-treated with benzathine penicillin (2.4 million units intramuscularly every week for three weeks). In penicillin-allergic patients, doxycycline or tetracycline should be given for 2 weeks. In pregnant patients, skin testing against penicillin should be performed. If the test is positive, the patient should be desensitized and treated with penicillin.

Latent Syphilis

a. In early latent disease (less than 1 year since documented exposure), the patient should receive a single dose of benzathine penicillin. The penicillin-allergic patient should receive doxycycline for 4 weeks.

b. In late latent disease (more than 1 year or unknown duration since exposure), the patient should receive three doses of benzathine penicillin. In penicillin-allergic patients, doxycycline should be given for 4 weeks. If symptoms of syphilis develop, if the patient's VDRL or RPR titer increases by a factor of 4, or if the initial titer is greater than 1:32 and fails to decrease to one quarter of that value over 12 to 24 months, a lumbar puncture should be performed to exclude neurosyphilis, and the patient should be re-treated.

Neurosyphilis or Ocular Syphilis. The preferred treatment is aqueous penicillin G, 12 to 24 million units daily in divided 4-hourly doses for 10 to 14 days. In the highly reliable patient, outpatient treatment with procaine penicillin (2.4 million units intramuscularly daily) plus oral probenecid (500 mg every 6 hours) for 10 to 14 days is a possibility. In the penicillin-allergic patient, desensitization is recommended.

KEY POINTS

About the Treatment of Syphilis

1. Penicillin is the drug of choice.
   a) Therapy must be prolonged (2 weeks) because of the slow rate of growth of the treponeme.
   b) Jarisch–Herxheimer reaction is common: 10% to 25% at most stages, 70% to 90% in secondary disease.
2. Primary or secondary syphilis. Intramuscular benzathine penicillin or, for the penicillin-allergic patient, doxycycline for 2 weeks.
3. Early latent syphilis (within 1 year of exposure). Intramuscular benzathine penicillin or, for the penicillin-allergic patient, doxycycline for 4 weeks.
4. Late latent syphilis. Intramuscular benzathine penicillin for 3 weeks, or, for the penicillin-allergic patient, doxycycline for 4 weeks.
5. Neurosyphilis. Intravenous aqueous penicillin G for 2 weeks, or intramuscular procaine penicillin plus probenecid for 2 weeks.
6. Late syphilis (other than neurosyphilis). Intramuscular benzathine penicillin for 3 weeks, or, for the penicillin-allergic patient, doxycycline for 4 weeks.

Late Syphilis. (other than neurosyphilis, that is gumma or cardiovascular syphilis)—Same as late latent syphilis. Patients with HIV and syphilis at any stage should be treated as if they have neurosyphilis. Aggressive serologic follow-up is recommended, and if titers fail to drop, re-treatment is usually recommended.

PAPULAR GENITOURINARY LESIONS

Syphilis, LGV, chancroid, and herpes can cause not only ulcers, but also papules. Condyloma acuminata (anogenital warts) are a common form of papule that are caused by the human papillomavirus (HPV). Lesions are flesh-colored to gray-colored, raised, and often pedunculated. They can be less than a millimeter to several square centimeters in size. Lesions are seen on the penile shaft and, in uncircumcised men, on the prepuce. In homosexual men, warts are commonly found in the perirectal region, and in women, they are distributed over the lower perineum and can involve the labia and clitoris. Early lesions can be visualized by treating the skin with 3% to 5% acetic acid for 3 to 5 minutes. Flat,

white plaques appear after this treatment. Infection with certain strains of HPV predispose to epithelial cancers, and infection of the cervix is a major risk factor for subsequent development of cervical cancer. Oncogenic viral strains produce early proteins that impair the function of epithelial cell p53 protein, a negative regulator of cell growth.

Multiple therapies are available. All regimens are palliative, and they include cryotherapy with liquid nitrogen, laser surgery, or topical therapy with 10% podophyllin, 0.5% podophyllotoxin (podofilox), or 5% 5-fluorouracil cream. Intralesional interferon has also been used with reasonable success. Given the complexity of therapy, the likelihood of relapse, and the risk of genital premalignant and malignant lesions, genital warts should be treated by a qualified specialist.

Prevention of HPV infection promises to lower the incidence not only of condyloma acuminata, but also of vervical cancer. A quadrivalent vaccine directed against the major HPV types associated with venereal warts (types 6 and 11) and cervical cancer (16 and 18) consists of recombinant type-specific HPV L1 capsid proteins. These proteins self-assemble into virus-like particles (VLPs) that are noninfectious and highly immunogenic. A randomized double-bind trial demonstrated a 90% reduction in the infection rate, and this

---

KEY POINTS

About Venereal Warts

1. Condyloma acuminata (anogenital warts) are caused by the human papilloma virus (HPV).
2. The papules vary in size and can be visualized by treatment with 3% to 5% acetic acid.
3. Genital warts predispose to epithelial cell cancers by altering the function of the p53 protein.
4. Palliative treatment is available:
   a) Cryotherapy with liquid nitrogen
   b) Laser surgery
   c) Topical therapy with 10% podophyllin, 0.5% podophyllotoxin (podofilox), or 5% 5-fluorouracil cream
   d) Intralesional interferon
5. A quadrivalent vaccine against HPV types 6, 11, 16, and 18 is efficacious and recommended for girls and women 9 to 26 years of age.
6. Molluscum contagiosum is a rarer form of venereal warts resulting from a poxvirus (seen mainly in patients with advanced AIDS).

vaccine is recommended for all girls and women 9 to 26 years of age.

A rarer form of venereal wart called molluscum contagiosum is caused by a poxvirus. The papules are usually discrete, firm, small, and umbilicated. In normal hosts, they often resolve spontaneously. However, in immunocompromised patients, they may persist and spread. This infection can be particularly troublesome in patients with advanced AIDS. Several patients have been successfully treated with cidofovir, but to date there has been no controlled clinical trial confirming the efficacy of this treatment.

FURTHER READING

Urinary tract infection

Bent S, Nallamothu BK, Simel DL, Fihn SD, Saint S. Does this woman have an acute uncomplicated urinary tract infection? *JAMA.* 2002;287:2701–2710.

Gupta K, Scholes D, Stamm WE. Increasing prevalence of antimicrobial resistance among uropathogens causing acute uncomplicated cystitis in women. *JAMA.* 1999;281:736–738.

Hooton TM, Scholes D, Gupta K, Stapleton AE, Roberts PL, Stamm WE. Amoxicillin–clavulanate vs ciprofloxacin for the treatment of uncomplicated cystitis in women: a randomized trial. *JAMA.* 2005;293:949–955.

Katchman EA, Milo G, Paul M, Christiaens T, Baerheim A, Leibovici L. Three-day vs longer duration of antibiotic treatment for cystitis in women: systematic review and meta-analysis. *Am J Med.* 2005;118:1196–1207.

Nicolle LE, Bradley S, Colgan R, Rice JC, Schaeffer A, Hooton TM. Infectious Diseases Society of America guidelines for the diagnosis and treatment of asymptomatic bacteriuria in adults. *Clin Infect Dis.* 2005;40:643–654.

Scholes D, Hooton TM, Roberts PL, Stapleton AE, Gupta K, Stamm WE. Risk factors for recurrent urinary tract infection in young women. *J Infect Dis.* 2000;182:1177–1182.

Vogel T, Verreault R, Gourdeau M, Morin M, Grenier-Gosselin L. Rochette L. Optimal duration of antibiotic therapy for uncomplicated urinary tract infection in older women: a double-blind randomized controlled trial. *CMAJ.* 2004;170:469–473.

Wilson ML, Gaido L. Laboratory diagnosis of urinary tract infections in adult patients. *Clin Infect Dis.* 2004;38:1150–1158.

Prostatitis

Collins MM, Meigs JB, Barry MJ, Walker Corkery E, Giovannucci E, Kawachi I. Prevalence and correlates of prostatitis in the health professionals follow-up study cohort. *J Urol.* 2002;167:1363–1366.

Game X, Vincendeau S, Palascak R, Milcent S, Fournier R, Houlgatte A. Total and free serum prostate specific antigen levels during the first month of acute prostatitis. *Eur Urol.* 2003;43:702–705.

Pelvic inflammatory disease

Ness RB, Soper DE, Holley RL, et al. Effectiveness of inpatient and outpatient treatment strategies for women with pelvic inflammatory disease: results from the Pelvic Inflammatory Disease Evaluation and Clinical Health (PEACH) Randomized Trial. *Am J Obstet Gynecol.* 2002;186:929–937.

McNeeley SG, Hendrix SL, Mazzoni MM, Kmak DC, Ransom SB. Medically sound, cost-effective treatment for pelvic inflammatory disease and tuboovarian abscess. *Am J Obstet Gynecol.* 1998;178:1272–1278.

Trent M, Ellen JM, Walker A. Pelvic inflammatory disease in adolescents: care delivery in pediatric ambulatory settings. *Pediatr Emerg Care.* 2005;21:431–436.

Sexually transmitted diseases

Centers for Disease Control and Prevention. Primary and secondary syphilis—United States, 2003-2004. *MMWR Morb Mortal Wkly Rep.* 2006;55:269–273.

Dunne EF, Markowitz LE. Genital human papillomavirus infection. *Clin Infect Dis.* 2006;43:624–629.

Mackay IM, Harnett G, Jeoffreys N, et al. Detection and discrimination of herpes simplex viruses, *Haemophilus ducreyi, Treponema pallidum,* and *Calymmatobacterium* (*Klebsiella*) *granulomatis* from genital ulcers. *Clin Infect Dis.* 2006;42:1431–1438.

Marra CM, Maxwell CL, Smith SL, et al. Cerebrospinal fluid abnormalities in patients with syphilis: association with clinical and laboratory features. *J Infect Dis.* 2004;189:369–376.

Villa LL, Costa RL, Petta CA, et al. Prophylactic quadrivalent human papillomavirus (types 6, 11, 16, and 18) L1 virus-like particle vaccine in young women: a randomised double-blind placebo-controlled multicentre phase II efficacy trial. *Lancet Oncol.* 2005;6:271–278.

Workowski KA, Berman SM. Sexually transmitted diseases treatment guidelines, 2006. *MMWR Recomm Rep.* 2006;55:1–94.

Skin and Soft Tissue Infections

10

Time Recommended to Complete: 1 day

Daniel P. Lew and Frederick S. Southwick

GUIDING QUESTIONS

1. Which are the two bacteria that most commonly cause skin infections?

2. Which skin and soft tissue infections require surgical intervention?

3. What are the clinical clues that help to differentiate cellulitis from necrotizing fasciitis?

4. What are the conditions that predispose to necrotizing fasciitis?

5. Which two organisms most commonly cause myonecrosis?

6. Which organisms cause indolent soft-tissue infections that fail to respond to conventional antibiotic treatment?

7. Should prophylactic antibiotics be given for bites by humans and animals?

8. When should tetanus toxoid vaccine and human tetanus immunoglobulin be given?

◼ SKIN AND SOFT TISSUE INFECTIONS

POTENTIAL SEVERITY

Can progress rapidly to shock and death. For deeper soft tissue infections, immediate antibiotic therapy is required, often accompanied by surgical debridement.

CLASSIFICATION OF SKIN AND SOFT TISSUE INFECTIONS

Skin and soft tissue infections are common presentations in acutely ill patients arriving in the emergency room. Cellulitis, a superficial, spreading infection involving subcuta-

neous tissue, is the most common skin infection leading to hospitalization. Two microorganisms are responsible for most cutaneous infections in immunocompetent patients:

1. Group A streptococcus (GAS)
2. *Staphylococcus aureus*, including community-acquired methicillin-resistant *S. aureus* (CA-MRSA)

The anatomic locations of skin and soft tissue infection are described in the next few paragraphs and illustrated in Figure 10.1. The symptoms and signs for these infections overlap; however, each infection has distinct clinical features.

The more superficial infections include impetigo, erysipelas, and folliculitis. As these infections penetrate deeper, they may become furunculosis (associated with hair follicles), hidradenitis (associated with sweat glands), and skin abscesses. Most of superficial localized infections (impetigo, folliculitis, furuncles) are caused by *S. aureus* or GAS. These infections rarely require hospitalization and often respond to local measures. Recurrence may be prevented by reducing specific microbial carriage. However, once these infections spread through subcutaneous tissues—as in the case of

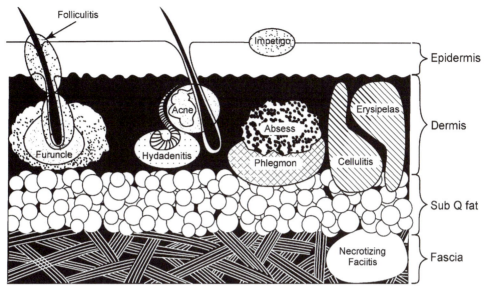

Figure 10–1. Schematic of the Anatomic Sites of Soft Tissue Infection. Adapted with permission from Saurat JH, Grosshans E, Laugier P, Lachapelle JM, editors. *Dermatologie et vénéréologie.* 2nd edition. Paris: Editions Masson; 1990: p. 109

KEY POINTS

About the Classification of Skin and Soft Tissue Infections

1. Superficial infections can usually be handled with outpatient treatment.
    a) Most superficial: impetigo, erysipelas, and folliculitis
    b) Deeper localized: furunculosis, hidradenitis, and skin abscesses
2. Deeper infections require hospitalization, parenteral antibiotics, and possibly surgical debridement.
    a) Cellulitis is the most superficial, can be treated with systemic antibiotics alone.
    b) Necrotizing fasciitis involves the fascia and requires emergent surgery.
    c) Myonecrosis also requires rapid surgical debridement; it is often fatal.

certain predisposing conditions, can result in deeper extension of infection, vascular thrombosis, and tissue necrosis. In addition to antibiotic therapy, these deeper infections require emergency surgical debridement.

The very severe form of deep tissue infection called necrotizing fasciitis is often caused by GAS. This infection is associated with thrombosis of vessels in the fascia and requires fasciotomy. Severe streptococcal infection may also involve muscles and, in this case, is defined as myonecrosis ("necrotizing myositis"). Necrotizing fasciitis and myonecrosis can lead to sepsis and irreversible septic shock. As a consequence of these severe forms of infection GAS is often popularized in the media as the "flesh-eating bacteria."

SEVERE SKIN AND SOFT TISSUE INFECTIONS

Cellulitis

Cellulitis is one of the more common infectious diseases and is managed by clinicians practicing in a wide variety of specialties. Cellulitis is an inflammatory process involving the skin and supporting tissues, with some extension into the subcutaneous tissues. The most common location is the extremities. Not only is the infection common, but some patients develop frequent recurrences of cellulitis.

cellulitis—they may become fulminant and, if not treated emergently with parenteral antibiotics, may prove fatal. Delay in therapy, or the presence of

PREDISPOSING FACTORS

Several predisposing factors increase the likelihood of cellulitis:

- Venous or lymphatic compromise secondary to surgery, previous thrombophlebitis, previous trauma, or right-sided congestive heart failure. These conditions represent the most common underlying cause leading to cellulitis.
- Diabetes mellitus results in progressive peripheral neuropathy and small vessel occlusion. These conditions lead to inadvertent trauma, poor wound healing, and tissue necrosis.
- Chronic alcoholism predisposes to cellulitis probably as a consequence of trauma to the skin and poor hygiene.

Not all patients with cellulitis have definable risk factors for the development of infection—about 50% of patients present without predisposing disease.

CAUSES AND CLINICAL MANIFESTATIONS

CASE 10.1

A 50–year-old white man arrived in the emergency room complaining of progressive warm erythema of his right leg. Three days earlier he had accidentally hit his right shin on a tree stump. Approximately 24 hours later, he noted increasing pain and erythema at the site of a small break in his skin. Erythema spread from his shin to his entire lower leg. He also noted fever and chills.

On physical exam, this patient appeared moderately ill. His right lower leg was diffusely red and edematous, except for a small region of his posterior calf. The margins of erythema were indistinct. His right inguinal nodes were enlarged and tender. There was no crepitation; however, the leg was very tender. A small skin break was noted on the right anterior shin.

Laboratory abnormalities included an elevated peripheral white blood cell (WBC) count of 15,500/mm³, with 75% polymorphonuclear leukocytes (PMNs) and 15% band forms. Two sets of blood cultures were positive for group A β-hemolytic streptococci.

As observed in case 10.1, cellulitis results in swelling of the involved area and macular erythema that is largely confluent (see Table 10.1). Upon examination, warmth and tenderness of the involved skin are usually found. Careful examination often reveals lymphangitis and tender regional lymphadenopathy. Presence of accompanying tinea pedis or other dermatologic abnormalities such as psoriasis or eczema should be sought, because these are preventable ports of entry. Treatment of these dermatologic disorders may reduce the frequency of recurrent cellulitis. In patients presenting in the emergency room, systemic findings must be sought. Systemic sepsis (including fever, chills, and myalgias) is seen in patients presenting with severe cellulitis.

In most patients, cellulitis is caused by β-hemolytic streptococci, including groups A, B, C, and G. The rapid onset of symptoms in case 10.1 was highly suggestive of GAS, which often progresses quickly once it gains entry through a break in the skin. *S. aureus* is also a common cause of cellulitis. In children, *H. influenzae* can produce facial cellulitis or erysipelas.

SPECIAL FORMS OF CELLULITIS

Erysipelas. Erysipelas is a distinct form of superficial cellulitis. It is associated with marked swelling of the integument, with sharp demarcation between involved and normal tissues, and often with prominent lymphatic

Table 10.1. Clinical Differentiation of Serious Soft Tissue Infections

Clinical finding	Cellulitis	Necrotizing fasciitis		Clostridial myonecrosis	Pyomyositis
		Type I	Type II		
Fever	+++	++	++++	+++	++
Systemic sepsis	+	++	++++	++++	+
Local pain	+++	++	++++	++++	++
Gas in tissue	−	++	−	++++	−
Obvious portal of entry	±	++++	±	++++	−
Diabetes mellitus	±	++++	±	−	−

Adapted with permission from www.UptoDate.com "Necrotizing infections of the skin and fascia" by Dennis L. Stevens

involvement. Erysipelas is almost always caused by GAS (occasionally by group C, G, or B). It is more common in young children and older adults.

Lesions present chiefly in the lower extremities, but a significant proportion of cases present with lesions in the face. Erysipelas lesions are painful, with a bright red edematous indurated appearance, particularly at the peripheral margins. The progression of this infection is similar to a forest fire, being most active and red at the leading edge.

Clostridial cellulitis. Clostridial cellulitis is a superficial infection most often caused by *Clostridium perfringens*. It is usually preceded by local trauma or recent surgery. Gas is invariably found in the skin, but the fascia and deep muscle are spared. This entity differs from clostridial myonecrosis, but thorough surgical exploration and debridement are required to distinguish between the two. Magnetic resonance imaging (MRI) or computed tomography (CT) scan and measurement of the patient's serum creatine phosphokinase concentration can also help to determine if muscle tissue is involved. However, imaging studies should not delay critical surgical therapy when crepitation is noted on examination or when clinical evidence shows progressive soft tissue infection.

KEY POINTS

About Cellulitis

1. An infection of the skin, with some extension to the subcutaneous tissues.
2. Predisposing factors include venous or lymphatic insufficiency, diabetes mellitus, and alcoholism.
3. Characteristics include erythema, edema, diffuse tenderness, indistinct border, lymphadenopathy.
4. Caused by streptococci and *Staphylococcus aureus*. *Haemophilus influenzae* is a possible cause in children.
5. Subclasses of cellulitis include
   a) erysipelas (more superficial; very sharp, raised border),
   b) clostridia cellulitis (associated with crepitation, no muscle involvement), and
   c) anaerobic cellulitis (foul smelling, more common in patients with diabetes).
6. Treat with penicillinase-resistant penicillin (oxacillin, nafcillin) or a first-generation cephalosporin (cefazolin). Use vancomycin for the penicillin-allergic patient or community acquired methicillin-resistant *S. aureus*.

Non-clostridial anaerobic cellulitis. Non-clostridial anaerobic cellulitis is the result of infection with mixed anaerobic and aerobic organisms that produce gas in tissues. Unlike clostridial cellulitis, this type of infection is usually associated with diabetes mellitus and often produces a foul odor. It must be distinguished from myonecrosis and necrotizing fasciitis by surgical exploration.

DIFFERENTIAL DIAGNOSIS OF CELLULITIS

The diagnosis of cellulitis is usually not difficult to make. Deep venous thrombosis can cause some of the same findings that characterize cellulitis, including fever, and it is the primary illness to consider when confronted with a patient with lower extremity changes suggestive of cellulitis. Radiation therapy can cause erythema and swelling of the skin and associated structures, and can be difficult to differentiate from cellulitis in some patients.

THERAPY AND NATURAL HISTORY OF CELLULITIS

A mild early cellulitis may be treated with low doses of penicillin—and if staphylococcal infection is suspected, a penicillinase-resistant penicillin (nafcillin or, for milder cases, dicloxacillin). For doses, see Table 10.2. A first-generation cephalosporin (cefazolin) also effectively covers GAS and methicillin-sensitive S. aureus (MSSA). Intravenous vancomycin (1 g twice daily) is an alternative for highly penicillin-allergic patients. Vancomycin is also the antibiotic of choice if CA-MRSA is suspected. Other antibiotics that can be used for MRSA soft tissue infection include linezolid and daptomycin.

Initial local care of cellulitis includes immobilization and elevation of the involved limb to reduce swelling, and a cool, sterile saline dressing to remove purulent exudate and reduce local pain. Resolution of local findings with treatment is typically slow and can require 1 to 2 weeks of therapy. Local desquamation of the involved area can be seen during the early convalescence.

Necrotizing Fasciitis

Necrotizing fasciitis is a rare, and often fatal, soft tissue infection involving the superficial fascial layers of the extremities, abdomen, or perineum. This deep-seated infection of the subcutaneous tissue results in progressive destruction of fascia and fat, but may spare the skin.

PREDISPOSING FACTORS AND CAUSES

Necrotizing fasciitis typically begins with trauma; however, the inciting event may be as seemingly innocuous as a simple contusion, minor burn, or insect bite. It can also result from bacterial superinfection in Varicella infection. An association between the use of nonsteroidal anti-inflammatory drugs and the progression

Table 10.2. Antibiotic Treatment of Skin and Soft tissue Infections

Drug	Dose	Relative Efficacy	Comments
Cellulitis, mild			
Dicloxacillin	250–500 mg PO q6h	First line	
Cefadroxil (or other first-generation oral cephalosporin)	0.5–1 g PO q12h	Alternative	Authors' preference because of convenience of dosing
Trimethoprim–sulfamethoxazole	1 double-strength tablet PO q12h	Alternative	For penicillin-allergic patients, or if community-acquired methicillin-resistant *S. aureus* (CA-MRSA) is suspected
Cellulitis, severe			
			See text for duration
Nafcillin or oxacillin	1–1.5 g IV q4h	First line	
Cefazolin	1–1.5 g IV q8h	First line	Inexpensive, less frequent dosing
Vancomycin	1 g IV q12h	Alternative	For penicillin-allergic patients, and CA-MRSA
Linezolid	600 mg IV q12h	Alternative	MRSA
Daptomycin	4 mg/kg IV q12h	Alternative	MRSA
Necrotizing fasciitis			
			See text for duration
Penicillin G, plus clindamycin	4×10^6 U IV q4h 600–900 mg IV q8h	First line	Penicillin dose for adults over 60 kg with normal renal function
Piperacillin–tazobactam	3/0.375 g IV q6h	Alternatives	Useful forms of monotherapy
Ticarcillin–clavulanate	3.1 g IV q4–6h		
Imipenem	500 mg IV q6h		
Meropenem	1 g IV q8h		
Ertapenem	1 g IV q24h		
Myonecrosis			
			See text for duration
Penicillin G, plus clindamycin	4×10^6 U IV q4h 600–900 mg IV q8h	First line	Penicillin dose for adults over 60 kg with normal renal function
Impetigo			
			Treat for 10 days; treatment prevents post-streptococcal complications
Erythromycin	250 mg PO q6h	First line	May cause gastrointestinal toxicity
Dicloxacillin	250 mg PO q6h	First line	
Cephalexin	250–500 mg PO q6h	Alternative	
Mupirocin	Apply q12h	Alternative	Polyethylene glycol ointment
Furuncles, skin abscesses			
Clindamycin	150 mg PO q6h	First line	Preferred if anaerobes are suspected
Dicloxacillin	250–500 mg PO q6h	First line	
Trimethoprim–sulfadiazine	1 double-strength tablet PO q12h	Alternative	First line if CA-MRSA is suspected

(Continued)

Table 10.2. (Continued)

Drug	Dose	Relative Efficacy	Comments
Amoxicillin–clavulanate	875 mg PO q12h	Alternative	Use in perirectal, perivaginal, or perioral abscesses
Bites by animals or humans			
Amoxicillin–clavulanate	875 mg PO q12h	First line	Prophylaxis, 3–5 days
Ampicillin–sulbactam	3 g IV once		Prophylaxis in emergency room
Clindamycin, plus	900 mg IV, followed by 300 mg PO q6h	Alternative	For the penicillin-allergic patient, no designated regimen of proven
ciprofloxacin	500 mg PO q12h		efficacy

or development of GAS necrotizing infection has also been suggested.

Necrotizing fasciitis has been classified into two groups based on bacteriology and clinical manifestations (see Table 10.1). Type I is a polymicrobial infection with a variety of gram-positive and gram-negative aerobic and anaerobic bacteria; four to five pathogenic bacteria are usually isolated. Infecting organisms can include *S. aureus*, GAS, *Escherichia coli*, *Peptostreptococcus*, *Clostridium*, *Prevotella*, *Porphyromonas*, and *Bacteroides* species. This infection is most frequently associated with diabetes mellitus. Type II is caused by a single organism, classically GAS (*Streptococcus pyogenes*). Necrotizing fasciitis caused by GAS was previously called "streptococcal gangrene" or "streptococcal toxic shock syndrome". In recent years, invasive infections caused by GAS, such as necrotizing fasciitis, have been increasing dramatically in number. Most cases are community-acquired, but a significant proportion may be nosocomial or acquired in a nursing home. Increasingly, CA-MRSA is also being reported as a cause of this infection. And in communities in which CA-MRSA is known to be prevalent, empiric antibiotic treatment should cover for this pathogen pending culture results.

The bacteria associated with necrotizing fasciitis depend on the underlying conditions leading to infection. Three important clinical conditions are associated with type I necrotizing fasciitis:

1. **Diabetes mellitus.** Necrotizing fasciitis with mixed flora occurs more often in patients with diabetes. These infections usually occur on the feet, with rapid extension along the fascia into the leg. Necrotizing fasciitis should be considered in diabetic patients with cellulitis who also have systemic signs of infection such as tachycardia, leukocytosis, marked hyperglycemia, or acidosis. Diabetic patients can also develop necrotizing fasciitis in other body areas, including the head-and-neck region and the perineum.

2. **Cervical necrotizing fasciitis.** Cervical necrotizing fasciitis can result from a breach of the integrity of the mucous membranes after surgery or instrumentation, or from an odontogenic infection. In the head-and-neck region, bacterial penetration into the fascial compartments can result in a syndrome known as Ludwig's angina (a rapidly expanding inflammation in the submandibular and sublingual spaces).

3. **Fournier's gangrene.** In the perineal area, penetration of the gastrointestinal or urethral mucosa can cause Fournier's gangrene, an aggressive infection. These infections begin abruptly with severe pain and may spread rapidly onto the anterior abdominal wall, into the gluteal muscles, and, in males, onto the scrotum and penis.

CLINICAL MANIFESTATIONS AND EARLY DIAGNOSIS

CASE 10.2

A 63–year-old black man presented to the emergency room with a 1-day history of mild swelling of his right foot and ankle that was extremely tender to palpation. He had a long history of alcohol abuse and a history of cirrhosis. He was afebrile at the time of presentation and was sent home with oral Keflex. Two days later, he returned complaining of fever and increased swelling. He was admitted to the hospital and intravenous clindamycin and gentamicin were started.

Despite the new therapy, his leg swelling and erythema failed to improve. On physical exam during the third hospital day, he appeared severely ill and septic. His temperature was 39.6°C, pulse was 120 beats per minute, and blood pressure was 90/70 mm Hg. Marked erythema was observed, along with edema of the right ankle that extended up the front and lateral regions of

the leg, half way to the knee. A new 1×1-cm patch of
dark reddish-purple skin was noted that was exquisitely
tender to touch. No lymphadenopathy was observed.

Laboratory studies revealed a WBC count of
25,000, with 90% PMNs. An emergency surgical explo-
ration revealed an area of necrotic fascia consistent
with necrotizing fasciitis. Intraoperative cultures grew
E. coli *and* Bacteroides fragilis.

Early diagnosis of necrotizing fasciitis is critical
because, as was observed in case 10.2, progression from an
unapparent process to a process associated with extensive
destruction of tissue may be remarkably rapid. Differentiating necrotizing infections from common soft tissue
infections such as cellulitis and impetigo is both challenging and critically important (see Table 10.1). A high
degree of suspicion may be the most important aid in early
diagnosis. Prompt diagnosis is imperative, because necrotizing infections typically spread rapidly and can result in
multi-organ failure, adult respiratory distress syndrome,
and death.

As noted in case 10.2, unexplained pain that increases
rapidly over time may be the first manifestation of necrotizing fasciitis. However, in some patients, signs and
symptoms of infection are not initially apparent. Erythema may be present diffusely or locally, but excruciating pain in the absence of any cutaneous findings is the
only clue for infection in some patients. Within 24 to 48
hours, erythema may develop or darken to a reddish-
purple color (as observed in case 10.2), frequently with
associated blisters and bullae. Bullae can also develop in
normal-appearing skin. The bullous stage is associated
with extensive deep soft tissue destruction that may
result in necrotizing fasciitis or myonecrosis; such
patients usually exhibit fever and systemic toxicity. In
addition to pain and skin findings, fever, malaise, myalgias, diarrhea, and anorexia may also be present during
the first 24 hours. Hypotension may be present initially
or may develop over time.

Necrotizing fasciitis must be distinguished from gas
gangrene, pyomyositis, and myositis. Frozen biopsy of
the skin and subcutaneous tissue has proven useful for
the early diagnosis of necrotizing fasciitis. However, any
of the abnormalities described above should be of sufficient concern to prompt consideration of surgical exploration. It is critical to proceed with surgery rather than
to delay so as to obtain an imaging study. Indeed, necrotizing fasciitis and myositis are diseases diagnosed by
surgeons in the operating room, leading often to extensive debridement. Imaging studies such as soft tissue
X-ray, CT scan, and MRI are most helpful if gas is

present in the tissue. However, in the absence of gas,
these imaging techniques cannot differentiate cellulitis
from fasciitis, and MRI tends to overestimate the extent
of deep tissue involvement.

TREATMENT

Intensive-care physicians and orthopedic surgeons are
often the first health care professional to evaluate
patients with such infections, and they therefore need to
be familiar with this potentially devastating disease and
its management. Prompt diagnosis, immediate administration of appropriate antibiotics, and emergent, aggressive surgical debridement of all compromised tissues are
critical to reduce morbidity and mortality.

Surgery. The primary indications for surgical intervention are severe pain, sepsis, fever, and elevated serum
creatine phosphokinase, with or without radiographic
findings. If necrotizing fasciitis is a possibility, the only
definitive method of diagnosis is surgical exploration.
After initial debridement, infection can continue to
progress if all necrotic tissue has not been removed. Surgical re-exploration is therefore often required and
should be performed as often as is necessary.

Antibiotics. Some recent studies have suggested that
clindamycin is superior to penicillin in the treatment of
experimental necrotizing fasciitis or myonecrosis caused
by GAS.

Clindamycin may be more effective because this
antibiotic is not affected by bacterial inoculum size or
stage of growth. It suppresses toxin production, facilitates
phagocytosis of *S. pyogenes*, and has a long post-antibiotic
effect. Most experts currently recommend administration
of combined therapy with penicillin G and clindamycin
(see Table 10.2). In communities in which CA-MRSA is
prevalent, empiric therapy with vancomycin should be
added pending culture results.

In patients with diabetes or Fournier's gangrene,
antibiotic treatment should be based on results of Gram
stain, culture, and sensitivity. However, early empiric
treatment is necessary: ampicillin (combined with clindamycin or metronidazole) or ampicillin–sulbactam are
appropriate. Broader gram-negative coverage may be
necessary if the patient was recently hospitalized or
has recently received antibiotic treatment. Ticarcillin–
clavulanate, piperacillin–tazobactam, or a carbapenem
(meropenem, imipenem, ertapenem) as monotherapy
provide the appropriate empiric coverage.

Additional measures. Because of intractable hypotension and diffuse capillary leak in patients with shock,
massive amounts of intravenous fluids (10 to 20 L daily),
plus vasopressors such as dopamine or epinephrine, are
often necessary to maintain tissue perfusion.

Several recent case reports and a case series suggest
a beneficial effect for intravenous administration of

KEY POINTS

About Necrotizing Fasciitis

1. This deep subcutaneous infection causes necrosis of the fascia and subcutaneous fat.

2. Causes include group A streptococci, community-acquired methicillin-resistant *Staphylococcus aureus* (CA-MRSA), or mixed infection with gram-positive and gram-negative aerobes and anaerobes.

3. Severe pain is often the earliest symptom; septic appearance and tachycardia are also suggestive.

4. Surgical exploration or punch biopsy are required for diagnosis.

5. Treatment must include
   a) aggressive and often repeated surgical debridement;
   b) systemic antibiotics (group A strep: penicillin and clindamycin; mixed infection: ticarcillin–clavulanate, piperacillin–tazobactam, or a carbapenem; CA-MRSA: vancomycin); and
   c) volume replacement and vasopressors.
   d) For seriously ill patients, intravenous administration of immunoglobulins should be considered.

high-dose immunoglobulins to neutralize circulating streptococcal toxins. It is the authors' opinion that in cases of severe infection this form of therapy is warranted. Unfortunately, even with optimal therapy, necrotizing fasciitis is associated with high (20% to 60%) mortality.

Myonecrosis

Myonecrosis (also called necrotizing myositis) is an uncommon infection of muscle that develops rapidly and is life-threatening. Early recognition and aggressive treatment are essential. Infections resulting in necrosis of muscle are almost entirely the result of infection by *Clostridium* species (gas gangrene). Spontaneous gangrenous myositis is another invasive infection caused by GAS, which often has features that overlap with those of necrotizing fasciitis. These infections typically evolve after contiguous spread from an area of trauma or surgery, or spontaneous spread from hematogenous seeding of muscle.

PREDISPOSING FACTORS AND CAUSES

Clostridial gas gangrene attributable to *C. perfringens* occurs after trauma involving deep, penetrating injury—

for example, knife or gunshot wound, or crush injury (classically occurring in war wounds). Other conditions associated with traumatic gas gangrene include bowel surgery and post-abortion with retained placenta. Clostridial gas gangrene may also be spontaneous and non-traumatic and is often associated with *C. septicum* (see case 10.3, later in this chapter). Many of the spontaneous cases occur in patients with gastrointestinal portals of entry such as adenocarcinoma.

Several other clinical entities may be associated with muscular injury and should be considered in patients presenting with myositis:

1. **Tropical myositis or pyomyositis.** *S. aureus*, and sometimes other organisms, can cause a primary muscle abscess (pyomyositis) in the absence of an apparent site of infection. Pyomyositis is more common in tropical areas.

2. **Necrotizing infections caused by *Vibrio vulnificus*.** *Vibrio* infections can involve the skin, fascia, and muscle and are most common among patients with cirrhosis, consumers of raw seafood, or inhabitants of coastal regions.

A number of viral infections, such as acute influenza type A, can also produce skeletal muscle injury also resulting in rhabdomyolysis.

PATHOPHYSIOLOGY OF CLOSTRIDIAL INFECTIONS

The initiating trauma introduces organisms (either vegetative or spore forms) directly into deep tissue. At the same time, through tissue damage, it produces an anaerobic environment with low oxidation-reduction potential and acid pH, which is optimal for growth of clostridial organisms. Necrosis progresses within 24 to 36 hours of the traumatic injury.

The rapid tissue destruction associated with clostridial infection is explained by the bacterium's ability to produce toxins. Its α-toxin has both phospholipase C and sphingomyelinase activity. This toxin induces platelet and PMN aggregation, resulting in blood vessel occlusion and rapid tissue necrosis, enhancing the anaerobic environment for clostridial growth. In addition, the α-toxin directly suppresses cardiac contractility. The theta-toxin is a cholesterol-dependent cytolysin, and in combination with the phospholipase activity of α-toxin, may cause lysis of red blood cells, WBCs, vascular endothelial cells, and myocytes. In addition, theta-toxin stimulates the production of multiple inflammatory cytokines that lead to blood vessel dilatation and hypotension.

Clostridia can also gain entry to the body by routes other than trauma. *C. septicum* most commonly spreads to soft tissue hematogenously. Infection with this pathogen usually accompanies a bowel lesion, particularly cecal carcinoma (see case 10.3, next). *C. sordellii* can be found in the vaginal flora and may become invasive after manual or

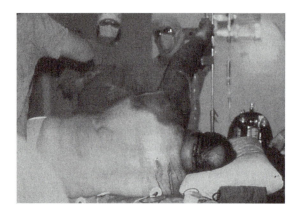

A.

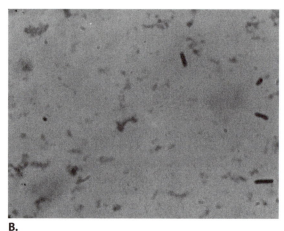

B.

Figure 10–2. Clostridia myonecrosis. **A.** Patient from case 10.3 undergoing surgical debridement. The skin over the left arm and shoulder had a brownish-red appearance. **B.** Gram stain of brown fluid obtained from the large blister on the patient's arm. Note the large gram-positive rods and the absence of inflammatory cells. *See color image on color plate 2*

pharmacologic abortion (RU486). Infection with *C. sordellii* is often accompanied by a unique constellation of findings: absence of fever, hemoconcentration because of increased vascular permeability, and a very high WBC count (leukemoid reaction), followed by shock. *C. septicum*, *C. sordellii*, and several other clostridia species have all caused severe infections following surgical placement of contaminated tissue allografts. Routine sterilization of tissue allografts may not remove *Clostridium* spores, explaining this potentially fatal complication.

CLINICAL MANIFESTATIONS AND DIAGNOSIS

CASE 10.3

A 54–year-old male truck driver presented to the emergency room with the sudden onset of severe left shoulder pain. On physical examination, severe tenderness of the left shoulder was elicited, and the patient was given a pain medication for presumed bursitis. Four hours later, the man returned to emergency room. He appeared septic and confused. His pulse was 125 beats per minute, and blood pressure was 80/50 mm Hg. A large blister was noted over the left deltoid, and the skin now had a bronze appearance. Aspiration revealed brownish fluid, and Gram stain demonstrated gram-positive rods and no PMNs (Figure 10.2).

Intravenous penicillin was initiated, but despite antibiotic therapy, edema and erythema marched down his arm. Within 1 hour they had spread to the elbow. The patient's hematocrit dropped from 45% to 23% over the

same period. Crepitus was readily palpated, and subcutaneous air in the arm and left chest wall was noted on X-ray. In the operating room, the arm was amputated, and the left chest wall debrided. In many areas, muscle was necrotic and had the appearance of cooked meat, failing to contract with electrical stimulation. Despite aggressive debridement, multiple blood transfusions and respiratory support, the patient developed irreversible shock and died 18 hours after admission. Blood cultures and tissue cultures were positive for C. septicum. Autopsy revealed an early carcinoma of the cecum.

As illustrated in case 10.3, the first symptom in traumatic or bacteremic gas gangrene is usually the sudden onset of severe pain at the site of infection. The mean incubation period may be less than 24 hours, but ranges from 6 hours to several days, probably depending on the size of the bacterial inoculum and the extent of vascular compromise. The skin over the infected area may initially appear pale, but quickly changes to bronze, and then to purplish-red. It becomes tense and exquisitely tender, with overlying bullae (Figure 10.2). An important local sign is the presence of crepitus. As observed in case 10.3, signs of systemic sepsis quickly develop. These include tachycardia and low-grade fever, followed by shock and multi-organ failure. When clostridial bacteremia occurs, it may be associated with extensive hemolysis. Gas within the soft tissue can be detected by physical examination, radiography, CT scan, or MRI. The presence of large gram-variable rods at the site of injury help to make a definitive diagnosis.

KEY POINTS

About Myonecrosis

1. Primarily caused by Clostridiim perfringens and C. Septicum (the latter associated with bowel cancer).
2. The clostrida α- and theta-toxin depress myocardial contractility, lyse white and red blood cells, and cause tissue necrosis and vasodilatation.
3. Skin becomes bronze-colored; bullae follow. Crepitus and extreme tenderness are noted on palpation. Sepsis, tachycardia, and hypotension are common.
4. Radiographs reveal subcutaneous gas.
5. Treatment must be rapid:
   a) Removal of all necrotic tissue, and amputation of the infected limb
   b) Intravenous penicillin and clindamycin
   c) Hyperbaric oxygen where available
6. Despite treatment, outcome is often fatal.

TREATMENT

Penicillin, clindamycin, metronidazole, and a number of cephalosporins have excellent activity in vitro against *C. perfringens* and other clostridia. As described earlier for streptococcal gangrene, the combination of penicillin and clindamycin is recommended. This combination would be expected both to reduce toxin production and to kill the organism (see Table 10.2)

Aggressive surgical debridement must be performed emergently, if there is to be any hope of improving survival and preserving tissue. It is critical that all necrotic tissue be resected and that the margins of resection contain bleeding healthy tissue. An extremity is clearly easier to debride than is the trunk. In case 10.3, the infection extended to the chest wall, making full debridement impossible. If anaerobic gas gangrene is diagnosed, and if hyperbaric oxygen facilities are available, that therapeutic modality should be considered. The fulminant nature of clostridia myonecrosis and the extensive associated toxin production make this infection particularly lethal. If early aggressive debridement of all infected tissue is not accomplished, a fatal outcome is to be expected.

BURN INFECTIONS

Pathology of burns

All burn wounds become colonized with microorganisms. Burn eschar is composed of dead and denatured

dermis in which a wide variety of microbes can flourish. The quantity of the organisms, their intrinsic virulence, and the degree to which they invade host tissues determine their significance.

Although microbial colonization should be expected, invasion of surrounding tissue is a dangerous sign. The organisms associated with invasive infection vary from institution to institution and also over time. Common pathogens include *Enterobacter cloacae*, *S. aureus*, *S. epidermidis*, *Enterococcus faecalis*, *E. coli*, *Pseudomonas aeruginosa*, *Klebsiella pneumoniae*, and *Acinetobacter baumannii*. Local and systemic fungal infections are becoming increasingly common. Mucormycosis (*Zygomycetes*), *Fusarium*, and *Candida* are among the more common fungi encountered. Aggressive wound care and extreme vigilance are required to control the concentration of organisms in the burn wound in an effort to protect patients from invasive burn wound sepsis.

Burn wound infections are generally classified as invasive or noninvasive based on tissue biopsy. If a burn wound is allowed to remain in situ and is treated with adequate debridement and topical antibiotics, after 2 to 3 weeks, the naturally occurring microorganisms that colonize the wound will promote separation of the eschar by producing bacterial collagenases. A layer of granulation tissue forms where the eschar separates, and the improved blood supply and wound hypermetabolism help to limit the proliferation of microbes.

When burn wound infections become invasive, the concentration of microorganisms rises to greater than 1 million per gram of tissue, and invading organisms are readily seen in biopsy specimens. Developing granulation tissue becomes edematous and pale, with subsequent occlusion and thrombosis of new blood vessels. Lack of bleeding is evident on surgical exploration of the wound. As the infection advances, the surface becomes frankly necrotic, and the infection spreads rapidly.

A very low threshold of suspicion should be applied to invasive burn wound sepsis. Attempts at early detection should be aggressive, and containment through extremely vigorous therapy is important. Fortunately, the advent of aggressive surgical removal of the burn wound has made burn wound sepsis a rare event.

Clinical Features

The presence of microorganisms in the wound and ongoing tissue necrosis in the burn eschar result in continuous elaboration of endogenous pyrogens. As a consequence, persistent fever almost always accompanies burns. Fever is therefore not usually a helpful sign for determining whether a burn patient has an invasive infection. Systemic antibiotics play little role in the prophylaxis of infections confined to the burn wound, because the avascular wound prevents adequate delivery of antibiotics to the bacteria. Fortunately, early burn excision has greatly diminished—although not eliminated—this problem. Topical antibacterial preparations have also reduced the extent of colonization.

When infections at all sites (lung, wound, and other) are combined, systemic infection is the most common cause of death in the burn patient. The high fatality rate associated with infection is explained by a combination of immune suppression, lung parenchymal damage from smoke inhalation, and the impossibility of immediately covering the wound to provide an effective barrier to infection, even though massive burns can be excised.

The burn patient manifests same signs of sepsis as other critically ill patients do, with the exception that the burn patient's "normal" hyperdynamic state mimics some of the typical signs of sepsis. Changes in status, rather than the presence or absence of specific abnormalities, are most helpful in deciding whether a burn patient has developed an invasive infection.

Treatment

Successful treatment of burn wound infections is extremely difficult. Appropriate systemic antibiotics may ameliorate some systemic manifestations, but they do little to treat the primary infection in the burn wound. Emergent excision of infected burn eschar is the primary treatment modality. Excision removes the source of infection, but it may lead to severe bacteremia during the operation. Specific antibiotic coverage is therefore necessary. Moreover, operations performed in patients with a deteriorating cardiovascular status and pulmonary function are extremely hazardous.

LESS SEVERE, MORE COMMON AND LOCALIZED SKIN INFECTIONS

Impetigo

Impetigo is a very superficial vesiculopustular skin infection that occurs primarily on exposed areas of the face and extremities. The infection is more frequent in warm, humid conditions and is common in children. Poverty, crowding, and poor personal hygiene promote impetigo, which is easily spread within families. Carriage of GAS and *S. aureus* predisposes to subsequent impetigo.

Impetigo resulting from infection with GAS, *S. aureus*, or both, cannot be distinguished clinically. In the typical case, vesiculopustules form that subsequently rupture and become crusted. Affected patients usually develop multiple red and tender lesions in exposed areas at sites of minor skin trauma such as insect bites or abrasions. Impetigo results in little or no systemic sepsis, but it may be accompanied by local lymphadenopathy. Post-streptococcal glomerulonephritis is a rare complication that can prevented by early antibiotic treatment.

Impetigo may be treated topically (see Table 10.2), but when multiple lesions are present, systemic oral therapy is appropriate. Although penicillin was the treatment of choice for impetigo in the past, this antibiotic is no longer recommended, because *S. aureus* almost universally produce β-lactamase that inactivates penicillin. Amoxicillin–clavulanate, erythromycin, cephalexin, dicloxacillin, and topical mupirocin ointment are effective and should therefore be used, provided that local strains of staphylococci do not harbor resistance to the selected agent. The preferred treatment is oral erythromycin (250 mg or, in children, 2.5 to 12.5 mg/kg every 6 hours for 10 days) or mupirocin ointment in a polyethylene glycol base applied locally. An alternative is oral cephalexin (250 mg every 6 hours or 500 mg twice daily for 10 days).

Folliculitis

Folliculitis is a pyoderma localized to hair follicles. Several factors predispose to the development of folliculitis. Individuals with nasal carriage of *S. aureus* have a higher incidence of folliculitis. Exposure to whirlpools, swimming pools, and hot tubs contaminated with *P. aeruginosa* because of inadequate chlorination can cause "whirlpool" folliculitis. Antibiotic administration and corticosteroid therapy predispose to *Candida* folliculitis.

The lesions of folliculitis are often small and multiple. They are erythematous and may have a central pustule at the peak of the raised lesion. Folliculitis does not cause systemic sepsis. Lesions may spontaneously drain or

ment of these lesions include obesity and corticosteroid therapy. Although defective neutrophil function has been sought in this condition, it is rarely found.

Furunculosis is a painful nodular lesion that usually drains pus spontaneously. Infections with CA-MRSA tend to be more rapid in onset and are often misinterpreted as spider bites. Systemic symptoms are uncommon, and the onset of a fever suggests a more deeply seeded infection.

Most patients with furuncles can be treated with warm compresses to promote spontaneous drainage. For carbuncles or furuncles in a patient with fever, antimicrobial therapy should be directed against *S. aureus*. Dicloxacillin is a reasonable first choice (see Table 10.2). Cephalexin or clindamycin can be used in penicillin-allergic patients. When CA-MRSA is suspected, oral trimethoprim–sulfamethoxazole is usually effective; however, continued progression of infection may warrant hospitalization and administration of intravenous vancomycin, daptomycin, or linezolid. Surgical drainage may be required in cases in which spontaneous drainage does not occur and antibiotic treatment does not achieve resolution of the lesion or lesions.

resolve without scarring. The pathogen most commonly responsible for folliculitis is *S. aureus*, but *P. aeruginosa*, and *Candida* species may also cause the disease.

Systemic antibiotics do not appear to be helpful in treating folliculitis. Topical therapies such as warm saline compresses and topical antibacterial or antifungal agents are usually sufficient. The monthly use of mupirocin ointment applied to the anterior nares bilaterally twice daily for 5 days each month reduces both the incidence of nasal colonization with *S. aureus* and the recurrence of either folliculitis or furunculosis in immunocompetent patients who carry *S. aureus* and who present with frequent recurrences of folliculitis. The primary complication of concern is recurrent folliculitis, but progressive infection attributable to *P. aeruginosa* can occur in immunocompromised hosts, and folliculitis is occasionally complicated by furunculosis.

Furunculosis and Carbuncles

Furunculosis is an inflammatory nodule that surrounds a hair follicle. It usually follows an episode of folliculitis. A carbuncle is a series of abscesses in the subcutaneous tissue that drain via hair follicles. *S. aureus* is the most common cause of both lesions.

Furuncles and carbuncles arise when areas of skin containing hair follicles are exposed to friction and perspiration. The back of the neck, face, axillae, and buttocks are commonly involved. Factors predisposing to the develop-

In the presence of recurrent or continuous furunculosis, chlorhexidine solution for bathing, attention to personal hygiene, appropriate laundering of garments, bedding, and towels, and careful wound dressing procedures are recommended. Elimination of nasal carriage of *S. aureus* should be attempted in patients with recurrent episodes of furuncles or carbuncles who have documented nasal carriage of the organism. Mupirocin nasal ointment or oral antibiotic regimens of rifampin (600 mg daily) plus dicloxacillin (500 mg every 6 hours) or ciprofloxacin (500 mg twice daily) for 10 days can be added to mupirocin nasal therapy, if an initial course of mupirocin is not effective. Low-dose clindamycin therapy is an alternative suppressive regimen.

Carbuncles are the most important complication of furunculosis, and surgical intervention may be necessary for debridement of affected tissues. Furuncles involving the nose and perioral area can be complicated by cavernous sinus infection attributable to venous drainage patterns. Bacteremia with development of distant secondary sites of infection can occur (particularly if the furuncle is manipulated) and can result in considerable morbidity and mortality.

Skin Abscesses

Skin abscess is a common infection that is usually managed in the ambulatory setting. The infection is characterized by a localized accumulation of PMNs, with tissue necrosis involving the dermis and subcutaneous tissue. Large numbers of microorganisms are typically present in the purulent material.

Skin abscesses and carbuncles are similar histologically, but like furuncles, carbuncles arise from infection of the hair follicles. Skin abscesses can arise from infection tracking in from the skin surface, but abscesses are usually located deeper than carbuncles (Figure 10.1). In contrast to carbuncles, abscesses can also be seen as a complication of bacteremia. Relatively minor local trauma, such as injection of a drug, can also be a risk factor. Skin abscess is the most common skin infection in intravenous drug abusers. Nasal or skin carriage of *S. aureus* further predisposes to the formation of skin abscess. Skin abscesses can be attributed to a variety of microorganisms and may be polymicrobial; however, the most common single organism is *S. aureus*.

The most common findings with a skin abscess are local pain, swelling, erythema, and regional adenopathy. Spontaneous drainage of purulent material also frequently occurs. Fever, chills, and systemic sepsis are unusual, except in patients with concomitant cellulitis. Patients may have single or multiple skin abscesses, and cellulitis around the skin abscess can occasionally occur. Skin abscess commonly involves the upper extremities in intravenous, drug abusers, but can be located at any anatomic site. Patients with recurrent episodes of skin abscess often suffer anxiety because of the discomfort and cosmetic effects of the infections.

Initial antibiotic therapy should always include coverage for *S. aureus* regardless of the anatomic area of involvement. Results of microbiologic studies, including Gram stain and routine culture should direct subsequent treatment. The initial antibiotic therapy is identical to that for furuncles and carbuncles, except for skin abscess in the oral, rectal, and vulvovaginal areas. Infections in these sites require broader-spectrum therapy, amoxicillin–clavulanate being a suitable option for oral therapy (see Table 10.2). At other sites, clindamycin can be considered for initial therapy if anaerobes are a possible cause. Surgical incision and drainage can be performed if the abscess feels fluctuant or has "pointed"; spontaneous drainage can obviate the need for surgery.

Although the results of testing will usually be negative, metabolic and immunologic screening should be performed in patients with recurrent furunculosis, carbuncles, or skin abscesses in the absence of another

---

KEY POINTS

About Skin Abscesses

1. Skin abscesses are localized infection of the dermis and subcutaneous tissue, usually deeper than carbuncles.

2. Can arise from local trauma, intravenous drug abuse, and bacteremic seeding.

3. *Staphylococcus aureus* is the most common cause.

4. Therapy is identical to that for furuncles and carbuncles, with these additions:
   a) Oral clindamycin may be considered if anaerobes are possibly involved.
   b) For concomitant cellulitis, use intravenous clindamycin, nafcillin, oxacillin, cefazolin, or vancomycin (the latter for community-acquired methicillin-resistant *S. aureus*).
   c) For infections in the perirectal, oral, or vulvovaginal areas amoxicillin–clavulanate is preferred.

5. Preventive measures:
   a) With recurrent furunculosis, carbuncles, or abscesses, exclude diabetes mellitus, neutrophil dysfunction, and hyperimmunoglobulin E syndrome.
   b) For patients at high risk for endocarditis, provide prophylactic antibiotics before incision and drainage of lesions.

predisposing factor. These tests should include determination of fasting blood glucose and, if values from the former test are high-normal or elevated, a hemoglobin A1c should be ordered. Neutrophil number and function, plus immunoglobulin levels also should be evaluated. Elevated levels of immunoglobulin E (IgE) in association with eczema defines a Job's (hyper-IgE) syndrome, a disease that is characterized by recurrent staphylococcal skin infections.

Most patients with skin abscess respond to therapy and do not develop serious complications. However, bacteremia can occur, and metastatic sites of infection, including endocarditis and osteomyelitis, can develop. Individuals at high or moderate risk for endocarditis should be given antimicrobial prophylaxis before potentially infected tissue is incised and drained. Parenteral administration of an anti-staphylococcal antibiotic (either oxacillin or cefazolin) is recommended as prophylactic therapy in this setting. Vancomycin should be given if the patient has previously been colonized or infected with MRSA (see Table 10.2).

RARER CAUSES OF INDOLENT SOFT TISSUE INFECTIONS

Chronic skin infections that are unresponsive to conventional antibiotics should stimulate a careful epidemiologic history. Commercial and sports fisherman may cut a finger on a fish spine, and that injury can result in an *Erysipelothrix* infection. This pleomorphic gram-positive rod causes painful erythematous lesions primarily of the hands and other exposed areas. Cultures and biopsies are often negative, because the pathogen remains deep in the dermis. Penicillin is preferred for treatment, although in the penicillin-allergic patient, clindamycin or ciprofloxacin have been found to be effective.

KEY POINTS

About the Causes of Indolent Soft Tissue Infections

- -

1. Waterborne pathogens and their treatments:
   a) Erysipelothrix (penicillin)
   b) *Mycobacterium marinum* (minocycline or clarithromycin)
2. Plant- and soil-borne pathogens and their treatments:
   a) Sporotrichosis (itraconazole)
   b) Nocardiosis (trimethoprim–sulfamethoxazole)

Mycobacterium marinum is another waterborne infection. This atypical mycobacterium is found in fresh and salt water, including aquariums. Individuals with cuts on the skin are susceptible to invasion by this organism. Infections usually begin as small papules, but gradually expand and fail to respond to conventional antibiotics. Surgical debridement in the absence of appropriate antibiotic treatment can result in worsening of the infection. Modified acid-fast organisms may be seen on biopsy. The organism can be grown at low temperature (28 to 30°C) using specific Middlebrook agar or Bactec broth. The microbiology laboratory should always be notified when atypical mycobacteria are suspected. Oral doxycycline or minocycline (100 mg twice daily), or oral clarithromycin (500 mg twice daily) for a minimum of 3 months is the treatment of choice.

Other atypical mycobacteria found throughout the environment that can also cause indolent soft tissue infections include *M. fortuitum*, *M. chelonae*, *M. abscessus*, and *M. ulcerans* (Australia and tropical countries). Gardeners who are cut by rosebush thorns are at risk for *Sporothrix schenckii* infection. This dimorphic fungus causes skin erythema, swelling, and lymphadenitis. In addition to rose thorns. soil contamination of any cut, and exposure to infected animals can result in sporotrichosis. Oral itraconazole (100 to 200 mg daily) for 3 to 6 months is the treatment of choice. Inoculation of soil into the skin as a consequence of trauma can also result in a Nocardia soft tissue infection that mimics sporotrichosis. Prolonged oral therapy with trimethoprim–sulfamethoxazole (5 mg/kg daily of the trimethoprim component, divided into two daily doses) or minocycline (100 mg twice daily) is usually curative.

Tetanus

Immunization policies have made tetanus an uncommon problem in the United States. Approximately 70 cases are reported annually, with most cases occurring in individuals over 60 years of age whose immunity is waning. The incidence is much higher in developing countries, where the mortality rates associated with tetanus are as high as 28 per 100,000 population.

In developed countries, most cases of tetanus are the sequelae of punctures or lacerations. *C. tetani* spores can contaminate these wounds and germinate in the anaerobic conditions created by a closed wound. The growing bacterium produces an exotoxin called tetanospasmin. This metalloprotease degrades a protein required for the docking of neurotransmitter vesicles that normally inhibit firing of the motor neurons. As a consequence, muscle spasms develop, and patients experience masseter muscle trismus ("lock jaw") and generalized muscle spasm, including arching of the back (opisthotonus), flexion of the arms, and extension of the legs. Spasms may be triggered by any sensory stimulus and are very painful. Spasm of the diaphragm and throat can lead to respiratory arrest and sudden death. Autonomic dysfunction can lead to hypertension or hypotension, and bradycardia or tachycardia. This symptom is the leading cause of death. Neonatal tetanus develops following infection of the umbilical stump and is most commonly reported in developing countries. Neonates present with generalized weakness, followed by increased rigidity. Mortality exceeds 90%.

Patients should receive intramuscular injections of human tetanus immunoglobulin 500 IU. Diphtheria-pertussis-tetanus vaccine (DPT, 0.5 mL) should also be administered intramuscularly. Intravenous metronidazole (500 mg every 6 hours) should be given for 7 to 10 days to eradicate *C. tetani* from the wound. Intravenous diazepam is recommended to control the muscle spasms, and tracheostomy should be performed after endotra-

cheal intubation, in anticipation of prolonged respiratory compromise. Sympathetic hyperactivity should be controlled with short-acting β-blockers, and hypotension should be treated with saline infusion combined with dopamine or norepinephrine. Intravenous magnesium sulfate (4 to 6 g over 15 to 20 minutes, followed by 2 g hourly) has also been shown to stabilize sympathetic hyperactivity. Severe muscle spasms can be controlled with benzodiazepines or pancuronium; however, use of these agents necessitates mechanical ventilation. Another alternative is intrathecal administration of the gamma-aminobutyric acid B receptor agonist baclofen (40 to 200 μg bolus, followed by 20 μg hourly, not to exceed 2 mg daily). This regimen may block muscle spasm without significant interference with respiratory function, but it is associated with an increased risk of developing bacterial meningitis as a consequence of prolonged placement of an intrathecal catheter. Two additional doses of DPT vaccine are recommended, one dose at the time of discharge and a third dose 4 weeks later. Mortality ranges from 6% in milder cases to 60% in severe disease.

The devastating consequences of this disease emphasize the importance of prevention. Tetanus toxoid vaccination provides complete immunity for at least 5 years. Routine boosters are recommended every 10 years. Tetanus spores can be inoculated into any wound; however, certain wounds are at higher risk. The high-risk group includes wounds contaminated with dirt, saliva, or feces; puncture wounds and unsterile injections; frostbite; bullet or shrapnel wounds; crush injuries; and compound fractures. If a patient with one of these wounds has not received immunization in the past 5 years or is immuno-compromised, passive immunization with human tetanus immunoglobulin and active immunization with a tetanus toxoid booster should be given.

Bites by Animals and Humans

ANIMAL BITES

Animal bites caused by pet dogs and cats are a common problem representing approximately 1% of visits to the emergency room. The incidence tends to be higher among children. Dog bites most frequently occur in young boys; cat bites more commonly occur in young girls and women. Dog and cat bites can result in soft tissue and bone infections, particularly on the hands. The teeth of cats are very sharp and commonly penetrate the skin and puncture the underlying bone, increasing the risk of osteomyelitis.

The organism most commonly associated with pet animal bites is *Pasteurella*, which is found in 50% of dog bites and 70% of cat bites. *P. canis* is most common in dog bites, and *P. multocida* is most common in cat bites. *S. aureus*, streptococci, *Capnocytophaga canimorsus*, and anaerobic bacteria are also frequently cultured from

---

KEY POINTS

About Tetanus

1. The disease is rare in the United States, but common in developing countries.

2. *Clostridium tetani* produces tetanospasmin and blocks normal inhibition of motor neurons.

3. Associated with severe muscle spasm, jaw trismus, opisthotonus, and respiratory failure.

4. Treatment includes administration of
   a) human tetanus immunoglobulin;
   b) tetanus toxoid vaccine;
   c) intravenous metronidazole;
   d) benzodiazepines and pancuronium, or intrathecal baclofen to control muscle spasm; and
   e) short-acting β-blockers, intravenous magnesium sulfate, and vasopressors for sympathetic instability.
   f) Intubation and tracheostomy are often required.

5. Prevention:
   a) Vaccination with tetanus toxoid every 10 years.
   b) Booster vaccination in cases of potentially contaminated wounds received 5 or more years after regular vaccination.
   c) Patient with high-risk wounds, or those who are immunocompromised should also receive human tetanus immunoglobulin.

<table>
</table>

KEY POINTS

About Animal Bites

1. Bites by pet animals are a leading cause of visits to the emergency room.
2. Animal bites are more common in children than in adults; dog bites are more common in boys than in girls; and cat bites are more common in girls and women than in boys and men.
3. *Pasteurella* species are important pathogens in dog and cat bites.
4. Recommended prophylaxis:
   a) Intravenous ampicillin–sulbactam followed by amoxicillin–clavulanate for 3 to 5 days.
   b) Intravenous clindamycin, followed by oral clindamycin, plus ciprofloxacin in penicillin-allergic patients.
5. Treatment includes
   a) the same antibiotic regimens as for prophylaxis, but more prolonged—10 to 28 days;
   b) rabies prophylaxis; and
   c) tetanus prophylaxis.

KEY POINTS

About Human Bites

1. Bites by humans are often associated with alcohol or other drugs; closed-fist injuries are most common.
2. Infections are usually polymicrobial, and often include *Eikenella corrodens*,
3. For prophylaxis and treatment, use ampicillin–sulbactam, ticarcillin–clavulanate, cefoxitin.
4. Avoid oxacillin, nafcillin, clindamycin, metronidazole, and many cephalosporins.
5. Duration of treatment depends on response rate, tissue damage, and bony involvement.

animal bite wounds. The resulting infections are usually polymicrobial.

Because of the high likelihood of infection, cat and dog bite wounds should not initially be closed. Antibiotic prophylaxis is usually recommended, consisting of a single parenteral dose of ampicillin–sulbactam (3 g), followed by oral amoxicillin–clavulanate (875 mg twice daily for 3 to 5 days). Alternative regimens in patients with penicillin allergy include clindamycin (900 mg intravenously, followed by 300 mg orally every 6 hours), plus ciprofloxacin (400 mg intravenously, followed by 500 mg orally twice daily). In children, clindamycin combined with trimethoprim–sulfamethoxazole is recommended.

The duration of intravenous and oral antibiotic treatment depends on the rate of response of the infection, the degree of tissue damage, and the likelihood of bone or joint involvement. Patients with defects in lymphatic or venous drainage and those who are immunocompromised or receiving corticosteroids re at higher risk of developing sepsis. These patients need to be followed closely. First-generation cephalosporins, dicloxacillin, and erythromycin should be avoided in these patients, because a number of bacteria that cause animal bite infections, including *P. multocida*, are resistant to these antibiotics. If the animal bite was unprovoked, rabies vaccination or quarantined observation of the animal are

the standard of care. Prophylaxis for tetanus must also be provided (see the earlier subsection specific to tetanus).

HUMAN BITES

Human bites most commonly arise as a consequence of closed-fist injuries during a fight. Human mouth flora can also be inoculated into the skin as result of nail-biting or thumb-sucking. Love nips and actual bites in association with altercations are also encountered. Alcohol, other drugs, or medical conditions leading to confusion are often associated with human bite injuries.

Multiple aerobes and anaerobes can be cultured from the human mouth, and infections associated with human bites are usually polymicrobial. Aerobic organisms include *S. viridans* and *S. aureus*. Important anaerobes include *Eikenella corrodens*, *Bacteroides* species, *Fusobacterium* species, and peptostreptococci. *Eikenella corrodens* is a particular concern, because this organism is resistant to oxacillin, nafcillin, clindamycin, and metronidazole, and variably resistant to cephalosporins.

Prophylaxis with amoxicillin–clavulanate is recommended. Treatment with intravenous ampicillin–sulbactam, ticarcillin–clavulanate, or cefoxitin is usually effective. As noted for animal bites, the duration of therapy depends on the rate of improvement, the degree of soft tissue damage, and the likelihood of bone involvement. In closed-fist injuries, bone and tendon involvement is common and usually warrants more prolonged antibiotic therapy for presumed osteomyelitis.

FURTHER READING

Albrecht MC, Griffith ME, Murray CK, et al. Impact of *Acinetobacter* infection on the mortality of burn patients. *J Am Coll Surg.* 2006;203:546–550.

Aldape MJ, Bryant AE, Stevens DL. *Clostridium sordellii* infection: epidemiology, clinical findings, and current perspectives on diagnosis and treatment. *Clin Infect Dis.* 2006;43:1436–1446.

Alsbjorn B, Gilbert P, Hartmann B, et al. Guidelines for the management of partial-thickness burns in a general hospital or community setting—recommendations of a European working party. *Burns.* 2007;33:155–160.

Anaya DA, McMahon K, Nathens AB, Sullivan SR, Foy H, Bulger E. Predictors of mortality and limb loss in necrotizing soft tissue infections. *Arch Surg.* 2005;140:151–157.

Aronoff DM, Bloch KC. Assessing the relationship between the use of nonsteroidal antiinflammatory drugs and necrotizing fasciitis caused by group A streptococcus. *Medicine (Baltimore).* 2003;82:225–235.

Atiyeh BS, Costagliola M, Hayek SN, Dibo SA. Effect of silver on burn wound infection control and healing: review of the literature. *Burns.* 2007;33:139–148.

Broder J, Jerrard D, Olshaker J, Witting M. Low risk of infection in selected human bites treated without antibiotics. *Am J Emerg Med.* 2004;22:10–13.

Fischer M, Bhatnagar J, Guarner J, et al. Fatal toxic shock syndrome associated with *Clostridium sordellii* after medical abortion. *N Engl J Med.* 2005;353:2352–2360.

Hart GB, Lamb RC, Strauss MB. Gas gangrene. *J Trauma.* 1983;23:991–1000.

Kainer MA, Linden JV, Whaley DN, et al. *Clostridium* infections associated with musculoskeletal-tissue allografts. *N Engl J Med.* 2004;350:2564–2571.

Lee MC, Rios AM, Aten MF, et al. Management and outcome of children with skin and soft tissue abscesses caused by community-acquired methicillin-resistant *Staphylococcus aureus. Pediatr Infect Dis J.* 2004;23:123–127.

Miller LG, Perdreau-Remington F, Rieg G, et al. Necrotizing fasciitis caused by community-associated methicillin-resistant *Staphylococcus aureus* in Los Angeles. *N Engl J Med.* 2005;352:1445–1453.

Naimi TS, LeDell KH, Como-Sabetti K, et al. Comparison of community- and health care–associated methicillin-resistant *Staphylococcus aureus* infection. *JAMA.* 2003;290:2976–2984.

Norrby-Teglund A, Muller MP, McGeer A, et al. Successful management of severe group A streptococcal soft tissue infections using an aggressive medical regimen including intravenous polyspecific immunoglobulin together with a conservative surgical approach. *Scand J Infect Dis.* 2005;37:166–172.

Santos ML, Mota-Miranda A, Alves-Pereira A, Gomes A, Correia J, Marcal N. Intrathecal baclofen for the treatment of tetanus. *Clin Infect Dis.* 2004;38:321–328.

Stamenkovic I, Lew PD. Early recognition of potentially fatal necrotizing fasciitis. The use of frozen-section biopsy. *N Engl J Med.* 1984;310:1689–1693.

Stevens DL, Bisno AL, Chambers HF, et al. Practice guidelines for the diagnosis and management of skin and soft-tissue infections. *Clin Infect Dis.* 2005;41:1373–1406.

Thwaites CL, Yen LM, Loan HT, et al. Magnesium sulphate for treatment of severe tetanus: a randomised controlled trial. *Lancet.* 2006;368:1436–1443.

Wong CH, Chang HC, Pasupathy S, Khin LW, Tan JL, Low CO. Necrotizing fasciitis: clinical presentation, microbiology, and determinants of mortality. *J Bone Joint Surg Am.* 2003;85-A:1454–1460.

Yeniyol CO, Suelozgen T, Arslan M, Ayder AR. Fournier's gangrene: experience with 25 patients and use of Fournier's gangrene severity index score. *Urology.* 2004;64:218–222

Osteomyelitis, Prosthetic Joint Infections, Diabetic Foot Infections, and Septic Arthritis

11

Time Recommended to Complete: 1 day

Daniel P. Lew

GUIDING QUESTIONS

1. How are acute and chronic bone infection distinguished?

2. What are the most frequent pathogens in osteomyelitis?

3. Is a bone biopsy necessary to guide treatment in osteomyelitis?

4. For how long should osteomyelitis be treated?

5. For how long should septic arthritis be treated?

6. Are oral antibiotics ever the appropriate treatment for osteomyelitis or septic arthritis?

7. What is the most common bacterial cause of polyarticular arthritis?

8. What are the indications for surgical debridement of a septic joint?

■ OSTEOMYELITIS

> ### POTENTIAL SEVERITY
>
> *A subacute to chronic infection that can cause severe disability if improperly managed.*

Osteomyelitis is a progressive infectious process that can involve one or multiple components of bone, including the periosteum, medullary cavity, and cortical bone. The disease is characterized by progressive inflammatory destruction of bone, by necrosis, and by new bone formation.

CLASSIFICATION

Classifying osteomyelitis is helpful because the different types of osteomyelitis have differing prognoses and are treated in different ways.

Acute Versus Chronic Osteomyelitis

Acute osteomyelitis evolves over several days to weeks; chronic osteomyelitis is disease characterized by clinical symptoms that persist for several weeks. Chronic osteomyelitis can also evolve over months or even years and is characterized by the persistence of microorganisms, by low-grade inflammation, by the presence of necrotic bone (sequestra) or foreign material (or both), and by fistulous tracts. The terms "acute" and "chronic" do not have a sharp demarcation, and they are often used somewhat loosely. Nevertheless, they are useful clinical concepts in infectious disease, because they describe two different patterns of the same disease, often caused by the same microorganisms but with different rates of progression.

Osteomyelitis of Hematogenous Origin or Attributable to a Contiguous Focus of Infection

Hematogenous osteomyelitis is the result of bacteremic spread with seeding of bacteria in bone. It is seen mostly in prepubertal children and in elderly patients. Osteomyelitis secondary to a contiguous focus of infection follows trauma, perforation, or an orthopedic procedure. As the name implies, infection first begins in an area adjacent to bone, eventually spreading to the bone. An important category of osteomyelitis resulting from contiguous spread is found in diabetic patients. Diabetic foot infection usually starts as an ulcer and commonly spreads to bone. It is secondary to neuropathy and associated with vascular insufficiency.

HEMATOGENOUS OSTEOMYELITIS OF LONG BONES AND VERTEBRAL BODIES

Pathogenesis

Hematogenous osteomyelitis most commonly occurs in children and usually results in a single focus of infection involving the metaphysis of long bones (particularly tibia and femur). In adults, hematogenous osteomyelitis most frequently involves the vertebral bodies These locations are favored because of their vascular supply.

In the case of the long bones, bacteria tend to lodge in small end vessels that form sharp loops near the epiphyses. In the case of vertebral bodies, small arteriolar vessels are thought to trap bacteria. The vertebral arteries usually bifurcate and supply two adjacent vertebral bodies, explaining why hematogenous vertebral osteomyelitis usually involves two adjacent boney seg-

ments and the intervening disc. In addition, the vertebra are surrounded by a plexus of veins lacking valves, called Batson's plexus. This venous system drains the bladder and pelvic region and, on occasion, can also transmit infection from the genitourinary tract to the vertebral bodies. The lumbar segments are most commonly infected, followed by the thoracic regions; the cervical region is only occasionally involved.

Microbiology

The bacteria responsible for hematogenous osteomyelitis essentially reflect their bacteremic incidence as a function of host age, so the organisms most frequently encountered in neonates include *Escherichia coli*, group B streptococci, and *Staphylococcus aureus*. Later in life, *S. aureus* predominates (see Table 11.1).

In elderly people, who are frequently subject to gram-negative bacteremias, an increased incidence of vertebral osteomyelitis attributable to gram-negative rods is found. Fungal osteomyelitis is a complication of intravenous device infections, neutropenia, or profound immune deficiency. *Pseudomonas aeruginosa* hematogenous osteomyelitis is often seen in intravenous drug abusers, and this organism has a predilection for the cervical vertebrae.

CASE 11.1

An 86-year-old white woman underwent cardiac catheterization 3 months before admission. Several days after her catheterization, she noted a fever that lasted for 2 to 3 days. Approximately 3 weeks after her catheterization, she began experiencing dull pain in the lumbosacral region that progressively worsened over the next two months. Pain was not relieved by over-the-counter pain medications, and it became so severe that she sought medical attention in the emergency room. She reported a 25-pound (11.3-kg) weight loss over the 3 months.

Physical examination showed a temperature of 36.4°C and pulse of 84 per minute. General appearance was that of an elderly woman complaining of back pain. A 2/6 systolic ejection murmur was noted along the left sternal border (previously described). Palpation over the L-S spine area elicited moderate tenderness. Motor and sensory exams of the lower extremities were within normal limits.

The patient's laboratory workup revealed an erythrocyte sedimentation rate (ESR) of 119 mm/h; a white blood cell (WBC) count of 8.1/mm³, with 52% polymorphonuclear leukocytes (PMNs), 12.8% lymphocytes, and 10.8% monocytes; and a platelet count of 537,000/mm³.

Table 11.1. The Microbiology of Osteomyelitis

Osteomyelitis type	Common Pathogens
Hematogenous spread (usually 1 organism)	
Infant (<1 year)	Staphylococcus aureus Coagulase-negative staphylococci Group B streptococci *Escherichia coli*
Children and adults (>16 years)	*S. aureus* Coagulase-negative staphylococci Gram-negative organisms: *E. coli* *Pseudomonas* spp. *Serratia* spp.
Contiguous spread (polymicrobial)	
Microbiology depends on the primary site of infection	*S. aureus* *Streptococcus pyogenes* *Enterococcus* Coagulase-negative staphylococci Gram-negative organisms Anaerobes
Diabetic foot (often polymicrobial)	
	S. aureus *Streptococcus* spp., including *Enterococcus* Gram-negative organisms: *Proteus mirabilis* *Pseudomonas* Anaerobes

A computed tomography (CT) scan showed marked decalcification of the L4-L5 vertebral bodies, with a "moth-eaten" appearance of the vertebral endplate in L5. A CT-guided aspirate grew no pathogens, but a repeat aspirate demonstrated an acute inflammatory reaction, with the culture was positive for S. aureus. Two blood cultures showed no growth.

Clinical Manifestations

The clinical features of hematogenous osteomyelitis in long bones include chills, fever, and malaise, reflecting the bacteremic spread of microorganisms. Pain and local swelling subsequently develop at the site of local infection. Patients with vertebral osteomyelitis complain of localized back pain and tenderness that may mimic an early herniated disk, but the presence of fever should always raise the possibility of infection. It should be pointed out, however, that fever may not be evident at the time of presentation (as noted in case 11.1), particularly in more chronic cases of osteomyelitis. The ESR is commonly elevated, and in a patient with back pain and a high ESR or C-reactive protein (CRP), vertebral osteomyelitis should be considered.

Diagnosis

In most cases, the peripheral WBC count is normal. If the infection has continued for a prolonged period, the patient may have a normochromic normocytic anemia (anemia of chronic disease). The diagnosis of osteomyelitis is usually made radiologically. Standard bone films generally show demineralization within 2 to 3 weeks of infection onset (Figure 11.1). On X-ray, a loss of 50% of the bone calcium is generally required before demineralization can be detected, which explains the low sensitivity early in the course of infection.

In long-bone infections, periosteal elevation may develop in addition to areas of reduced calcium (lytic

KEY POINTS

About the Pathogenesis, Microbiology, and Clinical Manifestations of Hematogenous Osteomyelitis

1. Bacteria are trapped in small end vessels
   a) at the metaphysis of long bone in children.
   b) in vertebral bodies in the elderly. Can also spread via Batson's venous plexus.
2. Microbiology reflects the causes of bacteremia:
   a) Neonates—*Escherichia coli*, coagulase-negative staphylococci, *Staphylococcus aureus*, group B strep, other streptococci
   b) Adults—*S. aureus*
   c) Elderly—Gram-negative organisms, *S. aureus*
   d) Immunocompromised—Fungi
   e) Intravenous drug abusers—*Pseudomonas aeruginosa*
3. Clinical manifestations:
   a) Long bones—Fever, chills, and malaise, plus soft tissue swelling and pain, usually children
   b) Vertebral osteomyelitis—Back pain and localized tenderness, plus high erythrocyte sedimentation rate or C-reactive protein

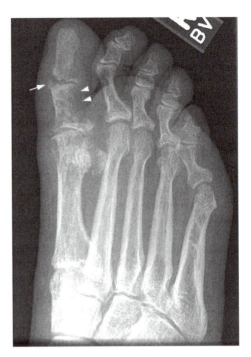

Figure 11–1. Plain radiograph showing changes of osteomyelitis of the great toe. The arrow points to fragmentation of the distal interphalangeal joint. Arrowheads outline the expected location of the medial margin of the proximal phalangeal bone. Multifocal areas of cortical destruction and ill-defined lytic areas are found throughout the distal first metatarsal and both first-toe phalanges. Picture courtesy of Dr. Maria T. Calimano and Dr. Andres R. Acosta, University of Florida Medical School

lesions), and soft tissue swelling is apparent. Later in the infection (and in chronic osteomyelitis), areas of increased calcification or bone sclerosis are also seen.

In vertebral osteomyelitis, early plain radiographs may reveal no abnormalities, and obvious changes may not develop for 6 to 8 weeks. At this time, the bone plate of the vertebra becomes eroded and appears irregular or "moth-eaten." Collapse of the disc space is usually seen as the infection progresses, and this event is most readily visualized on CT scan (Figure 11.2). Metastatic bone lesions can also cause erosions of the vertebral margin.

One critical finding helps to distinguish the latter two diseases. In osteomyelitis, infection almost always involves two adjacent vertebral bodies and the disc space. Most neoplastic processes involve a single vertebral body and do not extend across the disk space.

In both vertebral osteomyelitis and long-bone osteomyelitis, CT scan is helpful in defining the extent of bone damage and is more sensitive than plain films. In addition, CT imaging is commonly used to guide needle biopsy in vertebral osteomyelitis. If surgical debridement is being considered, CT scan is often used to help to decide the extent of debridement.

Magnetic resonance imaging (MRI) is also increasingly being used to detect sequestra. When long bones become necrotic, the bone marrow dies, producing a unique MRI signal. This diagnostic tool very effectively guides the orthopedic surgeon and allows for a more complete surgical debridement of a sequestrum. Magnetic resonance imaging has also proved to be more sensitive than CT scan for detecting early osteomyelitis. Decreased signal intensity of the disc and infected vertebral bodies is observed on T2-weighted images, and loss of endplate definition noted on T-1 images. Contrast enhancement of the infected regions is also observed (Figure 11.3). In addition, MRI is helpful in detecting the spread of vertebral infection to the epidural space (a rare event

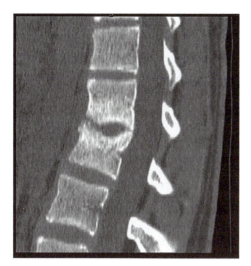

Figure 11–2. Sagittal computed tomography scan showing typical changes of vertebral osteomyelitis. Obliteration of the disc space is seen, together with marked irregularity and sclerosis of the cortical endplates. Picture courtesy of Dr. Maria T. Calimano and Dr. Andres R. Acosta, University of Florida Medical School

---

KEY POINTS

About the Diagnosis of Osteomyelitis

1. Plain films require 2 to 3 weeks to become positive (50% loss of bone calcium required); in vertebral osteomyelitis, bone loss can take 6 to 8 weeks. Radiographs may show
   a) periosteal elevation,
   b) areas of demineralization and loss of a sharp bony margin ("moth-eaten" look),
   c) soft tissue swelling, and
   d) late-stage areas of increased calcification or sclerosis.
2. Computed tomography (CT) scan is more sensitive.
3. Magnetic resonance imaging can detect early changes.
4. Bone scan can detect early disease, but false positives are common. Gallium is preferred for vertebral osteomyelitis.
5. Tissue sample for culture and histopathology should be obtained, except when blood cutures are positive.
   a) long-bone infection in children may be treated empirically.
   b) long-bone infection in adults usually requires operative culture.
   c) vertebral osteomyelitis requires CT-guided needle biopsy.

---

in the modern antibiotic era; see Chapter 6) and detecting contiguous soft tissue infection.

Bone scan may be useful in detecting early infection; however, in many circumstances, MRI has proved to be the study of choice in early osteomyelitis. Three-phase technetium bone scan is sensitive, but produces false positive results in patients with fractures or overlying soft tissue infection. False negative results are occasionally observed in early infection or when bone infarction accompanies osteomyelitis. Gallium imaging is more

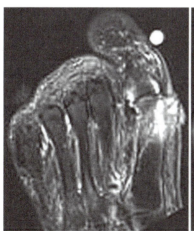

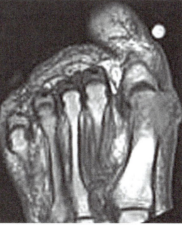

Figure 11–3. Changes of early osteomyelitis as detected by magnetic resonance imaging. *Left:* A T2 image shows increased signal in the bone marrow of the metatarsal and the surrounding soft tissue. *Right:* A T1 post-contrast image shows loss of the bone marrow fat signal and cortical margins in the metatarsal. Picture courtesy of Dr. Maria T. Calimano and Dr. Andres R. Acosta, University of Florida Medical School

specific and sensitive in cases of vertebral osteomyelitis, and demonstrates intense uptake in the disc space and adjacent vertebral bodies.

To define the microbiology, two to three blood samples for culture should be drawn during the acute presentation. However, blood cultures are positive only in a small percentage of cases, and in most patients, a deep-tissue sample should therefore be obtained for aerobic and anaerobic culture (and for fungal and mycobacterial culture, if appropriate), for Gram stain, and for histopathologic examination.

Children are often treated empirically, because any operative intervention near the epiphyseal plate can result in impaired bone growth. In the occasional adult with long-bone infection, debridement or incision and drainage of soft-tissue abscesses (or both) are usually required, and these procedures also allow for acquisition of deep-tissue samples for culture.

In vertebral osteomyelitis, the number of potential pathogens is large, and effective antimicrobial therapy needs to be guided by culture results. Needle biopsy under CT guidance is currently the procedure of choice for obtaining culture samples. Needle aspirates should be submitted in parallel for bacteriologic and pathologic evaluation. Pathology is particularly useful in patients with previous antibiotic therapy, in which cultures may be negative, and in patients with suspected mycobacterial or fungal disease. If the first biopsy is culture-negative, a second biopsy guided by CT scan should be obtained. In patients in whom the second sample fails to establish a diagnosis, the physician is faced with a choice: begin empiric therapy or request an open surgical biopsy for diagnosis.

Treatment

In long-bone infections, parenteral administration of an antimicrobial regimen may be begun as empiric therapy aimed at the clinically suspected pathogen or pathogens. Once the microorganisms are isolated, in vitro susceptibility testing can be performed as a guide to treatment.

The current standard of care is parenteral antimicrobial treatment for 4 to 6 weeks (see Table 11.2). The start of therapy must be dated from the day on which effective antimicrobial therapy, as judged by in vitro susceptibility, was begun or the day of the last major debridement.

Empiric coverage of vertebral osteomyelitis is generally not recommended. The choice of an antimicrobial drug should be guided by the results of blood cultures and of bone and soft tissue specimens obtained by biopsy or debridement before treatment. For patients who traveled to endemic areas, *Brucella* serology may occasionally be useful. Depending on pharmacologic

---

KEY POINTS

About the Treatment of Hematogenous Osteomyelitis

1. Empiric antibiotic therapy is usually avoided. Treatment usually continues for 6 weeks:

   a) *Staphylococcus aureus*, methicillin-sensitive: nafcillin or oxacillin; methicillin-resistant: vancomycin. A switch may be made to oral ciprofloxacin–rifampin if the *S. aureus* is sensitive.

   b) Streptococci: Penicillin G

   c) Enteric gram-negative organisms: oral ciprofloxacin

   d) *Serratia* or *Pseudomonas aeruginosa*: piperacillin–tazobactam or imipenem

   e) Anaerobes: clindamycin or metronidazole

2. Surgical debridement not necessary with early treatment. May be required

   a) to remove necrotic long bone.

   b) in vertebral osteomyelitis to treat instability, cord compression, drainage of soft tissue abscess.

---

characteristics, the selected drug may be administered by the oral or the parenteral route.

The indications for surgery in vertebral osteomyelitis are failure of medical management, formation of soft tissue abscesses, impending instability, or neurologic signs indicating spinal cord compression. In the latter case, surgery becomes an emergency procedure (see the discussion of spinal epidural abscess in Chapter 6). The neurologic status of the patient must therefore be monitored at frequent intervals. Eventual fusion of adjacent infected vertebral bodies is a major goal of therapy.

OSTEOMYELITIS SECONDARY TO A CONTIGUOUS INFECTION

Clinical Manifestations and Associated Primary Infections

In cases of osteomyelitis associated with a comminuted fracture, the situation and the clinical picture are more complex. Bacteria are often introduced at the time of trauma. Following initial corrective surgery, pain improves, and the patient progressively mobilizes the injured limb. As the patient begins to bear weight, pain reappears. A mild fever is noted, and the wound

Table 11.2. Antibiotic Treatment of Osteomyelitis in Adults

Microorganisms Isolated	Treatment of Choice	Alternatives
Staphylococcus aureus		
Penicillin-sensitive	Penicillin G (4–6 × 10⁶ U q6h)	2nd-generation cephalosporin (for example, cefuroxime), or clindamycin (600 mg q6h), or vancomycin[a]
Penicillin-resistant	Nafcillin or flucloxacillin (2 g q6h)	2nd-generation cephalosporin, or clindamycin (600 mg q6h), or vancomycin,[a] ciprofloxacin[a] (750 mg q12h), and oral rifampin (600–900 mg q24h)
Methicillin-resistant	Vancomycin (1 g q12h)	Teicoplanin[b] (400 mg q12–24h, first day q12h)
Various streptococci		
(group A or B β-hemolytic, *Streptococcus pneumoniae*)	Penicillin G (3 × 10⁶ U q4–6h)	Clindamycin (600 mg q6h), erythromycin (500 mg q6h), or vancomycin
Enteric gram-negative rods		
	Quinolone (ciprofloxacin,[d] 500–750 mg q12h IV or PO)	A wide-spectrum cephalosporin[c]
Serratia spp., Pseudomonas aeruginosa		
	Piperacillin[d] (2–4 g q4h), and initial gentamicin[e] (3 mg/kg daily)	A wide-spectrum cephalosporin, or a quinolone (with initial aminoglycosides)
Anaerobes		
	Clindamycin (600 mg q6h)	Amoxicillin–clavulanic acid (1.2 q6h to 2.2 q8h), or metronidazole for gram-negative anaerobes (500 mg q8h)
Mixed infection (aerobic and anaerobic microorganisms)		
	Amoxicillin–clavulanic acid (2.2 g q8h)	Imipenem[f] (500 mg q6h)

[a] For sensitive *S. aureus* strains, a switch from intravenous to oral therapy combining ciprofloxacin 500–750 mg q12h and rifampin 600–900 mg q24h is common practice.

[b] Teicoplanin is currently available only in Europe. The role of novel glycopeptides in osteomyelitis remains to be assessed.

[c] Third- or fourth-generation (ceftriaxone, ceftazidime, or cefepime according to sensitivity).

[d] Depends on sensitivities: piperacillin–tazobactam and imipenem are useful alternatives.

[e] Because of potential nephrotoxicity or ototoxicity, a regimen containing aminoglycosides is less often used, and only during the initial phase of treatment.

[f] In cases of aerobic gram-negative microorganisms resistant to amoxicillin–clavulanic acid.

becomes more erythematous, accompanied by a slight discharge. No other clinical signs point toward the diagnosis of osteomyelitis, and no radiographic examination or other imaging procedure is fully diagnostic.

Other forms of osteomyelitis resulting from contiguous spread include

1. Acute purulent frontal sinusitis spreading to the frontal bone and causing edema of the forehead (Pott's puffy tumor).
2. Dental root infection leading to local bony destruction.
3. Deep-seated pressure sores spreading to underlying bone, usually the sacrum. (This infection is usually polymicrobial.)

Causes

S. aureus remains the most frequently reported microorganisms in osteomyelitis secondary to contiguous spread (see Table 11.1). However, various types of streptococci, the Enterobacteriaceae, and *P. aeruginosa* (the latter mostly in the setting of chronic osteomyelitis, comminuted fractures, and puncture wounds to the heel) are also encountered. Osteomyelitis of the mandible and osteomyelitis secondary to pressure sores both frequently contain an abundance of anaerobic flora. Anaerobes also are common pathogens in osteomyelitis caused by human and animal bites (see Chapter 10). Sacral osteomyelitis is usually polymicrobial, with gram-negative microorgan-

KEY POINTS

About Osteomyelitis Resulting from Contiguous Spread

1. Clinical manifestations are subtle:
   a) Increasing pain
   b) Mild fever and minimal drainage
2. Imaging is often difficult to interpret.
3. Microbiology may reveal multiple organisms:
   a) *Staphylococcus aureus* most common
   b) Streptococci
   c) Enterobacteriaceae
   d) *Pseudomonas aeruginosa*
   e) Anaerobes

isms and anaerobes. In all these conditions, the inflammatory reaction may be mild, and the extent of bony destruction difficult to assess.

DIABETIC FOOT INFECTION (OSTEOMYELITIS SECONDARY TO NEUROPATHY OR VASCULAR INSUFFICIENCY)

Clinical Manifestations

Osteomyelitis secondary to neuropathy and vascular insufficiency is a special entity observed in patients with diabetes or vascular impairment (or both) and is located almost exclusively on the lower extremities. The disease starts insidiously in a patient who has complained of intermittent claudication, but sometimes has no pain because of neuropathy in an area of previously traumatized skin. Cellulitis may be minimal, and infection progressively burrows its way to the underlying bone—for example, toe, metatarsal head, tarsal bone.

Physical examination elicits either no pain (with advanced neuropathy) or excruciating pain (if bone destruction has been acute). An area of cellulitis may or may not be present. Crepitus can be felt occasionally, which points toward the presence of either anaerobes or Enterobacteriaceae. Physical examination must include careful evaluation of the vascular supply to the affected limb and of a concomitant neuropathy.

Causes, Diagnosis, and Treatment

As discussed earlier, the whole gamut of human pathogenic bacteria can be isolated, often in multiple combinations. *S. aureus* and β-hemolytic streptococci still predominate in acute soft tissue infections that spread into bone, but any other gram-positive or gram-negative aerobic or anaerobic bacteria may be involved—particularly in previously treated chronic, nosocomial, or more severe infections (see Table 11.1).

The ability to reach bone by gently advancing a sterile surgical probe, combined with plain X-ray, is the best initial approach to the diagnosis of osteomyelitis. If bone is detected on probing, treatment for osteomyelitis is recommended. If bone cannot be detected by probing and plain X-ray does not suggest osteomyelitis, the recommended treatment is a course of antibiotics directed at soft tissue infection. Because occult osteomyelitis may be present, radiography should be repeated in 2 weeks. Further studies such as nuclear magnetic resonance imaging are recommended in doubtful cases.

The prognosis for cure of osteomyelitis associated with vascular insufficiency is poor because of the impaired ability of the host to assist in the eradication of the infectious agent and the inability of systemic antibiotics to gain entry into the site of infection. Determining the extent of vascular compromise is important. This assessment can be made by measurement of transcutaneous oximetry (once

KEY POINTS

About Diabetic and Neuropathic Ischemic Osteomyelitis

1. The most common clinical presentation is a painless ulcer that extends to bone.
2. Acute cellulitis is usually attributable to *Staphylococcus aureus* or β-hemolytic streptococcus that may spread to bone.
3. Chronic ulcer with mild cellulitis and crepitation is often the result of infection by anaerobes or Enterobacteriaceae.
4. Probe the ulcer. If probe reaches bone, the patient has osteomyelitis.
5. Microbiology can include *S. aureus*, mixed gram-positive and gram-negative organisms, and anaerobes.
6. Treatment:
   a) Revascularization when possible. (Hyperbaric oxygen is of no benefit.)
   b) Amputation or debridement may be required.
   c) Antibiotics for 2 to 6 weeks, duration depending on the extent of amputation and soft tissue infection.

inflammation has been controlled) and of pulse pressures by Doppler ultrasonography. If serious ischemia is suspected, arteriography of the lower extremity, including the foot vessels, should be performed.

Treatment includes antimicrobial therapy, debridement surgery, or resection and amputation. The type of treatment offered depends on the oxygen tension in tissue at the infected site, the extent of osteomyelitis and duration of damage, the potential for revascularization, and the preferences of the patient. Revascularization often proves to be useful before amputation is considered. No convincing evidence has been developed to suggest that hyperbaric oxygen is useful for the treatment of diabetic osteomyelitis. Debridement and a 4- to 6-week course of antimicrobial therapy may benefit the patient with localized osteomyelitis and good oxygen tension at the infected site. In the presence of a well-defined pathogen (usually *S. aureus*), 6 weeks of therapy with an initial intravenous agent followed by a switch to an oral agent (if possible) can lead to a high cure rate. If these conditions do not exist, the wound often fails to heal, and resection of localized infected bone or amputation will ultimately be required.

Digital and ray resections, transmetatarsal amputations, and mid-foot disarticulations allow the patient to walk without a prosthesis. The patient should be treated with antimicrobial agents for 4 weeks when infected bone is transected surgically. Anti-infective therapy should be given for 2 weeks when the infected bone is completely removed, because some soft-tissue infection may remain. When the site of amputation is proximal to infected bone and soft tissue, the patient is given standard antimicrobial prophylaxis. In contrast, prolonged therapy is recommended for tarsal or calcaneal osteomyelitis, because the infected bone is debrided and not totally removed.

GENERAL PRINCIPLES FOR THE MANAGEMENT OF OSTEOMYELITIS

The many pathogenic factors, modes of contamination, clinical presentations, and types of orthopedic procedures related to osteomyelitis have precluded a very scientific approach to therapy, with well-controlled, statistically valid studies. Three critical principles govern the management of osteomyelitis.

- Adequate tissue for culture and histopathology
- Specific antimicrobial regimen
- Proper surgical management

Adequate Tissue for Culture and Histopathology

If there is one disease in which adequate sampling for bacteriology is important, it is osteomyelitis, because treatment will be given for many weeks, most often by a parenteral route, after initial culture results are obtained. Adequate sampling of deep infected tissue is thus extremely useful (as compared with superficial specimens obtained from ulcers or fistulae, which are often misleading). After clinical evaluation, a bone biopsy should be performed, and the sample obtained should be submitted for aerobic and anaerobic culture and histopathologic evaluation. Results of Gram stain and culture, ideally obtained before therapy, should be carefully analyzed.

Specific Antimicrobial Regimen

When possible, the patient should receive antimicrobial agents only after the results of cultures and susceptibility tests become available. However, if immediate debridement is required, and significant risk of precipitating bacteremia or spread of infection exists, the patient may receive empiric antimicrobial therapy after culture and before the bacteriologic data are reported. This antimicrobial regimen can be modified, if necessary, on the basis of culture and susceptibility results (see Table 11.2).

Experimental models have clarified some basic principles of antibiotic therapy. Except for the fluoroquinolones, which penetrate unusually well into bone, antibiotic levels in bone 3 to 4 hours after administration are usually quite low as compared to levels in serum. Maximal doses of parental antibiotics should therefore be used. Because revascularization of bone after debridement takes 3 to 4 weeks, prolonged antimicrobial therapy is required to treat viable infected bone and to protect bone that is undergoing revascularization. Parenteral therapy is generally recommended for 4 to 6 weeks. In cases of severe bone necrosis, parenteral therapy may be prolonged to 12 weeks. The start of this therapy is usually dated from the last major debridement. Early antibiotic treatment, given before extensive bone destruction has occurred, produces the best results.

Single-agent chemotherapy is usually adequate for the treatment of osteomyelitis resulting from hematogenous spread. Table 11.2 gives a conventional choice of antimicrobial agents for the most commonly encountered microorganisms. In recent years, new approaches to antimicrobial therapy have been developed experimentally and validated clinically. Thus, in hematogenous osteomyelitis of childhood, parenteral administration of antibiotics may be followed (with an equal success rate) by oral therapy for several weeks, provided that the organism is known, clinical signs abate rapidly, patient compliance is good, and serum antibiotic levels can be monitored. Another approach that is gaining acceptance because of its reduced cost is parenteral administration of antibiotics, first in hospital, and then on an outpatient basis. Outpatient parenteral therapy requires a team of dedicated nurses and physicians, plus minimal social living conditions.

Among new classes of drugs, fluoroquinolones have been one of the most important advances for the treatment of osteomyelitis. They have been shown to be effective in experimental infections and in several randomized and nonrandomized studies in adults. But although their efficacy in the treatment of osteomyelitis caused by most Enterobacteriaceae (which are very sensitive to fluoroquinolones) seems undisputed, their advantage over conventional therapy in osteomyelitis resulting from infection by *Pseudomonas* or *Serratia* species remains to be demonstrated. By contrast, an intravenous to oral switch involving ciprofloxacin (or levofloxacin) with rifampin for susceptible *S. aureus* has become common practice. Long-term oral therapy extending over months and, more rarely, years is aimed at palliation of acute flare-ups of chronic, refractory osteomyelitis. Local administration of antibiotics, either by instillation or using gentamicin-laden beads, has its advocates in both the United States and Europe, but the technique has not been submitted to critical, controlled studies. Antibiotic diffusion is limited in time and space, but may be of some additional benefit in osteomyelitis secondary to a contiguous focus of infection.

Proper Surgical Management

A combined antimicrobial and surgical approach should at least be discussed in all cases. At one end of the spectrum (for example, hematogenous osteomyelitis), surgery usually is unnecessary; at the other end (a consolidated infected fracture), cure may be achieved with minimal antibiotic treatment provided that the foreign material is removed. Proper surgical management includes drainage, thorough debridement, and obliteration of dead space. Ideally, specific antimicrobial therapy is initiated before debridement is undertaken. Debridement includes removal of all orthopedic appliances except those deemed absolutely necessary for stability. Indeed, without stability, bone healing will not occur. Often, debridement must be repeated at least once to ensure removal of all nonviable tissue.

Wound protection is also an important surgical management principle. Open wounds must be covered to prevent bacteria from re-infecting the bone. Posttraumatic infected fractures are especially difficult to treat. A variety of techniques have evolved for management of the exposed bone and any dead spaces created by the trauma and debridement. Examples include the use of local tissue flaps of vascularized tissue transferred from a distant site. Other experimental modalities that are occasionally employed include cancellous bone grafting and implantation of acrylic beads impregnated with one

---

KEY POINTS

About the General Management of Osteomyelitis

1. Adequate tissue must be obtained for culture and histopathology.
2. Empiric antibiotic therapy should usually be avoided.
   a) Once started, therapy must be prolonged for 4 to 6 weeks and sometimes for months.
   b) Outpatient parenteral therapy often utilized.
   c) Hematogenous osteomyelitis may be treated orally in children; in adults, ciprofloxacin plus rifampin may be also used for susceptible *Staphylococcus aureus*.
3. Surgery is often required for drainage, debridement, obliteration of dead space, and wound coverage.
4. Assessment of response and definitive cure are difficult. Relapse may occur.
   a) C-Reactive protein and symptomatic improvement are the best parameters. Imaging study improvement can be very delayed.
   b) Cure is the resolution of signs and symptoms for more than 1 year.

---

or more antibacterial agents. Finally, in patients with osteomyelitis, Ilizarov's fixation device allows major segmental resections, in combination with new bone growth, to progressively fill in the defect; however, the process is slow (months to years).

Assessment of Clinical Response

Assessing the response to therapy can be difficult, because bed rest or modification of physical activity by itself can temporarily improve symptoms. And despite appropriate antibiotic therapy, the radiologic and MRI changes of osteomyelitis can worsen for several weeks. Therefore, during antibiotic therapy, serial radiologic or MRI studies are not recommended. Clinical response and ESR or CRP are probably the most helpful objective criteria available for monitoring response to therapy.

Because of the protracted clinical course of osteomyelitis, cure is defined as the resolution of all signs and symptoms of active disease at the end of therapy, and after a minimal post-treatment observation period of 1 year. By contrast, failure is defined as a lack of apparent response to therapy, as evidenced by one or more of

1. persistence of drainage;
2. recurrence of a sinus tract or failure of a sinus tract to close;
3. persistence of systemic signs of infection (chills, fever, weight loss, bone pain); and
4. progression of bone infection shown by imaging methods—for example, radiography, CT, MRI.

■ INFECTIONS IN PROSTHETIC JOINTS

PATHOGENESIS AND MICROBIOLOGY

Infections following total replacement of the hip joint are divided into three categories that reflect the time course and pathogenesis:

1. Acute contiguous infections are recognized within the first 6 months after surgery and are often evident within the first few days or weeks. These infections result either directly from infected skin, subcutaneous tissue, and muscle, or from operative hematoma.
2. Chronic contiguous infections are diagnosed 6 to 24 months after surgery, usually because of persistent pain. In most cases, infection is believed to result from contamination at the time of surgery with microorganisms of lower pathogenicity. The infection progresses slowly to a chronic form before it is recognized.
3. Hematogenous infections, as discussed earlier, are diagnosed more than 2 years after surgery and arise from late transient bacteremia with selective persistence of the microorganisms in the joint.

Coagulase-positive and coagulase-negative staphylococci are the microorganisms most often isolated from infected prosthetic hip joints, accounting for three quarters of the bacteria cultured.

CASE 11.2

A 75–year-old white man with a history of diabetes mellitus for 38 years presented with fever and severe left knee pain over 10 days. He had suffered with osteoarthritis for many years, and 5 years earlier, he had had bilateral placement of hip prostheses followed 2 years later by replacement of both knees. Four

months before admission, he began to experience right knee pain that steadily worsened, until 10 days before admission, he began experiencing very severe pain accompanied by fever to 38.9°C and increased warmth and erythema of the right knee.

Physical findings included a temperature 39°C. In general appearance, the patient was pale and chronically ill appearing. Examination of the right knee revealed marked edema, erythema, and warmth, with decreased range of motion secondary to pain. No instability of the knee joint was noted.

Laboratory findings included a WBC count of 13,000/mm³, with 87% PMNs and 5% bands; a hematocrit of 29%; and an ESR exceeding 100 mm/h. Gram stain of knee aspirate showed many PMNs and gram-positive cocci in chains. Culture revealed group B streptococci.

CLINICAL MANIFESTATIONS AND DIAGNOSIS

Most patients have no elevation in temperature and present with a painful joint that is found to be unstable by physical examination or X-ray. Because of the difficulty of distinguishing loosening of the joint secondary to a noninfectious inflammatory process from that due to an infection, a positive culture of fluid aspirated from the artificial joint space or of bone from the bone–cement interface (or both) is required, as performed in case 11.2. Culture of a needle aspirate remains the diagnostic method of choice. Because the microorganisms responsible for these types of infections colonize the skin, Gram stain and quantitative cultures obtained from deep tissues are very useful for distinguishing colonization from infection.

TREATMENT

Classically, two approaches to treatment exist. With one-stage exchange arthroplasty, the infected components are excised, surgical debridement is performed, and a new prosthesis is immediately put into place. Several proponents of this technique use cement containing an antimicrobial drug—a factor that may contribute to the high success rate reported for the procedure. A second approach requires surgical removal of all foreign bodies, debridement of the bone and soft tissues, and a minimum of 4 weeks of parenteral antimicrobial therapy. Reconstruction is performed after the completion of therapy for "less virulent infections," but is delayed for several months for infections that are "more virulent."

KEY POINTS

About the Pathogenesis, Microbiology, Clinical Manifestations, and Diagnosis of Prosthetic Joint Infections

1. Prosthetic joint infections take three forms:
   a) Acute contiguous infection (less than 6 months after surgery)
   b) Chronic contiguous infection (6 to 24 months after surgery)
   c) Hematogenous spread (more than 24 months after surgery)
2. Microbiology:
   a) Three quarters of cases are caused by *Staphylococcus*.
   b) *S. aureus* produces a more acute presentation.
   c) Coagulase-negative staphylococci are most common, with a more insidious presentation.
3. Clinical manifestations are difficult to differentiate from mechanical loosening:
   a) Joint pain
   b) Fever often not present
4. Diagnosis by joint aspiration with quantitative culture and Gram stain is preferred.

KEY POINTS

About the Treatment of Prosthetic Joint Infections

1. In early acute infection, local debridement and prolonged antibiotic therapy are the treatment of choice. (A rifampin-containing antibiotic combination should be selected for susceptible staphylococci.)
2. When prosthetic loosening has occurred, removal of the prosthesis is usually required.
   a) The one-step procedure includes antibiotic-impregnated cement.
   b) Removal, debridements, and a minimum of 4 to 6 weeks of antibiotic therapy are followed by observation.
   c) With "less virulent" pathogens, the prosthesis is replaced after more than 3 months. With "more virulent" pathogens, replacement is done after up to 1 year.

In the early stages of infection, when the prosthesis is still firmly in place, it is possible to attempt to achieve a cure with only localized debridement and systemic antibiotics (usually a duration of 3 months for hip prosthesis and 6 months for a knee prosthesis), without removal of the prosthesis. Overall, however, this infection remains difficult to cure. Incidence of relapse is approximately 10% at 3 years and 26% after 10 years.

■ SEPTIC ARTHRITIS (EXCLUDING REACTIVE ARTHRITIS)

POTENTIAL SEVERITY

Delays in appropriate therapy can lead to irreversible joint damage.

Infectious arthritis is a serious condition because of its potential to lead to significant joint morbidity and disability if the condition is not detected and treated early.

PATHOGENESIS, PREDISPOSING FACTORS, AND MICROBIOLOGY

Septic arthritis primarily arises with hematogenous spread of bacteria to the synovial membrane lining the joint. An acute inflammatory reaction results in infiltration by PMNs. Bacteria and inflammatory cells quickly spread to the synovial fluid, leading to joint swelling and erythema. Cytokines and proteases are released into the synovial fluid and, if not quickly treated, cause cartilage damage and eventually narrowing of the joint space.

The causes of bacteremia leading to septic arthritis include urinary tract infection, intravenous drug abuse, intravenous catheters, and soft tissue infections. Patients with bacterial endocarditis, particularly when caused by *S. aureus* or *Enterococcus*, can present with septic arthritis. Patients with underlying joint disease are at higher risk for developing infection of the previously damaged joint. Patients with rheumatoid arthritis and osteoarthritis most commonly develop this complication. The use of new immunosuppressive agents to control rheumatoid arthritis can also predispose patients to septic arthritis caused by opportunistic pathogens. Patients with HIV infection also have a higher risk of septic arthritis and are more likely to be infected with a fungus or mycobacteria. Sometimes the predisposing factor is minor trauma or an upper respiratory infection. Unfortunately, a common medically induced cause is the intra-articular injection of corticosteroids leading to bacterial superinfection. Intravenous drug abusers have an increased risk of developing septic arthritis of their sternoclavicular joints.

S. aureus remains the most common cause of infectious arthritis. Other common causes include, in young adults, *Neisseria gonorrhoeae* (presenting sometimes as disseminated gonococcal infection) and gram-negative bacilli in elderly individuals (often secondary to urinary tract infection). Patients taking tumor necrosis factor inhibitors can develop joint infections with *Listeria monocytogenes* or *Salmonella*. Intravenous drug abusers most commonly suffer with septic arthritis caused by methicillin-resistant *S. aureus* or, less commonly, *P. aeruginosa*. Certain viruses such as parvovirus B19, hepatitis B virus, rubella, mumps, and HIV can be causes of acute arthritis. Mycobacterial and fungal infections commonly cause chronic monoarticular arthritis, often following the intra-articular administration of corticosteroids. Lyme arthritis caused by *Borrelia burgdorferi* is a diagnosis to be considered in the appropriate epidemiologic setting: it may occur as an acute transient arthritis or, more rarely, as a late chronic arthritis (see Chapter 13).

CASE 11.3

A 19–year-old black woman presented to her physician with a 3-day history of progressive swelling of her left knee. The knee was hot to the touch and painful to move. She denied any sexual contacts in the past year. She also denied fever or chills.

On physical examination, she was afebrile. No skin rashes were evident. The only positive finding was a swollen left knee that was erythematous and warm to touch. Fluid was readily palpable. Any movement of the knee caused moderate pain.

A laboratory workup found a peripheral WBC count of 7100/mm³, with 71% PMNs. Needle aspiration of the joint revealed a WBC count of 102,000/mm³, with 95% PMNs. Gram stain of the aspirate showed many PMNs and gram-positive cocci. Culture was positive for S. aureus. Blood cultures were negative.

CLINICAL MANIFESTATIONS, DIAGNOSIS AND TREATMENT

As illustrated by case 11.3, the primary manifestations of septic arthritis are swelling and pain in a single joint accompanied by fever. Elderly patients may be afebrile at the time of presentation. Connective tissue diseases usually present with bilateral joint involvement; any patient with monoarticular arthritis should therefore be considered to have septic arthritis until proven otherwise. In addition to being swollen, the infected joint is usually warm to the touch, and any movement of the joint is accompanied by exquisite pain. The most commonly involved joints in adults are the knee (40% to 50%) and hip (15% to 20%) followed by the shoulder, wrist, ankle, and elbow. In children, the hip joint is most commonly affected (60%), followed by the knee joint (35%). Nearly half of patients who develop septic arthritis have an underlying chronic joint disease such as rheumatoid arthritis or osteoarthritis. Damage to the synovial membrane probably increases the likelihood of bacterial invasion.

The critical diagnostic test is analysis of the synovial fluid. The synovial fluid leukocyte count is normally below 180/mm³, and a count that exceeds 200 is generally considered inflammatory. In acute infections, the count is often (but not always) over 50,000, with a

---

KEY POINTS

About Septic Arthritis

1. Usually results from hematogenous spread.

2. Primary causes are *Staphylococcus aureus* [including methicillin-resistant (MRSA) strains], gram-negative rods, and *Neisseria gonorrhoeae*.

3. Immunocompromised patients may be infected with *Listeria* or *Salmonella*.

4. Acute monoarticular arthritis is septic arthritis until proven otherwise.

5. Joint fluid usually shows more than 50,000 white blood cells per cubic millimeter (mainly polymorphonuclear leukocytes). Gram stain and culture are usually positive.

6. Therapy should include
   a) joint drainage, and
   b) systemic antibiotics for 3 to 4 weeks (nafcillin or oxacillin for *S. aureus*; a third-generation cephalosporin or fluoroquinolone for gram-negative organisms; vancomycin for MRSA).

predominance of PMNs. Gram stain reveals gram-positive microorganisms in 75% to 80% of patients, but that percentage is lower in the presence of gram-negative or *N. gonorrhoeae* infection. Blood cultures are positive in a significant proportion of cases. When *N. gonorrhoeae* infection is suspected, it may be useful to plate pharyngeal, rectal, cervical, or urethral specimens onto selected gonococcal media. The polymerase chain reaction (PCR) technique has been used with success to detect *B. burgdorferi* DNA and gonococcal arthritis. Analysis of the urine for gonococcal disease by PCR may also be helpful. Crystals should be sought, because crystal arthropathy may be inflammatory in the absence of infection or may even coexist with infection.

Therapy of infectious arthritis has two important components. The first is complete drainage and washing of the purulent exudate by arthroscopy when possible (example: the knee joint) or by surgery when arthroscopy is not possible (example: the hip joint)—in particular for *S. aureus* or gram-negative infection. If the activated polymorphonuclear leukocytes are allowed to remain in the joint space, these cells will continue to mediate a powerful inflammatory response that can lead to irreversible cartilaginous damage. The second component of therapy is administration of the most appropriate antibiotic based on Gram stain, bacterial culture results, or clinical presentation. The antibiotic regimens are identical to those used for osteomyelitis (see Table 11.2); however, the duration of treatment after appropriate drainage is usually shorter: 3 to 4 weeks.

Despite the development of more effective antibiotics, the outcome of septic arthritis has not improved. One third of patients experience significant residual joint damage. An adverse outcome is more likely in elderly patients and in patients with pre-existing joint disease or infection in a joint containing synthetic material.

■ DISSEMINATED GONOCOCCAL INFECTION

One to 3% of patients infected with *N. gonorrhoeae* develop disseminated disease, and the most common manifestation of this complication is monoarticular or polyarticular arthritis.

PATHOGENESIS AND PREDISPOSING FACTORS

Progression of localized gonococcal disease to disseminated disease requires that the bacterium gain entry into the bloodstream. The most important factor predisposing to bacteremia is delay in antibiotic treatment. Most patients who develop disseminated disease have a mucosal

infection that is asymptomatic. Women are more likely to have asymptomatic disease than men are, and women are three times more likely than men to develop disseminated disease. In women, dissemination often follows menstruation, and it is likely that during endometrial bleeding bacteria can more readily invade the bloodstream. Similarly, asymptomatically infected women who are postpartum are more likely to develop disseminated disease.

The terminal complement cascade plays an important role in killing *Neisseria* species, and patients that have congenital or acquired deficiencies (including patients with systemic lupus erythematosus) of the terminal complement components (C5–C8) have a higher risk of developing disseminated gonococcal and meningococcal infection. Bacterial virulence factors are also likely to play a role in dissemination. *N. gonorrhoeae* strains that fail to express the outer membrane protein II and that form transparent colonies on culture plates are more likely to disseminate. As compared with strains that cause urethritis, most strains associated with disseminated disease are penicillin-sensitive.

CLINICAL MANIFESTATIONS, DIAGNOSIS, AND TREATMENT

Disseminated gonococcal infection is primarily a disease of sexually active young adults or teenagers. Patients usually present with one of two syndromes:

KEY POINTS

About Disseminated Gonococcal Disease

1. Occurs most commonly in patients with asymptomatic mucosal infections.
   a) More common in women
   b) Higher incidence postpartum or following menstruation
   c) Higher incidence in patients with terminal complement deficiencies
2. Two clinical syndromes are associated with dissemination:
   a) Tenosynovitis, dermatitis, polyarthritis—tenosynovitis is pathognomic; pustular skin lesions range in number from 4 to 40, periarticular
   b) Purulent arthritis
3. Treat with intravenous ceftriaxone, followed by oral cefixime or a fluoroquinolone.

1. **Tenosynovitis, dermatitis, and polyarthritis syndrome.** The first manifestations of disease are fever, malaise, and arthralgias. Subsequently, inflammation of the tendons in the wrist, fingers, and (less commonly) the ankles and toes is noted. On examination, tenderness is noted over the tendon sheaths, and pain is exacerbated by movement. The development of tenosynovitis in a young person is virtually pathognomic for disseminated gonococcemia. Pustular, pustular–vesicular, and (less commonly) hemorrhagic or papular skin lesions accompany the onset of tenosynovitis. Lesions are often periarticular, relatively few in number (usually 4 to 10, rarely more than 40), and transient, spontaneously resolving over 3 to 4 days. If untreated, patients with this syndrome may progress to purulent arthritis.

2. **Purulent arthritis without skin lesions.** The purulent form of arthritis is similar to other forms of septic arthritis, with high numbers of PMNs being found in the synovial fluid.

Blood samples for culture should be drawn in all patients with suspected disseminated gonococcal disease. Cultures are positive in about half of all cases. Blood cultures are more frequently positive in patients with the tenosynovitis–dermatitis–polyarthritis syndrome. Culture and Gram stains of joint aspirates should also be performed, but are frequently unrevealing. Culture and Gram stain of cervical and urethral exudates and of skin lesion scrapings should also be obtained. Where PCR of the urine for gonococcus is available, this test may also be obtained.

Because of the increasing incidence of penicillin-resistant strains of *N. gonorrhoeae*, disseminated gonococcal infection is usually treated with parenteral ceftriaxone (1 g daily, intravenously or intramuscularly) that should be continued for 24 to 48 hours after clinical improvement. Patients can then be switched to an oral regimen such cefixime, ciprofloxacin, ofloxacin, or levofloxacin to complete 7 to 10 days of therapy if the strain is sensitive. Alternative regimens, including parenteral administration of other third-generation cephalosporins, a fluoroquinolone, or spectinomycin are also available (see Table 9.3). Management of purulent joint effusions is identical to that for other forms of septic arthritis. As compared with infection caused by *S. aureus* and gram-negative bacilli, *N. gonorrhoeae* infection seldom results in residual joint damage.

FURTHER READING

Caputo GM, Cavanagh PR, Ulbrecht JS, Gibbons GW, Karchmer AW. Assessment and management of foot disease in patients with diabetes. *New Engl J Med.* 1994;331) 854–860.

Gavet F, Tournadre A, Soubrier M, Ristori JM, Dubost JJ. Septic arthritis in patients aged 80 and older: a comparison with younger adults. *J Am Geriatr Soc.* 2005;53:1210–1213.

Katsarolis I, Tsiodras S, Panagopoulos P, et al. Septic arthritis due to *Salmonella enteritidis* associated with infliximab use. *Scand J Infect Dis.* 2005;37:304–305.

Lew DP, Waldvogel FA. Osteomyelitis. *N Engl J Med.* 1997;336:999–1007.

Lew DP, Waldvogel FA. Use of quinolones in osteomyelitis and infected orthopaedic prosthesis. *Drugs.* 1999;58 (Suppl 2): 85–91.

Lew DP, Waldvogel FA. Osteomyelitis. *Lancet.* 2004;364:369–379.

Lispky BA, Berendt AR, Deery HG, et al. Diagnosis and treatment of diabetic foot infections. *Clin Infect Dis.* 2004;39:885–910.

O'Brien JP, Goldenberg DL, Rice PA. Disseminated gonococcal infection: a prospective analysis of 49 patients and a review of the pathophysiology and immune mechanisms. *Medicine (Baltimore).* 1983;62:395–406.

Ross JJ, Shamsuddin H. Sternoclavicular septic arthritis: review of 180 cases. *Medicine (Baltimore).* 2004;83:139–148.

Schett G, Herak P, Graninger W, Smolen JS, Aringer M. *Listeria*-associated arthritis in a patient undergoing etanercept therapy: case report and review of the literature. *J Clin Microbiol.* 2005;43:2537–2541.

Shirtliff ME, Mader JT. Acute septic arthritis. *Clin Microbiol Rev.* 2002;15:527–544.

Zimmerli W, Trampuz A, Ochsner PE. Prosthetic-joint infections. *N Engl J Med.* 2004;351:1645–1654.

Parasitic Infections

12

Time Recommended to Complete: 2 days

Frederick Southwick, M.D.

GUIDING QUESTIONS

1. What is meant by a parasitic infection?

2. Why are parasitic infections increasing in incidence in the United States and Europe?

3. What patient population is particularly at risk for severe and life threatening parasitic infections?

What does the infectious disease specialist mean by parasitic infection?

Most infectious agents fulfill the definition of a parasite: an organism that grows, feeds, and shelters on or in a different organism and contributes nothing to the host. However, medical science has created the classification "parasite" to include a complex group of nonfungal eukaryotic human pathogens. Unlike fungi, parasites have no cell wall and are often motile. In addition, many parasites require two or more host species to complete their life cycle, and they reproduce both sexually and asexually. The host in which sexual reproduction takes place is called the "definitive host," and the one in which asexual reproduction occurs is called the "intermediate host."

Previously, parasitic infections were almost exclusively a health problem in developing countries with poor sanitation. However, with the current marked rise in international travel and increased military deployments to endemic areas, these infections are now increasingly being diagnosed in the United States, Europe, and other developed countries. The incidence of symptomatic parasitic infections has also increased because of the ever-increasing population of immunocompromised hosts. Organ transplant, cancer chemotherapy, and infection with HIV all lead to depressed cell-mediated and humoral immunity, allowing dormant parasites to reactivate and cause disease. More than ever before, thorough travel and exposure histories are critical steps in accurately diagnosing parasitic infections. An awareness of geography and environmental conditions and a familiarity with the life cycles of various parasites are all required for proper diagnosis and treatment.

■ BLOOD PROTOZOA

POTENTIAL SEVERITY

Hours can make the difference between life and death. Rapid diagnosis and treatment are critical.

MALARIA

GUIDING QUESTIONS

1. Which form of malaria is the most dangerous, and why?

2. Which disease does malaria most commonly mimic?

3. How is malaria diagnosed? Is there a particular time in the course of illness when diagnostic studies should be performed?

4. Why are many African Americans more resistant to some forms of malaria?

5. What are the current recommendations for malaria treatment, and what are the factors that dictate the regimen of choice?

6. When should chemoprophylaxis be begun, and how long after completion of a trip to an endemic area should preventive therapy be continued?

Prevalence

The combination of deteriorating political and economic conditions in the countries of sub-Saharan Africa and the development of chloroquine drug resistance in many parts of the world have resulted in a resurgence of malaria. Climate change and the increased resistance of mosquitoes to insecticides have also contributed to this trend. The worldwide annual incidence of malaria is between 300 and 500 million cases, causing between 1 and 2 million deaths. Areas with significant numbers of malaria cases include Africa, the Middle East, India, Southeast Asia, South America, Central America, and parts of the Caribbean.

Chloroquine resistance is now the rule in most countries. *Plasmodium falciparum* in Southeast Asia is frequently resistant not only to chloroquine, but also to pyrimethamine–sulfadoxine, mefloquine, and halofantrine. Areas in which *P. falciparum* remains sensitive to chloroquine include Central America and the Caribbean, in particular Haiti. In the United States, secondary cases have been reported around airports, and an outbreak of *P. vivax* was recently described in Palm Beach, Florida. Because the sensitivity patterns of malaria continue to change annually, the Centers for Disease Control and Prevention (CDC) should be consulted for the most up-to-date information (Web address: www.cdc.gov/travel).

Epidemiology and Life Cycle

Humans contract malaria after being bitten by the anophiline female mosquito. Only the female mosquito takes a blood meal, because blood is required for the development of the mosquito egg. Certain strains appear to be more efficient transmitters of disease. In particular *Anopheles gambiae* and *A. funestus* are thought to account for the high transmission rates in sub-Saharan Africa. These strains are not present in South America and Southeast Asia where transmission rates are lower. Clearly the larger the number of mosquito bites a person receives, the greater the risk of contracting malaria. Therefore, in addition to chemoprophylaxis (discussed later in this subsection), mosquito netting, long-sleeved shirts, long pants, insect repellant, and staying in a protected environment during the times of the day when mosquitoes are at their most active are all recommended as preventive measures.

The sporozoites introduced into the human bloodstream by the female anophiline mosquito quickly travel to the liver and invade hepatocytes (Figure 12.1). Sporozoites contain a specific protein thought to be critical for binding and entry into hepatocytes. This circumsporozoite protein binds to specific host-cell membrane receptors (heparin sulfate proteoglycans and

Life Cycle of Plasmodium

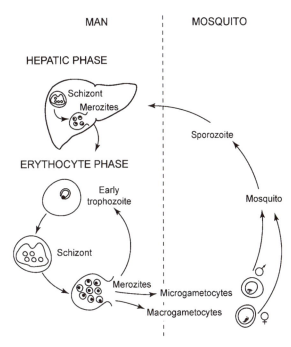

Figure 12–1. Life cycle of *Plasmodium*.

low-density lipoprotein receptor–related protein). Within the hepatocytes, most sporozoites mature to tissue schizonts. Some sporozoites become dormant, This dormant form, called a hypnozoite takes 6 to 11 months to activate into a tissue schizont. Each schizont-infected hepatocyte then produces 10,000 to 30,000 merozoites that are released into the bloodstream following cell lysis. Each merozoite can invade a single red blood cell and asexually replicate five times over 48 to 72 hours to produce 32 merozoites. The red blood cell then undergoes lysis, releasing the newly formed merozoites, which can infect additional red blood cells.

Under ideal conditions, a single sporozoite could theoretically account for the infection of nearly 1 million red blood cells (many of the free merozoites are intercepted by host macrophages, thus reducing the efficiency of red cell infection). As observed with sporozoite entry into hepatocytes, a specific protein on the merozoite surface (erythrocyte-binding antigen 175 in *P. falciparum* and Pv135 in *P. vivax*) binds to a specific red blood cell membrane receptor (glycophorin A in *P. falciparum* and Duffy factor in *P. vivax*) allowing attachment and entry. Once the merozoite enters the red blood cell, it matures to a trophozoite. This form looks like a signet ring and can readily be seen in parasitized red blood cells following Giemsa or

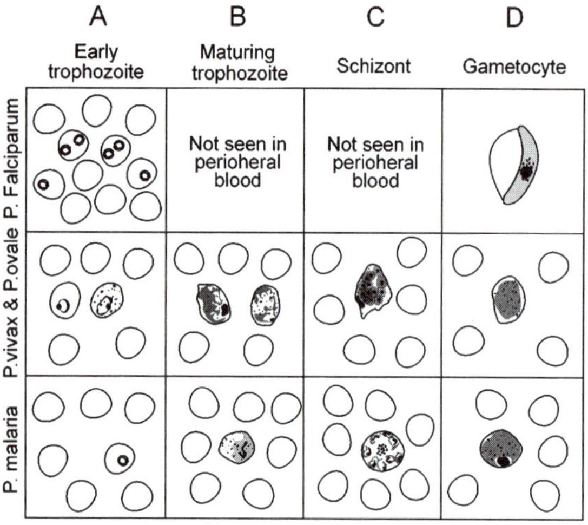

Figure 12–2. Typical blood smear findings for various forms of malaria. (Adapted from Schaechter M, Engleberg NC, Eisenstein BI, Medoff G, editors. *Mechanisms of Microbial Disease.* 3rd edition. Baltimore, Md.: Lippincott Williams and Wilkins; 1999)

Wright staining (Figure 12.2). As the trophozoite matures, it loses its signet ring morphology, becoming larger and subsequently developing into a red blood cell schizont, which then splits into multiple merozoites.

Upon entry into the red blood cell, some merozoites mature into sexual forms called gametocytes rather than into asexual forms. The male form is smaller and is called a microgametocyte; the larger female form is called a macrogametocyte. Because sexual mating does not occur in the human host, but only in the mosquito, the mosquito is considered the definitive host, and humans are considered the intermediate host.

Once fertilization occurs, a zygote is formed that subsequently develops into an oocyst. The oocyst then forms thousands of infectious sporozoites that gain entry into the mosquito salivary gland, where they are transmitted to the human host.

Life cycle Differences Between the Various Plasmodium Species

P. falciparum is the most common, and most dangerous, form of malaria. Unlike the sporozoites of other strains, all falciparum sporozoites that enter the liver remain active and develop into tissue schizonts that proceed to form thousands of merozoites. And unlike the merozoites of other strains, *P. falciparum* merozoites can infect red blood cells of all ages, explaining the high level of parasitized red blood cells observed in falciparum malaria. Moreover, in the non-falciparum forms of

malaria only a single merozoite gains entry into a given red cell; in falciparum malaria, multiple merozoites can infect and mature within a single red blood cell.

Once a merozoite has invaded a red blood cell, it rapidly matures, asexually divides, and within 48 hours, lyses the host cell. This rapid asexual reproduction produces a rapid rise in the percentage of infected host red blood cells, and as the percentage of parasitized red blood cells increases, the risk of death or serious complications also increases.

P. falciparum is more harmful to the host because invasion by this strain is uniquely associated with the formation of red blood cell membrane knobs that tightly adhere to the vascular endothelium. These knobs express erythrocyte membrane protein 1 on their surface, and this protein binds complement receptor 1 (CR-1) on uninfected red cells, causing red cell clumping ("rosetting"). These adherent red blood cells block blood flow in small blood vessels, causing severe hypoxic damage, particularly to the brain and kidneys. Because red blood cell adherence develops as the merozoite matures beyond the early trophozoite stage, other maturation stages of the parasite (with the exception of the banana-shaped gametocytes) are rarely seen in the peripheral blood (see Table 12.1 and Figure 12.2).

P. vivax is the next most common form of malaria. *P. malariae* is less common, and *P. ovale* is a rare human infection. When a female anophiline mosquito bites an infected human, gametocytes are taken in with the blood. *P. vivax* and *P. ovale* can form hypnozoites that can remain dormant within the liver for months before becoming active tissue schizonts. This behavior explains the ability of these strains to relapse 6 to 11 months after initial treatment. *P. malariae* has no dormant liver phase, but can persist as a low-level infection for up to 30 years. *P. vivax* and *P. ovale* merozoites bind only young red blood cells, having the highest affinity for reticulocytes. *P. malariae* tends to

---

KEY POINTS

About the Lifecycle of *Plasmodium falciparum*

P. falciparum is the most dangerous form of malaria because it

1. infects red blood cells (RBCs) of all ages and causes high levels of parasitemia.

2. induces the formation of knobs on the RBC surface that adhere to vessel walls and to uninfected RBCs, causing obstruction and local hypoxia.

3. can cause severe hemolysis, renal failure, central nervous system damage, and pulmonary edema.

Table 12.1. Differences in Malaria Strains

Strain	Characteristics
Plasmodium falciparum	No dormant phase in the liver Multiple "signet ring" trophozoites per cell High percentage (>5%) of parasitized red blood cells Development stages other than the early signet-ring trophozoite and mature gametocyte not seen
Plasmodium vivax and *Plasmodium ovale*	Dormant liver phase Single signet-ring trophozoites per cell Schuffner's dots in the cytoplasm Low percentage (>5%) of parasitized red blood cells All developmental stages seen Red blood cells often appear enlarged in the later stages
Plasmodium malariae	No dormant phase Single signet-ring trophozoite per cell Very low level parasitemia All developmental stages seen Red blood cells normal size

infect older red blood cells. The inability of these strains to infect a broad age range of red blood cells explains their low level of parasitemia. Furthermore, these three strains do not form knobs and do not obstruct the microcirculation, explaining their milder clinical manifestations.

In Malaysia, *P. knowlesi*, a form of malaria formerly thought to infect only monkeys, has been identified in humans. Its trophozoite stage is similar in morphology to that of *P. falciparum*, and its schizont stage is similar to that of *P. malariae*. The level of parasitism can be high, resulting in serious infections. *P. knowlesi* should be considered in individuals traveling to forested tropical regions where monkeys are known to be infected.

Genetic and Other Determinants of Susceptibility to Malaria

In areas in which malaria is endemic, the high prevalence of genetic traits that reduce susceptibility to malaria serves as remarkable examples of Darwinian evolution. Specific mutations that affect the surface proteins, cytoskeleton, and hemoglobin of red blood cells all interfere with *Plasmodium* invasion, survival, and spread, and thereby provide a survival advantage to the infected host. Absence of the Duffy blood group antigen blocks invasion by *P. vivax*. This strain of malaria must bind to this particular blood group antigen to gain entry into red blood cells. A significant number of black Africans are Duffy-negative and are resistant to *P. vivax*. Individuals with mutations in CR-1 demonstrate reduced rosetting in association with *P. falciparum* and have a decreased propensity to produce cerebral malaria. Individuals with hereditary ovalocytosis, elliptocytosis, and spherocytosis all have defects in specific

red blood cell cytoskeleton proteins, and these defects interfere with entry and release of the malaria parasite.

A broad range of hemoglobinopathies are protective against malaria. The high prevalence of sickle cell disease and sickle cell trait in Africa illustrates the frighteningly efficient selective powers of the deadly *P. falciparum* parasite. Parasite growth is slowed in cells with sickle cell hemoglobin (Hb S). In addition, when parasitized red blood cells that contain Hb S form membrane knobs and become trapped in small vessels, oxygen tension decreases, and the Hb S polymerizes, resulting in sickling of red blood cells. The polymerization of Hb S kills the *P. falciparum* parasite, preventing the infection from progressing. As a consequence, people with sickle cell trait and sickle cell disease are resistant to severe *P. falciparum* infection. Because the other strains of malaria do not form knobs and do not become trapped in blood vessels, Hb S does not protect against *P. vivax*, *P. ovale*, or *P. malariae*. A number of other hemoglobinopathies including Hb C, Hb E, α-thalassemia, and to a lesser extent, β-thalassemia reduce the severity of *P. falciparum*, accounting for their increased prevalence in endemic areas. Neonates are protected from severe malaria as a consequence of fetal hemoglobin, which interferes with the intracellular growth of *P. falciparum*.

In areas that have a high incidence of malaria, the indigenous population is continually exposed the parasite, resulting in a high level of immunity. In these regions, severe disease is rare. However, because the immune response to malaria is short-lived, immunity wanes in regions in which malaria has been controlled and the attack rate is low. Paradoxically, the percentage of patients developing severe disease increases in these regions.

KEY POINTS

About Genetics and Other Factors that Affect Susceptibility to Malaria

1. Surface proteins on red blood cells:
   a) Individuals negative for the Duffy blood group antigen are resistant to *Plasmodium vivax*.
   b) Complement receptor 1 mutations reduce the severity of *P. falciparum* infection.
2. Cytoskeleton defects in red blood cells are protective:
   a) Hereditary ovalocytosis
   b) Hereditary elliptocytosis
   c) Hereditary spherocytosis
3. Hemoglobinopathies confer resistance:
   a) Sickle cell disease and sickle cell trait are resistant to *P. falciparum*.
   b) Other hemoglobin mutations and fetal hemoglobin are also resistant to *P. falciparum*.
4. Low-level immunity increases the risk for severe disease:
   a) Population immunity wanes in areas with low attack rates.
   b) Tourists lack immunity.
   c) In pregnant women, the placenta is affected, resulting in low birth weight infants.

Tourists with no previous exposure to malaria are at highest risk for life-threatening disease (see case 10.1). Pregnant women and their fetuses are also at risk. *P. falciparum* binds to chondroitin sulfate A in the intervillous space of the placenta, causing hemolytic anemia, which leads to low birth weight infants.

Clinical Presentation

CASE 12.1

A married couple was sailing in the Caribbean near Jamaica with their three children. They lived primarily on their boat, but took several day trips to a small island off the coast of Jamaica. They noted some mosquito bites and ate some fruit while on the island. The man and the woman both suddenly came down with fever, chills, muscle aches, and loss of appetite. About 3 days into the illness, the man became jaundiced and began passing dark urine. The family sought treatment from a local Jamaican physician, who diagnosed hepatitis secondary to ingestion of a toxic food. Two days later, the man became comatose and died. The woman was referred to the university hospital for possible liver transplant. On further questioning, the medical staff learned that none of the children were sick despite eating the same diet. The family had begun a course of malaria prophylaxis. However, the parents had developed side effects from the chloroquine and had discontinued prophylaxis 2 weeks before the onset of their illness. Thin smears of the woman's blood revealed many signet-ring trophozoites, with a parasitemia level estimated to be 10%. She was treated with intravenous quinine and rapidly improved. In retrospect, her husband was determined to have died of untreated blackwater fever.

As described in case 12.1, the clinical manifestations of malaria are nonspecific. If the exposure history is not appreciated, the infection can be mistaken for other febrile illnesses. The incubation period is generally 9 to 40 days, but it may be prolonged in cases of non-falciparum malaria (6 to 12 months in *P. vivax*, and years for *P. malariae* and *P. ovale*).

The hallmark of all forms of malaria is fever. Fever can occur at regular 2 to 3-day intervals in *P. vivax* and *P. malariae*, or in a more irregular pattern with *P. falciparum*. Fever generally occurs soon after lysis of the red blood cells and release of the merozoites. Three classic stages of the febrile paroxysms have been described:

1. The initial "cold stage" occurs 15 to 60 minutes before the onset of fever. During this period, the patient feels cold and has shaking chills.
2. These symptoms are followed by the "hot stage," during which body temperature rises to between 39°C and 41°C. Fever is associated with lassitude, loss of appetite, and vague pains in the bones and joints. In nonendemic areas, these symptoms are most commonly mistaken for influenza. The clinician must always consider malaria in individuals who develop flu-like symptoms after returning from a developing country. Other symptoms associated with the fever include tachycardia, hypotension, cough, headache, back pain, nausea, abdominal pain, vomiting, diarrhea, and altered consciousness.
3. Usually within 2 to 6 hours, symptoms progress to the third "sweating" stage, at which time the patient develops marked diaphoresis, followed by resolution of the fever, profound fatigue, and a desire to sleep.

Other symptoms depend on the strain of malaria. In cases of *P. vivax*, *P. ovale*, and *P. malariae*, there are a few additional symptoms. However, depending on the prior immune status of the host, individuals with *P. falciparum* can develop a severe fatal illness similar to that described in case 12.1. Because *P. falciparum* infects red blood cells of all ages and induces the formation of knobs on the red blood cell surface that adhere to endothelial cells and obstruct small vessels, this parasite can cause severe damage, particularly to the kidneys, brain, and lungs. Tourists who have no immunity to *P. falciparum* and people who have undergone splenectomy can develop very high levels of parasitemia that result in profound hemolysis. The marked release of hemoglobin can exceed the metabolic capacity of the liver. The resulting rise in unconjugated bilirubin in the bloodstream produces jaundice. Hemoglobin also may be excreted into the urine, causing the urine to become dark. The combination of jaundice and hemoglobinuria has been called blackwater fever.

Severe malaria is commonly complicated by renal failure. Heavy infection with *P. falciparum* also results in obstruction of the small arteries in the central nervous system (CNS), leading to hypoxia. Hypoglycemia may also contribute to CNS dysfunction. Confusion and obtundation can rapidly progress to coma. Grand mal seizures may also develop. Pulmonary edema is a less common complication of *P. falciparum* infection, being the result of fluid leakage from pulmonary capillaries into the alveoli.

Diagnosis

Microscopic examination of a Giemsa-stained blood smear remains the primary way to identify malaria. In *P. falciparum*, blood smears are best taken just after the fever peak, when early ring forms are most abundant in peripheral red blood cells. At other times, *P. falciparum* becomes trapped in the capillaries and may not be found in the peripheral blood. In *P. vivax*, *P. malariae*,

> **KEY POINTS**
>
> **About Clinical Presentation in *Plasmodium* Infection**
>
> Always consider malaria in the traveler from a developing country who
> 1. presents with an influenza-like syndrome,
> 2. presents with jaundice, or
> 3. presents with confusion or obtundation.

> **KEY POINTS**
>
> **About Laboratory Diagnosis of Malaria**
>
> 1. The focus must be on differentiating falciparum malaria from other forms of the disease.
> 2. Blood smear remains the preferred method, but enzyme-linked immunoabsorbent assay and polymerase chain reaction methods are now available.
> 3. In falciparum malaria, signet-ring forms are most abundant on peripheral smear immediately after a fever spike.

and *P. ovale*, various stages of the parasite are present at all times, and therefore diagnostic smears can be taken at any time. Because parasites can be absent between attacks, the blood must be examined on 3 to 4 successive days before malaria can be ruled out. Presence of pigment in peripheral monocytes or neutrophils should encourage a continued search for parasites. Thin smears need to be examined for at least 15 minutes using a high-power oil objective microscope ($1000\times$ magnification). Thick smears are the most reliable method for detecting malaria. A 5-minute search will generally yield the diagnosis.

The clinician's primary goal is to differentiate potentially fatal *P. falciparum* from other, more benign forms of malaria (see Table 12.1). For this purpose, three new assays have been developed: an enzyme-linked immunoabsorbent assay (ELISA) for histidine-rich *P. falciparum* antigen, an immunoassay for species-specific parasite lactic dehydrogenase isoenzymes, and polymerase chain reaction (PCR) amplification of parasite DNA or mRNA.

Anemia, elevated levels of lactic dehydrogenase, and increased reticulocytes are associated with red blood cell hemolysis. An elevated unconjugated bilirubin level without a significant increase in hepatic enzymes is also observed when hemolysis is severe. A reduced white blood cell (WBC) count is noted in a high percentage of patients, and thrombocytopenia is common. Elevated serum creatinine, proteinuria, and hemoglobinuria are found in severe cases of *P. falciparum*. Hypoglycemia may also complicate severe cases of *P. falciparum*, requiring close monitoring of blood sugars during the acute illness.

Prophylaxis and Treatment

Drug treatment exploits unique targets in the parasite not found in host cells. The aminoquinolones, chloroquine, quinine, mefloquine, primaquine, and halofantrine inhibit proteolysis of hemoglobin in the food vacuole and inhibit the heme polymerase that *Plasmodium* requires for production of malaria pigment. Inhibition of these functions kills the organism. Pyrimethamine, sulfonamides, and dapsone are folate antagonists (see Chapter 1). Atovaquone inhibits parasite mitochondrial transport. Artemisinin derivatives bind iron in the malarial pigment to produce free radicals that damage parasite proteins. These derivatives are faster-acting than quinine, and they have activity against all stages of the intraerythrocytic life cycle.

In recent years, many areas of Africa, northern South America, India, and Southeast Asia have become populated with chloroquine-resistant *P. falciparum*. These strains contain an energy-dependent chloroquine efflux mechanism that prevents the drug from concentrating in the parasite. Resistance to mefloquine and halofantrine has also developed, being seen primarily in Southeast Asia.

Chemoprophylaxis should start 2 weeks before departure to an endemic area and continue until 4 weeks after return. Because of the continual changes in resistance patterns, up-to-date prophylactic and treatment regimens should be reviewed at the CDC's Web site (www.cdc.gov/travel). For areas with chloroquine-susceptible *P. falciparum*, chloroquine is the drug of choice. The adult dosage is 300 mg base (500 mg of chloroquine phosphate) orally per week. In areas of chloroquine-resistance, mefloquine 250 mg (228 mg base) orally per week, or doxycycline 100 mg orally per day, or primaquine 0.5 mg/kg base per day, or atovaquone 250 mg combined with proguanil 100 mg orally per day (in a combination tablet called Malarone), or chloroquine at the formerly mentioned dose combined with proguanil 200 mg per day.

A vaccine is not available, and the immune response required to protect the host against malaria is poorly understood, making development of an effective vaccine a formidable task.

All individuals without previous immunity who contract falciparum malaria should be hospitalized, because

their clinical course can be unpredictable. Patients with the *P. vivax*, *P. ovale*, and *P. malariae* strains can usually be treated as outpatients if follow-up will be reliable. The treatment for these three strains and for chloroquine-susceptible *P. falciparum* is the same: an initial dose of oral chloroquine 600 mg base (1000 mg chloroquine phosphate), followed 6 hours later by 300 mg base (500 mg phosphate), repeated on days 2 and 3. To prevent relapse of *P. vivax* or *P. ovale*, these infections also require treatment with oral primaquine 15.3 mg phosphate base (26.5 mg phosphate salt) daily for 14 days, or 45 mg base (79 mg salt) weekly for 8 weeks. This agent kills dormant hepatic hypnozoites, preventing their subsequent development into infective schizonts. Before the primaquine is administered, the patient should be tested for glucose-6-phosphate dehydrogenase deficiency, because patients with this deficiency are at risk of severe hemolysis during primaquine treatment.

Given the worldwide prevalence of chloroquine resistance, unless absolute assurance can be obtained that travel was only in regions with chloroquine-sensitive *P. falciparum*, patients should be presumed to have a resistant strain. Treatment of chloroquine-resistant *P. falciparum* is evolving and has become complex. Although artemisinin derivatives are not currently available in the United State, they have shown superior efficacy for severe chloroquine-resistant *P. falciparum* infection. They also reduce gametocyte carriage. Their use therefore decreases infectivity after treatment, and they can eliminate malaria transmission in endemic areas. These agents are short-acting, and they should be combined with one or more other classes of antimalarial agents. Dihydroartemisinin (6.3 mg/kg daily) combined with piperaquine (50 mg/kg daily) has produced superior response rates; however, trials of various combinations are ongoing. Monotherapy is discouraged because of the rapid development of resistance. Artemisinin manufacturing quality is not currently reliable, and these agents are therefore not recommended as standard therapy.

In the United States, quinine 650 mg every 8 hours for 3–7 days, plus doxycycline 100 mg twice daily for 7 days remains the recommended regimen. Atovaquone–proguanil (250 mg/100 mg tablets) four times daily for 3 days is equally efficacious. A single high dose of mefloquine (1250 mg) alone has been recommended as alternative therapy; however, this treatment frequently causes intolerable side effects, including vertigo (10% to 20%), gastrointestinal disturbances, seizures, and (less commonly) psychosis. In addition, mefloquine-resistant *P. falciparum* is increasing in frequency.

If a patient is too ill to take oral medicines, intravenous quinidine is the treatment of choice. This drug is three to four times more active than is intravenous quinine, and serum levels can be measured. Furthermore,

---

KEY POINTS

About Malaria Prophylaxis

- -

1. Determine if the traveler will be visiting areas with chloroquine-resistant strains (check www.cdc.org/travel).

2. Begin prophylaxis 2 weeks before travel to insure that no intolerable side effects develop.

3. Continue prophylaxis for 4 weeks after return.

KEY POINTS

About Choosing Chemotherapy for *Plasmodium* Infection

1. Determine whether the traveler came from a chloroquine-resistant area:
   a) For chloroquine-sensitive strains, use chloroquine.
   b) For resistant strains, use quinine or an equivalent regimen.
   c) Artemisinin derivatives have improved efficacy for severe disease, but manufacturing quality is unreliable. Monotherapy is discouraged. Not available in the United Kingdom or the United States.
2. Determine whether the patient is too ill to take oral medicines (requires intravenous quinidine).
3. Determine whether the patient has *Plasmodium vivax* or *ovale* (requires primaquine, if not deficient in glucose-6-phosphate dehydrogenase).
4. Refer to Web sites run by health authorities for the most current antimalarial regimens (Table 12.2).

KEY POINTS

About Managing Patients with *Plasmodium falciparum*

1. Levels of parasitemia above 5% constitute a medical emergency and require immediate institution of antimalarial treatment.
2. Hematocrit, blood sugar, volume status, cardiac rhythm, renal function, central nervous system function, and arterial oxygenation must all be closely monitored.
3. In the nonimmune host, the course of *P. falciparum* infection is not predictable.
4. The severity of organ damage and risk of death correlate with the level of parasitemia.

parenteral quinine is no longer available in the United States. Quinidine gluconate salt 10 mg/kg loading dose (maximum 600 mg) in normal saline should be infused slowly over 1 to 2 hours, followed by a continuous infusion of 0.02 mg/kg every minute until the patient is able to take oral medication. Given the rapid changes in malaria resistance patterns and newly reported clinical trials, health care providers should refer to excellent Web sites operated by recognized authorities that outline up-to-date treatment regimens (Table 12.2).

The risk of end-organ damage and death increases with the patient's level of parasitemia. Levels above 5% constitute a medical emergency, and patients with these levels require intensive treatment. Patients with no immunity and levels of *P. falciparum* parasitemia above 10% to 15% should be considered for exchange transfusion, a measure that can be life-saving. However, patients with levels of parasitemia of greater than 50% have survived without blood exchange. Volume status, renal function, and serum glucose must be carefully monitored. Respirator support may be required in cases of severe pulmonary edema. Intravenous steroids have been shown to be harmful in cases of cerebral malaria, and those agents should therefore be avoided. Because of the risk of arrhythmias associated with quinine, quinidine, mefloquine, and halofantrine, cardiac function should be monitored in patients treated with those agents.

Table 12.2. Online Sources of Current Guidelines for Antimalarial Therapy

U.K. Health Protection Agency, Committee on Malaria Prevention in U.K. Travellers
Infectious Diseases | Malaria | Treatment Guidelines www.hpa.org.uk/infections/topics_az/malaria/Treat_guidelines.htm
U.S. Centers for Disease Control and Prevention
Malaria | Diagnosis and Treatment | Treatment of Malaria (Guidelines for Clinicians) www.cdc.gov/malaria/diagnosis_treatment/tx_clinicians.htm
World Health Organization, Global Malaria Programme
Global Malaria Programme | Diagnosis and Treatment | Treatment | Treatment Guidelines www.who.int/malaria/treatmentguidelines.html (a detailed review of all aspects of malaria treatment)

BABESIOSIS

> ┊ POTENTIAL SEVERITY
>
> *Usually causes mild disease, but in splenectomized patients can be fatal.*

GUIDING QUESTIONS

1. *How is babesiosis contracted?*

2. *Why has the incidence of this infection increased in the United States?*

3. *How does life cycle of Babesia differ from that of Plasmodium, and how might these differences relate to the differences in clinical manifestations?*

4. *Which other infection do patients with babesiosis often contract at the same time, and why?*

5. *Is this blood protozoan treated in the same way as Plasmodium is?*

Prevalence, Epidemiology, and Life Cycle

Babesiosis was once thought to be a disease only of cattle and wild animals. However, in the last 30 years this organism has been found to occasionally infect humans. More than 100 cases of human babesiosis have been described, many occurring in Massachusetts on the islands of Nantucket and Martha's Vineyard. Other cases have been described throughout New England,

---

KEY POINTS

About the *Babesia* Lifecycle

1. The small nymph form (2 mm in diameter) of the deer tick, *Ixodes scapularis*, carries *Babesia* from white deer mice to humans.

2. In human red blood cells, the mature signet-ring trophozoite multiplies by binary fission forming characteristic tetrads.

3. Multiplication is asynchronous, and therefore hemolysis is never massive.

4. Babesiosis has no hepatic phase.

KEY POINTS

About *Babesia* Epidemiology

1. Endemic in areas where the deer population is abundant.

2. Requires the presence of the white deer mouse, which harbors the infectious deer tick (*Ixodes scapularis*) nymphs.

3. Human infections occur during the period of nymph feeding (May to September).

New York, Maryland, Virginia, Georgia, Wisconsin, Minnesota, Washington State, and California.

Like malaria, *Babesia* is a blood protozoan. It has a lifecycle similar to that of *Plasmodium*; however, *Babesia* is transmitted by the deer tick, *Ixodes scapularis*. Curiously, *Babesia* do not infect deer. However, the intermediate host, the white-footed deer mouse, is readily infected by *Babesia microti*, the primary strain causing human disease in the United States. In endemic areas, the percentage of these rodents infected by *Babesia* can reach 60%. During its larval and nymph phases, the tick lives on the deer mouse, where it obtains blood meals. The nymph can leave the deer mouse and attach to humans. After attachment, this tiny tick (2 mm in diameter) eats a blood meal and introduces the *Babesia* sporozoite. The sporozoites enter human red blood cells. The mature signet-ring-shaped trophozoite multiplies asexually by binary fission, forming characteristic tetrads. Subsequently, it lyses the host red blood cell. Because multiplication is asynchronous, massive hemolysis is not seen. Also, unlike *Plasmodium*, *Babesia* lacks a hepatic phase.

The rise in the incidence of babesiosis has been attributed to the decreased popularity of deer hunting and the associated increase in deer and deer tick populations. Also, migration to the suburbs in the United States has brought humans in closer proximity to the mouse reservoirs harboring the infectious *Ixodes scapularis* nymph. The infection is contracted by humans during the months of May through September when the nymphs are feeding.

Clinical Presentation

> ┊ CASE 12.2

A 65–year-old white female presented with intermittent fever for the preceding 2 months, associated with intermittent myalgias and fatigue. She had just returned from a 2-month summer vacation in Martha's Vineyard, Massachusetts. She denied any history of tick bites. One month earlier, she had been diagnosed with Lyme disease. However, despite appropriate treatment, her fevers did not resolve. Aside from a mild anemia, her routine blood tests were normal; however, Giemsa stain of her peripheral blood revealed occasional red blood cells containing ring forms, some in tetrads. Treatment with clindamycin and quinine caused a rapid resolution of her fever.

The symptoms of babesiosis are nonspecific, making the disease difficult to diagnose clinically. Generally, patients present 1 to 3 weeks after exposure with a flu-like illness. Fever, chills, myalgias, arthralgias, fatigue, and anorexia are most common. The illness presents during the summer months as a "summer flu." In endemic areas, the clinician should inquire about recent hiking in tick-infested locations, particularly those with tall grasses and brush. Patients often do not give a history of tick bites, having failed to detect the attached nymph because of its small size (the diameter of a small freckle). In the normal host, the disease may cause minimal symptoms and resolve spontaneously. However, in older patients or in those who have undergone splenectomy, infection can be more severe and persistent. Cases of adult respiratory distress syndrome and hypotension have been reported, and on rare occasions, patients have died. In Europe, cases have strictly involved splenectomized patients, and the clinical presentation has been more fulminant, being associated with severe hemolysis and death.

Patients with babesiosis may also have symptoms suggestive of Lyme disease, particularly the skin rash of erythema migrans. *Ixodes scapularis* is also the vector for *Borrelia burgdorferi*, and in one series of cases, 54% of patients with babesiosis also had antibodies against the Lyme spirochete, suggesting that these patients had dual infections.

Diagnosis and Treatment

Giemsa stain of thick and thin smears from the peripheral blood should be examined under an oil-immersion objective. Small ring forms, often grouped in tetrads (Figure 12.3) are the only form seen. Babesiosis is frequently mistaken for *P. falciparum*. The classic tetrad is not observed in *Plasmodium* infection, and the banana-shaped gametocytes observed in *P. falciparum* are never observed in *Babesia*. An indirect immunofluorescence antibody titer that measures antibody against *B. microti*, the primary form that causes

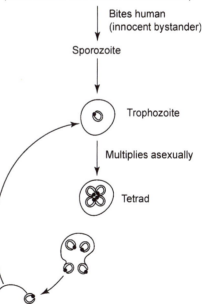

Figure 12–3. Life cycle of *Babesia*. The white-footed deer mouse is the main reservoir of this pathogen.

KEY POINTS

About the Clinical Presentation of Babesiosis

1. Presents as the "summer flu" 1 to 3 weeks after exposure.
2. History of hiking in tick-infested areas.
3. Often no history of tick bite, because the *Ixodes scapularis* nymph is mistaken for a small freckle.
4. More serious disease occurs in splenectomized patients and elderly individuals.
5. Patients with babesiosis may also have Lyme disease, because *Ixodes scapularis* transmits both infections.

babesiosis in the United States, is available through the CDC. Significant increases in antibody titer develop 3 to 4 weeks after the infection is contracted.

Treatment should be initiated in splenectomized patients and in other patients with serious disease. Clindamycin combined with oral quinine is the preferred regimen (see Table 12.3). Another equally effective regimen is azithromycin and atovaquone. This combination is associated with fewer adverse reactions than is clindamycin and quinine.

Chloroquine, often initiated when *Babesia* is mistaken for *P. falciparum*, is not effective. Similarly, doxycycline, pentamidine, primaquine, and pyrimethamine–sulfadoxine (Fansidar) are not efficacious.

KEY POINTS

About Diagnosis and Treatment of Babesiosis

1. Giemsa stain of the peripheral blood remains the best way to make the diagnosis.
2. Only ring forms are seen.
3. Frequently mistaken for *Plasmodium falciparum*.
4. Tetrad ring forms strongly support the diagnosis of babesiosis.
5. Many malaria regimens, including chloroquine and primaquine, are not effective in babesiosis.

Table 12.3. Antiparastic Therapy Dosingh

Parasite	Preferred therapy[a]	Alternative therapy[a]
Babesia		
	Intravenous clindamycin 1.2 g q12h, OR Clindamycin 600 mg q8h for 7–10 days, AND quinine 650 mg q8h for 7–10 days	Atovaquone 750 mg q12h for 7–10 days, AND azithromycin 600 mg daily for 7–10 days
Leishmania		
Visceral	Liposomal amphotericin B 3 mg/kg daily on days 1–5, 14, 21	Intravenous or intramuscular sodium stibogluconate 20 µg/kg daily for 28 days
Cutaneous	Intravenous or intramuscular sodium stibogluconate 20 mg/kg daily for	Intracutaneous sodium stibogluconate daily for 21 days Liposomal amphotericin B for unresponsive lesions
Trypanosoma cruzi (Chagas' disease)		
	Nifurtimox 8–10 mg/kg daily divided q6h for 90–120 days	Benznidazole 5 mg/kg daily for 60 days
Trichuris (whip worm)		
	Mebendazole 100 mg q12h for 3 days, OR Albendazole 400 mg q24h for 3 days	Ivermectin 200µg/kg daily for 3 days, OR Nitazoxanide 500 mg q12h for 3 days
Ascaris		
	Mebendazole 100 mg q12h for 3 days	Pyrantel pamoate 11 mg/kg (maximum 1 g) q12h for 3 days, OR Albendazole 400 mg once, OR Nitazoxanide 500 mg q12h for 3 days
Enterobius (pin worm)		
	Mebendazole 100 mg once, OR Albendazole 400 mg once, OR Pyrantel pamoate 11 mg/kg (maximum 1 g) once Repeat selected treatment after 2 weeks	
Strongyloides		
	Ivermectin 200 µg/kg daily for 2 days For disseminated disease, continue for 7 days (longer if immunocompromised)	Albendazole 400 mg q24h for 3 days

(Continued)

Table 12.3. (Continued)

Parasite	Preferred therapy[a]	Alternative therapy[a]
	Hook worm	
	Albendazole 400 mg once, OR Mebendazole 100 mg q12h for 3 days, OR Pyrantel pamoate 11 mg/kg (maximum 1 g) for 3 days	
	Trichinella	
	Steroids for severe symptoms, PLUS mebendazole 200–400 mg q8h for 3 days, THEN 400–500 mg q8h for 10 days	Albendazole 400 mg q12h for 8–14 days
	Echinococcus granulosus (hydatid cyst)	
	Aspiration or surgical excision, PLUS perioperative albendazole	Albendazole 400 mg q12h for 1–6 months
	Echinococcus multilocularis	
	Surgical excision or aspiration	
	Taenia solium (cysticercosis)	
	Albendazole 400 mg q12h for 8–30 days, repeated as necessary Concurrent steroids for central nervous system disease	Praziquantel 50–100 mg/kg daily divided q8h for 30 days Surgery
	Schistosomes (Schistosoma)	
S. mansoni	Praziquantel 40 mg/kg divided q12h over 1 day	Oxamniquine 15 mg/kg once (30 mg/kg once for East Africa; 30 mg/kg q24h for 2 days for Egypt and South Africa)
S. haematobium	Praziquantel as for *S. mansoni*	
S. japonicum and S. mekongi	Praziquantel 60 mg/kg divided q8h over 1 day	
	Clonorchis sinensis	
	Praziquantel 75 mg/kg divided q8h over 1 day	
	Fasciola hepatica	
	Triclabendazole 10 mg/kg once	
	Paragonimus westermani	
	Praziquantel 75 mg/kg daily divided q8h for 2 days	Bithionol 30–50 g/kg on alternate days for 10–15 doses
	Wuchereria bancrofti and Brugia malayi	
	Diethylcarbamazine 6 mg/kg once	Doxycycline 100 mg q12h for 3 weeks before diethylcarbamazine may reduce febrile reactions and kills adult worms
	Onchocerca volvulus	
	Ivermectin 150 µg/kg once Repeat every 6–12 months	
	Loa loa	
	Diethylcarbamazine 6 mg/kg once	

[a] All therapies are oral unless otherwise indicated.

■ TISSUE PROTOZOA

LEISHMANIASIS

Prevalence, Epidemiology, and Life Cycle

Leishmania has caused major epidemics in eastern India, Bangladesh, and East Africa. Urban outbreaks have been reported in the cities of northeastern Brazil. A small number of American military personnel contracted leishmaniasis during the Persian Gulf War in 1991 and in Afghanistan more recently. Indigenous cases have been reported occasionally in the United States, but most U.S. cases result from travel to a tropical country. Leishmaniasis has emerged as an opportunistic infection in patients with HIV or an organ transplant.

The *Leishmania* parasite is transmitted by the female phlebotomine sandfly. Sandflies breed in cracks in the walls of dwellings, in rubbish, and in rodent burrows. Because they are weak fliers, sandflies remain close to the ground near their breeding sites, resulting in localized

---

POTENTIAL SEVERITY

Visceral leishmaniasis is a chronic disease that can cause severe morbidity and death in debilitated and immunocompromised hosts.

GUIDING QUESTIONS

1. *How is leishmaniasis contracted, and where is this disease most commonly found?*

2. *Which form of immunity is most important for protecting against Leishmania, and are patients with HIV or an organ transplant at increased risk for developing leishmaniasis?*

3. *How do patients with visceral leishmaniasis usually present clinically, and which diseases can this infection mimic?*

4. *Where are lesions of cutaneous leishmaniasis usually located, and why?*

5. *What is the therapy approved by the U.S. Food and Drug Administration for visceral leishmaniasis?*

KEY POINTS

About the Epidemiology and Life Cycle of *Leishmania*

1. Contracted in tropical areas where the phlebotomine sandfly is common; rare in the United States Found in South America, India, Bangladesh, the Middle East, and East Africa.

2. Flagellated promastigote introduced by the sandfly is ingested by macrophages.

3. In the macrophage, *Leishmania* develops into a nonflagellated amastigote that lives happily within the macrophage phagolysosome.

4. This intracellular parasite is controlled by activation of the Th1 cell-mediated immune response that increases levels of interferon γ.

5. Leishmaniasis can be an opportunistic infection in patients with HIV or an organ transplant.

---

pockets of infectious insects. Humans and other animals infected with *Leishmania* serve as reservoirs. The sandfly bites the infected host and ingests blood containing the nonflagellated form called an amastigote. In the digestive tract of the insect, the amastigote develops into a flagellated spindle-shaped promastigote. When the infected sandfly takes its blood meal from an uninfected human, the promastigote enters the host's bloodstream. The promastigote then binds to complement receptors on macrophages and is ingested. Within the phagolysosome the promastigote differentiates into an amastigote. The amastigote is resistant to lysozyme damage and depends on the low pH of the phagolysosome for uptake of nutrients. The parasite multiplies by simple division and eventually is released to infect other cells.

Cell-mediated immunity plays an important role in controlling leishmaniasis. Interferon γ activates macrophages to kill the amastigote by inducing the production of nitric oxide. Resolution of leishmanial infection is associated with the expression of CD4+ T cells of the Th1 type, which secrete interferon γ and interleukin 2. Progression of infection is associated with *Leishmania*-induced expansion of CD4+ cells of the Th2 type that produce interleukin 4, a cytokine that inhibits the production of Th1 cells and the activation of interferon γ production.

Clinical Presentation

There are three forms of leishmaniasis: visceral, cutaneous, and mucosal. A single species can produce more than one syndrome, and each syndrome is produced by multiple different species.

VISCERAL LEISHMANIASIS (KALA-AZAR)

In different areas of the world, certain *Leishmania* species tend to be most commonly associated with the visceral form of the disease: *L. donovani* (in India), *L. infantum* (Middle East), *L. chagasi* (Latin America), and *L. amazonensis* (Brazil). After inoculation of promastigotes into the skin, a small papule may be noticed. *Leishmania* amastigotes subsequently silently invade macrophages throughout the reticuloendothelial system. Usually 3 to 8 months pass before the burden of organisms increases to a level that causes symptoms.

The onset of symptoms can be gradual or sudden. In subacute cases, the patient will experience slow but progressive enlargement of the abdomen as a result of hepatosplenomegaly. Increased abdominal girth is accompanied by intermittent fever, weakness, loss of appetite, and weight loss. This presentation can be mistaken for lymphoma, infectious mononucleosis, brucellosis, chronic malaria, and hepatosplenic schistosomiasis. In acute cases, an abrupt onset of high fever and chills mimics malaria or an acute bacterial infection. On physical examination, the spleen may be massively enlarged, hard, and nontender. Hepatomegaly is also present. The skin tends to be dry and thin, and in light-skinned individuals, it takes on a grayish tint. This characteristic accounts for the Indian name Kala-azar, which means "black fever." On laboratory examination anemia, leukopenia, and hypergammaglobulinemia are common.

The diagnosis is made when a biopsy of lymphatic tissue or bone marrow demonstrates amastigotes on Wright or Giemsa stain. Enzyme-linked immunoabsorbent assays usually demonstrate high anti-leishmanial antibody titers. However, this test frequently cross-reacts with antibodies to other pathogens. Patients with HIV infection frequently fail to develop antibody titers. Splenomegaly may not be present in these patients, and infection may disseminate to the lungs, pleura, gastrointestinal tract, or bone marrow (causing aplastic anemia). In patients with HIV, amastigotes may be identified in macrophages from bronchoalveolar lavage, pleural effusion, bone marrow aspiration, or even buffy coat samples of the peripheral blood.

CUTANEOUS LEISHMANIASIS

The cutaneous form of leishmaniasis is widespread, and it is a problem chiefly for farmers, settlers, troops, and tourists in the Middle East and Central and South America. The species most commonly associated with cutaneous disease are *L. major* and *L. tropica* (found in the Middle East, India, Pakistan, and Asia), and *L. mexicana, L. braziliensis, L. amazonensis,* and

---

> ### KEY POINTS
>
> ### About Visceral Leishmaniasis
>
> 1. Incubation period is 3 to 8 months.
> 2. Subacute onset presents with increased abdominal swellinig (because of massive splenomegaly and hepatomegaly), intermittent fever, and weight loss that can be mistaken for lymphoma or infectious mononucleosis
> 3. Acute onset presents with persistent high fever mimicking bactermia or malaria.
> 4. Anemia, leukopenia, and hypergammaglobulinema are common.
> 5. Diagnosis is made by biopsy and Giemsa stain showing amastgotes
> 6. Patients with HIV may have disseminated disease without splenomegaly.

L. panamensis (in Central and South America). *L. mexicana* has been reported in Texas.

After a sandfly bite, significant skin lesions generally take 2 weeks to several months to develop. Lesions usually develop on exposed areas. They are the result of amastigotes multiplying in mononuclear cells within the skin and causing a granulomatous inflammatory reaction. Single or multiple lesions may be found, with varying morphology. Lesions may be crusted and dry, or moist and exudative. Shallow and circular ulcers with sharp, raised borders may develop and progressively increase in size, becoming "pizza-like" in appearance as a result of the beefy red of the ulcer base being combined with a yellow exudate. Lesions may become secondarily infected with staphylococci or streptococci.

The diagnosis is made from a biopsy of the raised border of the skin lesion where *Leishmania*-infected macrophages are most abundant. Amastigotes are seen on Giemsa stain.

MUCOSAL LEISHMANIASIS

Mucosal leishmaniasis is a less common manifestation that is caused primarily by *L. braziliensis*. Only 2% to 3% of patients with skin lesions develop this complication. Organisms invade mononuclear cells in the mucosa. The nose is most commonly involved, resulting in nasal stuffiness, discharge, pain, or epistaxis. Later, the nasal septum is destroyed, and the nose collapses. Involvement of the genital mucosa and trachea have also been reported. Diagnosis is made by biopsy.

Treatment

The only drug approved in the United States for treatment of leishmaniasis is liposomal amphotericin B. For visceral leishmaniasis in immunocompetent patients, administer 3 mg/kg daily on days 1 to 5, 14, and 21. The course can be repeated if the parasite persists. For the immunocompromised host, the recommended regimen is amphotericin B 4 mg/kg daily administered on days 1 to 5, 10, 17, 24, 31, and 38. Relapses are common in HIV-infected hosts.

Outside the United States, pentavalent antimony continues be used; however, this treatment is associated with many side effects, including abdominal pain, anorexia, nausea and vomiting, and myalgias. Amylase and lipase levels often rise. Miltefosine, a phosphocholine analog has anti-leishmanial activity in vitro and in vivo, and acts by interfering with the parasite's cell-signaling pathways and membrane synthesis. This agent has successfully treated Indian visceral disease.

Treatment of cutaneous leishmaniasis depends on the location of the infection. The lesions can heal spontaneously, and so, if there is no mucosal involvement and if the lesions are located in areas of no cosmetic concern, they can be followed without therapy or treated topically with 15% puromycin and 12% methylbenzethonium chloride. Thermotherapy (warming the affected region with radiofrequency waves to $50°C$ for one treatment of 30 seconds) has proven effective in a high percentage of cases, and that approach compares favorably with 21 days of intralesional administration of pentavalent antimony. Patients with mucosal involvement, progressive lesions, or lesions in cosmetically sensitive areas require treatment with intravenous or intramuscular pentavalent antimony (20 mg/kg daily for 20 days, available through the CDC). Fluconazole (500 mg twice daily for 6 weeks) has been associated with modest response rates. Miltefosine has proved successful against some forms of cutaneous leishmaniasis, but other species are refractory.

TRYPANOSOMA CRUZI

GUIDING QUESTIONS

1. *Which insect is responsible for transmitting this disease, and is the disease commonly transmitted to tourists? Why, or why not?*

2. *How does this insect's toilet habits affect transmission to the human host?*

3. *Which organs are most commonly affected by chronic Chagas' disease?*

POTENTIAL SEVERITY

A chronic disorder that can lead to fatal cardiomyopathy.

Prevalence, Epidemiology, and Life Cycle

Chagas' disease caused by *Trypanosoma cruzi* is found throughout Central and South America. Between 16 and 18 million people worldwide are infected with *T. cruzi*, and nearly 0.5 million die from Chagas' disease annually. With improvement of substandard housing, the incidence of this disease among young people is decreasing.

The parasite is transmitted by reduviid bugs that suck blood from their host. This insect contains trypomastigotes in its gut. At the same time that it bites the host, it also defecates, depositing trypomastigotes on the skin. The human host then scratches the itchy bite, introducing the parasite into the wound and subsequently into the bloodstream. Mucous membranes, the conjunctiva, and breaks in the skin are common sites of entry. Once in the bloodstream, the trypomastigotes enter host cells and differentiate into amastigotes that multiply, filling the cell cytoplasm. They then differentiate again into trypomastigotes, and the cell ruptures, spreading the parasite to adjacent cells and into the bloodstream. Asymptomatic parasitemia is common. In endemic areas, the parasite can be transmitted by blood transfusions. Because the reduviid bug takes up residence in the cracks of primitive homes, this infection occurs almost exclusively among poor rural people. The disease is most commonly transmitted in young children. If one member of a family presents with acute disease, all pediatric family members should be screened for asymptomatic disease.

Chagas' disease has not been reported in tourists, because they are unlikely to be exposed to primitive living quarters. Vector control measures and educational programs have helped to reduce the incidence of disease. Insecticide impregnation of bed nets has proven to be an inexpensive and effective control measure.

Clinical Presentation

Acute Chagas' disease often causes minimal symptoms. About 1 week after the parasite enters the skin, an area of localized swelling called a chagoma develops, often in association with local lymph node swelling. Entry of the parasite via the conjunctiva causes periorbital edema (Romaña's sign). Onset of local edema is quickly followed by fever, malaise, anorexia, and edema of the face and legs. Occasionally, myocarditis or encephalitis may develop.

Years to decades after the primary infection 10% to 30% of individuals go on to develop chronic Chagas' disease. The heart is the organ that is primarily damaged. Severe cardiomyopathy results in thromboembolism, congestive heart failure, and life-threatening arrhythmias. Esophageal involvement can lead to megaesophagus associated with dysphagia, regurgitation, and aspiration pneumonia. Chagasic megacolon is another manifestation of chronic disease causing constipation and bowel obstruction that can lead to perforation and bacterial sepsis. In immunocompromised hosts such as organ transplant patients and patients with AIDS, *T. cruzi* can reactivate, presenting with manifestations of chronic Chagas' disease. Unlike normal hosts, immunocompromised patients are also at risk for developing *T. cruzi* brain abscesses.

Diagnosis

Acute disease can be diagnosed by examining Giemsa-stained blood or buffy coat smears. The trypomastigotes (whose length is approximately twice the diameter of a red blood cell) can readily be seen by microscopy.

KEY POINTS

About the Life Cycle of *Trypanosoma Cruzi*

1. Transmitted by the reduviid bug, which carries the trypomastigote in its feces.
2. The host allows the parasite to enter the bloodstream by scratching and rubbing infected insect feces into the skin.
3. The reduviid bug lives in the cracks of substandard housing.
4. The disease affects mainly poor rural people, not tourists.

KEY POINTS

About the Clinical Presentation of Chagas' Disease

1. Acute disease is associated ith localized areas of swelling called chagomas.
2. Chronic disease develops in 10% to 30% of cases decades after intial infection
3. Chronic disease affects
   a) the heart, causing a cardiomyopathy associated congestive heart failure, emboli, and arrhythmias; and
   b) The gastrointestinal tract, causing megaesophagus and megacolon.

In chronic disease, the diagnosis is made by detecting immunoglobulin G (IgG) antibodies. A number of sensitive serologic tests are available, but they frequently yield false positive results. In the United States, two ELISA tests have been approved by the U.S. Food and Drug Administration for detecting clinical disease. A recently developed ELISA has been shown to have high sensitivity and specificity, and may prove useful for screening the blood supply. The polymerase chain reaction (PCR) method has demonstrated promise, but it is not yet commercially available.

Treatment

T. cruzi is not sensitive to most antiparasitic drugs (see Table 12.3). Nifurtimox cures about 70% of acute cases. This drug causes gastrointestinal and neurologic side effects in many patients. Benznidazole has a similar cure rate. Peripheral neuropathy, granulocytopenia, and rash are the most common side effects with that agent. Treatment with these two agents is now recommended for chronic Chagas' disease. Recent studies have shown that treatment slows the progression of heart disease.

TRYPANOSOMA BRUCEI COMPLEX

POTENTIAL SEVERITY

Over weeks to months, this disease can progress to coma, followed by death.

T. brucei complex refers to several *Trypanosoma* subspecies that are spread by the blood-sucking tsetse fly. Unlike *T. cruzi*, which takes up residence within cells, *T. brucei* trypomastigotes multiply within the bloodstream, evading the humoral immune system indefinitely by changing their surface antigens every 5 days. This disease is confined to Africa. No more than a single case per year is imported to the United States. After the initial bite, the infection progresses slowly, with systemic symptoms of fever and lymph node swelling being noted weeks to months later. In the West African form, neurologic manifestations do not develop until months or years after the initial symptoms. In East African trypanosomiasis, systemic complaints may develop days after the insect bite, and CNS complaints may develop within weeks. Symptoms include somnolence, which explains the name "sleeping sickness" and choreiform movements, tremors, and ataxia mimicking Parkinson's disease. Coma and death frequently ensue.

The diagnosis is made by observation of trypomastigotes in Giemsa-stained thick and thin smears of peripheral blood. Trypomastigotes can also be found in the cerebrospinal fluid. The treatment for *T. brucei* is complex and depends on the species of the infecting parasite, whether the CNS is involved, and tolerance to the side effects of the treatment regimen. Potential medications include eflornithine; suramin alone or in combination with the arsenical tryparsamide; pentamidine; and the arsenical melarsoprol.

■ INTESTINAL HELMINTHS

GUIDING QUESTIONS

1. *What are the two ways by which intestinal helminths gain entry to the human host?*

2. *How does the life cycle of Ascaris differ from that of Trichuris, and how does the difference manifest itself clinically?*

3. *How is Strongyloides able to persist in the human host for three to four decades?*

4. *What are the conditions that precipitate Strongyloides hyperinfection syndrome, and why?*

5. *Which helminth most commonly causes iron deficiency anemia, and why?*

POTENTIAL SEVERITY

Infections are often asymptomatic. In the immunocompromised host, Strongyloides can progress to a fatal hyperinfection syndrome.

Helminths include the roundworms (nematodes), flukes (trematodes), and tapeworms (cestodes). These parasites are large, ranging in size from 1 cm to 10 m, and they often live in the human gastrointestinal tract without causing symptoms. Only when the infection is very heavy or the worm migrates to an extraintestinal site do patients seek medical attention. Transmission to humans results in most cases from contact with human waste. The diagnosis is generally made by examining the stool for eggs, larvae, or adult worms (Figure 12.4).

INTESTINAL NEMATODES (ROUNDWORMS)

Nematodes can be classified into two groups. Those that gain entry to the host by egg ingestion (*Trichuris*, *Ascaris*, and *Enterobius*), and those that are capable of producing larvae that penetrate the skin of their host (*Strongyloides* and hookworm). Roundworm life cycles can also be classified into two groups. One group, *Trichuris* and *Enterobius*, attach and grow in the intestine soon after being ingested. The second group, *Ascaris*, *Strongyloides*, and hookworm, first penetrate the venous system, enter the lungs, and migrate up the bronchi to the trachea, where they are swallowed. They then take up residence in the gastrointestinal tract (Figure 12.5). These differences in life cycle account for some of the unique clinical characteristics of the various species of nematodes.

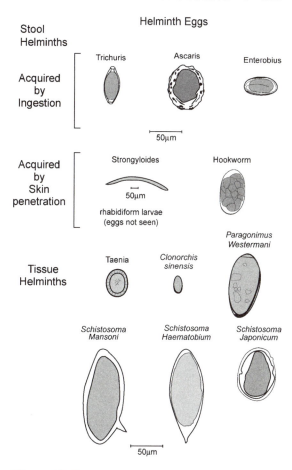

Figure 12–4. Stool helminths. All eggs drawn to scale. In *Strongyloides*, only the rhabditiform larvae are usually seen.

Nematodes Acquired by Ingestion

TRICHURIS TRICHIURA (WHIP WORM)

Trichuris trichiura is one of the most prevalent helminths. More than 2 million people are estimated to be infected in the United States. This parasite is most commonly found in the rural Southeast, particularly Puerto Rico, where the moisture and temperature favor egg maturation. Worldwide, this worm causes infection mainly in poor rural communities with poor sanitation. Humans are the principal host, and infection results from ingestion of embryonated eggs.

Under optimal conditions of shade and moisture, eggs excreted in the stool undergo embryonic development within 2 to 4 weeks. Then, when ingested by humans, the larvae break out of the eggshell and penetrate the intestinal villi of the small intestine. Over 3 to

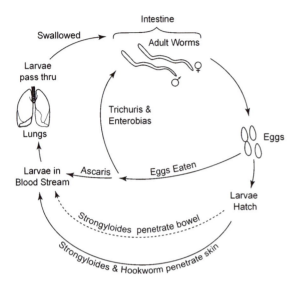

Comparative Life Cycles of
Intestinal Nematodes

Figure 12–5. Comparative life cycles of the intestinal nematodes. (Adapted from Schaechter M, Engleberg NC, Eisenstein BI, Medoff G, editors. *Mechanisms of Microbial Disease*. 3rd edition. Baltimore, Md.: Lippincott Williams and Wilkins; 1999)

10 days, they migrate down to the cecum, and over 1 to 3 months, they develop into egg-producing adults.

Most *Trichuris trichiura* infections are asymptomatic. Heavy infections can result in iron deficiency and abdominal pain and tenderness. Bloody diarrhea, growth retardation, and rectal prolapse are potential complications of a heavy infection.

Diagnosis is made by fecal smear. The ova has a classic lemon shape with plug-like ends (Figure 12-4). Mebendazole is a highly effective treatment and is seldom associated with side effects. Albendazole is also recommended as first-line therapy; ivermectin or nitazoxanide are efficacious alternatives (see Table 12.3).

ASCARIS

Ascaris is the most common helminthic infection of humans, being estimated to infect more than 1 billion humans worldwide. In the United States, infections are found predominantly in the southeast, where weather conditions favor egg embryonation.

Like *Trichuris*, *Ascaris* is a parasite of humans, the infection being contracted by ingesting material contaminated with human feces. Under proper temperature and moisture conditions, eggs develop into infective embryos within 5 to 10 days. When ingested, the parasites hatch in the small intestine. Embryos then penetrate the intestinal

wall and enter the venous bloodstream. On reaching the capillaries of the lung, they break into the alveoli, crawl up through the bronchi and trachea, and then are swallowed, re-entering the gastrointestinal tract, where they mature over a period of 2 months. Each mature gravid female can produce 200,000 eggs per day.

As in other roundworm infections, most patients with *Ascaris* are asymptomatic. However, patients with high worm burdens can experience obstruction of the small intestine, accompanied by vomiting and abdominal pain. Patients may vomit worms during such attacks or may pass them in their stool. Heavy infections may also be associated with malabsorption, steatorrhea, and weight loss. A single *Ascaris* worm can migrate up the biliary tree and obstruct the common bile duct, precipitating symptoms of cholecystitis, including epigastric abdominal pain, nausea, and vomiting. As the worms migrate into the lungs, some patients experience respiratory symptoms and develop pneumonia visible on chest radiographs, accompanied by peripheral eosinophilia (sometimes called Loeffler's syndrome). On occasion, worms can migrate to other sites in the body, causing local symptoms.

Because of the large number of eggs excreted daily, this infection is easily diagnosed by stool smear (Figure 12.4). *Ascaris* infection is effectively cured with mebendazole. Alternative treatments include pyrantel pamoate, albendazole, and nitazoxanide (Table 12.3). Improved sanitation is critical for controlling this infection. Hand-washing and boiling of water have been shown to prevent reinfection. Alternatively, all school-age children in endemic areas can be treated twice or three times per year to reduce the worm burden.

ENTEROBIUS (PINWORM)

Pinworm is the most common worm infection in countries within the temperate zone. This infection is very common in children of all socioeconomic groups in the United States. Between 20 and 40 million people are estimated to be infected. The eggs of this parasite resist drying and can therefore contaminate bed linens and dust. As a result, infection in one young child can lead to infestation of the entire family. After ingestion, the eggs hatch in the duodenum and jejunum, and the larvae mature in the cecum and large intestine. At night, gravid females migrate to perianal area, where they lay eggs and cause localized itching. When this area is scratched, eggs are trapped under fingernails and are subsequently ingested by the host, resulting in repeated autoinfection.

The major clinical manifestation is nocturnal itching of the perianal area that often interferes with sleep. This parasite rarely causes other symptoms. Because *Enterobius* rarely migrates through tissue, this infection is not associated with peripheral eosinophilia. Diagnosis is made by pressing adhesive cellophane tape onto the perianal area in the early morning. Small, white, thread-like

KEY POINTS

About Nematodes Acquired by Ingestion

1. Tend to cause minimal symptoms and are not life-threatening.
2. Contracted by contact with fecal material.
3. *Trichuris trichiura* can cause iron-deficiency anemia; excretes lemon-shaped ova.
4. *Ascaris* passes through the lung and can initially cause respiratory symptoms; can also cause biliary obstruction; excretes round, thick-walled ova.
5. *Enterobius* is common in children and readily spreads by dust and contaminated linens. Diagnosed when the adhesive cellophane tape test demonstrates worms in the anal area.
6. Mebendazole or albendazole is effective treatment.

KEY POINTS

About the Epidemiology and Life Cycle of *Strongyloides*

1. Endemic in warm areas, including the southeast United States.
2. Larvae in soil contaminated with fecal material penetrate the skin of bare feet.
3. Larvae enter the bloodstream, invade the lung, crawl up the bronchi to the trachea, are swallowed, and mature in the small intestine.
4. Adult worms deposit eggs in the bowel wall where the eggs hatch.
5. Larvae in the bowel can enter the bloodstream, causing autoinfection.
6. Infection can persist for 35 to 40 years.

worms and eggs become attached to the tape and can be easily identified using a low-power (100X) microscope. Two doses of mebendazole or albendazole taken 2 weeks apart is curative. All symptomatic family members should be treated simultaneously.

NEMATODES ACQUIRED BY SKIN PENETRATION

Strongyloides

PREVALENCE, EPIDEMIOLOGY, AND LIFE CYCLE

Strongyloides infection occurs less commonly than do infections involving the other roundworms; however, strongyloidiasis is widely distributed throughout the tropics and commonly infects people in the southern United States. Because *Strongyloides* can cause a fatal hyperinfection syndrome in the immunocompromised host, clinicians need to be familiar with this parasite.

The filariform larvae excreted in the feces are capable of penetrating the skin. Humans become infected as a result of skin exposure to feces or soil contaminated by feces. Walking barefoot on contaminated soil is the most common way of contracting this infection. After skin penetration, the larvae enter the bloodstream and lymphatics. Subsequently, they become trapped in the lungs, where they enter the alveoli and are coughed up and then swallowed, entering the gastrointestinal tract. The larvae mature in the upper gastrointestinal tract, where females are able to penetrate the bowel mucosa and deposit their eggs. Eggs hatch in the mucosa, releasing rhabditiform larvae that either mature within the intestine, forming filariform larvae capable of penetrat-

ing the bowel wall and causing autoinfection, or are passed in the feces. In warm moist soil, the excreted larvae can mature into the infectious form. Because *Strongyloides* can re-infect the human host, an initial infection can persist for 35 to 40 years. The intensity of the infection depends not only on the initial inoculum, but also on the degree of autoinfection. In the immunocompromised host, autoinfection can be intense and can cause severe disseminated illness.

CLINICAL PRESENTATION

CASE 12.3

A 60–year-old white man was admitted to the hospital for elective cardiac and renal transplantation. He had long-standing diabetes mellitus and had experienced multiple myocardial infarcts leading to severe ischemic cardiomyopathy. He had also developed end-stage diabetic nephropathy. Following transplantation, he received mycophenolate mofetil, tacrolimus, and high doses of methylprednisolone. One month after transplant, he suddenly developed fever and increasing shortness of breath, associated with a cough productive of clear watery sputum. Two days later, he began coughing up bloody sputum.

A social history found that this patient had never smoked. He had never traveled outside of northern Florida, having lived in the area his entire life.

Physical examination showed a blood pressure of 133/72 mm Hg, a pulse of 81 per minute, a respiratory rate of 20 per minute, and a temperature of 37.6°C. This patient appeared acutely ill, being short of breath on a Ventimask.

An examination of ears, nose, and throat was unremarkable. The patient's neck was supple, without lymphadenopathy.

Coarse breath sounds were heard bilaterally in the lungs, and the midline sternal wound was clean and without drainage. The heart showed normal S1 and S2, with no murmurs, rubs, or gallops. The abdomen was soft and nontender. No organomegaly was noted, and bowel sounds were normal.

Some leg edema was noted (3+ in the left lower leg, and 1+ in the right lower leg), but pedal pulses were intact. A neurologic exam uncovered no focal deficits. The patient was able to follow simple commands.

A laboratory workup showed a WBC count of 3700/mm^3, with 85%, neutrophils. 5.4% lymphocytes, 2% eosinophils, 0.6% basophils, and 4.4% monocytes. Hematocrit was 29%, and platelet count was 301,000/mm^3. Serum sodium was 137 mEq/L, and liver function tests were within normal limits. Arterial blood pH was 7.02, with a Paco$_2$ of 59 mm Hg, a Pao$_2$ of 51 mm Hg, an HCO$_3$ of 15 mEq/L, and oxygen saturation of 66% (Fio$_2$ 95%).

A chest radiograph revealed diffuse bilateral parenchymal opacities consistent with pulmonary edema (Fig. 12-6A). A computed tomography (CT) scan of the chest showed diffuse reticular interstitial infiltrates consistent with pulmonary edema (Fig 12-6B) and two subsequent bronchoscopy exams revealed no pathogens. Diffuse alveolar hemorrhage was observed.

Despite treatment with voriconazole, ganciclovir, and broad-spectrum antibiotics, the patient became hypotensive and remained hypoxic, dying 7 days after the onset of his acute respiratory illness. All blood cultures and sputum culture were negative for pathogens.

At autopsy numerous Strongyloides stercoralis filariform larvae were found to be present within the alveolar spaces, alveolar septa, and connective tissue (Figure 12.6C). Occasional filariform larvae were also seen within the sinuses of the hilar lymph nodes and were identified within the myocardial interstitium. Filariform larvae were seen within the walls of the esophagus, stomach, small bowel, and colon, with the heaviest infestation being observed in the colon.

As observed with other roundworm infections, most patients with *Strongyloides* have no symptoms when they harbor only a small number of worms. Heavier infestations can cause symptoms associated with the parasite's life cycle. When the filariform larvae first penetrate the skin,

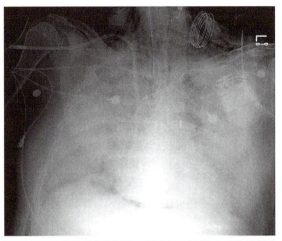

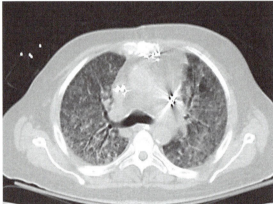

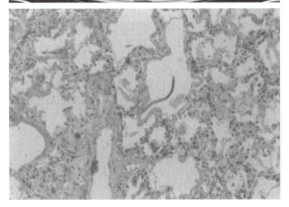

Figure 12–6. Strongyloidiasis hyperinfection syndrome. **A.** A chest radiograph demonstrates diffuse opacification of both lung fields. **B.** A computed tomography scan of the chest shows diffuse interstitial infiltrates consistent with pulmonary edema. **C.** Lung biopsy with hematoxylin and eosin staining shows inflammatory cells within the alveoli and a rhabditiform larva (middle of the field).

KEY POINTS

About the Clinical Presentation of *Strongyloides*

----

1. Many patients are asymptomatic.
2. Skin penetration can cause an itchy, erythematous rash.
3. Lung invasion can produce Loeffler's syndrome (cough, wheezing, pneumonia, and eosinophilia).
4. Heavy infection can cause abdominal pain and eosinophilia.
5. Treatment with high-dose steroids can cause a fatal hyperinfection syndrome (accelerated autoinfection).
6. Hyperinfection causes diffuse pneumonia, meningitis, abdominal pain, and gram-negative sepsis, hemoptysis, and skin rashes. Eosinophilia is absent.

KEY POINTS

About the Diagnosis and Treatment of Strongyloidiasis

----

1. Diagnosis is difficult. (Stools do not contain ova.)
2. Larvae are found in the stool; duodenal endoscopy may be required.
3. Peripheral eosinophilia may the only finding.
4. Treat asymptomatic infections.
5. Ivermectin is the drug of choice.

---

they can cause itching and a papular erythematous rash. Migration into the lungs can cause respiratory symptoms, pneumonia, and peripheral eosinophilia (Loeffler's syndrome). Once *Strongyloides* takes up residence in the gastrointestinal tract, the parasite can cause burning abdominal pain that mimics peptic ulcer disease or a colicky abdominal pain that mimics gallbladder disease. Abdominal pain may be associated with diarrhea and the passage of mucus. Malabsorption, nausea, vomiting, and weight loss may also be present. Because the female worm penetrates the bowel mucosa and the filariform larvae can migrate through the bowel wall, the host responds by producing eosinophils, and peripheral eosinophilia is a prominent finding in strongyloidiasis. When larvae penetrate the perianal area, a localized snakelike urticarial rash may be seen. A generalized urticarial rash may also be seen.

As illustrated by case 12.3, when asymptomatic individuals who harbor small numbers of organisms receive immunosuppressants such as high-dose corticosteroids, or develop depressed cell-mediated immunity because of severe malnutrition or AIDS, the level of autoinfection can increase markedly, resulting in a hyperinfection syndrome. Symptoms may include diffuse pulmonary infiltrates, severe abdominal pain, meningitis, and gram-negative sepsis, the latter manifestation being the result of filariform larvae compromising the integrity of the bowel wall. Other clinical manifestations can include hemoptysis and a skin rash. Periumbilical purpura, diffuse nonpalpable purpura, angioedema, or erythroderma mimicking a drug-related allergic eruption have all been described. As in case 12.3, eosinophilia is usually absent in the hyperinfection

syndrome. When an immunocompromised patient presents with this clinical constellation and was raised in the rural south or previously lived in a tropical region, hyperinfection with *Strongyloides* needs to be considered.

DIAGNOSIS AND TREATMENT

Because the eggs usually hatch in the gastrointestinal tract, *Strongyloides* ova are rarely seen on stool smear. Diagnosis depends on identifying rhabditiform larvae in the feces or duodenal fluid. Diagnosis requires expertise, because hookworm larvae can easily be misdiagnosed as *Strongyloides*. At least three stools need to be examined under a low-power (100X) microscope; if results are negative, endoscopy should be considered. The ELISA serum test is sensitive and specific, but it cannot differentiate recent from past infection. In the *Strongyloides*-infected immunocompromised host, the ELISA test may be negative. An important clue is the presence of peripheral eosinophilia, which may increase to between 10% and 20% of peripheral WBCs. However, lack of eosinophilia, particularly in the hyperinfection syndrome, does not exclude the diagnosis of strongyloidiasis.

Ivermectin for 2 days is curative in most cases. Albendazole can be given as alternative therapy. Because of the potential danger of severe autoinfection, all patients with *Strongyloides*, even asymptomatic patients, should be treated. Patients who develop the hyperinfection syndrome should be treated for a minimum of 7 days. However, despite treatment, the mortality associated with this syndrome remains high. Patients with a past history of *Strongyloides* or unexplained eosinophilia should therefore be thoroughly examined, tested, and treated before receiving immunosuppressive therapy.

Hookworm

PREVALENCE, EPIDEMIOLOGY, AND LIFE CYCLE

Hookworm (*Ancylostoma duodenale* and *Necator americanus*) has been estimated to infect nearly one quarter of the world's population. being found throughout the tropical and subtropical zones. Infection is prevalent in areas where untreated human feces are allowed to contaminate the soil, and people walk barefoot. *Necator americanus* ("New World hookworm") is found primarily in the Western hemisphere, but also in southern Asia, Indonesia, Australia, and Oceania. *Ancylostoma duodenale* ("Old World hookworm") is found predominantly in the Mediterranean region, northern Asia, and the west coast of South America. As a result of sanitary waste disposal policies in the United States, hookworm infection has a low prevalence, being found primarily in the southeast.

The life cycle of hookworm is very similar to that of *Strongyloides*. Like *Strongyloides*, the hookworm filariform larvae penetrate the skin, enter the bloodstream and lymphatics, pass into the lung, migrate up the bronchi to the trachea, are swallowed, and finally take up residence in the upper small intestine (Figure 12-5). They attach by means of a buccal capsule that is used to suck blood from the host. A single *Necator americanus* worm can remove 0.03 mL of blood daily, and a single *Ancylostoma duodenale* worm, 0.2 mL. Worldwide, hookworm is a major cause of iron deficiency anemia. It is responsible for an estimated blood loss of 7 million liters daily—the total blood volume of more than 1 million people!

The life cycle of the hookworm also differs from that of *Strongyloides* in several important ways, and the differences account for hookworm's milder clinical manifestations. The *Strongyloides* ova mature quickly, hatching in the bowel wall of the host; hookworm ova mature more slowly, requiring several days of incubation in warm, moist, shady soil. As a result, human hookworm infestation is confined to geographic areas with a warm climate. The longer maturation time for hookworm eggs also means that autoinfection does not occur and that infection by fresh feces is not possible.

CLINICAL PRESENTATION

When hookworm larvae penetrate the skin they can cause intense pruritus, sometimes called "ground itch." Itching is associated with local erythema and a papular rash at the site of penetration. As is observed with both *Ascaris* and *Strongyloides*, respiratory symptoms and patchy pneumonia associated with peripheral eosinophilia (Loffler's syndrome) can develop as the worm penetrates the lung. The abnormalities most commonly associated with hookworm are iron deficiency and protein malnutrition. These abnormalities depend both on the worm burden on the nutritional status of the patient. Other complaints may include abdominal pain, diarrhea, and weight loss.

DIAGNOSIS AND TREATMENT

Adult female worms release between 10,000 and 20,000 worms daily, making diagnosis by stool smear simple. The eggs are readily seen using a low-power (100×)

KEY POINTS

About Hookworm (*Necator americanus* and *Ancylostoma duodenale*)

1. Larvae from the soil penetrate the skin, causing a pruritic rash.
2. Larvae pass through the lung and can cause Loffler's syndrome.
3. Eggs hatch outside of the host in soil (no autoinfection).
4. Adult worms attach to bowel wall and suck blood.
4. Iron deficiency anemia is the most common manifestation.
5. The diagnosis is readily made from observation of ova in the stool.
6. Mebendazole is the treatment of choice.

---

microscope (Figure 12.4). Quantitation of the egg count allows for an estimate of the worm burden. Mebendazole for 3 days is usually curative (see Table 12.3).

■ TISSUE AND BLOOD HELMINTHS

GUIDING QUESTIONS

1. Which tissues do Trichinella, Echinococcus, and Taenia solium prefer to infect?

2. Why is Trichinella uncommon in the United States?

3. What is a hydatid cyst, and how is it treated?

4. Why does treatment with praziquantel often exacerbate the manifestations of neurocysticercosis?

TRICHINELLA

POTENTIAL SEVERITY

Usually asymptomatic, but heavy infections can lead to severe myocarditis, pneumonia, and encephalitis that can be fatal.

Prevalence, Epidemiology, and Life Cycle

Trichinosis is found worldwide, wherever contaminated meat is undercooked. *Trichinella* is a roundworm whose larvae are released from cyst walls in contaminated meat by acid–pepsin digestion in the stomach. Upon entering the small intestine, larvae invade the intestinal microvilli and develop into adult worms. Females then release larvae that enter the bloodstream and seed skeletal and cardiac muscle. The larvae grow in individual muscle fibers and eventually become surrounded by a cyst wall. Once encysted, the larvae can remain viable for many years. If the cyst-containing muscle tissue is ingested, *Trichinella* is able to take up residence in the new host.

The domestic animal that primarily becomes infected with *Trichinella* is the pig. In many countries, including the United States, pigs are fed with grain, which explaining the low incidence of trichinosis. In the United States, laws were enacted to prevent the feeding of uncooked garbage to pigs, and as a result, fewer than 100 trichinosis cases are reported annually. Most cases of trichinosis result from improperly processed pork, but undercooked bear, walrus, cougar, wild boar, and horse meat have also been sources of *Trichinella* infection.

Clinical Presentation

Symptoms correlate with the numbers of worms in tissues. Because the number of cysts ingested is often low, most infections are asymptomatic. Heavier infestations can result in diarrhea, abdominal pain, and vomiting during the intestinal phase, followed in 1 to 2 weeks by fever, periorbital edema, subconjunctival hemorrhages, and chemosis. Muscle pain, swelling, and weakness are common. The extraocular muscles are frequently involved first, followed by the neck and back, arms and legs. Occasionally, a macular or petechial diffuse body rash may be seen. These symptoms usually peak within 2 to 3 weeks, but they may be followed by a prolonged period of muscle weakness. Death is uncommon, but can result from severe myocarditis leading to congestive heart failure. Fatal encephalitis and pneumonia have also been reported.

Diagnosis and Treatment

An elevated peripheral eosinophil count associated with periorbital edema, myositis, and fever strongly suggest the diagnosis. Eosinophil counts are often very high. Serum creatine phosphokinase is also elevated, reflecting muscle damage. A specific diagnosis requires biopsy of a symptomatic muscle to demonstrate *Trichinella* larvae. Because exposure history and the clinical manifestations are usually distinct, a biopsy is rarely required. Antibody to *Trichinella* increases within 3 weeks and can be detected by ELISA.

Mebendazole is recommended for treatment. Myositis may be reduced by using a dosing regimen that starts with a lower dose for 3 days, and then follows with higher doses for 10 days (see Table 12.3). Albendazole can be given as alternative therapy. In critically ill patients, corticosteroids (prednisone 50 mg daily for 10 to 15 days) may be helpful, but no controlled trials have been conducted proving efficacy. Cooking meat above 55°C until all pink flesh is browned kills encysted larvae and prevents trichinosis.

ECHINOCOCCOSIS

POTENTIAL SEVERITY

Infections with Echinococcus multilocularis *usually lead to symptomatic disease; patients infected with* Echinococcus granulosus *may remain asymptomatic. Extensive disease causes significant morbidity and mortality.*

Prevalence, Epidemiology, and Life Cycle

Echinococcus is member of the cestode (tapeworm) family. Infections with *Echinococcus granulosus* are found worldwide, including in Africa, the Middle East, southern Europe, Latin America, and the southwestern United States. A second species, *Echinococcus multilocularis* is

---

KEY POINTS

About Trichinosis

1. Caused by ingesting larvae cysts, primarily from pork.
2. Uncommon in countries that don't feed pigs uncooked garbage.
3. Larvae infect skeletal and cardiac muscle.
4. Light infections are often asymptomatic.
5. Heavy infection causes abdominal pain and diarrhea, followed by fever, periorbital edema, muscle pain (ocular muscles first), and myocarditis, associated with marked eosinophilia and increased creatine phosphokinase.
6. Diagnosis is made by muscle biopsy, ELISA, or clinical signs.

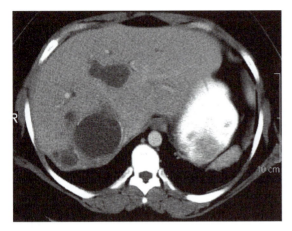

Figure 12–7. A computed tomography scan with both oral and intravenous contrast shows multiple echinococcal hepatic abscesses. (Picture courtesy of Dr. Pat Abbitt, University of Florida College of Medicine)

found in northern Europe, Asia, the northern United States, and the Arctic. Humans represent an inadvertent intermediate host, the infection being contracted by ingestion of food contaminated with viable parasite eggs. *Echinococcus* is carried in the feces of sheep, goats, camels, horses, and domestic dogs that live around live-stock. In the southwestern United States, most cases are contracted from sheep dogs. The primary host for *Echinococcus multilocularis* is the fox, and domestic cats and dogs become secondarily infected. Because eggs are partially resistant to drying and can remain viable for many weeks, food can become contaminated without coming in direct contact with infected animals.

Ingested eggs hatch in the intestine, forming oncospheres that penetrate the bowel wall, enter the bloodstream, and are deposited in various organs—most commonly the liver and lungs, and less frequently the brain, heart, and bones—where they encyst. The resulting hydatid cysts consist of a germinal membrane that produces multiple tapeworm heads and that also undergoes budding to form multiple, septated daughter cysts within the primary cyst (Figure 12.7). Cysts can survive in the host for decades.

CASE 12.4

A 33-year-old woman, an immigrant from Jordan, presented with a chief complaint of bloody cough and shortness of breath for a period of 2 weeks. At age 22, she had undergone a CT scan of the abdomen as part of a workup for polycystic ovaries. She was noted at that time to have a large liver cyst consistent with Echinococcus. Although she was asymptomatic, resection of the left lobe of the liver was performed that year. Despite surgical resection, she experienced recurrent cysts and on three occasions underwent percutaneous aspiration followed by injection of hypertonic saline. One month before admission and 6 years after her last aspiration and injection procedure, she began coughing up blood. At the same time, she noted shortness of breath. She received several courses of oral antibiotics, but failed to improve. Her coughing then became productive of gelatinous, foul-smelling serosanguinous fluid.

Pulmonary exam revealed decreased breath sounds and dullness to percussion at the right base. Bronchial breath sounds and E-to-A changes were noted in the right posterior mid-lung field. The liver was not palpable. A CT scan of the chest and abdomen revealed a fluid collection over the dome of the liver and an 8x5-cm abscess in the right lower lobe that contained an air–fluid level.

Clinical Presentation

Most patients with echinococcosis are asymptomatic, the infection being detected incidentally on an imaging study. Symptoms generally develop when the hydatid cyst reaches a size of 8 to 10 cm and begins compressing vital structures or eroding into the biliary tract or a pulmonary bronchus (as occurred in case 12.4). The cysts can also become superinfected, resulting in a bacterial abscess. Cyst leakage or rupture can result in an anaphylactic reaction, causing fever and hypotension. Cysts can also develop in the brain, heart, kidneys, eyes, and bones. Asymptomatic disease caused by *Echinococcus granulosus* rarely progresses; however, 90% of cases of asymptomatic *Echinococcus multilocularis* infection eventually progress to symptomatic disease.

Diagnosis and Treatment

Ultrasonography, CT scan, or magnetic resonance imaging reveal a characteristic hydatid cyst with a distinct septated structure representing daughter cysts (Figure 12.7). Often, tapeworm heads can also be visualized. The stage of infection can be classified based on ultrasound findings, but CT scan has been found to be the most effective diagnostic method for delineating the extent of disease. The diagnosis can be confirmed by ELISA, which is highly sensitive for liver cysts, but less sensitive for cysts in other organs.

Complete surgical resection of the hydatid cyst is often recommended in symptomatic disease. The cyst should be removed intact, taking great care to avoid a rupture, which will spread the infection by daughter cysts. To reduce the risk of spread, aspiration of the cyst is recommended—a procedure that involves removing a fraction of the contents and instilling a hypertonic saline solution (30% NaCl), iodophore, or 95% ethanol to kill the germinal layer and daughter cysts. Surgical resection should be performed 30 minutes after instillation of the solution. In cases with biliary communication, the foregoing cidal agents are not recommended because of the risk of inducing sclerosing cholangitis.

As compared with medical treatment alone, debulking of cysts does not improve outcome, but it may relieve symptoms in specific cases. Treatment in the perioperative period with three to four cycles of albendazole 400 mg twice daily for 4 weeks, followed by a 2-week rest period is generally recommended to limit the risk of intraoperative dissemination. The same medical therapy is recommended for patients with inoperable hydatid cyst (see Table 12.3). In selected cases, CT or ultrasound has been used to guide percutaneous needle aspiration drainage and instillation of cidal agents (hypertonic saline or ethanol) to sterilize the cyst, followed by re-aspiration after 15 minutes to remove the cidal agent ("PAIR"). The PAIR treatment is often curative, and it is becoming the treatment of choice. The efficacy of PAIR has not be confirmed by randomized trials, however.

KEY POINTS

About *Echinococcus*

1. Spread primarily by domestic dogs, who excrete eggs in their feces. Eggs survive in dust and contaminate food.
2. Eggs hatch in the intestine and oncospheres enter the bloodstream, where they migrate to the liver or lung, or (less commonly) to the brain, where they form hydatid cysts.
3. Hydatid cysts survive and grow over decades, causing symptoms when they reach 8 to 10 cm in diameter.
4. Diagnosis is made by computed tomography scan or ultrasonography.
5. Treatment involves administration of albendazole, combined with surgical resection preceded by instillation of an agent cidal to the germinal layer. Alternatively, percutaneous needle drainage and cidal agent instillation ("PAIR") may be curative.

CYSTICERCOSIS

POTENTIAL SEVERITY

Causes neurologic complications in a significant number of infected patients many years after the initial infection.

Prevalence, Epidemiology, and Life Cycle

Taenia solium is another cestode (tapeworm) common in Central and South America, Mexico, the Philippines, Southeast Asia, India, Africa, and southern Europe. Like *Echinococcus*, *Taenia* can be contracted by ingesting viable eggs or by eating raw or undercooked pork containing encysted larvae. Once ingested, the eggs hatch or the encysted larvae are released into the stomach, where they migrate into the intestine and develop into adult worms that can reach 8 m in length. Autoinfection can occur as a result of regurgitation of eggs into the stomach or accidental ingestion of eggs from the host's own feces.

Clinical Presentation

Adult intestinal worms rarely cause symptoms. However, larvae can penetrate the intestine, enter the bloodstream and eventually encyst in the brain, causing neurocysticercosis. Cysts may lodge in the cerebral ventricles (causing hydrocephalus), the spinal cord (resulting in cord compression and paraplegia), the subarachnoid space (causing chronic meningitis), or the cerebral cortex (causing seizures). Cysts may remain asymptomatic for many years, becoming clinically apparent only when the larvae die, an event associated with cyst swelling and increased inflammation. Larvae also encyst in other tissues (skin and muscle), but rarely cause symptoms. Eye involvement is also reported.

Diagnosis and Treatment

Computed tomography or nuclear magnetic resonance scan are the preferred diagnostic studies, demonstrating discrete cysts that may enhance following the administration of contrast media depending on the degree of surrounding inflammation. In CNS infection, multiple lesions are generally detected. Older lesions are often calcified (Figure 12.8). In the absence of cerebral edema, lumbar puncture can be performed. Analysis of the cerebrospinal fluid usually

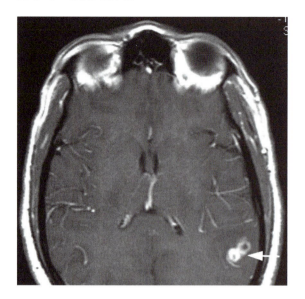

Figure 12–8. Computed tomography scan with contrast of the cerebral cortex, showing two typical ring-enhancing lesions of neurocysticercosis (arrow).

reveals lymphocytes or eosinophils accompanied by low glucose and elevated protein. Serologic tests detecting antibody directed against *Taenia solium* may be positive, particularly in patients with multiple cysts.

Treatment for neurocysticercosis is complex and controversial. Albendazole and praziquantel may kill living

---

KEY POINTS

About Cysticercosis (*Taenia solium* infection)

1. Contracted by ingesting eggs in fecally contaminated food or encysted larvae in undercooked pork.
2. Larvae enter the bloodstream, encysting primarily in the brain.
3. Symptoms develop after many years when the larvae die, causing increased inflammation.
4. Can cause seizures, hydrocephalus, paraplegia, and meningitis.
5. Diagnosis is made by computed tomography scan, magnetic resonance imaging, or serology.
6. Treatment involves administration of albendazole plus corticosteroids for symptomatic disease; surgical resection can be performed in selected patients.

---

cysts, but larval death results in increased inflammation and edema, and may exacerbate symptoms. A recent randomized trial and a meta-analysis suggested that in symptomatic patients with cortical lesions, albendazole combined with oral dexamethasone (2 mg three times daily) or oral prednisone (40 mg daily) enhances resolution of the lesions and reduces the incidence of seizures. Surgical resection of cysts may be required depending on the symptoms and on size and location of the offending cyst. Antiepileptic medications should be used to control seizures.

SCHISTOSOMIASIS

GUIDING QUESTIONS

1. *Why doesn't primary schistosomiasis occur in the United States?*
2. *How is schistosomiasis contracted?*
3. *Which Schistosoma strain causes swimmer's itch?*
4. *What is Katayama fever?*
5. *In late disease, how does egg deposition cause clinical symptoms?*

POTENTIAL SEVERITY

Usually a chronic disorder resulting in debilitating complications. Occasionally fatal during the early stage of infection as a result of a severe serum-sickness syndrome.

Prevalence, Epidemiology, and Life Cycle

Schistosoma mansoni, S. haematobium, and *S. japonicum* are members of the fluke (trematode) family. Schistosomes are estimated to infect between 200 and 300 million people worldwide. Primary infection does not occur in the United States because the critical intermediate host—a specific type of freshwater snail—is absent. However, approximately 400,000 imported cases occur in immigrants from Puerto Rico, South America (particularly Brazil), the Middle East, and the Philippines. *S. mansoni* is found primarily in South America, the Caribbean, Africa, and countries of the Arab Middle East. *S. haematobium* is found in Africa and the Middle East, and *S. japonicum* is found primarily in China and the

Philippines. Two other strains that have more recently been found to cause disease are *S. intercalatum* (Western and Central Africa) and *S. mekongi* (Indochina).

The parasite is contracted by exposure to fresh water containing infectious cercariae. The fork-tailed cercariae are able to swim to and penetrate the skin of people wading in stagnant infested freshwater pools or rice paddies. Once inside the host, cercariae lose their tails and mature into schistosomulae that enter the bloodstream. From the bloodstream, they penetrate the lung and liver, where over a period of 6 weeks, they mature to adult worms. The adult worms then migrate through the venous plexus to various sites, depending on the *Schistosoma* strain. *S. mansoni* worms take up residence in the inferior mesenteric veins responsible for venous drainage of the large intestine; *S. japonicum*, in the superior mesenteric veins that drain the small intestine, and *S. haematobium*, in the vesicular plexus that drains the urinary bladder.

Once resident in the host, the worms can live for decades, releasing eggs into the bowel or bladder. Improper handling of contaminated stool and urine leads to egg contamination of water. Eggs hatch in fresh water, forming miracidia whose cilia enable them to swim and infect freshwater snails. Each species of schistosome requires a specific freshwater snail intermediate, which explains the geographic distribution of each strain. The miracidia multiply within the snail, and within 4 to 6 weeks, they release large numbers of cercariae capable of infecting humans.

KEY POINTS

About the Life Cycle of *Schistosoma*

1. Cercariae swimming in fresh water can penetrate human skin.
2. Cercariae mature into schistosomulae that enter the bloodstream and migrate to the liver and lung, where they mature.
3. Mature worms migrate to the venous system of the small (*S. japonicum*) or large bowel (*S. mansoni*) or to the bladder venous plexus (*S. haematobium*).
4. The worms release eggs into stool or urine for many years, resulting in contamination of fresh water.
5. Freshwater snails are infected by miracidia, a necessary step in the production of cercariae and infection of humans.

CASE 12.5

A 32-year-old man was evaluated for a lesion of the urinary bladder. He had been well until 16 months earlier. Soon after returning from a 1-week vacation in Malawi, he had an episode of perineal pain associated with painful ejaculation and brown-colored ejaculate. His condition improved after treatment with ciprofloxacin.

Four months before the evaluation, this patient had begun experiencing urinary frequency, with intermittent passage of small blood clots in the urine. His symptoms failed to improve on ciprofloxacin treatment. An epidemiologic history noted frequent travel outside the United States. Most recently, the man had traveled to Malawi with his wife. While there, he had repeatedly swum in a lake that he was assured was "safe."

A laboratory workup showed a normal peripheral WBC count and differential. Urinalysis confirmed hematuria. Cytology found no malignant cells. A urogram and ultrasound demonstrated a round structure, 8 × 10 mm in diameter, adherent to the bladder wall. Cystoscopic examination disclosed multiple, slightly raised, polypoid lesions that were less than 5 mm in diameter. The lesions were erythematous, with focal yellow areas.

Low-power microscopic examination of material from a bladder biopsy revealed a polypoid inflammatory lesion of the bladder mucosa with dense inflammatory infiltrate surrounding clusters of eggs in the submucosa. At higher magnification, the granulomas were found to contain clusters of helminthic eggs surrounded by epithelioid histiocytes, chronic inflammatory cells, and eosinophils. The eggs were oval and had a terminal spine characteristic of S. haematobium (Figure 12.9). The man's wife was subsequently examined, and Schistosoma eggs were found in her urine. Both were treated with praziquantel, and the eggs disappeared from both patients' urine.

Clinical Presentation

The three stages of the disease correspond to the life cycle of the parasite in the human host.

The first stage occurs at the time of penetration and is commonly termed "swimmer's itch." A very itchy macular papular rash develops within 24 hours of the

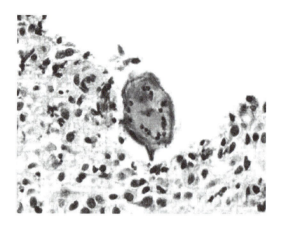

Figure 12–9. Bladder biopsy showing an egg of *Schistosoma haematobium.* (Picture from the N. Engl. J. Med 343:1105-1111, 2000)

cercariae penetrating the skin. The lesions spontaneously resolve as the organisms spread to the bloodstream. An avian schistosome is also able to penetrate the skin, but it is not capable of entering the bloodstream. This benign form of swimmer's itch is common in the Great Lakes of the north-central United States and in freshwater lakes in Europe.

The second stage of clinical disease occurs 4 to 8 weeks later, when the worms mature and begin releasing eggs. Patients develop a serum-sickness-like syndrome as they react with elevated levels of immunoglobulin E and peripheral eosinophilia to egg antigens. Fever, headache, cough, chills, and sweating are accompanied by lymphadenopathy and hepatosplenomegaly. This clinical constellation has been called "Katayama fever" and is most commonly associated with *S. japonicum.* The symptoms usually resolve spontaneously, but in heavy infections, this acute reaction can be fatal.

The third, chronic, stage results from granulomatous reactions to egg deposition in the intestine, liver, bladder, and (less commonly) the lung and CNS. Granulomatous reactions in the bowel can lead to chronic diarrhea, abdominal pain, and blood loss. Eggs may enter the portal venous system and gain entry to the liver, where chronic inflammation is followed by fibrosis leading to portal hypertension, splenomegaly, and bleeding esophageal varices. Because the hepatic parenchyma is seldom compromised, liver function tests are usually normal. Peripheral eosinophilia is commonly encountered. Hepatosplenomegaly with normal liver function tests, peripheral eosinophilia, and a history of residence in an endemic area should raise the possibility of chronic hepatic schistosomiasis. The development of

collateral venous channels in association with portal hypertension can result in egg deposition in the pulmonary arteries, causing pulmonary hypertension and right-sided congestive heart failure. Deposition of eggs in the CNS is less common and can cause seizures or, if eggs are deposited in the region of the spinal cord, transverse myelitis. In *S. haematobium,* eggs are deposited in the bladder wall, leading to hematuria, bladder obstruction, hydronephrosis, and recurrent urinary tract infections. Bladder cancer may also complicate chronic *S. haematobium* infection.

Diagnosis and Treatment

Demonstration of eggs in the stool or urine allows a specific diagnosis to be made. Quantitative egg counts are helpful in assessing the intensity of the infection. Urine is best collected between noon and 2 PM. Passing the urine through a 10-mm filter concentrates the eggs. Eggs may also be identified on tissue biopsies. Rectal biopsy is particularly helpful in diagnosing *S. mansoni.* The eggs of *S. mansoni, S. japonicum,* and *S. haematobium* have distinct morphologies, allowing them to be readily identified using a low-power (100X) microscope (Figure 12.4). In chronic disease, the egg burden may be low, making the diagnosis difficult. Anti-schistosome antibody tests are now available for detecting chronically infected patients; however, the specificity and sensitivity of these tests limit their value. Furthermore, the tests cannot be used in lifelong residents of endemic areas, because serology in these

---

KEY POINTS

About the Clinical Presentation of Schistosomiasis

1. Skin penetration causes "swimmer's itch."
2. A serum-sickness syndrome with eosinophilia and high immunoglobulin E levels may follow. This constellation of symptoms is called Katayama fever.
3. Granulomatous reaction to egg deposition leads to chronic diarrhea, portal hypertension and hepatosplenomegaly, and pulmonary hypertension in *Schistosoma mansoni* and *S. japonicum.*
4. Eggs deposited in the bladder can lead to hematuria, bladder obstruction, hydronephrosis, recurrent urinary tract infections, and sometimes bladder cancer in cases of *S. haematobium.*

individuals is frequently positive in the absence of active infection.

Praziquantel is effective treatment for all forms of schistosomiasis (see Table 12.3). Side effects of treatment are mild and include fever, abdominal discomfort, and headache.

OTHER, LESS COMMON TISSUE FLUKES

Other flukes that can infect humans undergo a life cycle similar to that of *Schistosoma*, requiring snails as the intermediate host. However, rather than gaining entry by penetrating the human skin, the cercariae take up residence in other food sources and become encysted. Infection is contracted when the human host eats cercariae contaminated food.

Clonorchis sinensis (Chinese liver fluke) infections result from the ingestion of raw or undercooked freshwater fish. Infections occur in China, Hong Kong, and Vietnam. Worms gain entry into biliary tract via the ampulla of Vater. Infection can be complicated by cholangitis and, later, by cholangiocarcinoma. Infections are effectively treated with praziquantel.

Fasciola hepatica, another liver fluke, is found in sheep-raising areas of the world, including South America, Australia, China, Africa, and Europe. Ingestion of vegetables contaminated with encysted cercariae is the most common route of infection. This fluke is treated with praziquantel or bithionol.

Paragonimus westermani (lung fluke) is contracted by eating raw or pickled crawfish or freshwater crabs. This parasite is found in Central and South America, West Africa, India, and East Asia. This parasite first enters the gastrointestinal tract and subsequently penetrates through the diaphragm, entering the pleural cavity and lungs, causing respiratory symptoms. Praziquantel is the treatment of choice.

KEY POINTS

About the Diagnosis and Treatment of Schistosomiasis

1. Characteristic eggs in the stool or urine (check between noon and 2 PM) or on tissue biopsy are diagnostic; consider rectal biopsy in *Schistosoma mansoni*.
2. Eggs may not be seen in chronic disease, anti-schistosome antibody may be helpful,
3. Praziquantel is the treatment of choice.

FILARIASIS (WUCHERERIA BANCROFTI AND BRUGIA MALAYI)

GUIDING QUESTIONS

1. *How is filariasis transmitted?*
2. *What is the key characteristic that helps to differentiate inflammatory filariasis from bacterial cellulitis?*
3. *Is elephantiasis an early or late manifestation of filariasis?*
4. *When during the day are blood smears most likely to be positive?*

POTENTIAL SEVERITY

A chronic debilitating infection that can cause severe disfiguring complications by blocking lymphatic drainage.

Prevalence, Epidemiology, and Life Cycle

Microfilaria is less common than many parasites, being estimated to infect approximately 120 million people. Several strains of worm can cause this disease. *Wuchereria bancrofti* is found throughout the tropics, and *Brugia malayi* is restricted to the southern regions of Asia. A third strain, *Brugia timori* is found only in Indonesia.

Infectious larvae are transmitted by the bite of a mosquito. Larvae pass from the skin into the lymphatic system, where, over several months, they mature near the lymph nodes. Adult worms (40 to 100 mm in length) can survive in the lymphatic system for 5 to 15 years. During this period, males and females mate, daily producing an average of 10,000 microfilaria (dimensions: 200 to 300 mm in length, and 10 μm in width). The microfilaria are released into the bloodstream. The time from initial insect bite to appearance of microfilaria in the infected human is usually 12 months. In *W. bancrofti*, the highest concentration of microfilaria in the blood is generally found in the middle of the night, explaining why midnight blood smears are recommended for diagnosis.

If a mosquito bites an infected human, the microfilaria are ingested and, over 10 to 14 days, they develop into infective larvae that can be transmitted to a new human host. The percentage of mosquitoes containing infective larvae has been estimated to be just 1% in endemic areas. Repeated mosquito bites are therefore generally required to contract this infection, which may explain why adults—particularly men—more commonly contract this infection.

Clinical Presentation

ASYMPTOMATIC FILARIASIS

Many individuals have asymptomatic infection. Peripheral eosinophilia and palpable lymphadenopathy may be the only clinical manifestations. Children usually experience no symptoms, despite high numbers of microfilaria in their blood.

INFLAMMATORY FILARIASIS

Adults more commonly react with strong allergic reactions to the invasion by worms that begins approximately 1 year after exposure. Fever, chills, vomiting, headache, and malaise may be associated with lymphangitis of an extremity, orchitis, epididymitis, or scrotal swelling. The affected extremity becomes hot, swollen, erythematous, and painful, mimicking cellulitis. These symptoms are associated with peripheral leukocytosis and an increased percentage of eosinophils (6% to 25%). Unlike cellulitis, which usually begins peripherally and moves up the limb, inflammatory filariasis begins centrally near the lymph nodes and extends peripherally. Attacks may occur monthly and do not respond to antibiotics. The granulomatous response in the lymphatic tissue is thought to be a host inflammatory reaction to dying worms. Death of the worms is associated with release of the rickettsial-like bacteria *Wolbachia* that live in a symbiotic relationship within the adult worms.

OBSTRUCTIVE FILARIASIS

Over time, chronic inflammation leads to fibrosis and permanent obstruction of lymphatic flow. This syndrome is the result of continuous microfilaria infection.

Persistent lymphatic obstruction and edema lead to marked skin thickening and deposition of collagenous material, eventually causing elephantiasis. Patients suffer with debilitating enlargement of the legs or massive enlargement of the scrotal tissue, making walking difficult. Cellulitis caused by streptococci or *Staphylococcus aureus* may periodically recur, requiring antibiotic treatment. Rupture of the lymphatics into the kidney or bladder can result in chyluria, and rupture into the peritoneum can cause chylous ascites.

Diagnosis and Treatment

Giemsa- or Wright-stained peripheral smears should be obtained at midnight in all cases except for those from the South Pacific. Identification of adult worms in the blood is definitive; however, in early and late disease, worms often are not seen. Antibody and antigen assays are highly sensitive and specific. An IgG4 antibody titer correlates with active disease. An ELISA for *W. bancrofti* circulating antigen is now the diagnostic test of choice, and titers correlate with adult worm burden. A PCR test for *W. bancrofti* has been developed, but it is not widely available. Biopsy of infected lymph nodes is generally not recommended, but when performed, may reveal adult worms in addition to granuloma. Ultrasonography of dilated lymphatics in the spermatic cord have revealed motile worms. In early infection and during the inflammatory stage, peripheral eosinophilia is commonly seen.

KEY POINTS

About the Clinical Presentation of Filariasis

1. Many people, particularly children, are asymptomatic.
2. Inflammatory filariasis is associated with periodic erythema, warmth, pain, and swelling that mimic cellulitis (associated with peripheral eosinophilia).
3. Obstructive disease results in chronic limb swelling (elephantiasis) because of lymphatic fibrosis.
4. Obstructive disease can lead to recurrent bacterial cellulitis.
5. Rupture of lymphatics can cause chyluria or chylous ascites.
6. Release of the rickettsial-like bacteria *Wolbachia* from the adult worms may be the major stimulus for inflammation.

KEY POINTS

About the Life Cycle of *Wuchereria bancrofti* and *Brugia malayi*

1. Transmitted by the bite of an infected mosquito.
2. Repeated mosquito bites are required.
3. Microfilaria live in the lymphatic system, and worms enter the bloodstream at midnight (except in the South Pacific).
4. Mosquitoes are infected by biting humans.

KEY POINTS

About the Diagnosis and Treatment of Filariasis

1. Midnight blood smear demonstrating worms yields a definitive diagnosis.
2. In early and late disease, worms may not be seen.
3. Ultrasound of dilated lymphatics may demonstrate worms.
4. Peripheral eosinophilia is common.
5. Enzyme-linked immunoabsorbent assay is sensitive and specific, and levels correlate with disease activity.
6. Diethylcarbamazine or ivermectin plus albendazole is used for treatment. Treatment can exacerbate symptoms.

During the chronic stages of disease, eosinophilia is generally not present. If worms cannot be identified, the diagnosis has to be made on clinical grounds.

Diethylcarbamazine in a single dose is the recommended therapy, but fails to kill adult worms (see Table 12.3). A reduction in the level of microfilaria in the blood is usually observed. Treatment may increase inflammation and may not halt progression to fibrosis and lymphatic obstruction. Ivermectin 200 to 400 mg/kg, combined with albendazole 400 mg, is another effective regimen that may more effectively kill the adult worms. For more severely infected patients, a 3-week course of doxycycline kills the symbiant *Wolbachia*, resulting in sterility of the adult worms. This treatment can be followed by diethylcarbazine or ivermectin plus albendazole. Normally, these agents exacerbate the host's inflammatory reaction as the microfilaria die, but doxycycline eradication of the *Wolbachia* eliminates this complication. Anti-inflammatory agents may be used to reduce the extent of inflammation, and elastic support stockings can be helpful in reducing moderate lymphedema.

DIROFILARIASIS (DOG HEARTWORM)

Humans are an accidental host in dirofilariasis. The disease is most commonly found in the southeastern United States and is transmitted by mosquitoes. After developing in the subcutaneous tissue, the young adult filaria migrate. In dogs, they migrate to the right side of the heart and right pulmonary vessels, where they survive. In humans, they migrate to the lung, but fail to develop. Their deaths produce local granulomatous

inflammation. Most human cases present as an asymptomatic pulmonary coin lesion mimicking an early neoplasm. Microscopic examination of the lung biopsy reveals a dead worm. Treatment of human cases is not necessary.

ONCHOCERCIASIS

The *Onchocerca volvulus* parasite is found primarily in Africa, where it infects approximately 20 million people. Cases are occasionally seen in Central and South America. The infection is transmitted by a black fly that swarms around the face, often biting around the eyes and depositing *Onchocerca* larvae onto the skin. These larvae penetrate and crawl through the skin and connective tissue. The worms initially cause an itchy erythematous rash. Later, fibrous skin nodules develop. Worms often migrate into the anterior chamber of the eye, causing inflammation and blindness. Because the offending black fly is commonly found near streams, this disease has been called "river blindness."

The diagnosis is made by skin snips or by visualizing worms in a slit lamp examination of the eyes. The treatment of choice is a single dose of ivermectin repeated at 3-month intervals until symptoms resolve (see Table 12.3). Fever, itching, and an urticarial rash may develop as result of dying microfilaria.

LOIASIS

The loa loa microfilaria is also transmitted by a fly, and the disease is found in Western and Central Africa. The microfilaria migrate through the skin, causing localized edema called Calabar swellings. Several hours before swelling occurs, local itching and pain are noted. Occasionally the microfilaria can be seen migrating through the subconjunctiva, causing intense conjunctivitis. Active microfilaria migration is associated with marked peripheral eosinophilia.

The diagnosis is made by daytime blood smear. Diethylcarbamazine or ivermectin are recommended as treatment (see Table 12.3). Diethylcarbamazine can precipitate encephalitis in heavily infected patients.

FURTHER READING

General

O'Brien D, Tobin S, Brown GV, Torresi J. Fever in returned travelers: review of hospital admissions for a 3-year period. *Clin Infect Dis.* 2001;33:603–609.

Malaria

Centers for Disease Control and Prevention. Local transmission of *Plasmodium vivax* malaria—Palm Beach County, Florida, 2003. *MMWR Morb Mortal Wkly Rep.* 2003;52:908–911.

Adjuik M, Babiker A, Garner P, Olliaro P, Taylor W, White N. Artesunate combinations for treatment of malaria: meta-analysis. *Lancet*. 2004;363:9–17.

Aronson NE, Sanders JW, Moran KA. In harm's way: infections in deployed American military forces. *Clin Infect Dis*. 2006;43: 1045–1051.

Baird JK, Hoffman SL. Primaquine therapy for malaria. *Clin Infect Dis*. 2004;39:1336–1345.

Bruneel F, Gachot B, Wolff M, Regnier B, Danis M, Vachon F. Resurgence of blackwater fever in long-term European expatriates in Africa: report of 21 cases and review. *Clin Infect Dis*. 2001;32:1133–1140.

Cockburn IA, Mackinnon MJ, O'Donnell A, et al. A human complement receptor 1 polymorphism that reduces *Plasmodium falciparum* rosetting confers protection against severe malaria. *Proc Natl Acad Sci U S A*. 2004;101:272–277.

Dondorp A, Nosten F, Stepniewska K, Day N, White N. Artesunate versus quinine for treatment of severe falciparum malaria: a randomised trial. *Lancet*. 2005;366:717–725.

Farcas GA, Soeller R, Zhong K, Zahirieh A, Kain KC. Real-time polymerase chain reaction assay for the rapid detection and characterization of chloroquine-resistant *Plasmodium falciparum* malaria in returned travelers. *Clin Infect Dis*. 2006;42:622–627.

Greenwood BM, Bojang K, Whitty CJ, Targett GA. Malaria. *Lancet*. 2005;365:1487–1498.

Kockaerts Y, Vanhees S, Knockaert D, Verhaegen J, Lontie M, Peetermans W. Imported malaria in the 1990s: a review of 101 patients. *Eur J Emerg Med*. 2001;8:287–290.

Kublin JG, Patnaik P, Jere CS, et al. Effect of *Plasmodium falciparum* malaria on concentration of HIV-1-RNA in the blood of adults in rural Malawi: a prospective cohort study. *Lancet*. 2005;365: 233–240.

Laufer MK, Thesing PC, Eddington ND, et al. Return of chloroquine antimalarial efficacy in Malawi. *N Engl J Med*. 2006;355: 1959–1966.

Marx A, Pewsner D, Egger M, et al. Meta-analysis: accuracy of rapid tests for malaria in travelers returning from endemic areas. *Ann Intern Med*. 2005;142:836–846.

McKenzie FE, Prudhomme WA, Magill AJ, et al. White blood cell counts and malaria. *J Infect Dis*. 2005;192:323–330.

Mount AM, Mwapasa V, Elliott SR, et al. Impairment of humoral immunity to *Plasmodium falciparum* malaria in pregnancy by HIV infection. *Lancet*. 2004;363:1860–1867.

Ochola LB, Vounatsou P, Smith T, Mabaso ML, Newton CR. The reliability of diagnostic techniques in the diagnosis and management of malaria in the absence of a gold standard. *Lancet Infect Dis*. 2006;6:582–588.

Price RN, Uhlemann AC, Brockman A, et al. Mefloquine resistance in *Plasmodium falciparum* and increased *PFMDR1* gene copy number. *Lancet*. 2004;364:438–447.

Reyburn H, Mbatia R, Drakeley C, et al. Association of transmission intensity and age with clinical manifestations and case fatality of severe *Plasmodium falciparum* malaria. *JAMA*. 2005;293: 1461–1470.

Shanks GD. Treatment of falciparum malaria in the age of drug resistance. *J Postgrad Med*. 2006;52:277–280.

Singh B, Kim Sung L, Matusop A, et al. A large focus of naturally acquired *Plasmodium knowlesi* infections in human beings. *Lancet*. 2004;363:1017–1024.

Smithuis F, Kyaw MK, Phe O, et al. Efficacy and effectiveness of dihydroartemisinin–piperaquine versus artesunate–mefloquine in falciparum malaria: an open-label randomised comparison. *Lancet*. 2006;367:2075–2085.

Williams TN, Mwangi TW, Wambua S, et al. Sickle cell trait and the risk of *Plasmodium falciparum* malaria and other childhood diseases. *J Infect Dis*. 2005;192:178–186.

Babesiosis

Hatcher JC, Greenberg PD, Antique J, Jimenez-Lucho VE. Severe babesiosis in Long Island: review of 34 cases and their complications. *Clin Infect Dis*. 2001;32:1117–1125.

Homer MJ, Aguilar-Delfin I, Telford SR 3rd, Krause PJ, Persing DH. Babesiosis. *Clin Microbiol Rev*. 2000:13:451–469.

Krause PJ. Babesiosis diagnosis and treatment. *Vector Borne Zoonotic Dis*. 2003;3:45–51.

Leishmania

Berenguer J, Gomez-Campdera F, Padilla B, et al. Visceral leishmaniasis (Kala-azar) in transplant recipients: case report and review. *Transplantation*. 1998;65:1401–1404.

Murray HW, Berman JD, Davies CR, Saravia NG. Advances in leishmaniasis. *Lancet*. 2005;366:1561–1577.

Reithinger R, Mohsen M, Wahid M, et al. Efficacy of thermotherapy to treat cutaneous leishmaniasis caused by *Leishmania tropica* in Kabul, Afghanistan: a randomized, controlled trial. *Clin Infect Dis*. 2005;40:1148–1155.

Rosenthal E, Marty P, del Giudice P, et al. HIV and *Leishmania* coinfection: a review of 91 cases with focus on atypical locations of *Leishmania*. *Clin Infect Dis*. 2000;31:1093–1095.

Schwartz E, Hatz C, Blum J. New world cutaneous leishmaniasis in travellers. *Lancet Infect Dis*. 2006;6:342–349.

Trypanosomiasis

Barcan L, Luna C, Clara L, et al. Transmission of *T. cruzi* infection via liver transplantation to a nonreactive recipient for Chagas' disease. *Liver Transpl*. 2005;11:1112–1116.

Barrett MP, Burchmore RJ, Stich A, et al. The trypanosomiases. *Lancet*. 2003;362:1469–1480.

Rassi A Jr, Rassi A, Little WC. Chagas' heart disease. *Clin Cardiol*. 2000;23:883–889.

Sinha A, Grace C, Alston WK, Westenfeld F, Maguire JH. African trypanosomiasis in two travelers from the United States. *Clin Infect Dis*. 1999;29:840–844.

Tobler LH, Contestable P, Pitina L, et al. Evaluation of a new enzyme-linked immunosorbent assay for detection of Chagas antibody in US blood donors. *Transfusion*. 2007;47:90–96.

Intestinal helminths

Bethony J, Brooker S, Albonico M, et al. Soil-transmitted helminth infections: ascariasis, trichuriasis, and hookworm. *Lancet*. 2006;367:1521–1532.

Crompton DW. *Ascaris* and ascariasis. *Adv Parasitol*. 2001;48:285–375.

Friis H, Mwaniki D, Omondi B, et al. Effects on haemoglobin of multi-micronutrient supplementation and multi-helminth chemotherapy: a randomized, controlled trial in Kenyan school children. *Eur J Clin Nutr*. 2003;57:573–579.

Juan JO, Lopez Chegne N, Gargala G, Favennec L. Comparative clinical studies of nitazoxanide, albendazole and praziquantel in the treatment of ascariasis, trichuriasis and hymenolepiasis in children from Peru. *Trans R Soc Trop Med Hyg.* 2002;96:193–196.

Gunawardena GS, Karunaweera ND, Ismail MM. Socio-economic and behavioural factors affecting the prevalence of *Ascaris* infection in a low-country tea plantation in Sri Lanka. *Ann Trop Med Parasitol.* 2004;98:615–621.

Strongyloidiasis

Keiser PB, Nutman TB. *Strongyloides stercoralis* in the immunocompromised population. *Clin Microbiol Rev.* 2004;17:208–217.

Ly MN, Bethel SL, Usmani AS, Lambert DR. Cutaneous *Strongyloides stercoralis* infection: an unusual presentation. *J Am Acad Dermatol.* 2003;49:S157–S160.

Marty FM, Lowry CM, Rodriguez M, et al. Treatment of human disseminated strongyloidiasis with a parenteral veterinary formulation of ivermectin. *Clin Infect Dis.* 2005;41:e5–e8.

Newberry AM, Williams DN, Stauffer WM, Boulware DR, Hendel-Paterson BR, Walker PF. Strongyloides hyperinfection presenting as acute respiratory failure and gram-negative sepsis. *Chest.* 2005;128:3681–3684.

Sarangarajan R, Ranganathan A, Belmonte AH, Tchertkoff V. *Strongyloides stercoralis* infection in AIDS. *AIDS Patient Care STDS.* 1997;11:407–414.

Siddiqui AA, Berk SL. Diagnosis of *Strongyloides stercoralis* infection. *Clin Infect Dis.* 2001;33:1040–1047.

Trichinosis

Centers for Disease Control and Prevention. Trichinellosis associated with bear meat—New York and Tennessee, 2003. *MMWR Morb Mortal Wkly Rep.* 2004;53:606–610.

Bruschi F, Murrell KD. New aspects of human trichinellosis: the impact of new *Trichinella* species. *Postgrad Med J.* 2002;78:15–22.

Gelal F, Kumral E, Vidinli BD, Erdogan D, Yucel K, Erdogan N. Diffusion-weighted and conventional MR imaging in neurotrichinosis. *Acta Radiol.* 2005;46:196–199.

Echinococcosis

Balik AA, Basoglu M, Celebi F, et al. Surgical treatment of hydatid disease of the liver: review of 304 cases. *Arch Surg.* 1999;134:166–169.

Dervenis C, Delis S, Avgerinos C, Madariaga J, Milicevic M. Changing concepts in the management of liver hydatid disease. *J Gastrointest Surg.* 2005;9:869–877.

Kadry Z, Renner EC, Bachmann LM, et al. Evaluation of treatment and long-term follow-up in patients with hepatic alveolar echinococcosis. *Br J Surg.* 2005;92:1110–1116.

Kern P, Bardonnet K, Renner E, et al. European echinococcosis registry: human alveolar echinococcosis, Europe, 1982–2000. *Emerg Infect Dis.* 2003;9:343–349.

McManus DP, Zhang W, Li J, Bartley PB. Echinococcosis. *Lancet.* 2003;362:1295–1304.

Stettler M, Fink R, Walker M, et al. In vitro parasiticidal effect of nitazoxanide against *Echinococcus multilocularis* metacestodes. *Antimicrob Agents Chemother.* 2003;47:467–474.

Cysticercosis

Del Brutto OH, Roos KL, Coffey CS, Garcia HH. Meta-analysis: Cysticidal drugs for neurocysticercosis: albendazole and praziquantel. *Ann Intern Med.* 2006;145:43–51.

Garcia HH, Pretell EJ, Gilman RH, et al. A trial of antiparasitic treatment to reduce the rate of seizures due to cerebral cysticercosis. *N Engl J Med.* 2004;350:249–258.

Garcia HH, Del Brutto OH. Neurocysticercosis: updated concepts about an old disease. *Lancet Neurol.* 2005;4:653–661.

Singhi P, Jain V, Khandelwal N. Corticosteroids versus albendazole for treatment of single small enhancing computed tomographic lesions in children with neurocysticercosis. *J Child Neurol.* 2004;19:323–327.

Schistosomiasis

Gryseels B, Polman K, Clerinx J, Kestens L. Human schistosomiasis. *Lancet.* 2006;368:1106–1118.

Ross AG, Bartley PB, Sleigh AC, et al. Schistosomiasis. *N Engl J Med.* 2002;346:1212–1220.

Talaat M, El-Ayyat A, Sayed HA, Miller FD. Emergence of *Schistosoma mansoni* infection in upper Egypt: the Giza governorate. *Am J Trop Med Hyg.* 1999;60:822–826.

Whitty CJ, Mabey DC, Armstrong M, Wright SG, Chiodini P. Presentation and outcome of 1107 cases of schistosomiasis from Africa diagnosed in a non-endemic country. *Trans R Soc Trop Med Hyg.* 2000;94:531–534.

Filariasis

Dunn IJ. Filarial diseases. *Semin Roentgenol.* 1998;33:47–56.

Ramzy RM, El Setouhy M, Helmy H, et al. Effect of yearly mass drug administration with diethylcarbamazine and albendazole on bancroftian filariasis in Egypt: a comprehensive assessment. *Lancet.* 2006;367:992–999.

Shah MK. Human pulmonary dirofilariasis: review of the literature. *South Med J.* 1999;92:276–279.

Tisch DJ, Michael E, Kazura JW. Mass chemotherapy options to control lymphatic filariasis: a systematic review. *Lancet Infect Dis.* 2005;5:514–523.

Turner JD, Mand S, Debrah AY, et al. A randomized, double-blind clinical trial of a 3-week course of doxycycline plus albendazole and ivermectin for the treatment of *Wuchereria bancrofti* infection. *Clin Infect Dis.* 2006;42:1081–1089.

Onchocerciasis

Hall LR, Pearlman E. Pathogenesis of onchocercal keratitis (river blindness). *Clin Microbiol Rev.* 1999;12:445–453.

Nguyen JC, Murphy ME, Nutman TB, et al. Cutaneous onchocerciasis in an American traveler. *Int J Dermatol.* 2005;44:125–128.

Udall DN. Recent updates on onchocerciasis: diagnosis and treatment. *Clin Infect Dis.* 2007;44:53–60.

Zoonotic Infections

Time Recommended to Complete: 2 days

Frederick Southwick, M.D.

GUIDING QUESTIONS

1. Why have zoonotic infections increased in frequency?

2. How is Lyme Disease contracted and what animal is responsible for spreading this infection?

3. What is the significance of erythema migrans and does this skin lesion require treatment?

4. Should patients with a positive Lyme Disease antibody titer and chronic fatigue be treated with antibiotics?

5. What activities are associated with the highest risk for Leptospirosis and why?

6. How is Rocky Mountain Spotted fever treated and how quickly should therapy be instituted?

7. What are morulae and in what disease are they most frequently seen?

8. What organism causes Cat Scratch Fever and how should this infection be treated?

9. Skinning of what animal carries a high risk of developing Brucellosis?

As a consequence of increased outdoor activities, increasing populations of deer in close proximity to urban areas, and the spread of housing to more rural settings, humans are increasingly coming in contact with animals and with disease-spreading insect vectors. As a consequence, the natural spread of infection from lower mammals to humans, termed "zoonotic infection," has greatly increased since the middle 1970s.

Zoonotic infections represent one of the most important classes of emerging infectious diseases. By combining new understandings of the genomic structures of pathogens with highly sensitive and specific polymerase chain reaction (PCR) detection methods, a number of newly discovered zoonotic diseases have been identified—for example, *Bartonella* and *Ehrlichia*.

■ SPIROCHETES

LYME DISEASE

> **POTENTIAL SEVERITY**
>
> *Can present acutely or result in a chronic disease that is occasionally life-threatening.*

Epidemiology

Lyme disease is the most common insect-borne infection in the United States. More than 10,000 cases are reported annually in United States between the months of May and September. Cases are concentrated in three areas of the country: the Northeast (Massachusetts to Maryland), the Midwest (primarily Wisconsin), and the far West (primarily California and Oregon). Lyme disease is also found in the temperate regions of Europe, Scandinavia, parts of the former Soviet Union, China, Korea, and Japan. Children and middle-aged adults are at greatest risk of acquiring this infection. A variant disease called "southern tick-associated rash illness" (STARI) that can cause an erythema migrans–like rash is found in Missouri and regions of the southeastern United States. This disease is caused by *Borrelia lonestari*.

Pathogenesis

Lyme disease is caused by the spirochete *Borrelia burgdorferi*, the longest and narrowest member of the *Borrelia* species at 20 to 30 μm in length and 0.2 to 0.3 μm in width. Like other spirochetes, it is microaerophilic and fastidious, but it can be grown in vitro using Barbour–Stoenner–Kelly medium. *B. burgdorferi* expresses a number of lipoproteins on its outer surface (called Osps—"outer surface proteins") that are thought to help the organism survive both within the tick and within mammals and birds. A fibronectin-binding protein, flagellar antigen, and two heat-shock proteins have also been described. The heat-shock proteins cross-react with human proteins and may play a role in the development of the rheumatologic complaints commonly associated with late Lyme disease.

Like *Babesia*, *B. burgdorferi* is transmitted the deer tick *Ixodes scapularis*. Other *Ixodes* species are responsible for transmission in the far western United States, Europe, and Asia. The increased incidence of Lyme disease since the end of the 1980s is thought to be the result of the rise in the deer population in suburban areas. Deer and other large mammals are the primary host for the adult tick, but do not play direct role in transmission of the spirochete. The adult *Ixodes* tick does not transmit Lyme disease to humans. As observed with *Babesia* (see Chapter 12), infection is spread to humans by the young *Ixodes* nymph.

These small ticks survive primarily on the white-footed mouse, but they can also be found on other rodents. They attach to humans who walk through brush or tall grass. Because the nymph is the size of a small freckle, it often is not detected and is allowed to remain attached for 36 to 48 hours, the period required to efficiently transmit infection. As the tick feeds, spirochetes escape from the salivary gland of the insect into the skin of human host. As observed with primarily syphilis, *B. burgdorferi* multiplies locally in the skin and after an incubation period of 3 to 32 days, begins forming a distinct, slowly expanding, circular erythematous lesion call erythema migrans. The organism then disseminates throughout the body.

During the dissemination stage, the organism can be cultured from blood and cerebrospinal fluid (CSF). Initially, the immune response is suppressed; however, over days to weeks, cell-mediated immunity is activated, and macrophages are stimulated to produce the proinflammatory cytokines, tumor necrosis factor, and interleukin 1. During this period, immunoglobulin M (IgM) and G (IgG) antibodies are slowly generated. Levels of (IgM) usually peak between 3 and 6 weeks after the initial infection; levels of IgG rise gradually over months. Sites of infection are infiltrated by lymphocytes and plasma cells, and evidence of small-vessel vasculitis is often apparent. However, despite these immune responses, *B. burgdorferi* can survive for years in the synovial fluid, nervous system, and skin of the untreated patient.

KEY POINTS

About the Epidemiology, Cause, and Pathogenesis of Lyme Disease

1. The most common insect-borne disease in the United States. Found in
   a) the Northeast United States, Wisconsin, California, and Oregon.
   b) temperate regions of Europe, Scandinavia, the former Soviet Union, China, Korea, and Japan.
2. Caused by *Borrelia burgdorferi*, a microaerophilic spirochete, that can be grown on Barbour–Stoenner–Kelly medium.
   a) Expresses lipoproteins on its surface help the organism survive in hosts.
   b) Produces fibronectin-binding protein, flagellar antigen, and two heat-shock proteins that cross-react with human proteins.
3. Transmitted by the nymph of the *Ixodes* tick. Moves from deer to white-footed mouse to humans.
   a) Size of a freckle, commonly missed.
   b) Must attach for 36 to 48 hours to transmit the spirochete.
4. Begins in the skin, and then disseminates.
5. Induces cell-mediated and humoral immunity. Can survive for years in joint fluid, the central nervous system, and skin of untreated humans.

Clinical Manifestations

Just as is observed in syphilis (see Chapter 9), Lyme disease has three stages:

1. Early localized infection ("primary Lyme disease").

Case 13.1 presented with erythema migrans, the hallmark of Lyme disease, noted in 90% of patients (Figure 13.1). The lesion begins within a month of exposure as a red macule or papule at the site of the tick bite. It then expands over days, forming a bright red flat border at the advancing edge. As the lesion expands, central clearing may develop, and in some cases, the site takes on the appearance of a target. However, in many patients, the lesion remains diffusely erythematous. Erythema migrans are usually large, reaching an average size of 15 cm (range: 3 to 70 cm). They are commonly located in moist, warm areas of the body where ticks prefer

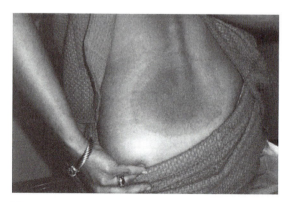

Figure 13–1. Erythema migrans. Note the dark erythematous center. *See color image on color plate 2*

to feed (axilla, behind the knees, and at the belt line). Despite their size, warmth, and bright color, the lesions are usually painless, but they can cause burning or itching.

2. Early disseminated disease ("secondary lyme disease").

Several days after the onset of erythema migrans, small annular satellite lesions may be observed, reflecting early dissemination. Also at this time, patients often experience a viral-like syndrome consisting of malaise, fatigue, myalgias, arthralgias, and headache. They may also develop generalized lymphadenopathy. Migratory joint, tendon, muscle, and bone pain are common complaints. In a significant percentage of patients, symptoms attributable to the nervous system and heart commonly develop at this stage.

Nervous system involvement. The spirochete often initially disseminates to the nervous system, causing a severe generalized headache that waxes and wanes. If the disease is not treated, about 10% of cases develop more serious neurologic manifestations. Frank meningitis can result in neck stiffness, and CSF lymphocytic pleocytosis (usually about 100 cells/mm^3), in elevated CSF protein with normal CSF glucose. Cranial nerve deficits can accompany meningitis, bilateral Bell's palsy being the most common cranial nerve dysfunction. Lymphocytic infiltration of small vessels supplying axons can lead to axonal degeneration and peripheral neuritis. The triad of meningitis,

---

KEY POINTS

About Primary and Secondary Lyme Disease

1. Hallmark of primary disease is erythema migrans:
   a) Macular expanding erythematous lesion, central clearing.
   b) Begins one month after the tick bite.
   c) Mean diameter 15 cm.
   d) Painless, can cause itching.
2. Dissemination is associated with small annular lesions and a flu-like illness.
   a) Central nervous system involvement can cause waxing and waning headache. Lymphocytosis of the cerebrospinal fluid (100 cells/mm^3), cranial nerve deficits (Bell's palsy), and peripheral neuritis is called Bannworth's syndrome.
   b) In cardiovascular involvement, spirochetes infiltrate the myocardium, causing conduction defects.

cranial nerve deficits, and radiculoneuritis has been termed Bannworth's syndrome. This syndrome is more commonly reported in Europe than in the United States.

Cardiovascular involvement. Among untreated patients, 5% to 8% develop cardiac manifestations within several weeks of the onset of illness. Spirochetes can directly infiltrate the myocardium, causing lymphocytic inflammation. Conduction defects are most common, and an electrocardiogram should be ordered in all patients with symptomatic Lyme disease. First-degree heart block is most common, but second-degree and complete heart block may also develop. However, complete heart block rarely persists for longer than 7 days and does not usually require placement of a pacemaker. More severe myocarditis accompanied by congestive heart failure is rare.

3. Late disease ("tertiary lyme disease").

Late disease develops months to years after primary infection. Some patients never experience symptoms from the earlier stages. Musculoskeletal complaints are most common at this stage, but neurologic complaints, skin disease, and generalized symptoms may also occur.

Musculoskeletal manifestations. Approximately 60% to 80% of untreated patients experience musculoskeletal symptoms. Migrating arthralgias or frank arthritis causing joint swelling most commonly involve the knees and other large joints. Less commonly, small joints may

be affected. Joint aspiration may reveal white blood cell (WBC) counts of 500 to 110,000 /mm^3, with a predominance of polymorphonuclear leukocytes (PMNs). The presence of spirochetes in the joint fluid can be detected by PCR in most patients, and arthritis usually resolves after antibiotic therapy.

Neurologic manifestations. Just as is observed in syphilis, *B. burgdorferi* may invade the cerebral cortex and cause a chronic encephalopathy associated with mood, cognitive, and sleep disorders. Subtle language disturbances have also been observed. The CSF may reveal elevated protein levels and increased titers of antibodies to *B. burgdorferi*. Patients may also develop peripheral neuropathies leading to paresthesias and radicular pain. Evaluation of these neurologic complaints can be complicated, and the neurocognitive complaints associated with fibromyalgia are often misdiagnosed as central nervous system Lyme disease. The response to antibiotic therapy is variable.

Other manifestations. Acrodermatitis chronica atrophicans can develop years after erythema migrans. It begins as a bright red skin lesion that later becomes atrophic, mimicking localized scleroderma. *B. burgdorferi* can be cultured from these lesions up to 10 years after their onset. A very difficult management problem arises from the small percentage of patients who experience persistent diffuse aches and pains. Some patients with Lyme disease develop a fibromyalgia-like syndrome; others may experience a chronic fatigue–like syndrome. The contribution of *B. burgdorferi* infection to these complaints remains controversial, and many patients with these complaints fail to improve after antibiotic therapy.

Diagnosis

Although *B. burgdorferi* can be grown in vitro, cultures are rarely positive because the number of organisms in skin lesions, blood, and CSF is very low. The diagnosis is based on clinical manifestations and a history of possible tick exposure in an endemic area, combined with serologic testing. In considering the diagnosis, it is important keep in mind that many patients with confirmed Lyme disease deny being bitten by a tick.

The Lyme disease enzyme-linked immunoabsorbent assay (ELISA) uses a sonicate of *B. burgdorferi* as the antigen and detects IgG and IgM antibodies directed against the spirochete. Acute and convalescent titers spaced 2 to 4 weeks apart should be collected. In early disease, a significant rise in antibody titer is detected in only 60% to 70% of patients. Negative titers at this stage therefore do not exclude Lyme disease. Also, antibiotic therapy can abort a full antibody response, further complicating serologic diagnosis. For these reasons, ELISA testing is not recommended for patients with classic erythema migrans, because the lesion is

---

KEY POINTS

About Late or Tertiary Lyme Disease

1. Symptomatic disease develops months to years after primary disease.
2. Musculoskeletal complaints are most common:
   a) Migrating arthritis and arthralgias
   b) Joint fluid contains 500 to 110,000 cells/mm^3, primarily polymorphonuclear leukocytes
   c) Patient usually improve with antibiotics
3. Central nervous system encephalopathy can cause mood, cognitive, and sleep disorders:
   a) Elevated protein and antibody against *Borrelia burgdorferi* in cerebrospinal fluid
   b) Response to antibiotics variable
4. Acrodermatitis chronica atrophicans, a chronic skin infection, contains spirochetes
5. Fibromyalgia-like or chronic fatigue–like syndrome may occur; controversial, antibiotics not helpful.

pathognomonic for Lyme disease. Titers for IgM begin to rise within 2 weeks, but a significant rise may not be detected for 6 to 8 weeks. Levels usually peak at 6 to 8 weeks and decline over 2 to 3 months. Titers for IgG rise later, being first detected at 6 to 8 weeks and peaking at 4 to 6 months. A significant IgG titer usually persists for life. False positive tests occur 3% to 5% of the time and are more common in patients with syphilis, leptospirosis, malaria, bacterial endocarditis, viral infections, and connective tissue diseases.

Western blot analysis is recommended to verify all positive ELISA tests. This test detects serum antibodies directed against specific polypeptide components of *B. burgdorferi*. Serum from infected patient most commonly contains antibodies directed against the 23 kDa OspC protein and the 41 kDa flagellar antigen, but may also cross-react with the Osp heat-shock proteins. Strict criteria for interpretation of Western blots have been established by the U.S. Centers for Disease Control and Prevention.

A number of other diagnostic tests have been described, but their usefulness has not been substantiated. Serologic tests are best utilized for the patient with suspected early disease who does not have erythema migrans or for the patient with symptoms of late disease. Negative serology in early disease may require follow-up testing because of the delay in the rise of antibody titers in some patients. In patients with suspected late disease, a negative IgG titer virtually excludes the diagnosis.

Treatment

For the treatment of early disease, amoxicillin or doxycycline for 21 to 28 days are equally effective (see Table 13.1). The ideal duration of therapy has not been determined, and many physicians opt for the longer course. Cefuroxime axetil is an effective alternative. Oral erythromycin (250 mg every 6 hours) and oral azithromycin (500 mg daily) have proved to be less effective.

For early disseminated disease with isolated palsies of the VIIth cranial nerve, multiple erythema migrans lesions, or carditis with first-degree heart block, both doxycycline and ceftriaxone are effective. A Jarisch–Herxheimer-like reaction may be observed in up to 15% of patients during the first 24 hours of therapy for disseminated disease. In patients with meningitis or other neurologic abnormalities, and in patients experiencing carditis with high-degree heart block, intravenous

Table 13.1. Antibiotic Treatment of Zoonotic Infections

Infection	Drug	Dose	Relative Efficacy	Comments
Lyme disease Early	Amoxicillin, or doxycycline Cefuroxime	500 mg PO q8h for 14–21 days 100 mg PO q12h for 14–21 days 500 mg PO q12h for 14–21 days	First line Alternative	
Early disseminated	Doxycycline, or ceftriaxone	100 mg PO q12h for 14–21 days 2 g IM q24h for 14–21 days		Jarisch–Herxheimer reaction common
Heart block or meningitis	Ceftriaxone, or penicillin G	2 g IV q24h for 14–28 days 4×10^6 U IV q4h for 14–28 days		
Chronic arthritis (duration 30–60 days)	Doxycycline, or amoxicillin, or Same as for heart block and meningitis	100 mg PO q12h for 28 days 500 mg PO q8h for 28 days		
Leptospirosis Severe (duration 5–7 days) Mild	Penicillin G, or ampicillin Ceftriaxone Doxycycline, or amoxicillin	1.5×10^6 U IV q6h for 5–7 days 0.5–1 g IV q6h for 5–7 days 1 g IV q24h for 5–7 days 100 mg PO q12h for 5–7 days 500 mg PO q8h for 5–7 days	Alternative	Jarisch–Herxheimer reaction common
Rocky Mountain Spotted Fever	Doxycycline Chloramphenicol	100 mg PO or IV q12h for 3 days after afebrile Children <45 kg: 2.2 mg/kg per dose q12h for 3 days after afebrile 500 mg PO or IV q6h for 3 days after afebrile	First line Alternative	Short-course doxycycline causes minimal harm to developing teeth For pregnant women
Typhus	Doxycycline Chloramphenicol Add rifampin in areas with resistant strains	100 mg PO or IV q12h for 3–5 days after afebrile Children: Same as Rocky Mountain Spotted Fever 500 mg PO or IV q6h for 3–5 days after afebrile 600–900 mg PO q24h for 3–5 days after afebrile	First line Alternative	
Ehrlichiosis and anaplasma	Doxycycline	100 mg PO or IV q12h for 3–5 days after afebrile Children: Same as Rocky Mountain Spotted Fever		Also preferred for children
Q fever	Doxycycline, plus hydroxychloroquine	100 mg PO or IV q12h 200 mg PO q8h		Add hydro- xychloroquine for endocarditis
Bartonella Lymphatic disease	Azithromycin, or clarithromycin, or doxycycline, or ciprofloxacin	500 mg PO once, then 250 mg 500 mg PO q12h 100 mg PO q12h 500 mg PO q12h		All equally effective
Severe disease	Azithromycin, plus rifampin	500 mg PO q24h 600 mg PO or IV q24h		Efficacy not proven

(Continued)

Table 13.1. *(Continued)*

Infection	Drug	Dose	Relative Efficacy	Comments
Brucellosis	Doxycycline plus rifampin	100 mg PO q12h 600–900 mg PO q12h	First line	See text for duration Single drug therapy not recommended
	Doxycycline plus gentamicin	100 mg PO q12h 5 mg/kg IV q24h	Alternative	

ceftriaxone for 30 days or high-dose penicillin is recommended. Patients with intermittent or chronic arthritis may be treated with a very prolonged course of doxycycline or amoxicillin for 30 to 60 days.

A rare but difficult management problem arises in the patient who complains of persistent symptoms despite appropriate therapy. Patients must be warned that symptoms can linger for up to 6 months after treatment. In the patient whose symptoms persist for more prolonged periods, objective evidence for relapse is rarely found. Repeat antibiotic therapy rarely relieves symptoms. The wisest course of action is re-evaluation rather than re-treatment, because the most likely explanation for a lack of response to therapy is misdiagnosis.

Prevention

Because of the extensive publicity surrounding Lyme disease, people often panic when they sustain a tick bite. In endemic areas, frantic calls to the physician's office are a frequent occurrence during the summer months. A logical approach to the management of tick bites will reduce unnecessary administration of antibiotics. Assessment of the risk of contracting Lyme disease requires a careful history of the nature of the tick bite. The questioner needs inquire about:

- **The size of the tick.** Lyme disease is primarily spread by the *Ixodes scapularis* nymph. This tick is very small, about the size of a small freckle. Larger ticks are unlikely to transmit Lyme disease.
- **Attachment.** If the tick fails to attach to the skin it cannot transmit disease. The likelihood of being bitten by a tick can be reduced by wearing long pants and shirts when walking in areas with brush and high grasses. In endemic areas, public health officials recommend that, upon returning from the outdoors, people perform a complete body check for ticks. Removing ticks before they attach is an excellent preventive measure. If an attached tick is discovered, the duration of attachment needs to be estimated. If attachment is less than a24 hours, the risk of disease transmission is low.
- **Engorgement.** If the tick is engorged with blood, prolonged attachment and an increased risk of disease transmission is suggested.

Prophylactic antibiotics consisting of a single dose of oral doxycycline (200 mg) within 72 hours of the tick bites can prevent the development of Lyme disease. The incidence of Lyme disease is approximately 1 in 100 in areas in which a high percentage of ticks harbor *B. burgdorferi*. In these locations, prophylaxis should be strongly considered. A more targeted approach of administering prophylactic antibiotics to the person who reports attachment of a small tick for more than 24 hours or who finds an engorged tick may prove more efficacious. In patients who do not fulfill these criteria, a careful explanation of the risk and natural progression of Lyme disease will usually calm the concerned caller.

LEPTOSPIROSIS

POTENTIAL SEVERITY

Can cause a life-threatening systemic illness. Early diagnosis and treatment reduce the severity of the disease.

Epidemiology

Leptospirosis is seldom diagnosed in the United States, except in Hawaii, where annual rates of 128 per 100,000 population have been reported. Leptospirosis is found throughout the world in temperate and tropical climates. Infection often follows hurricanes and flooding in Central and South America and Caribbean islands. In endemic areas, the incidence of leptospirosis is 5% to 20% annually.

The acute illness often causes nonspecific symptoms that never require medical attention, explaining the low incidence detected by passive surveillance studies. Dogs, livestock, rodents, amphibians, and reptiles can become infected. They often harbor *Leptospira* in their renal tubules, excrete the pathogen in the urine, and contaminate both soil and water, where the organism can persist for weeks to months. Humans at risk of becoming infected include trappers and hunters, dairy farmers, livestock workers, veterinarians, military personnel, and sewer workers. Infection has also been associated with outdoor activities in fresh water, including wading, swimming, whitewater rafting, kayaking, and canoeing. In cities, humans may be inadvertently exposed to infected rat and dog urine.

Pathogenesis

Leptospirosis is caused by *Leptospira interrogans*, a tightly spiraled spirochete with 18 or more coils per cell.

Like other spirochetes, it is narrow, 0.1 μm in width, and long, 6 to 12 μm in length, and is best visualized by darkfield microscopy. Leptospira are obligate aerobes and grow slowly. There are more than 200 serovars of *L. interrogans*, and different serovars have predilections for different animals.

These organisms gain entry to the human host through cuts, abrasions, and skin softened by prolonged water exposure. Mucous membranes and conjunctivae are other portals of entry. Inhalation of aerosolized droplets can lead to pulmonary invasion. Once in the host, the spirochetes spread to the lymphatic system and then enter the bloodstream, disseminating throughout the body. The organisms' outer wall is coated with lipopolysaccharide (LPS) that serves as a major antigenic stimulus. The spirochete releases a glycolipoprotein toxin that displaces long-chain fatty acids from host vascular endothelial cells, causing breakdown of the vessel walls and fluid leakage, allowing the organisms to escape from the bloodstream to the tissues. The host generates IgM and IgG antibodies directed against the *Leptospira* LPS. These antibodies are opsonins that enhance phagocytosis by macrophages in the reticuloendothelial system and enhance clearing of the organisms from the bloodstream.

Clinical Manifestations

CASE 13.2

A 25-year-old man presented to the hospital with complaints of fever and headache of 3 days' duration. His symptoms began 3 days after he completed a 12-day survival race with three teammates, in Sabah State on Borneo Island, Malaysia. The day before his admission, one of his teammates was admitted to the hospital with similar complaints.

Physical examination revealed a body temperature of 37.9°C and a pulse rate of 90 per minute (regular). Conjunctiva were hyperemic, but nonicteric. Lymph nodes were not palpable, and no skin eruption was seen. A neurologic exam was normal.

A laboratory workup showed a WBC count of 13,100/mm^3, with 91% neutrophils; a hemoglobin of 14.8 g/dL; a platelet count of 190,000/mm^3; and total bilirubin 0.5 mg/dL. Liver enzymes were 63 IU/L [aspartate aminotransferase (AST)] and 66 IU/L [alanine aminotransferase (ALT)]. Lactate dehydrogenase (LDH) was 420 IU/L; blood urea nitrogen (BUN), 12.5 mg/dL; and creatine, 0.9 mg/dL.

Minocycline was administered intravenously on the third hospital day, and fever subsided over 48 hours. The intravenous minocycline was continued for a week, followed by 2 weeks of oral doxycycline. Acute sera were negative for Leptospira *antibody, but convalescent serum 2 weeks later revealed a 1:160 titer of antibody directed against* L. interrogans *serovar hebdomadis.*

Further investigation revealed that 51 of 78 participants had developed symptoms consistent with leptospirosis. Activities had included jungle trekking, canoeing, kayaking, rafting, scuba diving, mountain biking, and cave exploring. Local rivers were flooded at the time of the race. (Adapted from Sakamoto M, Sagara H, Koizumi N, Watanabe H. Infect Agent Surveill Rep. *2001;22:5–6)*

The incubation period for leptospirosis is usually 5 to 14 days, but can be up to 30 days. The severity of illness varies greatly, and probably depends on the degree of exposure and the infecting serovar. Certain serovars from cows cause mild disease; others (contracted from rats) are more likely to cause severe disease. Classically, symptomatic disease occurs in two phases, the bacteremic phase and the immunologic phase; however, fewer than half of patients actually experience a biphasic illness. More than 90% of cases are self-limiting, but a small percentage experience a severe—sometimes fatal—illness called Weil's disease.

As illustrated in case 13.2, the onset of illness is usually sudden. Symptoms may include fever, rigors, sweating, headache, photophobia, and severe myalgias accompanied by marked tenderness of the calves, thighs, and mid back. Other manifestations can include epistaxis, cough, and sore throat. Severe abdominal pain can mimic an acute abdomen. Nausea, vomiting, and diarrhea may also develop. On examination, the vessels in the conjunctiva are often very prominent because of vascular dilatation. Transient skin rashes may be noted. Capillary fragility can result in macular, maculopapular, purpuric, urticarial lesions, or diffuse skin redness. During the acute phase, *Leptospira* can be cultured from the blood and CSF.

Resolution of fever may herald the onset of the second, immune, phase of the illness. This phase can last 4 to 30 days. Blood cultures turn negative at this time. Prominent conjunctivitis with or without hemorrhage is seen, accompanied by photophobia, retrobulbar pain, neck stiffness, diffuse lymphadenopathy, and hepatosplenomegaly. Aseptic meningitis with or without symptoms is characteristic of this stage and is immune-mediated. Lymphocytes ($<$500 mm^3) are seen in the CSF, together with moderate protein elevation (50 to 100 mg/mL and a normal glucose level.

Weil's disease can develop after the acute phase and consists of hemorrhage, jaundice, and renal failure.

KEY POINTS

About the Clinical Manifestations of Leptospirosis

1. Incubation period is 5 to 14 days, and severity depends on inoculum and serovar (rat serovars being more severe).

2. Two phases in fewer than half of patients:
   a) Bacteremic phase—Sudden onset; fever, rigors, headache, photophobia, and severe myalgias; dilated conjunctival vessels, marked tenderness calves, thighs, and mid back; macular rash
   b) Immunologic phase (after 4 to 30 days)—Conjunctivitis, photophobia, retrobulbar pain, neck stiffness, diffuse lymphadenopathy, hepatosplenomegaly, and aseptic meningitis with lymphocytosis in the cerebrospinal fluid.

3. Weil's disease is rare, severe; mortality 5% to 40%:
   a) High direct bilirubin, mild elevation in alkaline phosphatase, mild elevation in transaminase values, combined with a high creatine phosphokinase.
   b) Renal failure accompanied by thrombocytopenia
   c) Hemorrhagic pneumonia

Severe hemorrhagic pneumonitis may also develop. Jaundice is caused by vascular injury to the hepatic capillaries without significant hepatocellular necrosis. Transaminase levels seldom exceed 200 U/L, and an elevated prothrombin time is uncommon. Creatine phosphokinase (CPK, MM fraction) reflecting myositis is often disproportionately high in comparison with the serum transaminase values. Marked elevations in conjugated bilirubin are the hallmark of liver involvement and can reach levels of 80 mg/dL, associated with mild-to-moderate elevations of alkaline phosphatase.

The constellation of a high direct bilirubin, mild elevation in alkaline phosphatase, and mild elevation in transaminase values combined with a high CPK should always raise the possibility of Weil's disease. Liver biopsy reveals hypertrophy and hyperplasia of Kupffer cells, accompanied by cholestasis. The hepatic architecture usually remains intact, and little evidence of hepatic necrosis is seen. Acute renal failure is associated with oliguria and usually develops during the second week of illness at the same time that jaundice is noted. Thrombocytopenia may accompany renal failure in the absence of disseminated intravascular coagulopathy. Renal biopsy demonstrates acute interstitial nephritis, and immune-complex glomerulonephritis may also be seen. Pulmonary disease can develop in the absence of hepatic or renal involvement. This hemorrhagic pneumonia is generally associated with a bloody cough, and chest X-ray reveals nodular densities in the lower lobes. Histopathology reveals damage to the capillary endothelium and intra-alveolar hemorrhage. Cardiovascular collapse can develop suddenly. The mortality rate for severe leptospirosis ranges from 5% to 40%.

Diagnosis and Treatment

Even in endemic areas, the early clinical diagnosis of leptospirosis is difficult to make because the clinical manifestations are often nonspecific. *Leptospira* can be cultured in vitro on special media (Fletcher's, Ellinghausen's, or polysorbate 80). Significant growth may be detected after 1 to 2 weeks, but can take up to 3 months. Blood, CSF, and urine are positive during the first 7 to 10 days of illness, and urine remains positive during the second and third weeks of the illness.

The sensitivity of culture is low, and therefore the diagnosis must usually be made by measuring acute and convalescent antibody titers. The microscopic agglutination test is the most specific test and allows identification of serum antibodies to specific serovars.

Live leptospires are placed on a slide, and the highest serum dilution at which more than 50% of the spirochetes agglutinate on darkfield microscopy is defined as the positive titer. Antibody titers can be detected as early as 3 days into the illness, but usually take 2 weeks, and continue to rise for 3 to 4 weeks. A rise in titer by a factor of 4 or more is defined as serologic confirmation of leptospirosis. A single titer above 1:800 in combination with appropriate symptoms is considered indicative of active disease, and a single titer of 1:200 or a persistent titer of 1:100 is suggestive evidence. This test is technically demanding and potentially hazardous; it is performed only by CDC reference laboratories. An ELISA test for IgM antibodies is commercially available and has a sensitivity that varies from 100% to 77% and a specificity of 93% to 98%. Methods using PCR are under development, but are currently only experimental.

Penicillin G, ampicillin, or ceftriaxone are recommended for severe disease. In severe disease, penicillin treatment has been shown to reduce the duration of illness. As observed in the treatment of other spirochetes, therapy may be associated with a Jarisch–Herxheimer reaction. For mild leptospirosis, oral doxycycline or amoxicillin may be administered. When exposure in endemic areas is anticipated, prophylaxis with oral doxycycline (200 mg daily) has been shown to be efficacious (see Table 13.1).

KEY POINTS

About the Diagnosis and Treatment of Leptospirosis

1. Can be cultured from blood, cerebrospinal fluid, and urine. Low yield.
2. Serology is most helpful.
   a) Microscopic agglutination test (only in CDC reference labs): positive at 2 weeks, rises at 3 to 4 weeks (a rise by a factor of 4 or more is diagnostic), titer above 1:800 plus symptoms indicates active disease, 1:200 is suggestive.
   b) Enzyme-linked immunoabsorbent assay for immunoglobulin M antibodies is commercially available and has good sensitivity and specificity.
3. Treat with intravenous penicillin, ampicillin, or ceftriaxone for severe disease, oral doxycycline or amoxicillin for milder disease.
4. For prophylaxis in endemic areas use doxycycline.

RICKETTSIA AND RELATED INFECTIONS

The Rickettsiaceae family encompasses two genera: *Rickettsia* and *Ehrlichia*. These organisms are small gram-negative coccobacilli (coccal forms 0.3 μm in diameter, bacillary forms 0.3×1 to 2 μm) whose cell wall consists of a peptidoglycan layer sandwiched between two lipid membranes. They are all obligatory intracellular pathogens.

Rickettsia gains entry by inducing host cells to phagocytose them. Some strains—for example, *Rickettsia rickettsii*—produce a phospholipase that dissolves the confining phagolysosome membrane, allowing them to escape into the cytoplasm. Other strains multiply and survive within the phagolysosome by blocking the release of toxic enzymes into the phagolysosome (*Ehrlichia* species, for instance). All rickettsial diseases are spread to humans by arthropods: ticks, mites, lice, and fleas.

Clinically, the rickettsial family of diseases have been classified into four groups:

1. **The spotted fever group.** Includes *R. rickettsii* (Rocky Mountain spotted fever), *R. conorii*

(Boutonneuse fever), *R. australis* (Queensland tick typhus), *R. sibirica* (North Asian tick typhus), and *R. akari* (rickettsial pox).

2. **The typhus group.** Includes *R. prowazekii* (louse-borne or epidemic typhus and Brill–Zinsser disease), *R. typhi* (murine typhus), and *Orienta tsutsugamushi* (scrub typhus).

3. **The *Ehrlichia* group.** Consists of *E. chaffeensis* [human monocytotropic ehrlichiosis (HME)], *Anaplasma phagocytophilum* [human granulocytotropic anaplasma (HGA)], and the rarer human pathogens *E. ewingii*, *E. muris*, and *Neorickettsia sennetsu*.

4. **A final disease, Q fever.** That does not fall into any of the above categories. It is caused by *Coxiella burnetii*.

ROCKY MOUNTAIN SPOTTED FEVER

POTENTIAL SEVERITY

Untreated Rocky Mountain spotted fever can be fulminant and fatal.

Epidemiology

Rocky Mountain spotted fever (RMSF) is the most severe disease in the spotted fever group of rickettsial diseases. It occurs throughout the United States, Mexico, and Central and South America. Although first recognized in the Rocky Mountains, the disease is most commonly reported in the southeastern and south-central United States. Small endemic areas are also found in Long Island and Cape Cod. Cases have also been reported in urban parks.

The disease occurs in the late spring and summer, the seasons in which ticks feed. In the south, the dog tick (*Dermacentor variabilis*) is the primary vector, and in states west of the Mississippi the wood tick (*Dermacentor andersoni*) is primarily responsible for transmitting disease. A recent outbreak in Arizona was associated with the common brown dog tick (*Rhipicephalus sanguineus*).

Pathogenesis

After the tick has attached to the host for between several hours and a day, it injects the rickettsiae into the dermis. Once exposed to the warmer temperature

---

KEY POINTS

About the Epidemiology and Pathogenesis of Rocky Mountain Spotted Fever

1. Found throughout the United States, Mexico, and Central and South America.
   a) Most common in the southeastern and south-central United States; also found in the Midwest.
   b) Endemic in areas of Cape Cod and Long Island and in some urban parks.
2. Injected into the skin by dog and wood ticks in the late spring and summer.
3. Proliferates in the skin, disseminates via the bloodstream.
   a) Survives in the host cell cytoplasm; spreads cell-to-cell, producing plaques of necrotic cells.
   b) Causes hemorrhage in skin, intestine, pancreas, liver, skeletal muscle, and kidneys.

---

and mammalian blood, *R. rickettsii* activates and proliferates in the skin. The organism resides in the cytoplasm of host cells, where it divides by binary fission and spreads from cell to cell by a mechanism similar to that used by *Listeria monocytogenes*. Both organisms induce host-cell actin filament assembly to propel them to the periphery of the cell, where they are ingested by adjacent cells, forming plaques of necrotic cells.

R. rickettsii contains outer membrane proteins ("Omps") and lipoproteins that stimulate cell-mediated immunity, resulting in infiltration of lymphocytes and macrophages. After multiplying in the skin, the organism disseminates via the bloodstream, where it prefers to invade vascular endothelial cells. Damage to endothelial and vascular smooth muscle cells results in a vasculitis that can involve the lungs, heart, and central nervous system. Discrete areas of hemorrhage can be found in these organs and also in the skin, intestine, pancreas, liver, skeletal muscle, and kidneys. Hemorrhage often leads to platelet consumption and thrombocytopenia, but disseminated intravascular coagulopathy is rare. Increased vascular permeability and fluid leakage result in edema, low serum protein levels, hypovolemia, and shock. Decreased intravascular volume can induce antidiuretic hormone secretion and hyponatremia. In severe cases, shock can also precipitate acute tubular necrosis and renal failure.

Clinical Manifestations

> ### CASE 13.3
>
> *A 7–year-old girl arrived in the emergency room in Oklahoma with 2-day history of fever (39.3°C), malaise, abdominal pain, nausea, and vomiting. She was discharged with a diagnosis of viral gastroenteritis. Four days later, she was seen at a second emergency room with complaints of persistent fever, anorexia, irritability, photophobia, cough, diffuse myalgias, nausea, and vomiting.*
>
> *On physical exam she was noted to have hepatosplenomegaly and an erythematous papular rash with scattered petechiae on the trunk, arms, legs, palms, and soles. Laboratory findings included an elevated WBC count of 11,400/mm³, a low platelet count of 19,000/mm³, and elevated liver enzymes (AST: 279 IU/L; ALT: 77 IU/L). Intravenous doxycycline was initiated to treat suspected RMSF, and she was placed in intensive care. Her mental status declined, and she developed metabolic acidosis and respiratory failure, dying 6 days after her first visit to the emergency room.*
>
> *A serum sample drawn 2 days before her death revealed a 1:128 IgG anti–R. rickettsii antibody titer. Spotted-fever group rickettsiae were detected by immunohistochemical staining of autopsy specimens from brain, skin, heart, lung, spleen, and kidney. On questioning, the parents reported that their child played frequently in grassy areas near their home. They did not note any recent tick bite, but ticks had been frequently observed on the family's pet dogs and often were manually removed by members of the household. (Adapted from CDC Fatal cases of Rocky Mountain spotted fever in family clusters—three states, 2003. MMWR Morb Mortal Wkly Rep. 2004;53:407–410)*

As case 13.3 illustrates, the course of unrecognized and untreated RMSF can be fulminant. The incubation period is 2 to 14 days after a tick bite. The early symptoms and signs of this disease are nonspecific. Patients complain of fever, headache, malaise, myalgias, and nausea. Some patients experience severe abdominal pain, particularly children, suggesting the diagnosis of cholecystitis, appendicitis, or bowel obstruction—or as in case 13.3 with milder abdominal complaints mimicking viral gastroenteritis.

KEY POINTS

About the Clinical Manifestations of Rocky Mountain Spotted Fever

1. Incubation period is 2 to 14 days.
2. Acute onset of nonspecific symptoms: fever, headache, malaise, myalgias, and nausea. Abdominal pain may mimic cholecystitis or appendicitis.
3. Macular, petechial rash begins on ankles and wrists and spreads to trunk 5 days after symptoms begin,
   a) "Spotless" infection occurs in 10%—usually elderly and dark skinned individuals.
   b) Urticaria or pruritic rash makes the diagnosis unlikely.
4. Other symptoms include aseptic meningitis, conjunctivitis, fundoscopic hemorrhages, and acute respiratory distress syndrome in severe disease.
5. Death within 8 to 15 days if treatment is not initiated within 5 days.

A rash usually develops within 5 days of the onset of illness, and in case 13.3, a rash alerted the physicians to the possibility of RMSF. However, in up to 10% of patients, a rash may never appear. "Spotless" fever occurs more commonly in elderly and in dark skin individuals. Patients often seek medical attention before the rash develops, and therefore, as in the above case, the physician may fail to consider the diagnosis. Lesions are nonpruritic. They are usually first noted on the ankles and wrists, subsequently spreading centrally and to the palms and soles. Initially they are macular or maculopapular, subsequently becoming petechial. The presence of urticarial lesions or a pruritic skin rash makes RMSF unlikely.

As the disease progresses, headache may become an increasingly prominent complaint. Severe headache can be accompanied by neck stiffness and photophobia suggesting meningitis, and the CSF may contain lymphocytes or PMNs, together with elevated protein; however, low CSF glucose is unusual. Conjunctivitis may be noted, and fundoscopic examination may reveal manifestations of small-vessel vasculitis (flame hemorrhages and arterial occlusion), venous engorgement, and papilledema. Respiratory complaints may become prominent, and chest X-ray may reveal alveolar infiltrates or pulmonary edema, indicating the development of adult respiratory distress syndrome. In severe cases, gangrene of the digits can also develop as a consequence of occlusion of small arterioles.

Laboratory findings tend to be nonspecific. The peripheral WBC count can be normal, elevated, or depressed. Thrombocytopenia is common in more severe cases. Elevations in BUN and serum creatinine may be noted. Hyponatremia develops in patients with hypotension. Transaminase values and bilirubin levels may be elevated as well. As illustrated by case 13.3, if appropriate therapy is not given within the first 5 days of symptomatic disease, RMSF can progress and cause death within 8 to 15 days.

Diagnosis

Because of the rapid course of this disease and the inability of most laboratories to culture the organism, the diagnosis of RMSF is usually made based on epidemiology and clinical manifestations. A significant percentage of patients deny a tick bite, making the diagnosis particularly difficult. In the first few days, RMSF is most commonly mistaken for a viral syndrome. If penicillin or a cephalosporin is mistakenly prescribed during this period, the subsequent rash of RMSF may be mistaken for a drug allergy. Severe headache and abnormalities in the CSF may suggest viral meningoencephalitis. The development of petechial skin lesions may raise the possibility of meningococcemia or leptospirosis.

During the spring and summer months, patients in endemic areas must always be treated for Rocky Mountain spotted fever pending culture results. Skin biopsy is helpful in confirming the diagnosis. Immunofluorescence staining using antibodies specifically directed against *R. rickettsii* can be helpful (70% sensitivity and 100% specificity). If antibiotics for RMSF have been initiated, skin biopsy is not recommended, because the organisms are difficult to identify after treatment has been initiated. Acute and convalescent serum antibody titers can be measured by indirect immunofluorescence, latex agglutination, or complement fixation, and a significant rise in titer allows for a retrospective diagnosis. However, these tests are of no help in managing the acutely ill patient. The Weil–Felix test that detects cross-reactive antibodies to *Proteus vulgaris* are not only nonspecific, but also insensitive, and are no longer recommended.

Treatment

Because of the unpredictable course of RMSF, physicians in endemic areas should have a low threshold for initiating doxycycline or tetracycline therapy in patients who have a nonspecific febrile illness of more than 2 days' duration during the spring and summer. The disease responds rapidly to antibiotic therapy, and patients usually defervesce within 48 to 72 hours.

Therapy with doxycycline is the treatment of choice for adults and children alike (see Table 13.1). Short courses of doxycycline are reported to cause minimal damage to developing teeth, but the potential benefits of doxycycline far outweigh this potential toxicity. Chloramphenicol is recommended in pregnancy. Antibiotic therapy should be continued for at least 3 days after the patient has defervesced. The mortality in untreated patients varies depending on the strain and inoculum, but in one retrospective series, was 22% in untreated patients and 6% in patients who received treatment within 5 days of the onset of illness.

Other Spotted Fevers

A number of other rickettsial species cause skin rashes and fever in humans. *R. conorii* shares 90% DNA homology with *R. rickettsii* and many of the same proteins; it causes Mediterranean spotted fever ("Boutonneuse fever"). This tick-borne illness is found in southern Europe, Africa, and the Middle East, and is clinically very similar to RMSF. A black eschar called a *tache noire* may be noted at the site of the tick bite. This lesion is caused by vascular endothelial damage that leads to dermal and epidermal necrosis. A diffuse macular-papular rash develops within 3 to 5 days of the onset

---

KEY POINTS

About the Diagnosis and Treatment of Rocky Mountain Spotted Fever

1. Presumptive diagnosis must be made based on epidemiology and clinical manifestations.
2. Culture not recommended.
3. Skin biopsy with immunofluorescence staining has high specificity. Not recommended if antibiotics have been given.
4. Serology provides a retrospective diagnosis: indirect immunofluorescence, latex agglutination, or complement fixation.
5. Can be mistaken for viral syndrome, drug allergy, and meningococcemia.
6. Physicians in endemic areas should have a low threshold for treatment:
   a) Doxycycline for adults and children
   b) Chloramphenicol for pregnant women
7. Mortality has been reported as 22% untreated, 6% with treatment.

the site of the mite bite and abrupt onset of fever, chills, myalgias, and headache, followed by a rash that initially is maculopapular and later becomes papulovesicular. Lesions then scab over and heal without scars. The number of skin lesions varies, and they can involve the face, mucous membranes, palms, and soles. The disease spontaneously resolves within 2 to 3 weeks and is never fatal. Treatment with doxycycline or tetracycline is associated with resolution of symptoms within 24 to 48 hours. The diagnosis can be made by direct immunofluorescence staining of biopsy material from the eschar or by acute and convalescent antibody titers.

TYPHUS

POTENTIAL SEVERITY

Patients can become extremely septic, developing shock and organ failure, and dying.

This group of diseases received the name "typhus" because the illness caused by species of *Rickettsia* that clinically mimics typhoid fever (see Chapter 8).

Epidemiology, Pathogenesis, and Clinical Manifestations

R. prowazekii causes the most serious form of typhus. This disease has been called "louse-borne typhus" and "epidemic typhus." It is spread from person to person by body lice.

The louse harbors high concentrations of *Rickettsia* in its alimentary canal. When an infected louse bites a human and ingests a blood meal, it also defecates, releasing rickettsial organisms onto the skin. The unwitting host scratches the site and inoculates the infected feces into the wound or onto mucous membranes. This disease is most commonly encountered during periods of war and famine. During World War II, louse-borne typhus was common in Eastern European and North African concentration camps. Since the end of the 1980s, infections have been reported most commonly in Africa and less commonly in South and Central America. Rare cases have been reported in the eastern and central United States. Those cases are thought to have been transmitted by lice or fleas from flying squirrels.

The incubation period is approximately 1 week, after which the disease starts with the abrupt onset of

of the febrile illness; however, as observed with RMSF, some patients fail to develop a black eschar or rash.

R. africae also results in an eschar at the site of the tick bite, and for 60 years, this infection was mistaken for that caused by *R. conorii*. This disease, called African tick-bite fever, is found mainly in rural regions of Zimbabwe, South Africa, and the eastern Caribbean. The disease is usually mild, but can be associated with persistent neuropathy.

Rickettsialpox, caused by *R. akari*, is transmitted by a blood-sucking mite that normally lives on mice; however, on rare occasions, it also bites humans. When mouse populations are reduced by extermination campaigns, the mites are more likely to infest humans and cause disease. Rickettsialpox has been reported in urban areas of the United States, including Boston, Pittsburgh, and Cleveland, and it has also been seen in Arizona and Utah. This disease is not considered by many U.S. physicians, and it is often mistaken for chickenpox. The disease has also been reported in Mexico, where it may be initially mistaken for Dengue fever. Rickettsialpox is also found in South Africa, Ukraine, Croatia, and Korea.

The incubation period is 10 to 14 days and the illness is characterized by development of an eschar at

high fever, severe headache, and myalgias. The headache is retro-orbital and bifrontal, comes on suddenly, and is unremitting. As observed with severe RMSF, tissue necrosis develops as a result of small-vessel vasculitis, a process that involves multiple organs, including the lungs, liver, gastrointestinal tract, central nervous system, and skin. Skin rash is observed in 60% of patients and begins on the trunk, spreading outward over 24 to 48 hours. Lesions are initially macular, but quickly progress to a maculopapular form and then to petechiae. Peripheral gangrene can develop as a consequence of small-vessel occlusion. Central nervous system involvement can lead to drowsiness and confusion, and in severe cases, grand mal seizures and focal neurologic deficits can result. Louse-borne typhus has been associated with 30% to 70% mortality.

KEY POINTS

About the Epidemiology, Pathogenesis, and Clinical Manifestations of Typhus

1. Louse-borne typhus, caused by *Rickettsia prowazekii*, and is the most serious form.
   a) Person-person spread by lice, common during World War II.
   b) Now found in Africa and, less commonly, in South and Central America.
   c) Occasionally found in the eastern and central United States, transmitted by lice or fleas from flying squirrels.
   d) Causes small-vessel vasculitis, petechial skin rash on trunk, multi-organ failure, peripheral gangrene, and encephalitis; 30% to 70% mortality.
2. Brill–Zinsser disease is a reactivation of *R. prowazekii*, milder, but similar to primary disease.
3. Flea-borne typhus is caused by *R. typhi*. This milder form of typhus has worldwide distribution.
4. Scrub typhus is caused by *R. tsutsugamushi* and is transmitted by mite larvae (chiggers).
   a) Found in Japan, eastern Asia, Australia, and some Pacific islands.
   b) More gradual onset; black eschar at the chigger bite site in half of patients; rash common.

After primary infection, *R. prowazekii* can remain latent for decades, reactivating after physical or psychological stress, particularly in elderly people. This reactivated form of typhus is called Brill–Zinsser disease, and it is similar in clinical presentation to primary disease, except that the disease is milder. *R. typhi*, responsible for flea-borne (also called murine or endemic typhus) also causes a milder form of the disease and is found throughout the world. The prognosis for Brill–Zinsser disease and flea-borne typhus is much better than for primary louse-borne typhus, mortality being less than 5% for both diseases.

A third form of typhus called scrub typhus is caused by *R. tsutsugamushi*. This infection is transmitted by mite larvae (commonly called chiggers). These insects crawl on vegetation and then attach themselves to small mammals and humans as they pass through the brush. This disease is most often contracted by agricultural workers and military personnel in endemic areas. Scrub typhus is found in Japan, eastern Asia, Australia, and in the western and southwestern Pacific islands. The incubation period is similar to that of the other rickettsial diseases (6 to 21 days); however, the onset is usually gradual rather than sudden. Headache, high fever, chills, and anorexia are the most common symptoms. Diffuse lymphadenopathy, splenomegaly, conjunctivitis, and pharyngitis are common physical findings. Within 1 week of the onset of symptoms, a high percentage of patients develop a maculopapular skin rash. A black eschar may be noted at the site of the chigger bite in approximately half of patients.

Diagnosis and Treatment

The diagnosis of these febrile illnesses is presumptive and based on clinical and epidemiologic findings. Acute and convalescent antibody titers to the specific forms of *Rickettsia* can be performed, and the specific diagnosis made retrospectively. Immunofluorescence staining of the primary eschar (where available) can yield a more rapid diagnosis. The once-popular Weil–Felix *Proteus* agglutination test is no longer recommended because of its poor sensitivity and lack of specificity.

The treatment for all forms of typhus is identical to that for the spotted fever group: doxycycline or chloramphenicol (see Table 13.1). Therapy should usually be continued for 3 to 5 days after defervescence. In some regions in which antibiotic resistance has developed, oral rifampin (600 to 900 mg daily) may be more efficacious. Early treatment aborts the antibody response, and as a consequence, relapse may occur after treatment is completed. Patients respond well to re-treatment.

EHRLICHIA

| POTENTIAL SEVERITY |

Can cause severe, multisystemic disease that is usually not fatal.

There are two forms of ehrlichiosis: human monocytic ehrlichia, HME, caused by *Ehrlichia chaffeensis,* and human granulocyte anaplasma, HGA, caused by *Anaplasma phagocytophilum.*

Epidemiology

Both species of *Ehrlichia* are transmitted to humans by ticks, and the seasonal nature of these diseases is identical to those of other tick-borne illnesses. Most cases of human monocytotropic ehrlichiosis are associated with bites from the Lone Star tick (*Amblyomma americanum*). This tick also infests the whitetail deer, the natural reservoir for *E. chaffeensis.* This disease is very common in the southeast, and attack rates have been estimated to be 5 per 100,000 population; however, in certain endemic areas, incidences as high as 660 per 100,000 have been reported. In addition to hikers and outdoor workers, golfers are at risk for contracting this disease.

Human granulocytotropic anaplasma was first reported in 1994, and therefore the understanding of its epidemiology is evolving. To date, cases have been associated with tick bites from *Ixodes scapularis*, the same tick that transmits the pathogens that cause Lyme disease and babesiosis. Cases have been reported in California, Minnesota, Wisconsin, Massachusetts, Connecticut, New York, and Florida.

Pathogenesis

Once the organism is inoculated into the skin by the tick, it enters the lymphatic system and bloodstream. *E. chaffeensis* prefers to invade macrophages and monocytes; less commonly, it enters lymphocytes, and occasionally, polymorphonuclear leukocytes. Once phagocytosed by these cells, *E. chaffeensis* remains in the phagosomes, where it survives by inhibiting fusion of the lysosomes that release the toxic products that normally kill invading pathogens. In addition, this organism blocks the signal transduction pathways that enhance production of interferon γ and simultaneously upregulates cytokine genes important for generation of the inflammatory response. Finally, it induces clustering of transferrin receptors in the phagolysosome membrane, allowing it to compete effectively for iron, a vital nutrient for bacterial growth. As the bacteria divide by binary fusion, they cluster together, forming intracellular inclusions called morulae. *Anaplasma phagocytophilum* invades primarily PMNs (also called neutrophils or granulocytes) and uses strategies similar to those of *E. chaffeensis* to survive within those cells. Both pathogens not only invade peripheral leukocytes, but also infect the bone marrow, causing disruption of the normal maturation processes and blocking production of leukocytes, red blood cells, and platelets.

KEY POINTS

About the Diagnosis and Treatment of Typhus

1. Presumptive diagnosis must be made by clinical and epidemiologic findings.
2. Antibody titers are available; immunofluorescence staining of primary lesion is helpful.
3. Weil–Felix *Proteus* agglutination is no longer recommended.
4. Treat with doxycycline or chloramphenicol; patient may relapse, requiring re-treatment.

KEY POINTS

About the Epidemiology and Pathogenesis of Ehrlichiosis

1. Human monocytotropic ehrlichiosis is caused *Ehrlichia chaffeensis.*
   a) Transmitted by the Lone Star tick found on the whitetail deer.
   b) Common in the southeast United States; hikers, outdoor workers, and golfers are at risk.
2. Human granulocytotropic anaplasmosis is caused by *Anaplasma phagocytophilum.*
   a) Transmitted by *Ixodes*, the same tick that transmits Lyme disease and babesiosis.
   b) Found in California, Minnesota, Wisconsin, Massachusetts, Connecticut, New York, and Florida.

Clinical Manifestations

A 49–year-old white man presented to the hospital with a 2-week history of fever and malaise. Fever came on gradually and was associated with generalized headaches. He was given trimethoprim-sulfamethoxazole by his primary physician for presumed sinusitis, but he failed to improve. Fever increased to between 39.4°C and 40°C, the generalized headache persisted, and a nonproductive cough developed.

An epidemiologic history indicated that the patient was an avid hunter and had been hunting with his father on several occasions during the last 2 months. He reported extensive tick exposure. His father had died in the hospital from "influenza pneumonia" that had developed at the same time as his current illness.

In the emergency room, the patient was noted to have a fever of 39.4°C, a pulse of 96 beats per minute, a respiratory rate of 22 breaths per minute, and a blood pressure of 144/60 mm Hg. He appeared septic and somewhat lethargic and inattentive. Conjunctiva were injected with bilateral hemorrhages. Tender cervical lymphadenopathy was noted, but the neck was supple. A few hyperpigmented macular lesions over the anterior shins were observed, but there was no evidence of tick bites.

A laboratory workup showed a hematocrit of 34%, a platelet count of 61,000/mm³, and a peripheral WBC count of 3600/mm³, with 66% PMNs, 17% lymphocytes, and 16% monocytes. No morulae were noted in a blood smear. Serum sodium was 125 mEq/L; AST, 185 IU/L; ALT, 151 IU/L. Two blood cultures showed no growth. The CSF formula was 205 WBCs (2% PMNs, 78% lymphocytes, 20% monocytes), 0 red blood cells, total protein 139 mg/dL, and glucose 153 mg/dL. A chest X-ray was within normal limits.

The patient was treated with doxycycline and defervesced within 48 hours. One week after hospital discharge, his serum IgG and IgM titers came back positive for E. chaffeensis.

Case 13.4 represents a classic presentation of human monocytotropic ehrlichiosis. Both forms of ehrlichiosis have incubation periods of approximately 7 days. *Ehrlichia* varies in its severity, and fatality rates of approximately 5% have been reported in both diseases. Manifestations tend to be more severe in elderly and immunocompromised patients.

Like rickettsiosis, ehrlichiosis is a multisystem disease. Both forms of *Ehrlichia* present with the gradual onset of fever, chills, headache, myalgias, anorexia, and malaise. The monocytotropic form can result in respiratory insufficiency, renal insufficiency, and meningoencephalitis. It is very much possible that the patient's father in case 13.4 may have died of respiratory complications from ehrlichiosis. Neck stiffness, depressed mental status, coma, and seizures are accompanied by CSF lymphocytosis and elevated CSF protein. Case 13.4 had a depressed mental status and typical CSF findings. The granulocytotropic form can also be associated with respiratory insufficiency. Rhabdomyolysis has also been described. Meningoencephalitis has not been described in granulocytotropic anaplasma. Some patients with the HGA form have developed fatal opportunistic infections. Hypotension can develop with either infection and mimic other forms of gram-negative sepsis. A macular, maculopapular, or petechial rash is observed in 30% to 40% patients with HME, but in only 2% to 11% of patients with HGA.

Thrombocytopenia is a prominent finding in both diseases, and this finding combined with the epidemiology strongly suggested the diagnosis of ehrlichiosis in case 13.4. The platelet count is depressed (50,000 to 140,000/mm³) in most patients. Platelet counts can drop below 20,000/mm³ in severe disease and can be associated with gastrointestinal bleeding. Leukopenia (1300 to 4000/mm³) is also a frequent finding, peripheral neutrophil or lymphocyte counts (or both) being depressed in HME. In the granulocytotropic form, neutropenia predominates and is commonly associated with a left shift and relative lymphocytosis. As observed in case 13.4, elevated transaminase values (AST and ALT) are found in nearly all patients.

Diagnosis and Treatment

If the diagnosis of *Ehrlichia* is being considered, a Wright stain of the peripheral blood and a buffy coat smear should be carefully examined for the presence of morulae. These intracellular inclusions are seen in the peripheral monocytes of only a small percentage of patients with HME, but in HGA, granulocyte morulae can be identified in 25% to 80% of patients (Figure 13.2). The percentage of granulocytes containing morulae varies from 1% to 44%, with higher levels of intracellular invasion being seen in elderly patients.

In these diseases, culture techniques are impractical and insensitive, and PCR methods remain

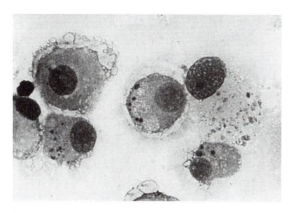

Figure 13–2. Morulae found in human granulocy-totropic anaplasma infection caused by *Anaplasma phagocytophilum. See color image on color plate 2*

experimental. As in rickettsiosis, serologic testing of acute and convalescent serum is the usual method for diagnosis. Antibodies usually take 2 to 3 weeks to reach detectable levels. Immunofluorescence assays are available through state laboratories and the CDC. Titers above 1:64, combined with a rise of at least a factor of four between acute and convalescent serum is considered diagnostic.

Doxycycline is the treatment of choice, and in vitro testing confirms that *Ehrlichia* and *Anaplasma* are sensitive to tetracyclines. Clinical experience suggests that either oral or intravenous chloramphenicol (500 mg four times daily) is also effective, even though in vitro testing has demonstrated no significant anti-*Ehrlichia* activity for this drug. Because of these concerns, doxycycline is preferred over chloramphenicol in children (see Table 13.1).

COXIELLA BURNETII

> POTENTIAL SEVERITY
>
> *Q fever is usually a self-limiting disease; however, the occasional patient who develops Q fever endocarditis often dies.*

Epidemiology

The main reservoirs for *C. burnetii*, the cause of Q fever, are farm animals: sheep, goats, and cows. Pet cats and dogs may also carry the organism. Mammals shed the

---

KEY POINTS

About the Clinical Manifestations, Diagnosis, and Treatment of Ehrlichiosis

1. Incubation period is 7 days, and mortality is 5% (mainly elderly and immunocompromised).
   a) Gradual onset of fever, chills, headache, myalgias, anorexia, and malaise.
   b) Severe monocytic form: respiratory insufficiency, renal insufficiency, and meningoencephalitis (with lymphocytosis noted in the cerebrospinal fluid).
   c) Severe granulocytic form: respiratory insufficiency, rhabdomyolysis, and neutropenia resulting in gram-negative sepsis.
   d) Macular, petechial rash in 30% to 40% of cases of the monocytic form, but in 2% to 11% of cases of the granulocytic form.
2. Diagnosis presumptive in most cases.
   a) Thrombocytopenia and leukopenia are common (neutropenia in granulocytic form).
   b) Moderate transaminase elevations are seen.
   c) Morulae are rare in peripheral blood smears in the monocytic form, common in the granulocytic form.
   d) Retrospective serology makes the diagnosis.
3. Treat with doxycycline. Chloramphenicol has no activity in vitro, and therefore doxycycline is also recommended for children.

---

pathogen in their urine, feces, and birth products. Transmission occurs most commonly in association with birthing, organisms being aerosolized from the placenta, and inhaled by humans. *C. burnetii* is resistant to drying and can survive for long periods in the environment, and wind-borne particles can be inhaled weeks after parturition. Q fever is rare in the United States, 20 to 60 cases being reported annually. Outbreaks occur worldwide, but may be missed because of the nonspecific symptoms and signs in this disease. Significant numbers of cases have been reported in Spain, France, England, Australia, and Canada. In some areas, the incidence of Q fever has been estimated to be 50 per 100,000 population.

Pathogenesis

C. burnetii is a small pleomorphic rod (0.3 to 1 μm), whose cell wall has many similarities to gram-negative rods. Although this pathogen was originally classified in the rickettsial family, DNA sequencing has indicated that the organism is more closely related to *Legionella* and *Francisella*, and is a proteobacteria. This organism is capable varying its LPS antigens in response to environmental conditions. In the external environment, the organism usually has phase II LPS antigens; however, on invading the host, a shift to phase I antigens occurs.

C. burnetii infects the host primary through the respiratory tract. Infectious particles are inhaled and are then phagocytosed by pulmonary macrophages, where they survive and grow within the acidic environment of the phagolysosome. The ability of the organism to hide within these acidic compartments may be the reason that curing chronic Q fever with antibiotics is so difficult. Pulmonary infection induces infiltration by mononuclear cells and can cause areas of focal necrosis and hemorrhage. Infection can spread to the liver, causing granuloma formation. In patients with damaged heart valves, *C. burnetii* can survive for prolonged periods and cause chronic infection.

Clinical Manifestations

The incubation period is approximately 3 weeks in most cases. Symptoms are often very mild or even absent. When symptoms are reported, most patients develop a self-limiting flu-like illness. Onset of fever is usually abrupt and is associated with headache and myalgias. Some patients complain of a nonproductive cough, and a few rales may be detected on pulmonary exam. Chest X-ray is suggestive of a viral pneumonia with mild bilateral lower lobe infiltrates. Occasionally, patients can develop acute respiratory distress syndrome or pleural effusions. Hepatitis may be asymptomatic or be associated with anorexia and malaise. Transaminase values are elevated, but jaundice is uncommon. Liver biopsy typically reveals doughnut-like granulomas consisting of a lipid vacuole surrounded by a fibrinoid ring. Other, less common manifestations include a maculopapular rash (10% of patients), myocarditis, and pericarditis (1%), and meningitis or encephalitis (1%).

A chronic infection persisting for longer than 6 months develops in about 5% of patients and primarily involves the heart, causing symptoms of subacute bacterial endocarditis. Conventional blood cultures are negative, however. Most cases of endocarditis develop in patients with valvular damage or a prosthetic valve. Vegetations are seldom seen on cardiac echo, and this negative result often delays the diagnosis. Embolic phenomena and digital clubbing may be observed in late stages of the infection. Valve replacement is commonly required as a consequence of severe valve dysfunction, and mortality in Q fever endocarditis is high (65% to 45%). Less commonly, chronic infection can develop in an aneurysm, vascular graft, liver, lungs, joints, or bone. If the infection is contracted during pregnancy, the mother may be asymptomatic. However, if untreated, infection is associated with a high rate of spontaneous abortion.

Diagnosis and Treatment

The organism can be readily grown using cell culture techniques; however, cultures are not performed in most facilities because of the danger to lab personnel and the need for a P3 containment facility. The PCR test for this illness has improved in specificity and sensitivity, and it is available in some locations. Immunofluorescence antibody testing remains the primary method of diagnosis. Anti-phase I and phase II IgG, IgM, and immunoglobulin A (IgA) antibody titers should be tested. Elevated IgG (above 1:200) and IgM (above 1:50) antibody titers against phase II antigens indicate acute disease. Elevated IgG (above 1:800) and IgA (above 1:100) antibody titers against phase I antigens are diagnostic of chronic Q fever.

Antibiotics are less effective in Q fever than in rickettsial diseases, and acute disease is usually

KEY POINTS

About Clinical Manifestations, Diagnosis, and Treatment of Q Fever

1. Incubation period is 3 weeks, usually causing an abrupt flu-like illness with cough.

2. Less commonly (10% of cases), a maculopapular rash appears. Other, rarer complications include
   a) severe respiratory comprise with acute respiratory distress syndrome;
   b) hepatitis with elevated transaminases, but minimal elevations in bilirubin;
   c) myocarditis and pericarditis;
   d) meningitis; and
   e) chronic endocarditis (negative echo early in the disease, high mortality).

3. Diagnosis is made by determining immunoglobulin G (IgG) and M (IgM) antibodies against phase I and II antigens (blood cultures negative):
   a) IgG (titer above 1:200) and IgM (titer above 1:50) anti-phase II antigens indicate acute disease.
   b) IgG (titer above 1:800) and IgA (titer above 1:100) anti-phase I antigens indicate chronic disease.
   c) Polymerase chain reaction is sensitive and specific (available in some locations).

4. Treatment not as effective as for rickettsial infections.
   a) Treat with doxycycline for 2 weeks for acute disease; fluoroquinolones may also be helpful.
   b) Treat with doxycycline and hydroxychloroquine for 18 months to 4 years or life for chronic endocarditis.

self-limiting, lasting 2 weeks. Tetracyclines have been shown to shorten the duration of fever in acute disease by 1 to 2 days. Oral or intravenous doxycycline is the treatment of choice (see Table 13.1), and fluoroquinolones are considered a reasonable alternative. In patients with Q fever endocarditis, cure rates have been improved by combining doxycycline with hydroxychloroquine. Therapy for endocarditis must be considerably prolonged—between 18 months and 4 years—to sterilize the valves. In some patients, antibiotics have been continued for life.

■ CAT SCRATCH DISEASE, BACILLARY ANGIOMATOSIS, AND OTHER DISEASES CAUSED BY BARTONELLA

POTENTIAL SEVERITY

Cat scratch disease and bacillary angiomatosis are usually localized diseases that seldom cause serious illness.

EPIDEMIOLOGY

Cat scratch disease is most commonly contracted by young people under the age of 21 years. This disease is distributed broadly throughout North America and is found worldwide. The incidence in the United States has been estimated to be between 9 and 10 per 100,000 population. Cat scratch disease is more common in warm humid climates.

As the name implies, all epidemiologic data point to the cat as the primary vector for disease. Young cats are most commonly implicated. Kittens have a very high incidence of asymptomatic bacteremia with *Bartonella*

KEY POINTS

About the Epidemiology of *Bartonella* Infections

1. Cat scratch disease is caused by *Bartonella henselae*:
   a) Transmitted primarily by young cats and, less commonly, by cat fleas.
   b) Common throughout North America; higher incidence in warm, humid areas.

2. Bacillary angiomatosis is caused by *B. henselae* and *B. quintana*:
   a) *B. quintana* is transmitted by human body lice.
   b) Spreads in areas with poor sanitation, among people with poor personal hygiene.

3. *B. bacilliformis* is transmitted by the sandfly in the Andes mountains of South America.

henselae, and they are more likely to scratch humans. In addition to cat scratches, this disease may be transmitted to humans by fleas, and the flea is also responsible for spread from cat to cat.

B. henselae not only causes cat scratch disease, it is one cause of bacillary angiomatosis. The other species that causes the latter disease, *B. quintana*, is also globally distributed. It is transmitted by human body lice (*Pediculus humanus*) and causes disease in areas where sanitation and personal hygiene are poor. A third pathogenic strain, *B. bacilliformis*, causes Oroya fever and Verruga peruana, diseases found only in the Andes mountains of South America, where the disease is transmitted by the sandfly. Other potentially pathogenic species of *Bartonella* have been identified; however, their relationship to disease is currently under active investigation.

PATHOGENESIS

Bartonella are pleomorphic gram-negative bacilli that take up Gram stain poorly. However, the organism binds silver and can be identified by Warthin–Starry stain. *Bartonella* enter the host through a break in the skin caused by a cat scratch or insect bite. The bacteria multiply at this site and subsequently spread to the local lymphatic system and adjacent lymph nodes. The bacteria contain flagella that allow them to move within the host. Flagellar and other surface proteins mediate attachment to red blood cells and endothelial cells. The attached bacteria can enter red cells, where they can multiply in vacuoles or in the cytoplasm. *Bartonella* are ingested by endothelial cells and multiply within a vacuole, forming intracellular clusters similar to the morulae of *Ehrlichia*. Certain species of *Bartonella*, including *B. bacilliformis*, *B. henselae*, and *B. quintana*, induce the formation of new vessels, and a *Bartonella* angiogenesis factor has been identified.

Because *Bartonella* grows in both the intracellular and extracellular environments of the host, it induces both a granulomatous reaction consisting of macrophages and histiocytes, and an acute inflammatory response consisting primarily of PMNs. This vigorous mixed immune response usually limits the spread of infection, which explains why most *Bartonella* infections remain localized. In individuals with depressed immunity, such as AIDS patients, this bacteria can cause bacteremia and disseminate throughout the body.

CLINICAL MANIFESTATIONS

CASE 13.5

A 21-year-old white man presented to the emergency room with a 2-hour history of severe right lower abdominal pain, nausea, vomiting, and loose stools. His temperature was 39.7°C; pulse, 133 per minute; and blood pressure, 101/40 mm Hg. His abdomen was soft and nontender; normal bowel sounds were heard. A warm, very tender mass, 1.5×1.5×6 cm, was palpated in the right inguinal area. Genitalia were normal, without ulcers. A computed tomography scan demonstrated a soft-tissue mass.

The patient's peripheral WBC count was 12,000/mm³ (54% PMNs, 34% bands), and his hematocrit was 43%. Urethral swabs were negative for Chlamydia *and gonococcus. Emergency surgical exploration revealed enlarged, matted right inguinal lymph nodes. Histopathology demonstrated an acute inflammatory response, and silver stain identified multiple rods.*

Three days following oral administration of ciprofloxacin, the patient defervesced. On further questioning, this college student reported that he had been playing with wild cats near his apartment over the 2 weeks before his admission, but said that he did not recall being scratched.

KEY POINTS

About the Pathogenesis of *Bartonella* Infections

1. Pleomorphic gram-negative rods. Takes up Gram stain only weakly; silver stain preferred.
2. Enters via breaks in the skin and spreads to the local lymphatics; rarely disseminates except in patients with AIDS.
3. Survives within host-cell intracellular vacuoles and extracellularly.
4. Produces an angiogenesis factor that stimulates the growth of new blood vessels.
5. Induces both a granulomatous and an acute inflammatory reaction that attracts polymorphonuclear leukocytes and prevents dissemination.

Cat Scratch Disease

Cat scratch disease usually presents as a single enlarged, warm, and painful lymph node near the site of skin inoculation. Lymph node swelling usually occurs within 2 weeks of inoculation. Case 13.5 developed unusually acute lymph node swelling that caused the sudden onset of severe pain, raising the possibility of a strangulated hernia and precipitating surgical exploration. The node can enlarge to between 8 and 10 cm in diameter; however, in most cases, the involved node expands to a diameter of 1 to 5 cm. Enlargement of a single node is the rule (85% of cases); however, as observed in case 13.5, some patients develop enlargement of a cluster of nodes or, less commonly, experience lymph node enlargement in two distinct anatomic sites. Generalized lymphadenopathy is rare.

The site of lymph node enlargement depends on the site of inoculation. Axillary node involvement is most common. Epitrochlear, supraclavicular, submandibular, and inguinal are other likely sites. In addition to being painful, warm, and erythematous, about 10% to 15% of the lymph nodes drain pus. The lymphadenopathy usually resolves over a period of 1 to 4 months, but can persist for several years if not treated with antibiotics.

On careful questioning, the patient may report a skin lesion in the region where the lymph node drains. Within 3 to 10 days after inoculation, a vesicular lesion develops that becomes erythematous and then papular. The skin lesions usually persist for 1 to 3 weeks, and by the time the patient seeks medical attention, the site of the scratch may be overlooked. However, if actively searched for, the primary lesion is detected in two thirds of patients. A primary lesion was not identified in case 13.5. When questioned, a significant percentage of patients do not recall a cat scratch, but nearly all patients provide a history of contact with a cat or (less commonly) a dog.

Low-grade fever and malaise accompany lymphadenopathy in about half of cases. Conjunctivitis occasionally develops when the eye is the portal of entry, and the combination of conjunctivitis and preauricular lymphadenopathy has been termed Parinaud's oculoglandular syndrome. Less common manifestations include optic neuritis, encephalopathy that can result in seizures and coma, lytic bone lesions, granulomatous lesions of the liver and spleen, pneumonia, erythema nodosum, and thrombocytopenic purpura.

Bacillary Angiomatosis

Bacillary angiomatosis develops predominantly in indigent patients with AIDS who also have body lice, the primary vector for spread of *B. quintana*. The disease is also seen in other immunocompromised patients and develops when the CD4 count drops below $100/mm^3$.

The skin lesions usually begin as cluster of small reddish papules that can enlarge to form nodules. Lesions appear vascular and bleed profusely when traumatized. They can be mistaken for Kaposi's sarcoma, pyogenic granuloma, cherry angiomas or hemangiomas. Skin biopsy reveals multiple small blood vessels, enlarged endothelial cells, and polymorphonuclear leukocyte infiltration. *B. henselae* has also been identified as a cause of bacillary angiomatosis. *B. quintana* can infect the liver and, less commonly, the spleen, resulting the formation of discrete blood-filled cystic structures. This disease has been called bacillary peliosis.

Bacteremic Illness

B. quintana can seed the bloodstream and cause trench fever. This disease was common during World Wars I and II, but is rare today, being seen primarily in homeless individuals with poor hygiene. Cases have been reported in the homeless in Seattle, Washington, and Marseilles, France.

Symptoms of fever, malaise, and bone pain involving the anterior shins usually begin 5 to 20 days after exposure. Splenomegaly is common, and in some patients, a maculopapular rash may be seen. Recurrent fever every 5 days (quintan fever) is the most common presentation, and it is the basis for the name of the organism. After the primary episode patients continue to have asymptomatic bacteremia lasting weeks to months. Both *B. quintana* and *B. henselae* can cause bacterial endocarditis, and these pathogens should be considered in cases of culture-negative bacterial endocarditis.

DIAGNOSIS

Bartonella grows slowly on fresh blood agar, rabbit-heart infusion agar, and chocolate agar. If *Bartonella* is suspected, the physician should contact the clinical microbiology laboratory to assure that all cultures are incubated for prolonged periods (at least 21 days) in 5% to 10% CO_2 and high moisture. Because the organism adheres to the sides of glass blood culture flasks, the liquid medium will not appear turbid. The slow rate of growth of this bacterium also impairs recognition by standard CO_2 detection methods. Staining of broth with Warthin–Starry stain or acridine orange has been used to overcome these limitations.

Biopsies of lymph nodes and skin lesions are generally not required for diagnosis, and the histopathology of mixed granulomatous and acute inflammatory reaction is not specific. Pallisading epithelioid cells are commonly seen, and a positive Warthin–Starry silver stain demonstrating black bacilli provides strong evidence for the diagnosis. However, organisms may be difficult to detect in chronically infected lymph nodes. Bacillary angiomatosis lesions demonstrate characteristic plump endothelial cells, neovascularity, and clusters of bacteria on silver staining.

An indirect immunofluorescence assay and enzyme immunosorbent assay are available to detect antibodies directed against *Bartonella*, and these tests have now replaced the cat scratch skin test. The skin test was previously considered to be a useful diagnostic tool, but it is no longer recommended. Unlike antibody titers (which have been ineffective at differentiating between species), PCR probes have proven to be more specific and are now commercially available.

TREATMENT

Azithromycin (standard 5 day course) is effective, and it is the treatment of choice in patients with lymph node

---

disease (See Table 13.1). Oral clarithromycin, oral doxycycline, or oral ciprofloxacin for 10 to 14 days may also be effective. In severe cases, intravenous azithromycin (500 mg daily) or gentamicin (5 mg/kg daily) combined with oral or intravenous rifampin (600 mg daily) are likely to be the most effective regimen. However, the efficacy of combined therapy has not been proven. In patients with bacteremia attributable to *B. quintana*, therapy should be continued for 4 to 6 weeks. and if endocarditis has developed, 6 months of therapy are advisable to reduce the risk of relapse. Patients with bacillary angiomatosis should be treated for 2 to 4 months, and 4 months of therapy is recommended for patients with bone, hepatic, or splenic lesions.

BRUCELLOSIS

POTENTIAL SEVERITY

This febrile illness is often difficult to diagnose, but seldom fatal.

Epidemiology

The bacteria that produce brucellosis are transmitted to humans primarily by infected wild and domestic animals. Direct animal contact, contact with animal products, or ingestion of unpasteurized dairy products are the most common ways in which humans can contract brucellosis. Cattle, buffalo, camels, yaks, goats, and sheep are the domestic animals most commonly responsible for disease transmission. In the wild, swine, fox, caribou, antelope, and elk have been implicated. Bacteria enter the host through abrasions or cuts, the conjunctiva, or the gastrointestinal tract. People at risk are farmers, hunters, and eaters of unpasteurized cheeses or other unpasteurized dairy products. The disease is found worldwide, being most common in the Mediterranean region, Arab Gulf basin, Indian subcontinent, Mexico, and Central and South America. In the United States, brucellosis is most frequently reported in the south and southwest. As a consequence of a rigorous farm animal screening and vaccination program, and pasteurization of all dairy products, the overall incidence of brucellosis in the United States is low, 0.05 per 100,000 population, with most cases being contracted by travelers who visit endemic areas.

Pathogenesis

Brucella are small aerobic gram-negative coccobacilli. The three strains that most commonly cause human disease are *B. abortis*, *B. suis*, and *B. melitensis*. The organism expresses LPS on its surface, and expression of the smooth form enhances intracellular survival, making an important contribution to virulence.

Brucella is a facultative intracellular pathogen. After entering the skin, the bacteria quickly attracts PMNs. These cells ingest the pathogen, where it easily survives within the phagolysosome by producing a superoxide dismutase to neutralize toxic oxygen byproducts. The bacteria subsequently invade the lymphatic system and bloodstream, disseminating primarily to organs with rich reticuloendothelial systems (liver, spleen, and bone marrow). Here, the bacteria are ingested by resident macrophages and survive in these cells by blocking phagosome–lysosome fusion, as is observed with *Ehrlichia*.

Clinical Manifestations

CASE 13.6

A 40–year-old white man was seen in the emergency room complaining of right-sided chest pain for 4 days. Pain was sharp and very severe, and was made worse by taking a deep breath. Pain was localized to the right chest, right upper quadrant, but occasionally radiated to the shoulder. The chest pain had been preceded by 2 weeks of a low-grade intermittent fever accompanied by sweating. He noted a mild cough with minimal yellow sputum production.

An epidemiologic history indicated that the patient periodically hunted wild pigs and had been hunting 5 weeks before his hospitalization. Past medical history included renal transplant surgery 4 years earlier; patient was on prednisone and azathioprine.

On physical examination a temperature of 36.7°C, a pulse rate of 102 per minute, a respiratory rate of 24 per minute, and a blood pressure of 126/94 mm Hg were recorded. He was ill appearing, breathing shallowly. No lymph nodes were palpable. Bilateral inspiratory rales were heard at the lung bases, with a small area of dullness in the right lower lung field. No abdominal organomegaly or tenderness was noted. Extremities showed 2 + edema. Chest X-ray showed a small right pleural effusion.

Laboratory results showed a hematocrit of 37.5% and a WBC count of 13,700/mm³, with 69% PMNs, 17% bands. Transaminases were 84 IU/L (AST) and 32 IU/L (ALT); alkaline phosphatase, 482 IU/L; total bilirubin, 2.4 mg/dL (1.5 mg/dL direct). Analysis of pleural fluid revealed a WBC count of 250/mm³, with 92% PMNs; LDH 741 IU/L; total protein 3.8 mg/dL;

KEY POINTS

About the Epidemiology and Pathogenesis of Brucellosis

1. Transmitted to humans by infected domestic and wild animals:
   a) Cattle, buffalo, camels, yaks, goats, and sheep
   a) Swine, fox, caribou, antelope, and elk

2. Most common in the Mediterranean region, Arab Gulf basin, Indian subcontinent, Mexico, Central and South America. Uncommon in the United States; seen mainly in the south and southwest.

3. Enters via a skin break or ingestion of unpasteurized dairy products (milk, cheeses).

4. Aerobic gram-negative coccobacilli has three pathogenic strains: *B. abortis*, *B. suis*, and B. melitensis.

5. Survives in phagolysosomes of polymorphonuclear leukocytes and macrophages by producing superoxide dismutase and blocking phagosome–lysosome fusion.

glucose 69 mg/dL; and pH 7.38. Two blood cultures were positive for B. suis. The patient was treated with doxycycline and rifampin for 6 weeks and fully recovered.

Fever, chills, malaise, anorexia, headache, and back pain usually develop 2 to 4 weeks after inoculation or ingestion of *Brucella*. In case 13.6, the history of intermittent low-grade fever and sweats was typical. These nonspecific symptoms can persist for weeks, making the diagnosis difficult to ascertain. As a result, brucellosis is among the listed infectious causes of fever of undetermined origin (see Chapter 3).

The physical exam is usually unimpressive; often, the only positive findings are lymphadenopathy and splenomegaly. As observed in case 13.6, approximately one third of patients develop a focal infection. Localized disease is more likely in patients who have had untreated infection for 30 or more days. Immunosuppression probably predisposed case 13.6 to develop a localized pleural infection as well as moderate hepatic involvement.

Septic arthritis is associated with mononuclear cells in the joint fluid. and *Brucella* can be cultured in half of

the cases. Sacroiliitis is particularly common. Osteomyelitis is rare and usually involves the vertebral bodies, mimicking tuberculous osteomyelitis. Granulomas are detected in bone marrow in up to 75% of cases. Infection of the marrow can lead to anemia, leukopenia, and thrombocytopenia.

The liver is probably always infected. Mild elevations of liver function tests are noted, and granulomas may be found on liver biopsy, particularly with *B. abortus*. Purulent abscesses are rare, but may be seen with *B. suis* and less commonly with *B. melitensis*. *Brucella* can often be recovered from the urine, but invasion of the kidney is rare. Orchitis is reported in up to 20% of men with brucellosis, the testes being infiltrated with lymphocytes and plasma cells.

Meningitis is the most frequent complication of the central nervous system and is associated with a CSF lymphocytic pleocytosis, elevated protein, and normal or depressed glucose. Encephalitis and brain abscess are rare. Endocarditis is rare, but can be fatal. Generally, valve replacement must be combined with prolonged antibiotic therapy. Pulmonary involvement is rare, but discrete granulomas can form, and bronchopneumonia occasionally occurs.

Diagnosis

Blood samples for culture should be drawn in all patients who are suspected of having brucellosis. Cultures are positive in up to 70% of patients. However, the organism is slow-growing, taking up to 35 days. However, blood cultures usually take 7 to 21 days to turn positive.

The clinical microbiology laboratory should be alerted so that cultures are held for beyond 7 days. Bone marrow culture is also a high-yield diagnostic test and should be considered in patients with negative blood cultures. Serology is the most common method for making the diagnosis. Serum agglutination titers measure IgG and IgM antibodies against the three major pathogenic *Brucella* strains, but do not detect *B. canis* (a rare cause of disease). A titer above 1:160 in the presence of appropriate symptoms is supportive of the diagnosis, as is a rise in the titer by a factor of four between acute and convalescent sera. ELISA methods for IgG and IgM are also available and demonstrate sensitivity and specificity similar to those of the serum agglutination tests.

Treatment

Because *Brucella* survives within phagocytes, antibiotics with good intracellular penetration are recommended (see Table 13.1). The treatment of choice is doxycycline and rifampin for 6 weeks. Single-drug

---

KEY POINTS

About the Clinical Presentation of Brucellosis

1. Incubation period is 2 to 4 weeks; symptoms include fever, chills, malaise, anorexia, headache, and back pain.
2. Important cause of fever of unknown origin; lymphadenopathy and splenomegaly are the only positive physical findings.
3. Focal infection is more common if treatment is delayed:
   a) Osteomyelitis and arthritis, particularly sacroiliitis, frequently occur.
   b) Hepatic involvement is common.
   c) Lymphocytic meningitis is a possibility.
   d) Endocarditis usually requires valve replacement.
   e) Positive urine culture is common; orchitis occurs in 20% of men.
   f) Bone marrow suppression can occur, with granulomas found.
   g) Pulmonary disease is rare.

therapy is not recommended because of the high likelihood of relapse. Doxycycline combined with intramuscular streptomycin or gentamicin (5 mg/kg) are useful alternatives. For children, trimethoprim sulfamethoxazole (10 to 12 mg/kg of the trimethoprim component daily, divided into two doses) and rifampin (20 mg//kg daily) are recommended. In cases of meningitis or endocarditis, a three-drug regimen consisting of doxycycline, rifampin, and trimethoprim–sulfamethoxazole has been used. Therapy for these diseases must be prolonged (several months to more than 1 year). In patients with endocarditis, replacement of the infected valve is usually required for cure.

FURTHER READING

Lyme Disease

Kalish RA, Kaplan RF, Taylor E, Jones-Woodward L, Workman K, Steere AC. Evaluation of study patients with Lyme disease, 10–20-year follow-up. *J Infect Dis.* 2001;183:453–460.

Klempner MS, Hu LT, Evans J, et al. Two controlled trials of antibiotic treatment in patients with persistent symptoms and a history of Lyme disease. *N Engl J Med.* 2001;345:85–92.

Krupp LB, Hyman LG, Grimson R, et al. Study and treatment of post Lyme disease (STOP-LD): a randomized double masked clinical trial. *Neurology.* 2003;60:1923–1930.

Nadelman RB, Nowakowski J, Fish D, et al. Prophylaxis with single-dose doxycycline for the prevention of Lyme disease after an *Ixodes scapularis* tick bite. *N Engl J Med.* 2001;345:79–84.

Smith RP, Schoen RT, Rahn DW, et al. Clinical characteristics and treatment outcome of early Lyme disease in patients with microbiologically confirmed erythema migrans. *Ann Intern Med.* 2002;136:421–428.

Steere AC, Dhar A, Hernandez J, et al. Systemic symptoms without erythema migrans as the presenting picture of early Lyme disease. *Am J Med.* 2003;114:58–62.

Varela AS, Luttrell MP, Howerth EW, et al. First culture isolation of *Borrelia lonestari,* putative agent of southern tick-associated rash illness. *J Clin Microbiol.* 2004;42:1163–1169.

Leptospirosis

Morgan J, Bornstein SL, Karpati AM, et al. Outbreak of leptospirosis among triathlon participants and community residents in Springfield, Illinois, 1998. *Clin Infect Dis.* 2002;34:1593–1599.

Nardone A, Capek I, Baranton G, et al. Risk factors for leptospirosis in metropolitan France: results of a national case-control study, 1999–2000. *Clin Infect Dis.* 2004;39:751–753.

Panaphut T, Domrongkitchaiporn S, Vibhagool A, Thinkamrop B, Susaengrat W. Ceftriaxone compared with sodium penicillin G for treatment of severe leptospirosis. *Clin Infect Dis.* 2003;36:1507–1513.

Ren SX, Fu G, Jiang XG, et al. Unique physiological and pathogenic features of *Leptospira interrogans* revealed by whole-genome sequencing. *Nature.* 2003;422:888–893.

Segura ER, Ganoza CA, Campos K, et al. Clinical spectrum of pulmonary involvement in leptospirosis in a region of endemicity, with quantification of leptospiral burden. *Clin Infect Dis.* 2005;40:343–351.

Suputtamongkol Y, Niwattayakul K, Suttinont C, et al. An open, randomized, controlled trial of penicillin, doxycycline, and cefotaxime for patients with severe leptospirosis. *Clin Infect Dis.* 2004;39:1417–1424.

Tansuphasiri U, Deepradit S, Phulsuksombati D, Tangkanakul W. Two simple immunoassays using endemic leptospiral antigens for serodiagnosis of human leptospirosis. *Southeast Asian J Trop Med Public Health.* 2005;36:302–311.

Rickettsial Diseases

Demma LJ, Traeger MS, Nicholson WL, et al. Rocky Mountain spotted fever from an unexpected tick vector in Arizona. *N Engl J Med.* 2005;353:587–594.

Kirk JL, Fine DP, Sexton DJ, Muchmore HG. Rocky Mountain spotted fever. A clinical review based on 48 confirmed cases, 1943–1986. *Medicine (Baltimore).* 1990;69:35–45.

Holman RC, Paddock CD, Curns AT, Krebs JW, McQuiston JH, Childs JE. Analysis of risk factors for fatal Rocky Mountain spotted fever: evidence for superiority of tetracyclines for therapy. *J Infect Dis.* 2001;184:1437–1444.

Jensenius M, Fournier PE, Fladby T, et al. Sub-acute neuropathy in patients with African tick bite fever. *Scand J Infect Dis.* 2006;38:114–118.

Jensenius M, Fournier PE, Raoult D. Rickettsioses and the international traveler. *Clin Infect Dis.* 2004;39:1493–1499.

Paddock CD, Greer PW, Ferebee TL, et al. Hidden mortality attributable to Rocky Mountain spotted fever: immunohistochemical detection of fatal, serologically unconfirmed disease. *J Infect Dis.* 1999;179:1469–1476.

Watt G, Kantipong P, Jongsakul K, Watcharapichat P, Phulsuksombati D, Strickman D. Doxycycline and rifampicin for mild scrub-typhus infections in northern Thailand: a randomised trial. *Lancet.* 2000;356:1057–1061.

Ehrlichiosis

Chapman AS, Bakken JS, Folk SM, et al. Diagnosis and management of tickborne rickettsial diseases: Rocky Mountain spotted fever, ehrlichioses, and anaplasmosis—United States: a practical guide for physicians and other health-care and public health professionals. *MMWR Recomm Rep.* 2006;55:1–27.

Dumler JS, Choi KS, Garcia-Garcia JC, et al. Human granulocytic anaplasmosis and *Anaplasma phagocytophilum. Emerg Infect Dis.* 2005;11:1828–1834.

Paddock CD, Childs JE. *Ehrlichia chaffeensis*: a prototypical emerging pathogen. *Clin Microbiol Rev.* 2003;16:37–64.

Wallace BJ, Brady G, Ackman DM, et al. Human granulocytic ehrlichiosis in New York. *Arch Intern Med.* 1998;158:769–773.

Q Fever

Fenollar F, Thuny F, Xeridat B, Lepidi H, Raoult D. Endocarditis after acute Q fever in patients with previously undiagnosed valvulopathies. *Clin Infect Dis.* 2006;42:818–821.

Parker NR, Barralet JH, Bell AM. Q Fever. *Lancet.* 2006;367:679–688.

Raoult D, Marrie T, Mege J. Natural history and pathophysiology of Q fever. *Lancet Infect Dis.* 2005;5:219–226.

Tissot-Dupont H, Vaillant V, Rey S, Raoult D. Role of sex, age, previous valve lesion, and pregnancy in the clinical expression and outcome of Q fever after a large outbreak. *Clin Infect Dis.* 2007;44:232–237.

Bartonella Infections

Brouqui P, Lascola B, Roux V, Raoult D. Chronic *Bartonella quintana* bacteremia in homeless patients. *N Engl J Med.* 1999;340:184–189.

Fournier PE, Lelievre H, Eykyn SJ, et al. Epidemiologic and clinical characteristics of *Bartonella quintana* and *Bartonella henselae* endocarditis: a study of 48 patients. *Medicine (Baltimore).* 2001;80:245–251.

Giladi M, Maman E, Paran D, et al. Cat-scratch disease-associated arthropathy. *Arthritis Rheum.* 2005;52:3611–3617.

Ridder GJ, Technau-Ihling K, Sander A. Boedeker CC. Spectrum and management of deep neck space infections: an 8-year experience of 234 cases. *Otolaryngol Head Neck Surg.* 2005;133:709–714.

Rolain JM, Lepidi H, Zanaret M, et al. Lymph node biopsy specimens and diagnosis of cat-scratch disease. *Emerg Infect Dis.* 2006;12:1338–1344.

Rolain JM, Brouqui P, Koehler JE, Maguina C, Dolan MJ, Raoult D. Recommendations for treatment of human infections caused by *Bartonella* species. *Antimicrob Agents Chemother.* 2004;48:1921–1933.

Brucellosis

Colmenero JD, Reguera JM, Martos F, et al. Complications associated with *Brucella melitensis* infection: a study of 530 cases. *Medicine (Baltimore).* 1996;75:195–211.

Hasanjani Roushan MR, Mohraz M, Hajiahmadi M, Ramzani A, Valayati AA. Efficacy of gentamicin plus doxycycline versus streptomycin plus doxycycline in the treatment of brucellosis in humans. *Clin Infect Dis.* 2006;42:1075–1080.

Pappas G, Akritidis N, Bosilkovski M, Tsianos E. Brucellosis. *N Engl J Med.* 2005;352:2325–2336.

Navarro E, Segura JC, Castano MJ, Solera J. Use of real-time quantitative polymerase chain reaction to monitor the evolution of *Brucella melitensis* DNA load during therapy and post-therapy follow-up in patients with brucellosis. *Clin Infect Dis.* 2006;42:1266–1273.

Solera J, Geijo P, Largo J, et al. A randomized, double-blind study to assess the optimal duration of doxycycline treatment for human brucellosis. *Clin Infect Dis.* 2004;39:1776–1782.

Bioterrorism

Time Recommended to Complete: 1 day

Frederick Southwick, M.D.

GUIDING QUESTIONS

1. What are the key characteristics of the ideal bioterrorist agent?

2. What can physicians do to help in the early phases of a bioterrorist attack?

3. What are the clinical clues that should raise the possibility of an anthrax attack?

4. How is bubonic plague normally transmitted, and what are the usual clinical manifestations of plague?

5. Which groups are normally at risk for developing tularemia?

6. How does the clinical presentation of smallpox differ from that of chickenpox?

POTENTIAL SEVERITY

Biologic weapons are intended to kill and terrorize their victims. Treatment must be immediate, and public health measures must be instituted quickly and efficiently to prevent additional casualties.

Bioterrorism was once called biologic warfare, a term that should now be avoided because it suggests that biologic agents are legitimate weapons for defeating a true or perceived enemy. In 1975, biologic weapons were rightfully condemned as inhumane and cowardly, and the civilized world agreed to ban them. Such agents cause great pain and suffering, and have the potential to kill large numbers of innocent bystanders. They subvert science conducted to save lives, to kill and maim instead.

The term "biologic weapons" is defined as the use of "microbial. . . agents. . . for hostile purposes or in armed conflict." "Ideal" biologic agents would be expected to

- reliably cause permanently debilitating or fatal disease in a high percentage of victims.
- be capable of being targeted precisely to the enemy, and not cause a worldwide epidemic that could harm friendly soldiers or civilians.
- be capable of being produced in large quantities at reasonable cost.
- be capable of being stored for prolonged periods without losing potency.
- be capable of being readily aerosolized to allow rapid delivery over a broad geographic area.

Only a limited number of biologic pathogens fulfill most of these criteria. Four agents are of particular concern today. However, new "advances" that create super pathogens genetically designed to fit the needs of the bioterrorist are likely to add new organisms to the "most wanted" list. Currently, experts usually list anthrax, plague, tularemia, and smallpox as the top four potential biologic weapons. Other organisms that could be used include *Clostridium botulinum* (botulinum toxins),

Brucella, *Coxiella burnetii* (Q fever), alpha viruses (Venezuelan equine encephalitis, Eastern and Western encephalitis), and viral hemorrhagic fevers (Ebolavirus and Marburg agent).

Medical personnel must be aware of the clinical manifestations, modes of transmission, appropriate diagnostic tests, and available treatment and prophylactic options for managing a biologic attack. The U.S. Army Medical Research Institute of Infectious Diseases (USAMRIID) recommends a 10-step approach:

1. **Maintain a high index of suspicion.** Whenever possible, these diseases should be treated in the early phase of illness, when symptoms tend to be nonspecific. Without a high index of suspicion, treatment may be delayed, and mortality greatly increased.

2. **Protect thyself.** Use of high-efficiency particulate air (HEPA) filters or even surgical masks is warranted when a contagious respiratory illness is suspected or an aerosolized pathogen has been released. All health care workers should be up-to-date with appropriate immunizations.

3. **Assess the patient.** History of recent symptoms; epidemiologic clues (see point 9); vital signs; pulmonary, cardiovascular, and skin examination; and assessment of motor function should all be quickly obtained.

4. **Decontaminate when necessary.** Patients usually present several days after exposure to biologic agents, making decontamination unnecessary. Decontamination is more commonly required after exposure to chemical agents. Bleach (0.1%) is an effective decontaminant that kills even the hardiest biologic agent, anthrax spores.

5. **Establish a diagnosis.** The approaches to diagnosis depend on the agent and are reviewed in this chapter. Where appropriate, nasal and throat swabs (use rayon rather than cotton swabs), blood, urine, and sputum cultures should be obtained, and environmental samples should be analyzed. Improved rapid diagnostic tests are currently under development, and samples should be provided to the Centers for Disease Control and Prevention (CDC: emergency contact number 1-770-488-7100), the USAMRIID (1-888 USARIID), or the Emergency Operations Centers Special Pathogens Branch (1-301-619-4728).

6. **Render prompt treatment.** Therapy is most effective in the prodrome period, when clinical signs may not allow for a specific diagnosis. Delay of treatment until the clinical manifestations are more developed often results in serious complications or death. In the proper setting, empiric therapy should be strongly considered in patients with an undifferentiated febrile illness or pneumonia. Doxycycline is particularly useful when a

bioterrorist agent is being considered, because this antibiotic treats anthrax, plague, tularemia, Q fever, and brucellosis. Fluoroquinolones also may have a potential role in empiric therapy.

7. **Practice good infection control.** For most agents, standard precautions provide adequate protection. The three exceptions are smallpox (requires strict airborne precautions), pneumonic plague (requires droplet precautions), and viral hemorrhagic fevers (require contact precautions).

8. **Alert the proper authorities.** Public health officials and the clinical lab should be immediately notified of a potential biologic attack. Rapid action on the part of public health officials to deliver stockpiles of appropriate medications, establish appropriate triage and management teams, and assess the extent of the attack will reduce casualties and save lives.

9. **Assist in epidemiologic investigation**. It is critical that all health care personnel have a fundamental knowledge of epidemiologic principles. Whenever possible, an occupational and travel history, immunizations, exposure to contaminated food or water, and history of friends or coworkers becoming ill should be obtained and provided to public health personnel.

10. **Maintain proficiency**. During a time of increased threat, health care personnel are inundated with facts concerning various biologic agents, but knowledge and proficiency can wane over time. It is critical that each person maintain "proficiency in dealing with this low probability, but high consequence problem."

(Adapted from the USAMRIID's handbook called *Medical Management of Biological Casualties*. Visit www.usamriid.army.mil/education for additional training.)

ANTHRAX

Anthrax is a natural infection of animals, primarily herbivores. Humans can contract the disease from infected animals or animal products. With the advent of domestic animal vaccinations, this disease is now seldom encountered in developed countries. As a consequence, most health professionals are unfamiliar with the clinical manifestations of this potentially deadly organism.

The United States, the former Soviet Union, and Iraq have all manufactured anthrax spores capable of being disseminated as aerosols. For the first time in history, anthrax spores were used in 2001 as a biologic weapon against U.S. citizens. That attack underscored the importance of early recognition and treatment of pulmonary and cutaneous anthrax.

MICROBIOLOGY AND PATHOGENESIS

Bacillus anthracis is a gram-positive rod that can be easily grown on conventional nutrient media. On blood agar plates, the nonhemolytic colonies are gray-white in color with ragged edges. Colonies adhere tightly to the media and cannot easily be displaced by a culture loop. When this bacterium encounters unfavorable environmental conditions, it readily forms endospores. The spores are highly resistant to adverse conditions and are able to survive extreme temperatures, high pH and salinity levels, and disinfectants.

When spores are inhaled, their small size allows them to reach small bronchioles and alveoli, where macrophages phagocytose and carry them to the hilar and perihilar lymph nodes. Under the favorable environmental conditions in a host, the spores then germinate, and bacteria begin to quickly multiply.

The bacteria produce three exotoxins: protective antigen, lethal factor, and edema factor. Protective antigen binds to specific receptors on the cell surface and forms a channel that facilitates the entry of edema and lethal factor. These two agents result in cell swelling and death. Lethal factor is a protease that cleaves specific MAP (mitogen-activated protein) kinase kinases, blocking cell signals important for neutrophil chemotaxis, macrophage cell survival, and immune cell cytokine production. As a result, the host's immune system is paralyzed, and the bacteria continue to grow rapidly and quickly entering the bloodstream to cause overwhelming bacteremia, shock, and meningitis.

EPIDEMIOLOGY

Most cases of anthrax in the United States occur as a result of contact with animal products imported from Asia, the Middle East, and Africa. Wool, goat hair, and animal hides are the most common sources of infection. A case of inhalation anthrax contracted from contaminated hides was recently reported in Pennsylvania. Cases have also been traced to shaving-brush bristles, wool coats, yarn, goat-skin bongo drums, and heroin preparations.

The largest outbreak of anthrax in recent years occurred in Sverdlovsk (now Yekaterinburg), Russia, in 1979. The approximately 96 inhalation cases resulted in 64 deaths. The accidental release of anthrax spores from a germ-warfare facility was suspected, and recent polymerase chain reaction (PCR) analysis of tissue samples from 11 victims confirmed that suspicion.

The deliberate introduction of anthrax spores into letters sent through the United States Postal Service in 2001 caused 11 cases of inhalation and 11 cases of cutaneous anthrax. Postal workers were at particular risk, because of spores released from sealed envelopes during mail processing. Cross contamination of mail also

---

KEY POINTS

About the Pathogenesis and Modes of Spread of Anthrax

1. *Bacillus anthracis* is an aerobic gram-positive rod, nonhemolytic on blood agar plates.

2. Under poor nutrient conditions, *B. anthracis* forms spores:

   a) Spores resist heat, high salinity, alkaline pH, and many disinfectants.

   b) When aerosolized, spores enter the lung, are ingested by macrophages, and are transported to the mediastinum.

3. Spores germinate in the mediastinum, and the bacteria produce three exotoxins:

   a) Protective antigen binds to host cell receptors, and allows entry by lethal factor and edema factor.

   b) Lethal factor and edema factor paralyze the immune system and cause cell edema and death.

4. Natural transmission of the disease occurs through infected animal products—for example, wool, goat hair, animal hides.

5. Spores can be purposely aerosolized as a bioterror weapon. "Weaponized" anthrax was transmitted by mail in 2001. Postal workers and other mail handlers are at high risk.

---

occurred. As a consequence of those events, all mail recipients have been instructed to avoid opening suspicious mail. If powder is found in an envelope, the letter should be gently set down, the room quickly vacated, and appropriate authorities immediately notified. These events of 2001 emphasize the importance of training public health and law enforcement personnel on the proper handling of potentially contaminated samples and on decontamination and prophylaxis.

CLINICAL MANIFESTATIONS

CASE 14.1

A 63-year-old man was taken by his wife to the emergency room with four-day history of fever, myalgias, and malaise. His wife reported he had no complaints of sore throat, rhinorrhea, and other upper respiratory tract symptoms. He awoke confused and disoriented on the morning of admission. This man's prior medical history included mild hypertension and placement of a coronary stent for atherosclerotic heart disease.

An epidemiologic history indicated that the patient was employed as a photo editor for a major tabloid newspaper in Florida, where he spent most of the day reviewing photographs submitted by mail

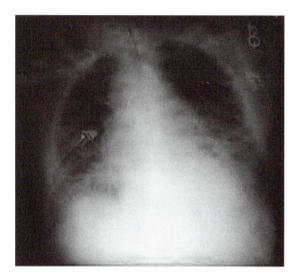

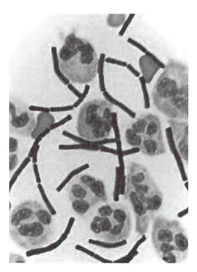

Figure 14–1. Pulmonary anthrax with dissemination to the meninges. **A.** This chest radiograph shows a widened mediastinum. **B.** Gram stain of the cerebrospinal fluid demonstrates boxcar-like gram-positive rods. *See color image on color plate 3*

or over the Internet. On physical examination, he was found to be lethargic and disoriented. His temperature was 39°C; blood pressure, 150/80 mm Hg; pulse, 110 beats per minute; and respirations, 18 per minute. An ear, nose, and throat exam showed no pharyngeal erythema or exudate, and no nuchal rigidity was noted. Bibasilar rhonchi without rales were heard in the lungs, but no heart murmurs, rubs, or gallops were noted. Abdomen was soft and nontender, with no organomegaly. The patient's skin was clear, and a neurologic exam revealed no focal deficits.

The patient's laboratory workup showed a hematocrit of 46% and a peripheral white blood cell (WBC) count of 9400/mm³, with 77% polymorphonuclear leukocytes (PMNs), 15% lymphocytes, and 8% monocytes. A chest x-ray revealed basilar infiltrates and a widened mediastinum [Figure 14.1(A)]. Cloudy fluid from a lumbar puncture contained red blood cells (1375/mm³), WBCs (4750/mm³, with 81% PMNs and 19% monocytes), 666 mg/dL protein, and 57 mg/dL glucose, A Gram stain of the cerebrospinal fluid (CSF) revealed many PMNs and many large gram-positive bacilli, both single and in chains [Figure 14.1(B)]. Cultures of blood and CSF grew B. anthracis.

Despite administration of high-dose penicillin, the patient suffered grand mal seizures, hypotension, acidosis, and renal failure. On the third hospital day, he died of an asystolic cardiopulmonary arrest. Autopsy revealed no pulmonary parenchymal consolidation. Other findings included 50 mL gross blood in the mediastinum and several enlarged lymph nodes (1 cm to 2 cm). On cross-sectional examination, the lymph nodes were hemorrhagic. (Adapted from Bush LM, Abrams BH, Beall A, Johnson CC. Index case of fatal inhalational anthrax due to bioterrorism in the United States. N Engl J Med. 2001;345:1607–1610)

It is critical that health care personnel be familiar with the clinical manifestations of anthrax. In patients with a febrile illness or cutaneous lesions of unclear cause, an exposure and occupational history may be particularly helpful in focusing on the possibility of anthrax. During the 2001 bioterror attack in the United States, early recognition of the index case (case 14.1) in South Florida by an infectious disease specialist led to rapid institution of antibiotic prophylaxis and saved many lives. Unfortunately, several other physicians failed to recognize the early manifestations of inhalation anthrax in postal workers, and those patients were discharged from the emergency room only to return later with full-blown fatal disease. The earlier recognition of several cutaneous anthrax cases could have alerted the authorities in New York in a more timely manner that a bioterror attack had also been launched in that state.

Inhalation Anthrax (Woolsorters' Disease)

It is important that clinicians be aware of the biphasic presentation of inhalation anthrax. Recognition and treatment during the first phase can be life saving.

Case 14.1 in all likelihood inhaled spores from a contaminated letter sent to his newspaper, and a flu-like illness was present for 4 days before the onset of fulminant mediastinal involvement, with bacteremia and meningitis. Because the patient failed to seek medical attention during the early phase of his illness, his fatal outcome could not have been prevented.

FIRST PHASE

From 1 to 5 days after inhalation of spores, the patient has symptoms suggestive of a viral syndrome: nonproductive cough, malaise, fatigue, myalgia, and mild fever. Occasionally, the sensation of chest heaviness is reported. Rhonchi may be heard on examination, but aside from fever, no other abnormal physical findings are observed. As noted in case 14.1, pharyngitis and rhinitis do not usually accompany inhalation anthrax.

Unless a careful exposure and occupational history is obtained, and inhalation anthrax is included in the differential diagnosis, patients are often sent home with antipyretics for a presumed viral syndrome. It is during this period that spores are being transported by pulmonary macrophages from the lung parenchyma to the mediastinal lymph nodes. At this stage, antibiotic treatment should prevent progression to the second phase.

SECOND PHASE

Within 2 to 4 days, symptoms temporarily resolve, but are rapidly followed by the second, more severe, stage of the disease. At this time, the spores have germinated in the mediastinal lymph nodes, and protective antigen, lethal factor, and edema factor are being produced by rapidly multiplying anthrax bacilli. Necrosis and hemorrhagic inflammation quickly develop, causing the sudden onset of severe respiratory distress with dyspnea, cyanosis, and diffuse diaphoresis accompanied by fever, tachycardia, and tachypnea. On pulmonary auscultation, moist, crepitating rales are evident, and findings consistent with pleural effusions may be apparent. Chest x-ray demonstrates a widened mediastinum without a definite parenchymal infiltrate. Pleural effusions are often also revealed [Figure 14.1(A)].

KEY POINTS

About Inhalation Anthrax

1. First phase presents as a viral-like syndrome. No pharyngitis or rhinitis, but chest heaviness may be described. Treatment can abort the second lethal phase.

2. Second phase follows after a brief asymptomatic period and can include:

   a) Sudden onset of severe respiratory distress, fever, tachycardia, and tachypnea.

   b) Rales on chest exam. Chest radiograph shows a widened mediastinum often with pleural effusions.

   c) Thoracentesis reveals hemorrhagic fluid that is positive for *Bacillus anthracis* on Gram stain and culture.

   d) Confusion in half of cases, and cerebrospinal fluid contains polymorphonuclear leukocytes and is positive for *B. anthracis* on Gram stain and culture.

   e) In the terminal stage, blood cultures are positive for anthrax bacilli. Death follows within 24 hours and can occur "in mid-sentence."

The combination of a widened mediastinum accompanied by pleural effusions should immediately raise the possibility of inhalation anthrax. Thoracentesis reveals hemorrhagic fluid, and Gram stain and culture are both usually positive. As described in case 14.1, confusion followed by lethargy and coma may develop in about half of all cases as a consequence of meningitis. On lumbar puncture, the CSF contains PMNs and large boxcar-like gram-positive rods [Figure 14.1(B)]. In the terminal stages of the illness, blood cultures are usually positive for *B. anthracis*. Death usually occurs within 24 hours and may be accompanied by septic shock. Death can be very sudden, and patients have been reported to die "in mid-sentence."

Cutaneous Anthrax

Skin disease is the most common manifestation of anthrax. Between 1 and 7 days after spores are inoculated into the skin, a small papule develops. Over the next 3 to 4 days, the lesion progresses to a vesicle, 1 cm to 3 cm in diameter. Erythema and non-pitting edema often surround the vesicle. Initially, the vesicular fluid is serous and contains large numbers of

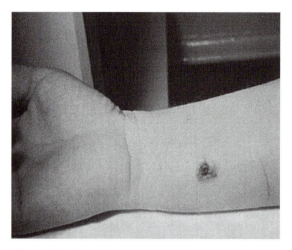

Figure 14–2. Cutaneous anthrax. Note the black eschar and edematous margins of this 7-day-old lesion. *See color image on color plate 3*

organisms. The vesicle subsequently ruptures, and a black eschar becomes evident at the base of the ulcer (Figure 14.2). The name "anthrax" (Greek for coal) refers to this characteristic black eschar.

Despite the erythema and swelling, lesions are not painful, but they may be mildly pruritic. Lymphangitis, lymphadenopathy, fever, and malaise may accompany infection of the skin. After several weeks, the skin lesion dries, and a permanent scar is formed. Lesions occur primarily on exposed regions of the body. The arms are the most frequent site of infection; the face and neck are also commonly involved. A single lesion is usually found, although multiple sites

---

KEY POINTS

About Cutaneous Anthrax

1. Usually a single lesion develops on an exposed area of the body, an arm being most common.
2. Develops 1 to 7 days after inoculation; begins as a papule.
3. Progresses over 3 to 4 days to a vesicle filled with organisms; margin is edematous.
4. Lesion then ruptures and forms a black eschar.
5. Not painful, but often itches.
6. Spontaneously heals over several weeks, leaving a scar.

---

may become infected as a result of simultaneous inoculations.

Gastrointestinal Anthrax

Gastrointestinal infection has not been reported in the United States, and it is not an expected clinical consequence of a bioterrorist attack. This disease occurs primarily in developing countries, usually after ingestion of contaminated meat. The incubation period is usually 3 to 5 days. Patients initially have nausea, vomiting, anorexia, and fever. These symptoms are rapidly followed by acute abdominal pain, hematemesis, and bloody diarrhea. Findings on examination suggest an acute surgical abdomen, and moderate leukocytosis with immature band forms is seen. Rapid progression to toxemia and shock leads to death within 2 to 5 days after the initial onset of symptoms.

An oropharyngeal form of anthrax has also been described. Inflammatory lesions that resemble the cutaneous lesions develop on the posterior pharynx, hard palate, or tonsils. Tissue necrosis and edema are accompanied by sore throat, dysphagia, fever, regional lymphadenopathy, and toxemia.

DIAGNOSIS

A careful epidemiologic history is the single most important means of reaching the diagnosis. In cases of natural infection, a history of contact with herbivores or products from these animals, particularly if the products come from outside the United States, should raise the possibility of anthrax. In the setting of a possible bioterrorist attack, employment history and a history of being present in a contaminated area are important clues. By the time Gram stains and cultures of blood and CSF are positive, the illness has progressed to the second fatal phase. Diagnosis must therefore be presumptive, and the threshold for treatment low to prevent progression from mildly symptomatic to life-threatening disease.

For epidemiologic purposes, samples from the nose and face can be obtained using rayon-tipped swabs. Cultures from these sites are specific, but insensitive, and, in the individual patient, cannot be used to decide whether to begin treatment. Nasal samples can be used to determine the physical perimeters of exposure, and the resulting data can used to determine who should receive prophylactic antibiotics. The physical appearance of the skin lesions is characteristic, and Gram stains and cultures of the ulcer base are frequently positive. Enzyme-linked immunosorbent assays (ELISAs) are available that measure antibody titers against lethal and edema toxin. A rise in multiple titers by a factor of four over 4 weeks or in a single titer to 1:32 is considered positive.

KEY POINTS

About the Diagnosis of Anthrax

1. Epidemiologic history is important, and the diagnosis is often presumptive.
2. Nasal swabs are helpful for determining the physical parameters of exposure, but not for deciding individual treatment or prophylaxis.
3. Gram stain and culture of skin lesions are often positive.
4. Positive cultures of blood and cerebrospinal fluid usually accompany a fatal outcome.
5. Enzyme-linked immunosorbent assays for antibodies against lethal toxin and edema toxin are available.

TREATMENT

Although penicillin has been recommended as the treatment of choice for naturally occurring anthrax, penicillin-resistant natural strains have been reported. Penicillin-resistant strains of anthrax have also been genetically engineered as bioterrorist weapons, and the military protocol recommends intravenous ciprofloxacin (400 mg twice daily) or doxycycline (200 mg loading dose, followed by 100 mg twice daily) as first-line therapy (see Table 14.1). Penicillin is recommended as an alternative once sensitivities have been obtained. Because penicillin treatment induces β-lactamase activity, penicillin should be combined with an additional antibiotic. Other antibiotics that demonstrate activity against anthrax—and that may be combined with any of the above agents in the seriously ill patient—include rifampin, vancomycin, imipenem, clindamycin, and clarithromycin. Treatment should be continued for 60 days, with a switch to oral antibiotics as the patient's clinical condition improves. Excision of skin lesions is contraindicated because of the increased risk of precipitating bacteremia. However, after appropriate antibiotic therapy, excision and skin grafting may be necessary.

Before antibiotics became available, cutaneous disease resulted in a mortality of 10% to 20%. With appropriate antibiotic treatment, fewer than 1% of patients die. Despite appropriate antibiotics and respiratory support, inhalation anthrax is frequently fatal. In the 2001 U.S. bioterrorist attack, half of the patients who contracted inhalation anthrax survived, proving that rapid institution of antibiotics can be life-saving in early second-phase pulmonary anthrax. Gastrointestinal disease is also associated with high mortality (25% to 100%).

PROPHYLAXIS

A killed vaccine derived from a component of the anthrax exotoxin is available and is recommended for all industrial workers at risk for exposure to contaminated animal products. As a result of increased concerns about biologic warfare and bioterrorism, military personnel are now vaccinated. To date, surveillance studies have not detected any serious or unexpected adverse reactions. The vaccination (BioThrax), which is available through the CDC (telephone: 770-488-7100; Web: http://cdc.gov), is administered in six doses at two-week intervals.

In cases of suspected exposure to *B. anthracis*, antibiotic prophylaxis and vaccination are recommended. The regimen of choice is an oral fluoroquinolone or, if fluoroquinolones are contraindicated, doxycycline (see Table 14.1). Prophylaxis should be continued until exposure is excluded. If exposure is confirmed, prophylaxis should be continued for 4 weeks in individuals who have received three or more doses of the vaccine, and for 60 days in the unvaccinated patient.

KEY POINTS

About the Treatment and Prevention of Anthrax

1. The treatment threshold must be very low in the setting of a bioterrorist attack.

   a) Give intravenous ciprofloxacin, levofloxacin, or doxycycline.

   b) Combination therapy is recommended for the seriously ill patient: add rifampin, vancomycin, imipenem, clindamycin, or clarithromycin to the basic regimen.

   c) Avoid excision of skin lesions, which carries a danger of precipitating bacteremia.

   d) Continue therapy for 60 days; newly germinating spores can cause relapse.

2. All individuals suspected of exposure should receive prophylaxis:

   a) Give a fluoroquinolone (ciprofloxacin, levofloxacin, or ofloxacin) or alternatively doxycycline for 60 days.

   b) Vaccine based on inactivated exotoxin is given to military personnel and workers at risk of exposure; 6 doses required for immunity, followed by annual booster.

   c) Decontaminate exposed areas and personal items with 0.5% hypochlorite.

Table 14.1. Antibiotic Treatment of Bioterror Bacterial Agents

Disease	Drug	Dose	Relative efficacy	Comments
Anthrax, prophylaxis				
				Duration: 60 days
	Ciprofloxacin	500 mg PO q12h	First line	Also for cutaneous disease
	Levofloxacin	500 mg PO q24h		
	Doxycycline	100 mg PO q12h		Also for cutaneous disease
Anthrax, treatment				
	Ciprofloxacin, or doxycycline	400 mg IV q12h 200 mg, then 100 mg IV q12h	First line	Duration: 60 days
	In serious disease can be combined with:			
	Penicillin G, or	4×10^6 U IV q4h		Only if anthrax is confirmed penicillin-sensitive
	rifampin, or vancomycin, or imipenem, or clindamycin, or clarithromycin	600 mg PO or IV q24h 1 g IV q12h 500 mg IV q6h 600–900 mg IV q8h 500 mg PO q12h		
Plague, prophylaxis				
	Doxycycline	100 mg q12h		Duration: 7 days
Plague, treatment				
				Duration: 10–14 days
	Streptomycin, or gentamicin, or doxycycline	15 mg/kg IM q12h 5 mg/kg IV q24h 200 mg, then 100 mg IV q12h	First line	Equally effective
	Ciprofloxacin	400 mg IV q12h	Alternative	Likely to be effective, but little clinical experience
	Chloramphenicol	500 mg IV q6h		Treatment for meningitis
Tularemia, prophylaxis				
	Ciprofloxacin	500 mg PO q12h		Duration: 2 weeks
	Doxycycline	100 mg PO q12h		
Tularemia, treatment				
	Gentamicin	5 mg/kg IV q24h	First line	Duration: 10–14 days
	Streptomycin	10–15 mg/kg IM q12h	Alternative	
	Doxycycline	200 mg, then 100 mg IV q12h		

Notably, in the 2001 bioterrorist attack in the United States, only 44% of exposed individuals adhered to the recommended 60-day regimen. Failure to complete the regimen was not accompanied by any adverse outcomes. However, because spores may remain in the body for prolonged periods before germinating, prophylaxis needs to be prolonged, and patients should be closely observed after completion of antibiotics. Within the first several days, exposed skin should be washed extensively with soap and water, and personal items should be decontaminated with 0.5% hypochlorite (one part household bleach to 10 parts water).

■ PLAGUE

Like anthrax, plague is primarily a disease of animals. The causative organism, *Yersinia pestis*, primarily infects rodents. In the United States, the most common reservoirs are squirrels and prairie dogs. An outbreak associated with cats was also reported in the southwestern United States. The disease is transmitted to humans by infected rodent fleas. Approximately 10 human cases are reported annually in the southwestern United States during the late spring, summer, and early fall. Disease outbreaks frequently occur in developing countries throughout the world.

Y. pestis was used as a biologic weapon during World War II when the Japanese released plaque-infected fleas in China. However the spread of the disease proved to be unpredictable and ineffective. Subsequently both the United States and the former Soviet Union developed reliable and effective methods of aerosolizing this agent.

MICROBIOLOGY AND PATHOGENESIS

Y. pestis is a gram-negative bacillus that grows aerobically on standard nutrient plates including blood and MacConkey agar. The organism grows slowly, often requiring 48 hours to become apparent, and the colonies are small and grayish.

When an infected flea bites a human, it regurgitates thousands of organisms into the skin, where they are phagocytosed by PMNs and monocytes. *Y. pestis* is usually killed by PMNs, but is able to survive and replicate within monocytes, evading the host's immune system. Infected monocytes carry the organism to lymph nodes, where the pathogen actively replicates, causing marked acute inflammation and tissue necrosis. Regional lymph nodes become enlarged, forming buboes. *Y. pestis* can also quickly enter the bloodstream. Like other gram-negative bacteria, it produces endotoxin and also possesses other virulence factors including a coagulase and a fibrinolysin.

CLINICAL MANIFESTATIONS

Natural infection resulting from flea bites causes bubonic plaque. The incubation period is usually 2 to 8 days, ending with the abrupt onset of fever, chills, weakness, and headache. Within hours, the patient notes an enlarged extremely painful cluster of regional lymph nodes termed a "bubo." Marked swelling is noted, and pain is so severe that the patient avoids moving the infected area. Buboes are usually egg-shaped swellings 1 cm to 10 cm in length. Within 2 to 4 days, the patient dies of septic shock. Thrombosis of small vessels can develop, causing peripheral tissue necrosis and gangrene that may require amputation. In some patients, no bubo appears, and the patient presents in a moribund state caused by high-grade bacteremia. Meningitis may develop in a small percentage of patients.

If bioterrorists were to aerosolize *Y. pestis*, the primary clinical presentation would be pneumonic plague. After an incubation period of 2 to 4 days, fever, chills, and myalgias suddenly begin. Within 24 hours, patients begin coughing up blood as bacterial production of

---

KEY POINTS

About the Epidemiology and Pathogenesis of Plague

1. Usually spread by rodent fleas; cases are occasionally seen in the southwestern United States.
2. The former Soviet Union and the United States developed methods to aerosolize the bacillus.
3. Ingested by PMNs and monocytes, able to replicate in monocytes.
   a) Produces acute inflammation and tissue necrosis.
   b) Spreads to regional lymph nodes, forming fluctuant buboes.
   c) Readily enters the bloodstream.

KEY POINTS

About the Clinical Manifestations of Plague

1. In the flea-transmitted form of the disease, incubation of 2 to 8 days is followed by
   a) fever, chills, weakness, and headache; and
   b) bubo formation (very painful).
   c) Within 2 to 4 days, septic shock leads to peripheral gangrene and death.
2. Pneumonic form more likely in a bioterrorist attack.
   a) Incubation period is 2 to 4 days, leading to chills, fever, myalgias.
   b) Within 24 hours, bloody sputum production and chest pain begin, followed by dyspnea and cyanosis.
   c) Death follows within 18 hours if antibiotic treatment is not started.

coagulase and fibrinolysin leads to tissue necrosis. Sputum can also be mucopurulent or watery. Chest pain, abdominal pain, nausea, vomiting, and diarrhea are other common symptoms. If antibiotics are not begun within 18 hours, the outcome is fatal. Patients experience increasing dyspnea, stridor, and cyanosis, followed by respiratory arrest and circulatory collapse.

DIAGNOSIS

The possibility of a biologic attack with *Y. pestis* should be considered if large numbers of patients begin presenting to the emergency room with hemoptysis and severe, rapidly progressive pneumonia. Sputum Gram stain frequently reveals gram-negative rods. A presumptive diagnosis can also be made by finding bacilli on peripheral blood smear. Chest x-ray demonstrates bilateral bronchopneumonia. Definitive diagnosis is made by sputum and blood cultures that often take more than 48 hours because of the organism's slow growth rate. A rapid ELISA antigen test (takes 15 minutes) has been developed that is highly sensitive and specific. Detection by PCR is under development and, in fleas, is specific and highly sensitive (can detect as few as 11 organisms).

TREATMENT

If pneumonic plague is not considered and if conventional antibiotic treatment for community-acquired pneumonia is mistakenly begun, the infection will quickly progress, resulting in death. Streptomycin, gentamicin, and doxycycline (see Table 14.1 for doses) are the treatments of choice and should be continued for 10 to 14 days. Ciprofloxacin is another potentially effective regimen, but clinical experience with that agent is limited. Chloramphenicol is recommended for the treatment of meningitis.

Surgical debridement of buboes should not be performed, because of the risk of spreading the infection to others. Needle aspiration of lymph nodes may provide some relief and also provide material for culture and Gram stain. The lymph nodes usually slowly shrink on antibiotic therapy. The overall mortality for pneumonic plague is 60%; however, if appropriate therapy is delayed for more than 24 hours, then mortality is nearly 100%. The fatality rate for bubonic plague is 14%, but with early therapy, all patients should survive.

PROPHYLAXIS

Person-to-person spread of *Y. pestis* does occur. Patients with pneumonic plague can cough and aerosolize the organism, leading to secondary cases of

---

KEY POINTS

About the Diagnosis, Treatment, and Prevention of Plague

1. The disease is readily diagnosed by Gram stain of sputum or lymph node aspirate; cultures usually require 48 hours. A sensitive PCR method is under development.

2. Treat with streptomycin, gentamicin, or doxycycline for 14 days; delaying beyond 24 hours can lead to death.

   a) Ciprofloxacin may be effective.

   b) Use chloramphenicol for meningitis.

3. Prophylaxis:

   a) Take respiratory (droplet) precautions for pneumonic plague for 48 hours after the start of antibiotic treatment.

   b) Give doxycycline for 7 days after respiratory exposure.

   c) Vaccine is under development.

---

pneumonia. Patients with pulmonary disease therefore require strict isolation with droplet precautions for at least 48 hours after the start of antibiotic therapy. People who have had face-to-face contact with patients with plague pneumonia should receive oral doxycycline prophylaxis (100 mg twice daily) for 7 days or for the duration of potential exposure plus 7 days. In patients with bubonic plague, only standard precautions are required, and prophylaxis is unnecessary. Contacts should be observed for 7 days.

A vaccine is not currently available. Production of a licensed killed vaccine was discontinued in 1998. The vaccine was effective for prevention of the bubonic, but not the inhalation disease. A new recombinant protein vaccine that has been shown to be effective for inhalation disease in animals, has been developed and could be approved by the U.S. Food and Drug Administration in the near future.

■ TULAREMIA

Francisella tularensis is another zoonotic pathogen that, under natural conditions, incidentally infects humans. Infection is usually contracted following contact with rabbits, muskrats, beaver, squirrels, and birds. A case was also reported following a pet hamster bite. Hunters develop the disease after skinning, dressing, and eating infected animals. Less commonly, the infection can be spread to humans by ticks, biting flies, and mosquitoes. Aerosol droplets of contaminated water or mud can be produced by lawn-mowing and other gardening activities.

Tularemia is most commonly encountered in temperate climates during the summer months (insect transmission) and during hunting season. The United States (and possibly other countries) has weaponized this agent. Dry and wet forms have both been created. Like *B. anthracis* and *Y. pestis*, *F. tularensis* is most efficiently delivered in lethal doses by aerosol.

MICROBIOLOGY AND PATHOGENESIS

Francisella is a small aerobic gram-negative coccobacilli that does not routinely grow on standard media; it requires either cysteine or cystine for growth. Glucose–cystine blood agar supports growth; however, a selective medium is often required to isolate this pathogen from normal skin and mouth flora. The cell wall of this bacterium has a capsule with high fatty acid content that resists serum bactericidal activity. *Francisella* produces no known exotoxins, but it expresses a lipopolysaccharide (LPS) endotoxin that is one one-thousandth as potent as LPS from *E. coli*.

Like most natural infections, tularemia begins when *F. tularensis* bacteria gain entry to the body through a small break in the skin. The organism is phagocytosed by monocytes, where it is able to survive intracellularly. *F. tularensis* can also grow in hepatocytes and endothelial cells.

As the organisms grow and lyse cells, they induce an acute inflammatory reaction, and tissue necrosis is followed by granuloma formation. Cell-mediated immunity plays a critical role in controlling this intracellular pathogen. Only 10 to 50 bacteria are required to cause skin and pulmonary infection, making this organism extremely dangerous to laboratory workers.

CLINICAL MANIFESTATIONS

The clinical picture of tularemia is very similar to that of plague. The incubation period is usually 3 to 5 days, ending with the abrupt onset of high fever, chills, malaise, myalgias, chest discomfort, vomiting, abdominal pain, and diarrhea. A severe generalized headache is often a prominent complaint.

Natural disease most commonly takes the ulceroglandular form. At the site of bacterial entry, a painful ulcer with raised borders develops, associated with painful regional adenopathy. Approximately 20% of patients may develop a febrile illness without lymphadenopathy and may become hypotensive. Watery diarrhea may be a prominent complaint, with the disease being mistaken for *Salmonella* typhoid fever.

The pneumonic form is rare under natural circumstances, but can occur in sheep shearers, farmers, and laboratory workers. The pneumonic form would be the expected presentation after an aerosol bioterrorist attack. The clinical presentation is identical to that of pneumonic plague, with the exception that the cough is usually dry and hacking rather than productive. Hemoptysis can occur, but is rare. In some patients, respiratory

---

KEY POINTS

About the Mode of Spread and Pathogenesis of Tularemia

1. *F. tularensis* is a gram-negative coccobacilli usually spread cutaneously from infected rabbits, muskrats, beaver, squirrels, and birds.
2. An aerosolized form can be manufactured.
3. Growth in culture requires a cystine-supplemented medium.
4. Cell wall has a high fatty-acid content; produces a lipopolysaccharide endotoxin that is considerably less potent than that produced by *Escherichia coli*.
5. As an intracellular pathogen, induces acute inflammation and granuloma formation.
6. A low inoculum (10 to 50 organisms) can cause disease (very dangerous).

KEY POINTS

About the Clinical Manifestations of Tularemia

1. Clinically similar to plague; incubation period of 3 to 5 days.
   a) Abrupt onset of fever, headache, malaise, myalgias, abdominal pain, and diarrhea.
   b) Ulceroglandular form presents as a painful ulcer with raised borders and associated regional lymphadenopathy.
   c) About 20% of patients present with typhoid fever–like illness without lymphadenopathy.
2. Bronchopneumonia would be expected in a bioterrorist attack: similar to plague except that cough is dry, hacking; hemoptysis is rare.

complaints may not be prominent, and primary complaints may mimic typhoid fever.

DIAGNOSIS

Presentation of a large number of patients with severe bronchopneumonia associated with a nonproductive cough should raise the possibility of a bioterror attack involving *F. tularensis*. Chest x-ray demonstrates changes consistent with a bronchopneumonia in 50% of cases after inhalation. Pleural effusions may be noted in 15% of those with pneumonia. Aspiration of the pleural fluid usually reveals lymphocytes, suggesting tuberculosis. Gram stain of sputum and wounds are usually negative. The organism can be identified in lymph nodes by silver stain. Blood cultures and tissue sample cultures may be positive, but the organism must be grown using medium containing a sulfhydryl compound. The organism should be handled in a biosafety level 3 containment facility because of the risk to laboratory personnel.

The diagnosis is usually made by testing for antibodies to the organism. Two weeks are required before significant antibody titers (above 1:160) develop.

TREATMENT

Effective treatment regimens include streptomycin and gentamicin (see Table 14.1). In a presumed bioterror attack, gentamicin would be preferred over streptomycin, because a streptomycin-resistant strain was developed in the 1950s and may have been obtained by other countries. (That strain was sensitive to gentamicin.) Doxycycline is another alternative for treatment.

The mortality from tularemia pneumonia is 30%, making weaponized *Francisella* a less deadly agent than either anthrax or plague.

PREVENTION

Person-to-person transmission is not reported with tularemia. Standard precautions are therefore sufficient. Prophylaxis should be administered within 24 hours of exposure. Ciprofloxacin or doxycycline for 2 weeks is recommended (see Table 14.1). An investigational live-attenuated vaccine given by scarification is available. The vaccine provides significant protection against the inhalation and typhoidal forms of the disease.

■ SMALLPOX

Endemic smallpox was eradicated in 1977. As a result, smallpox vaccinations were discontinued for civilians in 1980 and for military recruits in 1989, leaving a high percentage of the world's population without immunity to this deadly virus. Although only two repositories of the *Variola* virus are known (the CDC in Atlanta and the Research Institute of Viral Preparations in Moscow), stockpiles of the virus may be in the hands of others.

EPIDEMIOLOGY

Smallpox is spread person-to-person and has no other animal reservoirs. The incubation period before symptomatic illness is 7 to 17 days (average: 12 days). The period of communicability begins with the onset of rash and continues until all scabs separate from the skin, 3 to 4 weeks after the onset of illness. The virus is shed from lesions in the oropharynx and on the skin, producing airborne droplets and skin fragments that can be inhaled. Patients are most infectious if they are coughing or have the hemorrhagic form of disease. The communicability of smallpox is low as compared with chickenpox and measles; secondary cases occur most commonly in household contacts and hospital personnel. The virions are relatively resistant to drying and to many disinfectants; they can remain infectious for months at room temperature. Autoclaving, chlorine preparations, iodophores, and ammonia inactivate them.

KEY POINTS

About the Diagnosis, Treatment, and Prevention of Tularemia

1. Gram stain of sputum and skin ulcers is usually negative; culture requires a special medium.
2. May be identified in lymph nodes by silver stain.
3. Diagnosis is usually presumptive; antibody titers rise after 2 weeks.
4. Treatment:
   a) Gentamicin is the drug of choice; doxycycline and streptomycin are alternatives.
   b) Respiratory precautions are not required.
5. Prophylaxis:
   a) Treat within 24 hours of exposure with ciprofloxacin or doxycycline for 14 days.
   b) A vaccine is under development.
6. Mortality rate is 30% (lower than for pulmonary anthrax or plague).

KEY POINTS

About the Epidemiology of Smallpox

1. Humans are the only reservoir for the disease.
2. Incubation period is 7 to 17 days.
3. Patients are infectious from the onset of rash until scabs separate from the skin.

   a) Person-to-person transmission occurs by inhalation of droplets or skin particles shed by a patient.

   b) Spread within households and to hospital personnel.

   c) Virions can survive in the environment, but are inactivated by chlorine, ammonia, iodine, and heat.

A number of factors make *Variola* a potentially dangerous biologic weapon:

- Infection can be aerosol-spread, and the virions can survive in the environment.
- Person-to-person transmission facilitates continued spread after an initial attack.
- Routine vaccination was discontinued, creating large susceptible civilian and military populations.
- The potency of stored vaccine may be declining.
- The disease causes severe morbidity and mortality.
- Health care personnel have no clinical experience with the disease, and delays in diagnosis, treatment, and prevention would therefore be expected.

VIROLOGY AND PATHOGENESIS

Variola is a large, double-stranded DNA virus. It replicates in the cytoplasm of host cells that release new viral particles by bud formation on the cell surface. Virus-containing airborne droplets and dust particles are inhaled. The virus then spreads from the upper respiratory tract to the regional lymph nodes, where it enters the bloodstream, causing transient viremia before it invades virtually all body tissues. Epithelial cells are particularly susceptible, accounting for the prominent skin lesions.

Initially, edema develops at infected sites in the skin, accompanied by perivascular infiltration with mononuclear and plasma cells, causing the formation of macular skin lesions. Subsequently, the epithelial cells undergo ballooning degeneration, and spherical inclusion bodies containing clusters of virions (Guarnieri bodies) form in the cell cytoplasm. These changes are accompanied by the formation of papular skin lesions. Cell necrosis follows, accompanied by the formation of skin vesicles. Viral replication then ceases, and the skin lesions become crusted and dry, eventually healing and forming prominent scars.

CLINICAL MANIFESTATIONS

The first clinical manifestations of the disease are nonspecific and consist of the acute onset of fever, rigors, malaise, headache, backache, and vomiting. Delirium develops in approximately 15% of cases, and a transient erythematous rash may appear. This clinical prodrome lasts 2 to 4 days and is caused by high-level viremia. During this period, virus can be readily cultured from the blood.

Next, the exanthem becomes apparent. Lesions begin on the face, hands, and forearms, subsequently spreading to the lower extremities and, over the following week, to the trunk [see Figure 14.3(A)]. The distribution of skin lesions is centrifugal—that is, lesions are first seen on the distal extremities and face and then progress to the trunk). Initially, macules are seen that subsequently form papules, and then progress to pustular vesicles [see Figure 14.3(B)]. After about 2 weeks, the lesions form dry scabs that fall off, leaving scars. The skin lesions progress in a synchronous fashion—that is, at any one time, all skin lesions are at a similar stage.

The clinician must be able to differentiate smallpox from chickenpox (varicella virus), a common, naturally

KEY POINTS

About the Pathogenesis of Smallpox

1. *Variola* is a double-stranded DNA virus.
2. Replicates in the cytoplasm of host cells. Infectious particles bud from the cell surface.
3. The virus enters the lung in airborne droplets, spreads to regional lymph nodes, and then to the bloodstream.

   a) Disseminates to all tissues.

   b) Epithelial cells are particularly susceptible; skin develops perivascular infiltration.

   c) Ballooning degeneration and inclusion body formation is followed by cell necrosis.

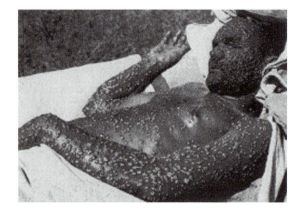

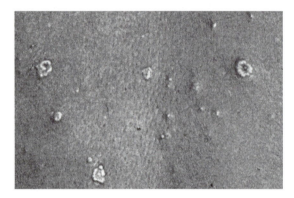

Figure 14–3. Smallpox. **A.** Adult with severe smallpox skin lesions. (Picture from www.coldcure.com;). **B.** View of individual raised skin lesions, all at a similar stage of progression. (Picture from Henderson DA. Smallpox: clinical and epidemiologic features. *Emerg Infect Dis.* 1999;5:537–539) *See color image on color plate 3*

occurring infection. Three clinical characteristics are most helpful in differentiating the two diseases:

- First, chickenpox is usually not associated with a significant prodrome. Patients often feel well before the onset of skin lesions.
- Second, the lesions of chickenpox and of smallpox begin in different locations. In chickenpox, lesions are first seen on the trunk, and they often spare the face. Subsequently, lesions spread to the arms and legs. That is, the distribution of chickenpox lesions is centripetal—that is, first seen on the central trunk and later on the distal extremities and face—rather than centrifugal (like smallpox).
- Third, the morphology of the skin lesions differs. Skin lesion development is asynchronous in chicken-

pox: macules, papules, vesicles, and scabs can all be seen at the same time on an individual patient. Chickenpox lesions are also irregular in shape and size, and are usually superficial. Smallpox lesions have smooth borders, are of similar size, and often extend to the dermis. The vesicles of smallpox feel shot-like; chickenpox vesicles are soft and collapse easily.

A series of criteria for the presumptive diagnosis of smallpox are available on the CDC Web site: visit http://www.bt.cdc.gov/agent/smallpox/diagnosis/eval-poster.asp.

DIAGNOSIS

Full-blown disease can be readily diagnosed clinically. The diagnosis can be confirmed by viral culture on chorioallantoic membrane. Diagnostic techniques using PCR are under development and will allow for more rapid diagnosis.

A particular problem from an epidemiologic standpoint is the potential for failure to recognize relatively mild cases of smallpox in people with partial immunity. These patients may shed virus from the oropharynx in the absence of skin lesions.

TREATMENT AND PROGNOSIS

Currently, no treatment for smallpox other than supportive care is available. Cidofovir is active against poxviruses and may be considered for treatment. In animal studies, the tyrosine kinase inhibitor imatinib has been shown to reduce the spread of the closely related *Vaccinia* virus. Imatinib blocks the Abl family of tyro-

---

KEY POINTS

About the Clinical Manifestations of Smallpox

1. Febrile prodrome over 2 to 4 days is associated with high-level viremia. (No prodrome with chickenpox.)
2. Skin lesions are centrifugal (begin on the extremities later moving to the trunk) with smallpox versus centripetal (begin on the trunk and later involve the extremities) with chickenpox.
3. Synchronous development with smallpox versus asynchronous development with chickenpox.
4. Lesions progress in unison from macular to papular to vesicular to crusting, feel shot-like, and leave scars; chickenpox lesions are softer and usually do not scar.

sine kinases, whose activity is required for extracellular release of the virus. Two additional antiviral drugs are under development. One interferes with a specific host signal transduction pathway required for viral spread, and the other blocks synthesis of a vital poxvirus protein. The overall mortality for smallpox is 30% in unvaccinated and 3% in vaccinated patients. Mortality is highest in very young and very old patients.

PREVENTION

The identification of a smallpox case represents a public health emergency, and public health officials should be notified immediately. Vaccination of all exposed individuals as quickly as possible is recommended, and vaccination within 7 days is protective.

The vaccine contains *Vaccinia* virus (cowpox virus) and is administered by intradermal inoculation using a bifurcated needle. Successful vaccination should result in vesicle formation at the site of inoculation, followed by scarification. Immunity has recently been shown to be lifelong. Side effects include low-grade fever and axillary adenopathy. Disseminated *Vaccinia* occurs in approximately 3 in 10,000 vaccinations. The vaccine is contraindicated in people with HIV infection, immunosuppression, or a history or presence

of eczema, or in people who are in close contact with individuals having one of the foregoing conditions. Other complications reported during the recent vaccination of 38,000 first responders included myocarditis or pericarditis, cardiac ischemic events and postvaccinal encephalitis. *Vaccinia* immune globulin (VIG) may be protective, but the large volume required for intramuscular administration (0.6 mL/kg—for example, 42 mL in a 70-kg person) make it an impractical tool for mass prophylaxis.

Infected patients must be strictly isolated. Placement in a negative air-pressure room, with the door closed, is recommended. Masks, gowns, and gloves must be worn when entering the room. Transport of the patient should be limited. All surfaces and supplies must be treated as contaminated. Large numbers of patients would quickly overwhelm isolation facilities and would necessitate separate temporary isolation facilities.

FURTHER READING

General

United States, U.S. Army Medical Research Institute of Infectious Diseases (USAMRIID). Medical management of biological casualties: handbook. Frederick, Md.: USAMRIID; Feb 2001.

Anthrax

Centers for Disease Control and Prevention. Inhalation anthrax associated with dried animal hides—Pennsylvania and New York City, 2006. *MMWR Morb Mortal Wkly Rep.* 2006;55:280–282.

Guarner J, Jernigan JA, Shieh WJ, et al. Pathology and pathogenesis of bioterrorism-related inhalational anthrax. *Am J Pathol.* 2003;163:701–709.

Holty JE, Bravata DM, Liu H, Olshen RA, McDonald KM, Owens DK. Systematic review: a century of inhalational anthrax cases from 1900 to 2005. *Ann Intern Med.* 2006;144:270–280.

Jernigan DB, Raghunathan PL, Bell BP, et al. Investigation of bioterrorism-related anthrax, United States, 2001: epidemiologic findings. *Emerg Infect Dis.* 2002;8:1019–1028.

Jernigan JA, Stephens DS, Ashford DA, et al. Bioterrorism-related inhalational anthrax: the first 10 cases reported in the United States. *Emerg Infect Dis.* 2001;7:933–944.

Kyriacou DN, Stein AC, Yarnold PR, et al. Clinical predictors of bioterrorism-related inhalational anthrax. *Lancet.* 2004; 364: 449–452.

Lanska DJ. Anthrax meningoencephalitis. *Neurology.* 2002;59: 327–334.

Sejvar JJ, Tenover FC, Stephens DS. Management of anthrax meningitis. *Lancet Infect Dis.* 2005;5:287–295.

Shepard CW, Soriano-Gabarro M, Zell ER, et al. Antimicrobial postexposure prophylaxis for anthrax: adverse events and adherence. *Emerg Infect Dis.* 2002;8:1124–1132.

Vietri NJ, Purcell BK, Lawler JV, et al. Short-course postexposure antibiotic prophylaxis combined with vaccination protects against experimental inhalational anthrax. *Proc Natl Acad Sci U S A.* 2006;103:7813–7816.

KEY POINTS

About the Diagnosis, Treatment, and Prevention of Smallpox

1. Disease can be readily diagnosed clinically and can be confirmed by viral culture.

2. Minimally symptomatic patients may spread disease; they need to be recognized and isolated.

3. Infected patients should be strictly isolated: use negative-pressure rooms and masks, gloves, and gowns.

4. Cidofovir may prove helpful; imatinib slows spread in animal studies.

5. Vaccine is protective if given within 7 days of exposure.

   a) Live *Vaccinia* virus is given by intradermal inoculation.

   b) Contraindicated in HIV infection, immunosuppression, history or presence of eczema.

   c) *Vaccinia* immune globulin is protective, but impractical for large numbers of patients.

Plague

Chanteau S, Rahalison L, Ralafiarisoa L, et al. Development and testing of a rapid diagnostic test for bubonic and pneumonic plague. *Lancet.* 2003;361:211–216.

Drancourt M, Roux V, Dang LV, et al. Genotyping, Orientalis-like *Yersinia pestis*, and plague pandemics. *Emerg Infect Dis.* 2004;10:1585–1592.

Gage KL, Dennis DT, Orloski KA, et al. Cases of cat-associated human plague in the Western US, 1977–1998. *Clin Infect Dis.* 2000;30:893–900.

Morris SR. Development of a recombinant vaccine against aerosolized plague. *Vaccine.* 2007;25:3115–3117.

Tularemia

Centers for Disease Control and Prevention. Tularemia associated with a hamster bite—Colorado, 2004. *MMWR Morb Mortal Wkly Rep.* 2005;53:1202–1203.

Centers for Disease Control and Prevention. Tularemia transmitted by insect bites—Wyoming, 2001–2003. *MMWR Morb Mortal Wkly Rep.* 2005;54:170–173.

Dennis DT, Inglesby TV, Henderson DA, et al. Tularemia as a biological weapon: medical and public health management. *JAMA.* 2001;285:2763–2773.

Feldman KA, Enscore RE, Lathrop SL, et al. An outbreak of primary pneumonic tularemia on Martha's Vineyard. *N Engl J Med.* 2001;345:1601–1606.

Smallpox

Casey CG, Iskander JK, Roper MH, et al. Adverse events associated with smallpox vaccination in the United States, January–October 2003. *JAMA.* 2005;294:2734–2743.

Hammarlund E, Lewis MW, Hansen SG, et al. Duration of antiviral immunity after smallpox vaccination. *Nat Med.* 2003;9: 1131–1137.

Moore ZS, Seward JF, Lane JM. Smallpox. *Lancet.* 2006;367: 425–435.

Reeves PM, Bommarius B, Lebeis S, et al. Disabling poxvirus pathogenesis by inhibition of Abl-family tyrosine kinases. *Nat Med.* 2005;11:731–739.

Smee DF, Bailey KW, Wong MH, Wandersee MK, Sidwell RW. Topical cidofovir is more effective than is parenteral therapy for treatment of progressive vaccinia in immunocompromised mice. *J Infect Dis.* 2004;190:1132–1139.

Talbot TR, Stapleton JT, Brady RC, et al. Vaccination success rate and reaction profile with diluted and undiluted smallpox vaccine: a randomized controlled trial. *JAMA.* 2004;292: 1205–1212.

Yang H, Kim SK, Kim M, et al. Antiviral chemotherapy facilitates control of poxvirus infections through inhibition of cellular signal transduction. *J Clin Invest.* 2005;115:379–387.

Yang G, Pevear DC, Davies MH, et al. An orally bioavailable antipoxvirus compound (ST-246) inhibits extracellular virus formation and protects mice from lethal orthopoxvirus Challenge. *J Virol.* 2005;79:13139–13149.

Serious Viral Illnesses in the Adult Patient

15

Time Recommended to Complete: 1 day

Sankar Swaminathan M.D.

GUIDING QUESTIONS

1. Who is likely to become ill with one of these serious adult viral illnesses?

2. What are the presenting features and laboratory tests that are useful in making a diagnosis?

3. What are the major complications of each of these diseases?

4. What are the treatments available for each viral illness?

5. Which patients should be treated?

6. What are the preventive measures that are available?

7. How does the avian influenza virus differ from other influenza viruses, and why should we worry?

■ VARICELLA IN THE ADULT

Varicella virus [also called varicella-zoster virus (VZV)] is a double-stranded DNA herpesvirus that causes two diseases: varicella (chickenpox) and zoster (shingles). Chickenpox is a manifestation of primary infection; zoster is caused by reactivation of latent infection.

EPIDEMIOLOGY

Approximately 3 to 4 million cases of chickenpox and 500,000 cases of zoster occurred each year in the United States before the introduction of the VZV vaccine in 1995. Since then, dramatic reductions in chickenpox incidence have been reported.

Chickenpox is primarily a disease of childhood. Nevertheless, 10% of the adult population is estimated to be at risk for infection, and 10% of cases occur in patients over the age of 13 years. For unclear reasons, chickenpox occurs more frequently in adults who reside in tropical regions. The virus circulates exclusively in humans, and no other reservoirs of infection are known. The disease becomes epidemic in the susceptible population in winter and early spring, affecting both sexes and all races equally. Transmission occurs via the respiratory route and requires close contact even though the virus is highly infectious, with attack rates of 70% to 90% in susceptible family members.

In contrast, zoster affects primarily elderly people. Zoster is caused by reactivation of latent VZV in people who previously had chickenpox. Zoster occurs in up to 1% of people over 60 years of age, and 75% of cases occur in those over the age of 45 years. The development of zoster is not associated with exposure to other people with chickenpox or zoster, although patients with zoster may themselves be capable of transmitting the virus to susceptible individuals. Zoster occasionally occurs in younger individuals, particularly those who are immunosuppressed.

PATHOPHYSIOLOGY AND CLINICAL MANIFESTATIONS

Chickenpox is popularly felt to be a benign childhood rite of passage. Nevertheless, from 1990 to 1994, approximately 100 deaths each year in the United States were attributed to chickenpox and its complications. Deaths continue to occur in healthy adults and children despite the availability of a vaccine. The overall risk of death is about 15 times higher in adults than in children, being estimated at more than 3 per 10,000 cases. Most deaths in adults are a result of the development of visceral complications as discussed later in this subsection.

The disease begins with infection by the respiratory route. The virus then replicates at local sites (which have not been clearly identified) and infects the reticuloendothelial system. Viremia ensues, followed by diffuse seeding of the skin, internal organs, and nervous system. Replication of the virus occurs in the corium and dermis, leading to degenerative changes and the formation of multinucleated giant cells, producing the characteristic diffuse vesicular rash. A mild prodrome of fever and malaise of 3 to 5 days usually precedes the rash.

The rash initially appears on the face and trunk and spreads outward. It may also be present on the oral mucosa. It begins as small erythematous papules less than a centimeter in diameter that rapidly evolve into vesicles. As viral replication proceeds and infiltration by polymorphonuclear leukocytes occurs, the lesions appear purulent. A hallmark of chickenpox is that lesions at all stages of development—maculopapules, vesicles, and scabs—are all found together. As they evolve, the lesions appear umbilicated in the center. Successive crops of lesions occur over several days, with complete healing by 10 to 14 days in uncomplicated cases. The virus establishes lifelong latent infection in the dorsal root ganglia.

Reactivation of VZV can result in zoster, also known as herpes zoster and shingles. Zoster presents as a localized eruption along the course of one or more dermatomes, most commonly the thoracic or lumbar. The rash, which is often preceded by localized pain, begins as erythematous papules that evolve into vesicles. The vesicles may coalesce into large, confluent blisters with a hemorrhagic component. Healing occurs over the course of 2 weeks, although permanent skin changes such as discoloration and scarring may occur.

When zoster affects the first branch of the trigeminal nerve, herpes zoster ophthalmicus may occur, with involvement of the cornea and potentially sight-threatening complications. Involvement of other branches of the trigeminal or facial nerves may result in unusual presentations with intra-oral vesicles. The constellation of lesions in the external auditory canal, loss of taste, and facial palsy is termed Ramsay Hunt syndrome.

KEY POINTS

About the Epidemiology, Pathogenesis, and Clinical Manifestation of Chickenpox

1. Chickenpox infected 3 to 4 million people annually (10% adults) in the United States before vaccine availability; zoster, 500,000 annually.

2. Highly infectious, spreads person-to-person by air droplets; zoster represents reactivation.

3. Double-stranded DNA virus; enters via the respiratory tract, and then disseminates.

4. Chickenpox primarily infects the skin:
   a) Preceded by a mild prodrome.
   b) Lesions have a centripetal distribution beginning on the trunk and later spreading to the extremities.
   c) Lesions at all stages (maculopapules, vesicles, scabs) are present at the same time.
   d) Lesions are pruritic.

5. Zoster is the result of viral reactivation from the nerve ganglion.
   a) Involves a single dermatome.
   b) Pain precedes the rash.
   c) Zoster ophthalmicus involves the cornea; can be sight-threatening.
   d) Combination of facial palsy, loss of taste, and lesions in external auditory canal is called Ramsay Hunt syndrome.

DIAGNOSIS

The diagnosis of chickenpox can usually be made on clinical grounds, based on the characteristics described earlier. Since the eradication of all known natural human reservoirs of smallpox and the discontinuation of universal vaccination, the clinical diagnosis of chickenpox has been relatively straightforward. Nevertheless, the possibility of smallpox as a biologic weapon and resumption of vaccination of larger segments of the population may necessitate considering smallpox or disseminated *Vaccinia* in the differential diagnosis of a diffuse vesicular rash in an adult.

A diffuse vesicular eruption, Kaposi's varicelliform eruption, occasionally occurs in patients with eczema. This syndrome may be caused either by vaccination with *Vaccinia* virus or by herpes simplex virus. The diagnosis can be made on the basis of the history and identification of the virus in vesicle fluid. Occasionally, enteroviral infection may cause diffuse cutaneous vesicular lesions that mimic early chickenpox. These lesions are often found on the palms, soles, and oral mucosa and do not progress like those of chickenpox.

The diagnosis of zoster may sometimes be more difficult, with the primary alternative diagnosis being herpes simplex virus. Culture of the virus from unroofed vesicles remains the most reliable method of differentiating viral agents in this situation, although polymerase chain reaction (PCR)–based tests are also highly specific and sensitive. Antibody-based assays performed on lesion scrapings or vesicle fluid may also be useful if available.

COMPLICATIONS

CASE 15.1

A 36–year-old mother of two presented to the emergency room with complaints of shortness of breath. She had noted the onset of the skin lesions and low-grade fever 2 days before admission. Her son was recovering from a recent bout of chickenpox. Aside from the rash, she had been feeling well until the day of admission, when she began experiencing a dry cough and increasing shortness of breath.

On exam, this woman had a temperature of 38.5°C and a respiratory rate of 30 breaths per minute. She appeared in moderate respiratory distress. Her extensive skin rash primarily involved the trunk and face. Lesions varied in character, some being vesiculopustular, and others, nodular. A few crusted lesions were also noted. Pulmonary exam revealed a few rales. A chest X-ray revealed bilateral lower lobe infiltrates with a fine reticulonodular pattern. Arterial blood gas registered a pH of 7.45, a $Paco_2$ of 35 mm Hg, and a Pao_2 of 70 mm Hg on room air.

Intravenous acyclovir was begun. New crops of skin lesions were noted over the first 24 hours; however, the patient then defervesced, and her respiratory status slowly improved. She did not require intubation, and she was discharged on oral acyclovir.

The major complications of varicella result from involvement of the pulmonary and nervous systems. Varicella pneumonitis is more common in adults and immunocompromised patients than in children. It has been estimated that as many as 1 in 400 adults with chickenpox have some pulmonary involvement, although most cases appear to be subclinical. When clinical varicella pneumonitis occurs in adults, it is often associated with high morbidity and mortality. Fortunately case 15.1 responded quickly to acyclovir and did not suffer severe respiratory compromise. The disease can be particularly severe in pregnant women during the later stages of pregnancy, possibly because of both the respiratory impairment resulting from a gravid uterus and the immunologic changes associated with pregnancy. Smoking and the presence of a large number of skin lesions have been identified as risk factors for the development of varicella pneumonia. Tachypnea, dyspnea, and fever with nodular or interstitial markings on chest X-ray are typically observed. Development of encephalitis in association with chickenpox in adults is relatively uncommon, occurring in up to 0.1% to 0.2% of patients, with mortality being as high as 20%. Seizures are common and are accompanied by headache, fever, and progressive obtundation.

The major complications of zoster are also neurologic. Involvement of the central nervous system (CNS) can almost always be demonstrated in relatively asymptomatic patients with zoster when the cerebrospinal fluid (CSF) is examined. The most common

---

KEY POINTS

About the Complications Associated with Varicella Infection

1. Pneumonia in adults can be fatal.
   a) Severity is increased in pregnant women and smokers.
   b) Severity often correlates with extent of the skin lesions.
2. Encephalitis is a rare complication associated with seizures, headache, obtundation, and 20% mortality.
3. Zoster is associated with multiple complications:
   a) Postherpetic neuralgia occurs in up to 50% of cases. More common in patients more than 50 years of age.
   b) Guillain–Barré syndrome, transverse myelitis, and encephalitis are occasionally seen.
   c) Ophthalmic-branch keratitis, iridocyclitis, blindness, and granulomatous cerebral angiitis are also possible.
4. Dissemination in immunosuppressed patients is often fatal.

complication is postherpetic neuralgia, especially in people over 50 years of age. As many as half of these patients will have persistent severe pain in the area where the lesions appeared. Encephalitis, transverse myelitis, and Guillain–Barré syndrome can also occur in association with an episode of zoster. A specific complication, particularly of ophthalmic zoster, is the subsequent development of granulomatous cerebral angiitis, which may result in stroke. Ophthalmic zoster may also result in keratitis, iridocyclitis, and (in severe cases) loss of vision.

Chickenpox and zoster are often more severe in the immunosuppressed patient. Bone marrow transplant recipients and children with hematologic malignancies are especially prone to visceral dissemination, with associated high mortality, and they require early and aggressive antiviral therapy.

TREATMENT

The mainstay of treatment for VZV is acyclovir and related nucleoside analogs that inhibit the viral DNA polymerase. Oral acyclovir therapy is recommended for adults and adolescents with chickenpox. Treatment reduces the total number of lesions and shortens the duration of lesion formation by about 1 day. Whether treatment reduces the likelihood of the serious complications described earlier in adults is unknown. The recommended adult dosage is 800 mg five times daily.

The minimum inhibitory concentration of acyclovir for VZV is 2 to 6 mmol/L, which is difficult to achieve by oral administration. Intravenous treatment is indicated in cases of varicella pneumonia and should be considered in other cases of visceral or CNS involvement. The usual dosage is 5 to 10 mg/kg every 8 hours. Prompt infectious disease consultation should be obtained in all cases of complicated varicella or varicella in the immunocompromised patient.

Antiviral treatment of zoster reduces acute neuritis and accelerates healing. Treatment in the immunosuppressed patient prevents dissemination. Ophthalmic zoster is usually treated with oral acyclovir or with the more bioavailable agents valacyclovir and famciclovir. Treatment of cutaneous zoster may also reduce the incidence or duration of postherpetic neuralgia, but the data supporting these effects has been questioned. Nevertheless, oral famciclovir and valacyclovir are approved for this indication and are more convenient than acyclovir because they are administered less frequently. Concurrent administration of corticosteroids to treat postherpetic neuralgia is also controversial, but some studies claim improvement in quality of life when steroids are added to antiviral therapy.

PREVENTION

A live attenuated varicella vaccine has been available since 1995. It is close to 100% effective in preventing serious disease, and it has a low incidence of side effects. Immunity has been persistent over the period since initial licensure. Varicella vaccination is recommended for all susceptible individuals over the age of 12 months. Although rates of zoster are lower in vaccinees, the vaccine strain may actually reactivate more frequently, but subclinically. Further, a decrease in circulating wild-type virus may result in less frequent natural boosting of immunity and therefore lead to an increased incidence of zoster in previously infected individuals. Vaccination also becomes more important as its acceptance rate increases, because the likelihood of infection during childhood decreases, increasing the risk of adult disease. The most recent recommendations are that all children

---

KEY POINTS

About the Treatment and Prevention of Varicella and Zoster Infections

1. Acyclovir is recommended for adolescents and adults with chickenpox. Those with serious infection should receive high-dose intravenous therapy.
2. Antiviral treatment (acyclovir, famciclovir, or valacyclovir) is recommended for all cases of zoster.
   a) Reduces acute neuritis and accelerates healing.
   b) Prevents dissemination in the immunocompromised host.
   c) May reduce postherpetic neuralgia.
   d) Efficacy of concurrent treatment with corticosteroids to reduce postherpetic neuralgia is controversial.
3. Live attenuated vaccine is highly efficacious for chickenpox.
   a) Recommended for all susceptible individuals over the age of 12 months.
   b) Impact on zoster has not been clarified.
4. Zoster vaccine was released in 2006.
   a) It reduces the attack rate by 50%, and
   b) it reduces postherpetic neuralgia.
5. Varicella-zoster immune globulin is effective at preventing active disease.
   a) Give within 96 hours of exposure.
   b) Recommended for all exposed pregnant women and immunocompromised patients.

receive two doses of varicella vaccine before the age of 4 to 6 years, with the first dose at 12 to 15 months of age. Adults without evidence of prior infection should also be vaccinated, and children and adults who have received only 1 dose in the past should receive a second catch-up dose. The vaccine should not be administered to pregnant women.

In 2006, a zoster vaccine was approved for use in patients over 60 years of age who have not previously had zoster. The vaccine achieved an approximately 50% reduction in the incidence of zoster and a 67% reduction in postherpetic neuralgia, suggesting that the vaccine may lessen the likelihood of complications even if zoster occurs.

Varicella-zoster immune globulin is effective in preventing disease in susceptible individuals when administered within 96 hours of exposure. Its use should be considered in all immunocompromised patients and in susceptible pregnant women who have been exposed.

■ EPSTEIN–BARR VIRUS

EPIDEMIOLOGY

Infection with Epstein–Barr (EBV) is ubiquitous, with 90% to 95% of all adults displaying serologic evidence of a past infection. In the United States, approximately 50% of children are seropositive by 5 years of age, with a second period of seroconversion occurring in early adulthood. Infection occurs earlier in developing countries and in certain areas of the United States. Most cases of EBV infection are transmitted by the presence of virus in oropharyngeal secretions of asymptomatic shedders. Blood transfusions and transplantation of solid organs or bone marrow may also be associated with EBV transmission.

PATHOPHYSIOLOGY AND CLINICAL MANIFESTATIONS

CASE 15.2

An 18–year-old college freshman presented to the student health office with fever and sore throat for 1 week. His temperature was 38.9°C, his tonsils were enlarged, and he had diffuse nontender lymphadenopathy. The possibility of mononucleosis was raised, and titers for viral capsid antigen (VCA) immunoglobulins G (IgG) and M (IgM) were 1:20 and 1:80 respectively at that time. Over the next week, he became increasingly ill, developing scleral icterus and fever to 40.6°C.

On physical examination, the student was noted to have a tender, enlarged liver and palpable spleen. Multiple petechiae were noted on both lower legs. Laboratory workup showed elevated liver transaminases: 550 IU/L aspartate aminotransferase, 1000 IU/L alanine transaminase, 4000 IU/L lactate dehydrogenase (LDH), and bilirubin 6.0 mg/dL (total) and 4.8 mg/dL (direct). His hematocrit was 25%, and his white blood cell (WBC) count was 860/mm³, with 3% polymorphonuclear leukocytes (PMNs), 19% bands, 70% lymphocytes, and 10% monocytes. Numerous atypical lymphocytes were seen on smear. Platelets measured 23,000/mm³, and his erythrocyte sedimentation rate was 12 mm/h. Repeat serology revealed a VCA IgM of 1:160 and a VCA IgG of 1:640. Glucocorticoid therapy was considered; however, over the next 2 weeks, the fever spontaneously resolved, liver function tests returned to normal, hematocrit increased to 35%, WBC count improved to 3000/mm³ (with 70% PMNs), and platelets rose to 100,000/mm³. The young man's spleen remained enlarged, and he was warned to avoid contact sports for the next few months.

Epstein–Barr virus is associated with a variety of clinical disorders arising from various pathogenic mechanisms. Infection during childhood is often asymptomatic or associated with nonspecific symptoms. Infection during adolescence or adulthood more commonly results in the syndrome of acute infectious mononucleosis, characterized by a vigorous humoral and cellular immune response to rapidly proliferating EBV-infected B cells. The most common signs and symptoms of mononucleosis include fever, sore throat, malaise, and lymphadenopathy. The pharyngitis may be exudative and severe. As noted in case 15.2, the enlarged lymph nodes are usually not tender. Other findings, in order of decreasing likelihood, include splenomegaly, hepatitis, palatal petechiae, jaundice, and rash. The rash, when seen, is nonspecific and may be transient. Administration of ampicillin during early EBV-associated mononucleosis very commonly results in a maculopapular rash.

Many aspects of the clinical syndrome of acute infectious mononucleosis—for example, fever, lymphadenopathy, splenomegaly, atypical lymphocytosis—are the result of vigorous T cell and natural killer (NK) cell proliferation and a cytokine response by the immune system rather than a result of direct viral infection, replication, and cytolysis. A few individuals develop a chronic active infection characterized by ongoing lytic EBV replication and multiple organ system disease such as pneumonitis, hepatitis, pancytopenia, and iritis.

Individuals with a rare, inherited immunodeficiency linked to the X chromosome and known as X-linked lymphoproliferative syndrome or Duncan syndrome are prone to overwhelming lethal primary infection with EBV. Survivors are at risk for the subsequent development of lymphoma and agammaglobulinemia. The genetic defect in these patients has been mapped to a small cytoplasmic protein (Sap) that is implicated in regulation of T and NK cell signaling.

After resolution of primary infection, EBV persists for life as a latent infection in B cells and as a lytic infection in the oropharynx. Persistent EBV infection is controlled by a virus-specific immune response and most humans remain asymptomatic. However, immunosuppression associated with HIV infection, transplantation, or congenital immunodeficiency can result in uncontrolled oligoclonal or monoclonal B cell proliferation of latently infected cells. Uncontrolled lytic infection in the oropharynx is manifested as oral hairy leukoplakia in immunosuppressed hosts.

Persistent, latent EBV infection is also associated with development of Burkitt's lymphoma, nasopharyngeal carcinoma, certain types of Hodgkin's disease, gastric adenocarcinoma, and leiomyosarcomas in immunosuppressed hosts. Infection of NK cells by EBV has recently been associated with hypersensitivity to mosquito bites and the development of NK cell leukemia.

COMPLICATIONS

Serious and life-threatening complications of EBV infection occasionally occur. These include autoimmune hemolytic anemia, erythrophagocytic syndrome, thrombocytopenia, splenic rupture, and neurologic syndromes. The neurologic syndromes, although rare, include encephalitis and Guillain–Barré syndrome. The most common causes of death from EBV-associated mononucleosis in healthy adults are neurologic complications, splenic rupture, and airway obstruction. It should be emphasized that mononucleosis-associated encephalitis is rare and usually benign. Nevertheless, any of these complications may be the presenting sign of mononucleosis and "atypical" cases are not unusual.

DIAGNOSIS

Diagnosis of mononucleosis is usually based on clinical suspicion confirmed by laboratory testing. The clinical diagnosis in the typical adolescent or young adult is usually not too difficult. However, many cases occur in which few or none of the classic signs are evident at initial presentation.

Other causes of the infectious mononucleosis syndrome that should be considered in the young adult are cytomegalovirus, acute HIV infection, human herpes-

KEY POINTS

About the Epidemiology, Pathogenesis, and Clinical Manifestation of Epstein–Barr Virus

1. Spread by oral secretions, with 95% of adults carrying the virus.
2. Infects B cells, and illness manifestations are the result of vigorous T cell and natural killer (NK) cell inflammatory response.
3. Fever, sore throat, and lymphadenopathy are the classic triad of mononucleosis.
4. Acute complications of the infection include splenic rupture, neurologic syndromes, and airway obstruction. Less commonly, hepatitis, hemolytic anemia, thrombocytopenia, and neutropenia sometimes occur.
5. Complications of chronic infection include hairy leukoplakia, B cell lymphoma, NK cell lymphoma, gastric adenocarcinoma, and leiomyosarcoma.

virus 6, toxoplasmosis, cat scratch disease, and lymphoma. Laboratory confirmation of EBV infection is achieved primarily by serologic testing. Heterophil antibodies directed against sheep erythrocyte agglutinins are positive in about 90% of cases during the primary infection. Commercially available monospot testing for heterophil antibodies is less sensitive in children, and sequential monospot testing or determination of EBV-specific antibodies is indicated when clinical findings are suggestive of EBV infection, and the initial monospot is negative. The presence of IgM antibodies to VCA is the most sensitive and specific indicator of acute infection. The antibodies are usually detectable at initial presentation, along with IgG VCA antibody (see Table 15.1). By 4 to 8 weeks, the IgM VCA antibodies decline and disappear, but IgG VCA antibodies persist for life. Antibodies to Epstein–Barr viral nuclear antigens (EBNAs) do not develop until approximately 4 weeks after onset of symptoms, but they persist for life. Seroconversion to anti-EBNA positivity is therefore indicative of recent EBV infection. Although antibodies to EBV early antigens are often elevated during acute infection, they may persist for variable periods. These antibodies are occasionally detectable in healthy convalescent patients many years after infection, and they are therefore of limited utility in diagnosing acute infection.

At the time of presentation, VCA IgM antibody is positive, and VCA IgG and early lytic antigen (EA) antibody are also usually positive. As convalescence proceeds, EBNA antibodies become detectable, and VCA IgM antibody disappears. The EBNA and VCA IgG

Table 15.1. Typical result patterns in serologic testing for Epstein–Barr virus during various stages of infection.

Clinical status	VCA IgM Ab	EA Ab	VCA IgG Ab	EBNA Ab
Susceptible	-	-	-	-
Acute infection	+	+	+	-
Early convalescence	+	+	+	+
Late convalescence	-	+	+	+
Previous infection	-	+	+	+
		(low)		

VCA = viral capsid antigen; IgM = immunoglobulin M; Ab = antibody; IgG = immunoglobulin G; EA = early lytic antigen; EBNA = Epstein–Barr virus nuclear antigen.

KEY POINTS

About the Diagnosis of Epstein-Barr Virus

1. The heterophil antibody agglutination test is positive in 90% of primary disease.
2. The monospot test may be negative, especially early in the course of the disease.
3. Monospot is also less sensitive in children and often needs to be repeated.
4. Titer of immunoglobulin M (IgM) antibody to viral capsid antigen (VCA) is the most sensitive and specific test.
   a) Titer is often elevated at the time of presentation.
   b) Declines quickly and has disappeared by 4 to 8 weeks; a positive titer indicates recent infection.
   c) An elevated immunoglobulin G VCA titer persists for life.
5. The Epstein–Barr nuclear antigen begins to rise after 4 weeks, and so a rising titer indicates recent infection.
6. Antibodies to early Epstein–Barr viral antigens (EA) are usually not helpful.
7. The differential diagnosis includes acute HIV infection.
8. Quantitative PCR testing of the viral load may be helpful for predicting the risk of subsequent lymphoproliferative disease in transplant patients with Epstein–Barr virus infection.

---

antibodies remain detectable for life, and EA antibodies are also usually detectable, although at low titers.

Quantifying the EBV DNA load in peripheral blood by PCR identifies immunosuppressed patients who have or who are at high risk for developing EBV-associated B cell lymphomas. Although an elevated EBV DNA load in blood is clearly associated with the development of post-transplant lymphoproliferative disease (PTLD), the predictive value of such a finding is not uniformly high, given that only approximately 50% of bone marrow transplant patients with elevated EBV DNA develop PTLD. An increasing EBV DNA load may be predictive of the development of PTLD, underscoring the need for serial monitoring in high-risk patients.

THERAPY

Treatment of EBV-associated diseases is closely linked with the underlying pathogenesis of the disease. The usual treatment for EBV-associated malignancies involves cancer chemotherapy and radiation therapy as opposed to antiviral strategies, and those options are not discussed here.

Infectious Mononucleosis

More than 95% of infectious mononucleosis cases resolve uneventfully without specific therapy, and so supportive treatment is generally indicated. Acetaminophen can be used to reduce fever. Use of concomitant antibiotics for possible bacterial pharyngitis should be judicious, with support from positive bacterial culture results, because a high incidence of allergic reactions to antibiotics such as ampicillin is observed during acute infectious mononucleosis.

The use of corticosteroids for uncomplicated infectious mononucleosis remains controversial. Corticosteroids have been shown to reduce fever and shorten the duration of constitutional symptoms. However, adverse drug complications can arise from even short courses of corticosteroids, and corticosteroid use is probably best avoided in routine infectious mononucleosis, given its self-limiting nature. Corticosteroids are generally reserved for infectious mononucleosis cases complicated by potential airway obstruction from enlarged tonsils, severe thrombocytopenia, or severe hemolytic anemia. These complications result from the excessive immune response rather than from uncontrolled viral infection, and a short course of corticosteroids (1 mg/kg prednisone daily) with tapering over 1 to 2 weeks can be effective for treating the excessive tonsillar proliferation or autoimmune symptoms. Corticosteroids might also be used for other autoimmune complications occasionally associated with infectious mononucleosis—for example, CNS involvement, myocarditis, or pericarditis. Unless contraindicated, administration of corticosteroids concurrently with acyclovir is the author's general practice.

In general the combination of acyclovir and corticosteroids for uncomplicated infectious mononucleosis inhibits oral viral replication, but provides no clinical benefit. In rare, complicated cases of primary EBV infection and infectious mononucleosis in which the patient is immunosuppressed or severely ill, acyclovir or ganciclovir treatment may be rational, given the safety profile of these drugs, their ability to inhibit EBV replication in vitro and in vivo, and anecdotal reports of clinical response in unusual cases in which excessive EBV replication may have been pathogenic.

Splenic rupture is a rare, but potentially fatal, complication of infectious mononucleosis, occurring in approximately 0.1% of cases. Splenic rupture is more common in men, and approximately half of cases are spontaneous (not associated with trauma or other contributory factors). In one review of 55 cases of splenic rupture associated with infectious mononucleosis, all cases occurred within 3 weeks after the start of the illness. Another case–control study that combined physical, ultrasound, and laboratory examinations of patients with infectious mononucleosis found that physical examination was an insensitive method of detecting splenomegaly (17%), but that all patients were found to have splenomegaly for the first 20 days, and the severity of laboratory abnormalities did not correlate with splenic enlargement.

Although various strategies to minimize the risk of splenic rupture have been advanced, incorporating the results of physical exam and ultrasound imaging, no studies have validated the utility of any approach. It therefore seems prudent to recommend that the patient avoid, for a minimum of 4 weeks after the onset of illness, contact sports or activities (such as weightlifting) that raise intra-abdominal pressure.

Patients recovering from infectious mononucleosis may shed virus in their saliva for a period of several months after recovery despite being clinically well (see "Epidemiology" earlier in this subsection). Furthermore, it is clear that all latently infected humans may intermittently shed EBV in saliva. It is therefore difficult for seronegative subjects to avoid the risk of acquiring EBV infection. It appears that intimate sexual contact is more likely to transmit EBV infection.

Chronic Active EBV Infection

Occasionally, patients have an unusual clinical course following infectious mononucleosis with severe illness and evidence of chronic active EBV infection, as described earlier. These patients typically have extremely high antibody responses to EBV early antigens, lack antibodies to EBNA-1, and exhibit severe disease with end-organ involvement or evidence of increased viral load in affected tissues. Clinical responses and failures with acyclovir or corticosteroids have both been noted in anecdotal reports of these unusual patients with chronic active EBV infection.

CHRONIC FATIGUE SYNDROME

Infection with EBV has also been implicated as a cause of fatigue syndrome. However, seroepidemiologic studies have argued against a pathogenic role for EBV in chronic fatigue syndrome. In addition, a placebo-controlled study with acyclovir has shown no efficacy for patients with chronic fatigue syndrome.

ORAL HAIRY LEUKOPLAKIA

Oral hairy leukoplakia is an unusual lesion of the tongue found in HIV-infected patients. Vigorous EBV lytic replication is present in the excessively proliferating epithelium. This is the only instance in which disease appears to be a direct consequence of lytic EBV replication, and oral acyclovir therapy (3.2 g daily) can temporarily reverse the lesions. However, because nucleoside analogs have no effect on persistent, latent EBV infection, lytic EBV replication and oral hairy leukoplakia frequently recur upon withdrawal of therapy.

KEY POINTS

About Therapy of Epstein–Barr Virus

1. Patients with acute mononucleosis are generally given supportive care.
   a) Avoid antibiotics when possible.
   b) Ampicillin almost always causes a rash.
   b) Use prednisone for airway obstruction, thrombocytopenia, or hemolytic anemia.
   c) Acyclovir or ganciclovir may be helpful in very severe cases.
2. Chronic active infection with Epstein–Barr virus (EBV)
   a) involves very high antibodies to early antigens and no EBNA antibody production;
   b) produces severe end-organ involvement; and
   c) may benefit from antiviral therapy.
3. In chronic fatigue syndrome, antiviral therapy is of no benefit.
4. Oral hairy leukoplakia can result from lytic EBV infection in HIV-infected patients.
   a) Acyclovir can control the infection.
   b) Relapse often occurs when treatment is discontinued.

■ HANTAVIRUS

CASE 15.3

In 1993, a 19-year-old male marathon runner who had been in excellent health presented to a local emergency room in New Mexico complaining of fever, myalgia, chills, headache, and malaise. He had no dyspnea or cough. His fiancée had died 2 days earlier of a respiratory illness that was not characterized. The patient had a temperature of 39.4°C, a blood pressure of 127/84 mm Hg, a heart rate of 118 per minute, and a respiratory rate of 24 per minute. The remainder of his physical exam was normal.

Laboratory examination revealed a hematocrit of 49.6%, a WBC count of 7100/mm³, with 66% segmented neutrophils and 10% band forms; a platelet count of 195,000/mm³; a creatinine level of 1.1 mg/dL; a serum lactate dehydrogenase level of 195 IU/L; and an oxygen saturation of 91% on room air. Urinalysis and chest x-ray were both normal.

The patient was discharged after treatment with acetaminophen, antibiotics, and amantadine; but, 2 days later, he returned to a clinic complaining of persistent symptoms, now including vomiting and diarrhea. He was discharged with no change in diagnosis or therapy. Over the following day, a cough productive of blood-tinged sputum developed, and the young man's respiratory distress worsened. He suffered cardiopulmonary arrest and could not be resuscitated.

A chest x-ray during the terminal illness revealed diffuse alveolar and interstitial infiltrates.

Case 15.3, which is taken from the description of the outbreak of Hantavirus pulmonary syndrome (HPS) in the Four Corners region of New Mexico, Arizona, Colorado, and Utah in 1993, dramatically illustrates almost every characteristic of this devastating illness spread by rodents.

EPIDEMIOLOGY

Hantaviruses are carried by chronically infected rodents, which shed the virus in their saliva and urine. Humans become infected when they inhale aerosols of these infected fluids. Risk factors thus include cleaning or entering buildings that harbor rodents. Certain mice also harbor hantavirus strains and readily enter human dwellings in many

areas of the United States. Since 1993, cases of HPS have been reported in New England, the Midwest, and other areas of the United States. Dozens of cases occur annually.

PATHOPHYSIOLOGY AND CLINICAL MANIFESTATIONS

As already described, HPS begins with fever and myalgias that may be associated with abdominal complaints. Initially, the patient does not appear extremely ill. Over the next few days, respiratory symptoms develop. These are initially mild, and cough and dyspnea may be minimal. Fever, tachycardia, mild hypotension, and hypoxia are usually present. Hemoconcentration, presence of immature white blood cells, mild thrombocytopenia, increased partial thromboplastin time, and lactate dehydrogenase are all typical. A pulmonary vascular leak syndrome occurs, and hypoxia, shock, and pulmonary edema may develop rapidly. Little inflammation is seen in autopsies or biopsies of affected lung.

DIAGNOSIS

Hantavirus serology is almost always positive in patients at the time of admission. Virus can also be demonstrated in tissue by PCR-based methods and by

---

KEY POINTS

About Hantavirus

1. Spread by rodents that shed the virus in their saliva and urine; virus is inhaled as an aerosol.
2. Found in the Four Corners area (New Mexico, Arizona, Colorado, Utah), New England, and the Midwest.
3. Starts as a mild febrile illness with abdominal pain, and proceeds to fulminant respiratory failure.
   a) Virus causes a pulmonary capillary leak syndrome with acute respiratory distress syndrome (ARDS).
   b) Severe hypoxia, hemoconcentration, and increased partial thromboplastin time and LDH are typical.
4. Serologies, polymerase chain reaction, and immunohistochemical staining are all available for diagnosis.
5. If supportive care and cautious fluid administration assist the patient to survive the ARDS, full recovery is possible.

immunohistochemical staining. If HPS is suspected, infectious disease consultation should be obtained immediately, and the Centers for Disease Control and Prevention (CDC) should be notified.

THERAPY AND PREVENTION

If the patient can be supported through the period of hypoxia and shock, recovery can be complete. It is important to realize that in HPS the vascular permeability of the lung is abnormal; fluid administration should be performed with this fact in mind. Intravenous ribavirin has been used in experimental treatment protocols; however, efficacy has not been demonstrated to date.

Prevention of HPS consists of personal precautions to avoid inhalation of aerosolized material contaminated by rodents, and general measures to reduce rodent infestation.

■ SEVERE ACUTE RESPIRATORY SYNDROME

EPIDEMIOLOGY

In March 2003, the World Health Organization (WHO) orchestrated a worldwide effort to control a sudden outbreak a progressive respiratory illness termed Severe Acute Respiratory Syndrome (SARS). This epidemic first arose in Guangdong Province, China, and quickly spread. In February 2003, an infected business man traveling from China stayed in a hotel in Hong Kong and infected 10 other individuals staying on the same floor. These individuals in turn spread the illness to five different countries, including Hong Kong, Singapore, Vietnam, Thailand, and Canada. The illness was spread primarily through air droplets in closed spaces including airplanes. Family members and hospital personnel who failed to maintain respiratory precautions were primarily affected. The virus is also shed in the stool, and in one regional outbreak, infection spread through an apartment complex as consequence of a defective sewage system.

CAUSE AND PATHOGENESIS

The causative agent of SARS was quickly identified as a single-stranded RNA coronavirus. This virus has characteristics similar to those of the influenza and measles viruses. However, before the SARS outbreak, coronaviruses were known to be among the most common causes of adult viral upper respiratory infection (URI), producing clinical symptoms and signs identical to those caused by rhinoviruses. The SARS strain has a unique genomic sequence, being most closely related to bovine and avian coronaviruses and distantly related to other human coronaviruses. This enveloped virus does not withstand drying, but may remain infectious in a warmer, moist environment. On average, the virus survives on surfaces and hands for approximately 3 hours.

The virus attaches to cells in the respiratory tract and enters the cytoplasm, where it multiplies. It is then released from dead cells or extruded from living cells. The severe tissue damage associated with SARS infection is thought to be largely a result of the host's overly vigorous immune response to the virus. Coronavirus is spread primarily by respiratory droplets produced by coughing. Epidemiologic studies suggested that a small subset of SARS patients were particularly efficient at spreading the virus to others; they have been called "super spreaders." These individuals had severe infection and were suspected to be producing small droplets that more efficiently aerosolized and remained in the air for prolonged periods.

CLINICAL MANIFESTATIONS

The infection attacks primarily adults aged 25 to 70 years who are healthy. Children are generally spared, although a few cases have been suspected in children under the age of 15 years. The incubation period typically lasts 2 to 7 days, but can take as long as 10 days. The illness usually begins with a severe febrile prodrome (fever being defined as temperature above 38.0°C for epidemiologic purposes). This fever is often high and can be associated with chills and rigors. Fever is accompanied by headache, malaise, and myalgias. During this phase of the illness, respiratory symptoms are mild. Rash and neurologic symptoms and signs are usually absent. Gastrointestinal symptoms are also usually absent at this stage, although diarrhea has been reported in some cases. The lower respiratory phase of the illness begins 3 to 7 days after the onset of symptoms. Patients begin to experience a severe, dry, nonproductive cough, accompanied by dyspnea and hypoxemia. Respiratory distress is often severe, with 10% to 20% of patients requiring intubation and mechanical ventilation.

Laboratory findings may include a decreased absolute lymphocyte count. The total peripheral WBC count is usually normal or decreased. At the peak of the respiratory illness, 50% of patients develop leukopenia and thrombocytopenia (50,000 to 150,000/μL). Muscle and hepatic enzymes are often elevated early in the respiratory phase, reflecting the onset of rhabdomyolysis and hepatitis. Levels of creatine phosphokinase can be as high as 3000 IU/L, and hepatic transaminases usually are 2 to 6 times normal. Serum LDH is elevated in 70% to 80% of patients. Renal function usually remains normal.

Chest x-ray is usually normal during the febrile prodrome, but changes dramatically during the respiratory phase. The initial abnormalities seen are focal interstitial infiltrates that quickly progress to more generalized, patchy, interstitial infiltrates. In the late stages, these interstitial infiltrates develop into areas of dense consolidation. At autopsy, lung pathology may reveal pulmonary edema, hyaline membranes, and desquamation of type 2 pneumocytes. In later stages, fibroblast proliferation is observed in the interstitium and alveoli.

DIAGNOSIS

For epidemiologic purposes, the diagnosis must be made quickly based on clinical criteria. For this purpose, the WHO created a series of case definitions (See Table 15.2).

Real-time reverse transcriptase PCR tests have been developed to rapidly and sensitively identify the SARS coronavirus in clinical samples. However, in the absence of ongoing worldwide SARS transmission, the probability that a positive test will be a false positive is high. In addition, sample collection technique is extremely important to maximize sensitivity and specificity. Therefore testing should be ordered only after informed consent is obtained from the patient and preferably after consultation with state public health authorities and the CDC. A reliable enzyme-linked immunoabsorbent assay has been developed to measure SARS antibody titers in patient serum. However, detectable antibody titers are generally not observed until the second week of the illness.

TREATMENT AND OUTCOME

No specific treatment for SARS is available. At the present time, meticulous supportive care is all that medical science has to offer. A number of specific therapies have been attempted without clear benefit. Antibiotics may prevent bacterial superinfection and should be considered later in the disease course based on Gram stain findings (see Chapters 1 and 4). Oseltamivir, intravenous ribavirin, and combined ribavirin and corticosteroids have not been shown to be of benefit. Some patients have worsened as corticosteroids have been tapered.

In the 2003 outbreak, the overall fatality rate was 11% worldwide. A poorer prognosis was associated with older age: patients above the age of 60 years had a 43% mortality. A high serum LDH or high peripheral neutrophil count is also associated with a worse outcome.

PREVENTION

Given the unavailability of curative therapies, infection control practices are critical for preventing the spread of this deadly infection. All suspected cases must be placed in strict respiratory isolation. Hospitalized patients should be placed in negative pressure rooms. Respirator masks (N-95) should be worn in combination with gowns, gloves, and protective eyewear. Health care workers are at particularly high risk if present during intubation of an infected patient. In the Toronto outbreak, one

Table 15.2. World Health Organization Case Definitions for Severe Acute Respiratory Syndrome (SARS)

Case type	Characteristics
Suspected	Fever above 38°C, PLUS cough or difficulty breathing, PLUS residence in an area with recent local transmission of SARS within 10 days of the onset of symptoms.
Probable	A suspected case with radiographic findings of pneumonia or with acute respiratory distress syndrome (ARDS), OR a suspected case with a positive test for SARS, OR a suspected case with an unexplained respiratory illness leading to death with autopsy demonstrating ARDS pathology without a defined cause.

KEY POINTS

About Severe Acute Respiratory Syndrome

1. Caused by a unique strain of coronavirus that is spread by aerosolized droplets and is excreted in stool. Beware of "super spreaders."
2. Attacks mainly people over the age of 15 years. Most cases occur in people 25 to 70 years of age,
3. Incubation period is 2 to 7 days. Illness occurs in two stages:
   a) Febrile prodrome
   b) Respiratory phase with infiltrates and hypoxia
4. Diagnosis based on clinical criteria.
5. Only current treatment is meticulous supportive care.
6. Mortality is 11% overall, and 43% in people over 60 years of age.
7. Strict respiratory isolation and standard contact isolation are used to prevent transmission.

case of SARS was mistakenly diagnosed as congestive heart failure, and respiratory precautions were not instituted.

Possibly infected patients who do not require hospitalization should be instructed not leave home until they have been asymptomatic for 10 days. They should use separate utensils, towels, and sheets. Contacts may leave home as long as they are asymptomatic. Travel to areas where the WHO has determined the presence of multiple active cases of SARS should be avoided.

INFLUENZA

VIROLOGY AND EPIDEMIOLOGY

Influenza virus is a major cause of morbidity and mortality worldwide. Influenza A and B both cause epidemic illnesses, and influenza A can cause pandemics such as the 1918–1919 pandemic in which at least 20 million people died. (Some estimates suggest that the number may have even reached 100 million.) Influenza routinely causes epidemics every 1 to 3 years. The number of cases always increases in the winter months.

The influenza virus, an enveloped RNA virus, has eight gene segments that encode proteins. Two of these genes, the hemagglutinin (HA) and neuraminidase (NA) genes, are important mediators of pathogenicity and immunogenicity. Virus binding and infection requires HA, and virion release requires NA. The antibody responses to HA and NA are critical for protection against infection.

Influenza strain nomenclature consists of the type (A or B), the geographic source of the initial isolate, the isolate number, the year of isolation, and the HA and NA gene subtypes. Thus a strain of influenza A virus that was isolated in Hong Kong in 1968 is designated A/Hong Kong/03/68[H3N2].

The influenza virus changes the structure of its HA and NA proteins by genetic mutation—a process known as antigenic drift. Antigenic drift produces variant strains against which human populations have less protective antibody. Occasionally, influenza A virus acquires a completely different set of antigens by a process known as antigenic shift. The unique strains produced by antigenic shift can infect large segments of the population, because cross-reactive or protective antibodies are lacking, thus leading to a pandemic. The virus is thought to undergo antigenic shift by reassortment (exchange of segments of genome with avian influenza species). The process of reassortment and production of virulent human influenza species may occur in pigs, which can be infected with human and avian species of influenza alike.

Influenza attack rates are highest in the very young, but the greatest morbidity and mortality are seen among elderly patients. Influenza is also particularly dangerous to people with underlying pulmonary disease or those who are immunocompromised. In the United States, influenza annually causes about 15 million excess cases of respiratory illnesses in young people and about 4 million cases in older adults. The virus is efficiently transmitted by aerosols of respiratory secretions generated by coughing, sneezing, and talking.

In 1997, direct transmission of avian influenza from birds to humans was documented in Hong Kong. Sporadic cases of bird-to-human transmission have been occurring since 2003, primarily in Southeast Asia. Although occasional human-to-human transmission has been reported, efficient spread of avian strains among humans has not yet occurred. Recent data derived from

---

KEY POINTS

About the Virology and Epidemiology of Influenza

1. Influenza is caused by an enveloped RNA virus that is classified by specific surface proteins:
   a) Hemagglutinins (HA)
   b) Neuramidases (NA)
2. Influenza A and B both cause epidemics; influenza A also causes pandemics.
3. Epidemics occur every 1 to 3 years, mainly in the winter.
4. "Antigenic drift" refers to changes in hemagglutinin and neuraminidase proteins resulting from genetic mutation.
5. "Antigenic shift" refers to reassortment (exchange of genomic segments with other virus strains).
   a) Occurs in influenza A.
   b) Produces pandemic-causing viral strains.
   c) Reassortment may occur in pigs.
6. Virus is spread by aerosolized respiratory secretions.
7. In the United States, 15 million infections occur annually in young people and 4 million in older adults.
8. Avian influenza ("bird flu") is a concern:
   a) The 1918 pandemic strain may have evolved from an avian strain.
   b) The H5N1 strain has recently caused human disease in Southeast Asia (direct spread from birds; human-to-human spread is minimal).

sequencing of isolates obtained from formalin-fixed, paraffin-embedded lung tissue from 1918 influenza cases and a frozen sample from a victim buried in permafrost since 1918 have shed light on the nature of the 1918 pandemic strain. The sequences suggest that the 1918 strain was derived from an avian strain by adaptation to a human host rather than by reassortment. Experiments in mice also suggest that the 1918 strain possesses strong and unique virulence determinants. These findings have raised the possibility that the H5N1 avian influenza strains sporadically infecting humans today could mutate to become more infectious and transmissible among humans while retaining a high level of lethality.

PATHOPHYSIOLOGY AND CLINICAL MANIFESTATIONS

The onset of influenza is abrupt. The patient can often say exactly when they fell ill with fever, headache, shaking chills, and myalgias. The fever may be quite high. It remains elevated for at least 3 days and usually resolves within 1 week. Fever and systemic symptoms predominate in the clinical picture, but a dry cough is invariably present and usually persists after the fever is gone. Rhinorrhea, cervical adenopathy, and non-exudative pharyngitis are common. Recovery can be prolonged, taking up to 3 weeks or even longer; during this period, the patient experiences cough and persistent fatigue.

Once influenza virus infects the respiratory epithelium, it kills the host cell as it replicates. The virus multiplies rapidly, producing large numbers of infectious viruses in the respiratory secretions and causing diffuse inflammation and damage. In severe cases, extensive necrosis occurs. Pulmonary function is abnormal even in normal hosts and may remain abnormal for a period of weeks after recovery.

Human cases of avian influenza differ from typical human influenza in several ways. Although experience with H5N1 avian influenza remains limited, the disease typically presents with fever, cough, and respiratory failure, often accompanied by diarrhea. Almost all cases report close contact with poultry, and the virus has predominantly infected children. Lymphopenia and abnormalities on chest x-ray are common. Mortality has been high among hospitalized cases, although the full clinical spectrum of infection is not well established. Unlike most previous influenza strains, H5N1 is particularly virulent in children over the age of 12 years with no underlying diseases (those that would be predicted to have a strong immune system). Within 6 to 29 days of the onset of fever, many of these patients develop a respiratory distress syndrome and die of respiratory failure. Of the 23 cases reported from Southeast Asia in 2004, 18 (78%) died. The initial cases were reported in China, Thailand, and Vietnam. Subsequently, cases were reported in Azerbaijan,

Djibouti, Egypt, Indonesia, Iraq, Laos, Nigeria, and Turkey. The WHO is tracking new cases, and up-to-date information can be obtained by visiting http://www.who.int/csr/disease/avian_influenza/en/.

COMPLICATIONS

The major complications of influenza are viral pneumonia and secondary bacterial pneumonia.

In influenza pneumonia, rapid progression to dyspnea and hypoxia occurs. The clinical and radiographic picture is that of ARDS, and antibiotics are ineffective. Mortality in this situation is very high. The lungs are hemorrhagic, and there is diffuse involvement, but little inflammation. This complication was a major cause of death among young adults during the 1918 pandemic, but is rarely seen today. However, recent experience with avian influenza virus suggests that, if the H5N1 strain adapts to humans, the incidence of this complication could greatly increase.

KEY POINTS

About the Pathogenesis and Clinical Manifestations of Influenza

1. Infects the respiratory epithelium, causing cell necrosis and acute inflammation.

2. Is characterized by abrupt onset of high fever, shaking chills, headache, myalgias, pharyngitis, and rhinorrhea.

3. Several complications are possible:
   a) Viral pneumonia [can progress to fatal acute respiratory distress syndrome (ARDS) and pulmonary hemorrhage]
   b) Superinfection with *Staphylococcus aureus*, *Haemophilus influenzae*, or *Staphylococcus pneumoniae*
   c) Reye's syndrome (associated with use of aspirin)

4. Avian influenza attacks children.
   a) Severe disease occurs in children more than 12 years of age.
   b) Symptoms include diarrhea and severe cough, in addition to fever.
   c) Lymphopenia occurs, with prominent infiltrates on chest x-ray.
   d) Acute onset of ARDS that develops 6 to 29 days after onset of fever leads to 78% mortality.
   e) Cases have been seen in Southeast Asia, the Middle East, Turkey, and Nigeria.

In some cases of influenza pneumonia, patients initially appear to be recovering from the virus, but then suddenly relapse with fever and typical signs of bacterial pneumonia (see Chapter 4, case 4.1). As a consequence of damage to the tracheobronchial epithelial lining, secondary bacterial pneumonia develops, with *Staphylococcus aureus*, *Haemophilus influenzae*, and *Streptococcus pneumoniae* being the most common offenders (see Chapter 4).

As noted with varicella virus, use of aspirin during influenza has been associated with the development of Reye's syndrome. Reye's syndrome is characterized by fatty infiltration of the liver and changes in mental status, such as lethargy or even delirium and coma. No specific treatment for Reye's syndrome is available other than correction of metabolic abnormalities and reduction of elevated intracranial pressure.

DIAGNOSIS

The most useful characteristic distinguishing influenza from other respiratory illnesses is the predominance of the systemic symptoms. In addition, the epidemic nature of the disease in the community is helpful in making a diagnosis. When influenza is circulating in a community, an adult displaying the symptoms described earlier is highly likely to have influenza. Rapid antigen tests are now available, and some can detect both the A and B types of influenza in throat and nasal swabs. However, the sensitivity of these tests is somewhat variable, depending on the source and quality of the specimen and on other factors, possibly being as low as 60%.

TREATMENT

Amantadine and rimantadine inhibit influenza A virus infection by binding to a virus membrane protein. These drugs were long used for prevention and treatment of influenza A. However, influenza A is now widely resistant to both amantadine and rimantadine, and the U.S. Advisory Committee on Immunization Practices therefore recommends that amantadine and rimantadine not be used for the treatment or chemoprophylaxis of influenza A in the United States.

Two NA inhibitors, zanamivir and oseltamivir are highly effective in inhibiting type A and B influenza alike. Zanamivir has to be administered by inhalation; oseltamivir is given orally. Both agents can be used for prophylaxis and treatment, and they are most effective when administered soon after the onset of infection. Recently, rare but serious psychiatric and neurologic side effects have been associated with oseltamivir, particularly in pediatric patients. These side effects include panic attacks, delusions, delirium, convulsions, depression, loss of consciousness, and suicide.

KEY POINTS

About the Diagnosis and Treatment of Influenza

1. Commercial immunodetection methods are available for early diagnosis; viral culture is confirmatory.
2. Amantadine and rimantadine should no longer be used because of widespread resistance.
3. Neuraminidase inhibitors zanamivir and oseltamivir are effective for types A and B influenza alike.
   a) Give these agents early.
   b) Resistance to oseltamivir has been reported for the H5N1 strain of avian influenza.
   c) Oseltamivir associated with neurologic and behavioral side effects, particularly in children.

Both oseltamivir and zanamivir are active against H5N1 avian influenza in animal and in vitro models. Resistance to oseltamivir has already been documented. Whether widespread resistance to oseltamivir will present a significant obstacle in the management of an avian influenza outbreak is unknown.

PREVENTION

Influenza vaccine is a trivalent inactivated vaccine directed against types A and B influenza. The strains selected for each year's vaccine are based on the strain that was circulating worldwide the previous year. The effectiveness of the vaccine depends to some degree on the success of the match between the vaccine and the circulating strains. Vaccination decreases both disease severity and the infection rate. The groups that should be targeted for influenza vaccination include:

A. Groups at increased risk for influenza complications;

1. People 65 years of age or older
2. Residents of nursing homes or other chronic care facilities
3. All people with chronic pulmonary or cardiovascular disease (including asthma)
4. All children under 18 years of age on chronic aspirin therapy
5. Women who will be in the second or third trimester of pregnancy during the influenza season

B. Those at increased risk of transmitting influenza to high-risk individuals:

1. Health care personnel
2. Employees of nursing homes or other chronic care facilities who have patient contact
3. Home care providers and household contacts of people at high risk

A live attenuated influenza vaccine (LAIV) that is administered as a nasal spray is also available. This vaccine is approved for use in patients 5 to 49 years of age. The LAIV is considered as equally efficacious as inactivated vaccine. Side effects are generally minor and consist mainly of cough and rhinorrhea, which may be more common in adults than children. An increased risk of respiratory side effects has been noted in younger children. Because of the potential risks of a live vaccine, LAIV should not be administered to immunocompromised patients. Because of the potential risk of shedding and transmission of LAIV, health care workers should avoid contact with severely immunocompromised patients for 7 days after vaccination. The "Populations That Should Not Be Vaccinated with Live Attenuated Influenza Vaccine" below shows a complete list of patients in whom LAIV is contraindicated.

The U.S. Advisory Committee on Immunization Practices has recommended a broader policy for the administration of the vaccine (see the box Populations That Should Be Vaccinated).

POPULATIONS THAT SHOULD NOT BE VACCINATED WITH LIVE ATTENUATED INFLUENZA VACCINE

- Children under the age of 5 years or adults over the age of 50 years
- People with asthma, reactive airway disease, or other chronic disorders of the pulmonary or cardiovascular systems; people with other underlying medical conditions, including metabolic diseases such as diabetes, renal dysfunction, and hemoglobinopathies
- People with known or suspected immunodeficiency diseases or who are receiving immunosuppressive therapies
- People with a history of Guillain–Barré syndrome
- Pregnant women
- People with a history of hypersensitivity, including anaphylaxis, to any of the components of LAIV or to eggs

- Children or adolescents receiving acetylsalicylic acid or other salicylates (because of the association of Reye's syndrome with wild-type influenza virus infection)

Because of the potential for a pandemic originating from avian influenza, extensive efforts to produce effective vaccines against currently circulating strains are underway. Unfortunately, the vaccines that have been produced to date have been poorly immunogenic, and may require multiple immunizations to achieve adequate protection. Research on various strategies to improve and expand on current methods is continuing. Possible strategies include alternative routes of administration, adjuvants, recombinant DNA vaccines, and passive immunization.

HERPES SIMPLEX VIRUS
EPIDEMIOLOGY

Herpes simplex virus (HSV) is a ubiquitous human pathogen with two distinct types, HSV-1 and HSV-2. The HSV-1 type causes primarily orolabial lesions; HSV-2 causes genital lesions. More than 90% of adults worldwide exhibit serologic evidence of infection with HSV-1. The prevalence of HSV-2 infection is considerably lower, but ranges from at least 10% to as high as 80% depending on the population studied. As sexual activity (number of sexual partners and other STDs) increases the likelihood of HSV-2 infection also increases. Transmission of HSV usually occurs person-to-person, by direct contact with infected secretions or mucosal surfaces.

PATHOPHYSIOLOGY AND CLINICAL MANIFESTATIONS

Once HSV enters a mucosal or skin surface, it replicates in the epithelium and infects a nerve ending. It is then transported to the nerve ganglion where it establishes a latent infection that persists for the lifetime of the host. The trigeminal and sacral ganglia are the most common sites of HSV-1 and HSV-2 latency. Viral replication occurs in the ganglion during the initial infection.

Initial infection with HSV-1 is often subclinical and many people never experience clinical reactivation, although they are clearly seropositive. Others experience gingivostomatitis (especially small children). The lesions are usually ulcerative and exudative, and may involve extensive areas of the lips, oral cavity, pharynx, and perioral skin. Healing occurs over a period of several days to 2 weeks, usually without scarring. Secondary episodes result in fever blisters—the typical vesicular and ulcerative lesions. These occur most commonly at the vermilion border of the lips, but may also occur at other sites on the face or in the mouth. Many environmental factors may trigger a recurrence, such as sunlight exposure, stress, and viral infections. Secondary episodes are usually much less severe.

In both women and men, HSV-2 causes genital herpes. Lesions may be vesicular, pustular, or ulcerative, involving the penis in men and vagina and cervix in women. Typical symptoms are pain, itching, dysuria, and vaginal or urethral discharge. Upon primary infection, symptoms tend to be more severe in women. Primary infection can be associated with an aseptic meningitis and mild systemic symptoms such as fever. Occasionally, inflammation is severe enough to lead to temporary bladder or bowel dysfunction.

Both HSV-1 and HSV-2 can also affect many other sites in the body where they have been inoculated. "Whitlow" is an HSV infection of the fingers, resulting from the inoculation of virus into abraded skin. This condition may be seen in health care workers and others who have been exposed to the virus either from autoinoculation or person-to-person transmission. The lesions are vesicular and pustular, with local erythema, pain, and drainage. They are often mistaken for bacterial infections, resulting in unnecessary drainage and antibiotics. "Herpes gladiatorum" is the name given to HSV infection acquired by wrestlers, in whom the virus is inoculated into breaks in the skin during wrestling competition.

COMPLICATIONS

A potentially dangerous consequence of HSV infection of the cornea is HSV keratitis. This infection may be caused by either HSV-1 or HSV-2, but more commonly by HSV-1. Once HSV keratitis has occurred, the patient remains at risk for recurrences. This infection is one of the most common causes of blindness in the United States. Symptoms consist of tearing, pain, erythema, and conjunctival swelling. Dendritic corneal lesions are easily visualized by fluorescein staining (See Chapter 5, Figure 5-2). Involvement of deeper structures or corneal scarring can lead to blindness.

Annually, HSV encephalitis occurs in approximately 1 of 250,000 to 500,00 population. A preponderance of these cases are attributable to HSV-1; concurrent skin lesions are usually not present. Although HSV encephalitis may be the result of primary infection, most patients can be shown to have been previously infected. The disease is characterized by fever, altered mentation, and focal neurologic signs. Personality changes and bizarre behavior are common, and many patients experience seizures. The disease process typically affects the temporal lobe and is

---

KEY POINTS

About the Epidemiology, Pathogenesis, and Clinical Manifestations of Herpes Simplex Virus

1. Type 1 (HSV-1) causes herpes labialis; more than 90% of people worldwide have been infected.
2. Type 2 (HSV-2) causes genital herpes; incidence varies from 10% to 80%, depending on sexual activity.
3. Transmitted from person to person by contact with infected surfaces or mucosa.
4. Viral replication occurs in nerve ganglia; virus periodically reactivates causing recurrent infection.
   a) HSV-1 resides in the trigeminal ganglion.
   b) HSV-2 resides in the sacral ganglion.
5. Lesions are vesiculopustular and moderately painful.
6. Less common forms of skin infection also occur:
   a) Herpetic whitlow is usually found in health care workers; can be mistaken for a bacterial infection.
   b) Herpes gladiatorum develops in wrestlers at sites of skin abrasion.
7. Complications can be serious:
   a) Herpes encephalitis (HSV-1) can manifest with personality changes, obtundation, and seizures. Mortality is 15%.
   b) Herpes keratitis is a leading cause of blindness.
   c) Cutaneous dissemination can occur in eczema patients, and bronchopneumonia is a possibility in debilitated patients.

---

usually unilateral. It may progress in a fulminant manner with frank hemorrhagic necrosis of the affected areas of the brain. With antiviral treatment, mortality has been reduced, but remains above 15%, and most survivors exhibit long-term cognitive impairment.

Widespread cutaneous dissemination (eczema herpeticum) can be seen in people with eczema. Visceral dissemination of HSV is rare in the normal host, but herpetic tracheobronchitis is often seen in debilitated, intubated hospitalized patients, in whom it may occasionally progress to pneumonitis.

DIAGNOSIS

The clinical diagnosis of labial or genital herpes is usually not difficult; however, the typical vesicle on an erythematous base, the "dewdrop on a rose petal," is not always present. Culture of vesicle fluid is highly

KEY POINTS

About the Diagnosis and Treatment of Herpes Simplex Virus

1. The diagnosis is made clinically, or with immunofluorescence and viral culture. For encephalitis, a polymerase chain reaction test of the cerebrospinal fluid is useful.

2. Primary skin infections can be treated with acyclovir, famciclovir, or valacyclovir.

3. Treatment of recurrent episodes is more controversial. Treat during the prodrome; suppressive therapy can be used for recurrent genital herpes.

4. Use high-dose, intravenous acyclovir for encephalitis or disseminated disease.

sensitive and specific. Direct staining for HSV antigens can also be used to diagnose infection. Staining of lesion scrapings and examination for giant cells (the Tzanck test) is quick, but nonspecific and insensitive. The diagnosis of HSV encephalitis can be difficult, especially early in the course of the illness. A mild lymphocytic CSF pleocytosis is common, as are red blood cells and an elevated protein level. However, none of these findings are diagnostic. A PCR test of the CSF for HSV is highly sensitive and specific—the optimal laboratory test to confirm the diagnosis. Magnetic resonance imaging of the brain and electroencephalography often show abnormalities localizing to the temporal areas even early in the disease.

TREATMENT

First episodes of all types of HSV infection benefit from treatment. For both orolabial and genital herpes, oral acyclovir, famciclovir, and valacyclovir are all effective. Treatment of recurrent episodes of HSV-1 or HSV-2 is somewhat unsatisfactory. Although treatment may somewhat reduce duration of symptoms, especially in HSV-2, the results are not dramatic. Some patients find that early institution of therapy (as soon as prodromal symptoms such as tingling or itching appear) can be helpful. For patients with frequent and severe recurrent genital herpes, suppressive therapy can be helpful. Any of the three antivirals mentioned earlier can be used. For HSV encephalitis, treat every 8 hours with intravenous acyclovir 10 mg/kg, for a minimum of 14 days. Disseminated HSV infection, particularly in the immunosuppressed host, a usually requires high-dose intravenous acyclovir therapy.

■ CYTOMEGALOVIRUS

EPIDEMIOLOGY

Human cytomegalovirus (CMV) is a common infection worldwide. Prevalence of the infection varies greatly based on socioeconomic factors, but no clear link to hygienic practices exists. In the United States, from 40% to 80% of children are infected by puberty. Young children may be a major source of infection for adults; caretakers of young children may have a risk of infection that is 20 times normal. Person-to-person spread can occur by contact with almost any human body fluid or substance: blood, urine, saliva, cervical secretions, feces, breast milk, and semen. The virus is therefore also spread by sexual contact and by blood transfusion and organ donation.

PATHOPHYSIOLOGY AND CLINICAL MANIFESTATIONS

Most human CMV infections are thought to be subclinical, but primary infection in the normal host occasionally results in a mononucleosis syndrome. Approximately 10% of mononucleosis cases are thought to be caused by CMV, which is the major cause of heterophil (monospot)–negative mononucleosis. Mononucleosis caused by CMV is more common in slightly older adults, but it can be difficult to distinguish clinically from EBV-associated mononucleosis. Pharyngitis and cervical adenopathy have been suggested to be less common with CMV, but both may be observed with CMV mononucleosis. Fever in CMV mononucleosis lasts on average for more than 3 weeks. Rash is present in about 30% of patients, and ampicillin provocation of rash has been noted. Other complications of CMV infection in the normal host include hepatitis, pneumonitis, and Guillain–Barré syndrome. Many of the laboratory findings of EBV mononucleosis are also seen in CMV infection.

In the immunocompromised host, infection with CMV produces most of the morbidity and mortality associated with the virus. Infection produces severe disease in multiple organs, causing retinitis, hepatitis, pneumonitis, gastrointestinal disease (gastric and esophageal ulcers and colitis), and polyradiculopathy. Further details of preventive strategies in these patients are discussed in Chapter 16.

DIAGNOSIS

Viral culture is not useful for diagnosing CMV infection in the normal host. Virus may be shed for long periods in the urine and intermittently by persons infected in the past. The most reliable test is a rise in CMV IgG titer to about four times baseline value.

KEY POINTS

About Cytomegalovirus Infection

1. Infection with cytomegalovirus (CMV) is common worldwide. In the United States. 40% to 80% of children are positive.

2. Young children are the primary source of infection for adults.

3. The virus is transmitted by blood, urine, saliva, cervical secretions, semen, feces, and breast milk.

4. Many infections are subclinical, and CMV is a leading cause of heterophil-negative mononucleosis.

5. In the immunocompromised host, the virus causes retinitis, hepatitis, pneumonitis, gastrointestinal disease (gastric and esophageal ulcers and colitis), and polyradiculopathy.

6. The diagnosis can be made by noting a rise in immunoglobulin G titer (to four times normal levels), the existence of IgM anti-CMV titer in the normal host, or quantitative PCR.

7. The disease is self-limiting in the normal host. The immunocompromised patient should be treated with ganciclovir or foscarnet.

Detection of IgM is also strong evidence for acute infection, although IgM can occasionally be seen in normal hosts during virus reactivation. Quantitative PCR of viral DNA is also widely available. Diagnosis of the various manifestations of CMV disease in the immunocompromised host is discussed in Chapter 16.

TREATMENT

Antiviral treatment of CMV infection is almost never required in the normal host. Spontaneous resolution, even after a lengthy illness, is almost invariable. However, corticosteroids may be used for the same autoimmune or hematologic complications as are seen in EBV infection. Treatment with ganciclovir or foscarnet may be considered in those rare cases in which CMV appears to be causing specific organ-system disease (such as esophagitis) in the normal host. These agents should be used in the immunocompromised patient (See Chapter 16).

FURTHER READING

Varicella Virus

Heininger U, Seward JF. Varicella. *Lancet.* 2006;368:1365–1376.
Jumaan AO, Yu O, Jackson LA, Bohlke K, Galil K, Seward JF. Incidence of herpes zoster, before and after varicella-vaccination-associated

decreases in the incidence of varicella, 1992–2002. *J Infect Dis.* 2005;191:2002–2007.
Oxman MN, Levin MJ, Johnson GR, et al. A vaccine to prevent herpes zoster and postherpetic neuralgia in older adults. *N Engl J Med.* 2005;352:2271–2284.
Shafran SD, Tyring SK, Ashton R, et al. Once, twice, or three times daily famciclovir compared with aciclovir for the oral treatment of herpes zoster in immunocompetent adults: a randomized, multicenter, double-blind clinical trial. *J Clin Virol.* 2004;29:248–253.

Epstein–Barr Virus

Balfour HH Jr, Holman CJ, Hokanson KM, et al. A prospective clinical study of Epstein–Barr virus and host interactions during acute infectious mononucleosis. *J Infect Dis.* 2005;192:1505–1512.
Crawford DH, Macsween KF, Higgins CD, et al. A cohort study among university students: identification of risk factors for Epstein–Barr virus seroconversion and infectious mononucleosis. *Clin Infect Dis.* 2006;43:276–282.
Candy B, Hotopf M. Steroids for symptom control in infectious mononucleosis. *Cochrane Database Syst Rev.* 2006;3:CD004402.
Fafi-Kremer S, Morand P, Brion JP, et al. Long-term shedding of infectious Epstein–Barr virus after infectious mononucleosis. *J Infect Dis.* 2005;191:985–989.
Petersen I, Thomas JM, Hamilton WT, White PD. Risk and predictors of fatigue after infectious mononucleosis in a large primary-care cohort. *QJM.* 2006;99:49–55.
Swaminathan S, Wang F. Antimicrobial therapy of Epstein–Barr virus infections. In: Yu V, Merigan TC, Barriere S, et al., eds. *Antimicrobial Therapy and Vaccines.* Baltimore, Md.: Williams & Wilkins; 2002. [For current update, visit http://www.antimicrobe.org/v02rev.asp]
Waninger KN, Harcke HT. Determination of safe return to play for athletes recovering from infectious mononucleosis: a review of the literature. *Clin J Sport Med.* 2005;15:410–416.

Hanta Virus

Jenison S, Hjelle B, Simpson S, Hallin G, Feddersen R, Koster F. Hantavirus pulmonary syndrome: clinical, diagnostic, and virologic aspects. *Semin Respir Infect.* 1995;10:259–269.

Severe Acute Respiratory Syndrome

Donnelly CA, Fisher MC, Fraser C, et al. Epidemiological and genetic analysis of severe acute respiratory syndrome. *Lancet Infect Dis.* 2004;4:672–683.
Huang J, Ma R, Wu CY. Immunization with SARS-CoV S DNA vaccine generates memory CD4+ and CD8+ T cell immune responses. *Vaccine.* 2006;24:49054913.
Peiris JS, Guan Y, Yuen KY. Severe acute respiratory syndrome. *Nat Med.* 2004;10:S88–S97.
Lau SK, Woo PC, Li KS, et al. Severe acute respiratory syndrome coronavirus-like virus in Chinese horseshoe bats. *Proc Natl Acad Sci U S A.* 2005;102:14040–14045.

Influenza

Brownstein JS, Wolfe CJ, Mandl KD. Empirical evidence for the effect of airline travel on inter-regional influenza spread in the United States. *PLoS Med.* 2006;3:e401.

Kandun IN, Wibisono H, Sedyaningsih ER, et al. Three Indonesian clusters of H5N1 virus infection in 2005. *N Engl J Med.* 2006;355:2186–2194.

Monto AS. The threat of an avian influenza pandemic. *N Engl J Med.* 2005;352:323–325.

Shinya K, Ebina M, Yamada S, Ono M, Kasai N, Kawaoka Y. Avian flu: influenza virus receptors in the human airway. *Nature.* 2006;440:435–436.

Taubenberger JK, Reid AH, Lourens RM, Wang R, Jin G, Fanning TG. Characterization of the 1918 influenza virus polymerase genes. *Nature.* 2005;437:889–893.

Tumpey TM, Basler CF, Aguilar PV, et al. Characterization of the reconstructed 1918 Spanish influenza pandemic virus. *Science.* 2005;310:77–80.

Cytomegalovirus

Gandhi MK, Khanna R. Human cytomegalovirus: clinical aspects, immune regulation, and emerging treatments. *Lancet Infect Dis.* 2004;4:725–738.

Razonable RR, Brown RA, Wilson J, et al. The clinical use of various blood compartments for cytomegalovirus (CMV) DNA quantitation in transplant recipients with CMV disease. *Transplantation.* 2002;73:968–973.

Staras SA, Dollard SC, Radford KW, Flanders WD, Pass RF, Cannon MJ. Seroprevalence of cytomegalovirus infection in the United States, 1988–1994. *Clin Infect Dis.* 2006;43:1143–1151.

Infections in the Immunocompromised Host

16

Time Recommended to Complete: 1 day

Reuben Ramphal, M.D., and Frederick Southwick, M.D.

GUIDING QUESTIONS

1. How should an immunocompromised host be classified, and why?

2. Which pathogens most commonly infect neutropenic patients?

3. Which pathogens are responsible for infection in patients with defects in cell-mediated immunity?

4. How should bone marrow transplant patients be classified with regards to their host immune deficiencies?

5. Do all immunocompromised hosts with fever require empiric antibiotics?

POTENTIAL SEVERITY

Rapid evaluation and empiric antibiotics are required in the febrile neutropenic patient. High-grade life-threatening bacteremia is common.

■ DEFINITION OF THE IMMUNOCOMPROMISED HOST

Medical advances in the management of malignancies and organ failure have given rise to a population of patients now commonly called immunocompromised hosts. An immunocompromised host is a patient with leukemia, lymphoma, or solid tumors who is receiving cytotoxic chemotherapy or other chemotherapy, or who has received a bone marrow transplant (including a stem cell transplant), or a solid organ transplant. Additionally, patients in whom immunosuppressive agents and immune modulators are being applied for inflammatory

disorders are adding to this expanding population whose major host defense mechanisms are in some way not functioning optimally to combat environmental and endogenous organisms. Immune system failures result in incidences of infection not only by normally accepted human pathogens and human saprophytes, but also by environmental organisms of low intrinsic virulence.

One of the most striking examples of the immunocompromised host is the patient with AIDS who advances from susceptibility only to virulent organisms such as *Mycobacterium tuberculosis* that are controlled by cell-mediated immunity, to susceptibility to organisms such as *Pneumocystis jiroveci* that are relatively avirulent, and later, as immunity wanes even further, susceptibility to saprophytic mycobacteria, latent viruses, and parasites. Many of the ideas discussed in this chapter—with the exception of the other major defect that is seen following cytotoxic chemotherapy, loss of mucosal barriers and circulating neutrophils—apply to the AIDS patient, although these patients are not formally discussed here, but in Chapter 17.

Another type of immunocompromised host that should be kept in mind is the patient with an immunodeficiency syndrome that has a genetic basis. Most of these patients become apparent in childhood, presenting with histories of recurrent sinopulmonary or skin infections, most often attributable to bacterial agents. The management of these patients is best handled in the pediatric literature.

Thus, in the truest sense, the population under discussion should be called the "medically or iatrogenically compromised host," because the compromise results mainly from treatment of an underlying disease. Careful attention must also be paid to the splenectomized patient whose ability to clear encapsulated bacteria is compromised in the absence of opsonic antibody and who is susceptible to overwhelming sepsis caused mainly by pneumococcus and *Haemophilus influenzae*.

CLASSIFICATION OF THE IMMUNOCOMPROMISED HOST

Immunocompromised patients can be divided into three main groups (although overlaps in these populations exist, as will be discussed later in this chapter):

1. Patients whose major defect is caused by cytotoxic therapy or irradiation, or both, with the major defect being neutropenia and mucosal barrier damage
2. Patients whose major defect is suppression of cell-mediated immunity resulting from the administration of immunosuppressive agents to control organ rejection or inflammation
3. Patients with both types of major defect

It is absolutely essential that these distinctions be made at the initial patient encounter, because important decisions about diagnostic approaches—and the need for immediate empiric therapy and its type—have to be made based on this assessment. Stated another way, a distinction must be drawn between "neutropenia" and "immunosuppression" as the cause of the host compromise, because these conditions predispose to different types of infections.

Figure 16.1 shows the categorization of common medically compromised patients. Some defects are temporary, until repair mechanisms return to full functionality (for example, the bone marrow recovers, mucosal regeneration is complete, or immunosuppressive

agents are stopped), and some will be lifelong (for example, immunosuppression may be permanently required to maintain organ function or to control inflammation).

A full understanding of these classifications and their application to specific populations will provide a firm foundation for managing the immunocompromised host.

■ NEUTROPENIA AND MUCOSITIS

CASE 16.1

A 51–year-old white man received high induction with cytosine arabinoside for relapse of acute lymphocytic leukemia. Two days after completion of his 7-day course of chemotherapy, his absolute neutrophil count was 0/mm³. One day later, he developed a fever and was started on ticarcillin-clavulinate and gentamicin. Over the next 48 hours, he remained febrile, and he developed a black skin lesion (2 × 2 cm) on his right thigh. The lesion was dark black, necrotic in appearance, and mildly painful to touch. Tissue biopsy revealed sheets of gram-negative rods. Four of four blood cultures drawn at the onset of fever were positive for Pseudomonas aeruginosa, Escherichia coli, *and* Klebsiella pneumoniae. *His antibiotic regimen was switched to ceftazidime and gentamicin. Over the next week, his neutrophil count increased, and he defervesced.*

PATHOGENESIS

Neutropenia is defined as an absolute neutrophil count below 500/mm³. It is often accompanied by mucosal damage. As a result, bacteria from the mouth and lower gastrointestinal (GI) tract are able

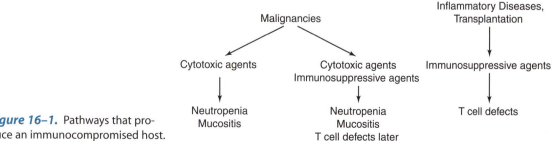

Figure 16–1. Pathways that produce an immunocompromised host.

KEY POINTS

About the Classification of
Immunocompromised Patients

- -

1. Neutropenia is defined as a neutrophil count below 500 mm³.
   a) Risk of infection increases as the cell number decreases below this threshold.
   b) Reduced count is typically caused by cancer chemotherapy that depresses the bone marrow.
2. Cell-mediated immune deficiencies are
   a) associated with corticosteroids, and
   b) follow immunosuppression for organ transplantation.
3. Mixed defects are seen chiefly in bone marrow transplant patients, who
   a) are neutropenic in the early stages, and
   b) have depressed cell-mediated immunity after the bone marrow repopulates.

---

to pass through the damaged mucosal barrier unchecked by the host's first line of defense: the neutrophil. Normally, any bacteria passing through the mucosa are phagocytosed and killed by toxic oxygen byproducts, proteases, and small bactericidal cationic proteins within the closed environment of the phagolysosome.

The risk of infection increases as the cell number decreases, with the incidence of infection being inversely related to how far the number of neutrophils falls below the threshold of 500/mm³. The risk of serious infection is considerably higher when the neutrophil count is less than 200/mm³. The duration of neutropenia is also an important determinant of infection risk. The incidence of infections is low if

neutropenia lasts only 7 to 10 days. However, neutropenia that continues for more than 10 days is associated with a high risk of infection.

MICROBIOLOGY

The infecting organisms usually come from among those found on the skin or in the oral cavity and GI tract, plus any introduced by cross-contamination from environmental sources. For example, environmental cross-infection can occur if organisms are ingested in food at a time when the gut has been denuded by cytotoxic chemotherapy.

1. **Bacteria**. Table 16.1 lists the bacteria most commonly reported, with their probable sources. Gram-positive pathogens have increased in frequency in recent series describing neutropenic bacteremia, probably as a consequence of the increased use of long-lasting indwelling venous catheters and the overuse of fluoroquinolones. The most frequent gram-positive bacteria are coagulase-negative staphylococci, *Staphylococcus aureus*, and *Streptococcus viridans*. Enterococci and *Corynebacterium* are increasingly being cultured. Gram-negative pathogens are second in frequency, and as seen in case 16.1, they usually originate from the GI tract. As in that case, severe neutropenia is commonly accompanied by polymicrobial bacteremia. The most frequently encountered organisms are *E. coli*, *Klebsiella* species, *Pseudomonas aeruginosa*, and less commonly, *Enterobacter*, *Proteus*, *Acinetobacter*, *Stenotrophomonas*, and *Citrobacter*. Remarkably, despite their presence in large numbers in the GI tract, anaerobic gram-negative rods such as *Bacteroides* are not frequent causes of bacteremia in neutropenic patients. However, bacteremia with anaerobes is occasionally seen in association with severe mucositis.

2. **Fungi**. Bacteria are not the only members of the human or environmental flora that infect the

Table 16.1. Sources of Bacteria Commonly Infecting Neutropenic Patients

Skin	Oral cavity	Gut
Coagulase negative staphylococci	*Streptococcus viridans*	*Escherichia coli*
Staphylococcus aureus	Oral anaerobes	*Klebsiella* spp.
		Other enteric bacteria
		Gut anaerobes
		Enterococci
		Pseudomonas aeruginosa

neutropenic patient. Organisms that are present in lower numbers and that are resistant to antibacterial agents—for example, yeasts and moulds—also play a significant role in infections in the neutropenic patient. However, it should be borne in mind that certain fungi are held in check by cell-mediated immunity, and these pathogens infect patients with compromised cell-mediated immunity.

Fungal infections usually develop after broad-spectrum antibiotics have had time to reduce the competing bacterial flora. In patients with no prior history of fungal infection, these pathogens are not usually seen for at least 7 days into a febrile neutropenic episode. Hence, fungal infections are often called "superinfections," because they occur while patients are receiving antibacterial agents.

Occasionally, when a patient has received antibiotics in the recent past and the level of fungal colonization in the gut is high, fungi may emerge as primary pathogens early in neutropenia before antibiotics are given, or they may infect a central venous catheter from the skin. Some fungi may be acquired early by inhalation from the environment, but may not become symptomatic until much later, after the organism has multiplied sufficiently in the lung and has invaded lung parenchyma and blood vessels, thus appearing to be a superinfection. Fungi that may appear early in neutropenia include *Candida* species (*albicans, tropicalis, krusei, glabrata*, and others) and occasionally *Aspergillus* species. Certain fungi that are

cause severe infections in other populations—*Mucor* species, for example—are only infrequently encountered in the neutropenic patient.

Pathogens Encountered in Patients with Suppression of T Cell Functions

The number of patients with suppression of T cell function is progressively increasing. Initially, patients receiving corticosteroids were the major group of patients falling into this category. Increasingly, patients with connective tissue disease including lupus erythematosus and rheumatoid arthritis are being treated with new cytokine antagonists to control their disease. These agents also impair cell-mediated immunity. Most of the patients in this category have undergone organ transplantation. To prevent organ rejection, they receive agents directed against T cells.

Post-transplant infections fall into two groups:

- Infections occurring during the first postoperative month.
- Infections occurring during the subsequent 1-6 months.

During the first month, patients become infected with the same hospital-acquired pathogens as other hosts do. Pathogens of particular concern during this period include *Legionella* species and other gram-negative bacilli such as *P. aeruginosa*; gram-positive organisms, particularly antimicrobial-resistant species such as vancomycin-resistant enterococci (VRE) and methicillin-resistant *S. aureus*; and fungi, such as *Aspergillus* species and azole-resistant *Candida* species. Because these patients often receive broad-spectrum antibiotics during their postoperative recovery, they are also at risk for *Clostridium difficile* colitis.

During the first month, transplant patients are also at risk of developing infections transmitted by the donor organ or organs. In some instances, the donor had an acute infection (with *S. aureus* or pneumococci) or gram-negative bacteremia before death. Before organs are harvested, adequate therapy must be assured. Still, bacteria can occasionally survive in a vascular aneurysm or other protected sites. Or the donor may have an asymptomatic low-grade infection that becomes apparent only when the organ is transplanted into an the immunocompromised recipient. Recent examples have included West Nile virus, lymphocytic choriomeningitis virus, rabies, leishmaniasis, and Chagas' disease.

The period from 1 to 6 months post-transplant is associated with the widest variety of potential opportunistic infections. Immunosuppression is at its highest during this period to prevent acute rejection.

KEY POINTS

About Infections Associated with Neutropenia and Mucositis

1. Risk is inversely related to the number of neutrophils below 500/mm^3.

2. Infecting organisms primarily come from among those found on the skin and in the oral cavity and gastrointestinal tract.

3. Bacteria include *Staphylococcus epidermidis, Staph. aureus, Streptococcus viridans*, enterococci, enteric gram-negative organisms, and *Pseudomonas;* anaerobes are less common.

4. Fungal infections develop after antibiotic therapy has had time to reduce the bacterial flora (usually after 7 days or more); *Candida* and *Aspergillus* species are the most common.

BACTERIA

Mycobacteria are of particular concern. Post-transplant patients harboring latent *M. tuberculosis* can develop miliary tuberculosis (see Chapter 4). Atypical mycobacteria may become more invasive and cause symptomatic infection. *L. monocytogenes* can be contracted by eating contaminated foods, and transplant patients should be instructed in how to avoid foods contaminated with this deadly pathogen. *Listeria* is the third most frequent cause of community-acquired bacterial meningitis, and it almost exclusively infects people with depressed cell-mediated immunity (see Chapter 6). *Nocardia* species can result in cavitary or nodular pulmonary infections, plus bacteremia and brain abscess. These patients are also at increased risk for *L. pneumophila*.

FUNGI

Fungal infections in patients with suppressed T cell function are often life-threatening and may be difficult to diagnose. *Cryptococcus neoformans* is the most common fungal pathogen encountered in the transplant population. The sites primarily infected are the lungs and the meninges. In the meninges, the organism causes a lymphocytic meningitis (see Chapter 6). The filamentous fungi that are most likely to cause disease are *Aspergillus* species, *Fusarium* species, and the *Mucor* and *Rhizopus* groups. Depending on geographic location, *Histoplasma capsulatum* and *Coccidioides immitis* are also important pathogens in these patients. Increasingly, the dematiaceous ("black") fungi are being reported as a cause of infections. On the other hand, *Candida* rarely causes infection in this population, probably because these fungi are controlled primarily by neutrophils.

The role of filamentous fungal infections in organ transplantation cannot be overemphasized. When such infections occur, cure is extremely difficult in the face of continued immunosuppression, and death is a common outcome.

VIRUSES

The most important arms of the host defense mechanisms against viral infections are the T cells and antibodies. In most instances, cell-mediated and humoral immunity function together to prevent and control active viral infections. The patient with T cell defects following immunosuppression is likely to have antibodies against many viruses, unless total ablation of existing T cells and reconstitution with immunologically naive cells has been carried out. Reconstituted donor populations usually contain memory cells to make antibody, but the response may be blunted. Transplant patients therefore tend to be more susceptible to viruses that are latent in the body rather than to infections with new viruses. Loss of cell-mediated immunity allows latent viruses to reactivate. Additionally, patients may acquire reactivation infections from transfused blood components or a transplanted organ. The virus that most commonly reactivates is cytomegalovirus (CMV). A CMV infection can also be acquired from blood transfusion or transplantation with an infected organ. The risk of infection depends on the recipient and donor CMV antibody (Ab) status:

- **High Risk**—CMV Ab– recipient, CMV Ab+ donor
- **Intermediate Risk**—CMV Ab+ recipient, CMV Ab+ or Ab– donor
- **Lowest Risk**—CMV Ab–recipient, CMV Ab–donor

Diagnosis of active CMV infection utilizes two tests that are also used to monitor response to therapy: the CMV antigen test always correlates with active replication, and a CMV polymerase chain reaction (PCR) test can detect latent and active infection (a higher copy number is indicative of active invasive infection).

Epstein–Barr virus less commonly causes symptomatic disease. However, the virus actively replicates in 20% to 30% of transplant recipients and can cause a

---

KEY POINTS

About Infections in Patients with Defective Cell-Mediated Immunity

1. Can contract the same community-acquired pathogens as normal hosts.
2. Have an increased risk of bacterial infections with *Mycobacterium* species, *Listeria monocytogenes*, *Nocardia* species, and *Salmonella* species.
3. Fungal infections are often life-threatening and may be difficult to diagnose.

   a) *Cryptococcus* is most common.

   b) *Aspergillus* species, *Fusarium* species, and the *Mucor* and *Rhizopus* groups are other common possibilities.

   c) Histoplasmosis and coccidiomycosis should be considered depending on geographic location.

   d) Reports of dematiaceous fungi ("black mold") infection are increasing.
4. Reactivation of old viral infections is a major concern.

   a) Cytomegalovirus is most common. Can be the result of reactivation, blood transfusion, or transplantation with an infected organ.

   b) Epstein–Barr virus is less common.
5. Other possible pathogens include *Pneumocystis*, *Toxoplasma*, disseminated *Strongyloides*.

lymphoproliferative syndrome. Less common viruses that can become active include herpes simplex, herpes zoster, HHV-6, and hepatitis B and C viruses.

OTHER PATHOGENS

Latent parasites can become active as a consequence of reductions in cell-mediated immunity. *Pneumocystis jiroveci*, a pathogen common in AIDS, can also result in severe, hypoxic pneumonia in transplant patients. Therefore, during the period of peak immunosuppression, these patients should receive prophylactic trimethoprim–sulfamethoxazole (see Chapter 17). Toxoplasmosis is another latent pathogen that can reactivate in the central nervous system causing brain abscesses and encephalitis (see Chapter 17). Patients with low level *Strongyloides* infection can develop disseminated strongyloidiasis in association with immunosuppression (see Chapter 12). To prevent this often fatal complication, all patients with unexplained eosinophilia should undergo stool sampling and an enzyme-linked immunoabsorbent assay to exclude *Strongyloides* before they receive an organ transplant.

Pathogens Associated with Mixed Deficits Found in Bone Marrow Transplantation

Bone marrow transplantation involves three phases of immunosuppression:

1. **Phase I (days 0 to 30 post transplant)**. During this neutropenic phase, patients are managed in a manner similar to that of other neutropenic patients.
2. **Phase II (days 30 to 100 post transplant)**. During this phase of (primarily) compromised cell-mediated immunity, the patient is managed in a manner similar to that of other organ transplant patients with compromised cell-mediated immunity. Infection with CMV is particularly common at this stage, and acute graft-versus-host disease is also frequently encountered during this period.
3. **Phase III (beyond day 100 post transplant)**. Bone marrow transplant patients often continue to have defects in cell-mediated immunity, plus depressed humoral immunity, resulting in continued susceptibility to CMV, herpes zoster virus, and lymphoproliferative disorders related to infection with Epstein–Barr virus. These patients are also at increased risk of infections with encapsulated *S. pneumoniae* and *H. influenzae* bacteria. Predisposing factors for these infections include functional hyposplenism after total body irradiation, and chronic graft-versus-host disease. This later disorder renders B cells dysfunctional, resulting in decreased production of immunoglobulin G2 (IgG2) and specific pneumococcal antibodies.

KEY POINTS

About Infections Associated with Mixed Deficits Found in Bone Marrow Transplantation

1. Three phases of immunosuppression follow transplantation:
   a) Phase I (days 0 to 30): Neutropenia
   b) Phase II (days 30 to 100): Primarily depressed cell-mediated immunity and graft-versus-host disease
   c) Phase III (beyond day 100): Depressed cell-mediated and humoral immunity, chronic graft-versus-host disease
2. Major infections seen are the same as are seen with neutropenia (early) and solid organ transplant (later).
3. Problems with encapsulated bacteria (*Haemophilus influenzae* and *Streptococcus pneumoniae*) are also a possibility.

Clinicians should have a low threshold of suspicion for starting coverage for encapsulated organisms when these patients develop an worsening of fever, particularly fever accompanied by rigor (see Chapter 6).

DIAGNOSIS AND TREATMENT

Overall Approach in Immunocompromised Hosts

In approaching the febrile compromised host or even a compromised host who has a site of infection, generalizations about the medical urgency required for treatment should be avoided until the patient has been properly classified. **The guiding principle is the type of infecting organism; hence, empiric therapy and the need for urgency is governed chiefly by the type of host compromise. Not every compromised host requires empiric antibiotic therapy.** The questions and algorithm that follow are therefore suggested.

THE FEBRILE NEUTROPENIC PATIENT

If neutropenia is the consequence of recent cytotoxic chemotherapy, then the onset of significant fever (temperature above 38.3°C) warrants emergent diagnostic studies and antibiotic therapy. The progression of infection in neutropenic patients can be rapid, and infection cannot be readily differentiated from noninfectious causes of fever. The usual manifestations of infection are often absent. Skin infections lack erythema, warmth, and purulence. Conventional chest x-ray may appear normal in bacterial pneumonia, and in bacterial meningitis, the cerebrospinal fluid may contain minimal polymorphonuclear leukocytes.

Initial workup for a fever should include

- physical examination looking for sites of infection in lungs, skin, and mucous membranes;
- biopsy and culture of any skin lesions;
- culture of blood, urine, and any other suspicious sites; and
- chest x-ray with high resolution computed tomography. in neutropenic patients with fever, computed tomography may detect infiltrates in half of patients with "normal" conventional radiographs. If an infiltrate is detected, bronchoscopy with lavage should be performed to differentiate among the wide variety of potential pathogens.

Empiric antibiotic therapy should be initiated emergently. The regimen depends on the severity of disease. Low severity is defined as

- a temperature below 39°C and a non-septic appearance;
- an absolute neutrophil and monocyte count below 100/mm3, with neutropenia for less than 7 days and recovery expected by less than 10 days;
- a normal chest x-ray;
- nearly normal liver and renal function;
- no evidence for intravascular device infection;
- malignancy in remission;
- no neurologic deficits;
- no abdominal pain;
- no comorbid conditions (hypotension, vomiting, diarrhea, evidence for deep organ infection); and
- a low severity score (below 21—see Table 16.2).

In these patients, oral antibiotics can be administered. Ciprofloxacin (500 mg twice daily) plus amoxicillin–clavulanate (875 mg twice daily) is the recommended regimen.

Intravenous antibiotics should be given to more severely ill patients who do not meet the above criteria. (Intravenous administration can also be used for low-severity cases.) A number of regimens can be used (see Table 16.3), and all have resulted in comparable response rates and reductions in mortality. The specific empiric regimen must take into account the antibiotic resistance patterns of the local institution and the patient's prior history of infections and antibiotic treatment. Specific doses for each regimen are given in Table 16.3.

In multiple studies, monotherapy has been shown to be comparable to dual therapy. Monotherapy can be initiated with cefepime, imipenem, or piperacillin–

Table 16.2. Scoring Index[a] for Identification of Low-Risk Febrile Neutropenic Patients at the Time of Presentation of Fever

Characteristic	Score
Extent of illness[b]	
No symptoms	5
Mild symptoms	5
Moderate symptoms	3
No hypotension	5
No chronic obstructive pulmonary disease	4
Solid tumor or no fungal infection	4
No dehydration	3
Outpatient at the time fever onset	3
Age below 60 years[c]	2

[a] Highest score is 26. A score of less than 21 indicates low risk for complications and morbidity.

[b] Choose one item only.

[c] Does not apply to children under the age of 16 years.

Hughes WT, Armstrong D, Bodey GP, et al. 2002 Guidelines for the Use of Antimicrobial Agents in Neutropenic Patients with Cancer. *Clin Infect Dis.* 2002;34:730–751.

tazobactam. Dual therapy regimens without vancomycin have all proven to be therapeutically equivalent, and they include cefepime combined with gentamicin, tobramycin, or amikacin; ticarcillin–clavulanate or piperacillin–tazobactam combined with an aminoglycoside; imipenem plus an aminoglycoside; or piperacillin–tazobactam plus ciprofloxacin (see Table 16.2).

A recent study demonstrated reduced toxicity and a suggestion of superior response rates in patients receiving a β-lactam antibiotic combined with ciprofloxacin as compared with a β-lactam combined with an aminoglycoside. When dual therapy is desired, and the patient has not previously received a fluoroquinolone, ciprofloxacin combined with a β-lactam antibiotic should be strongly considered. Aminoglycosides should be avoided if the patient is receiving other nephrotoxic or ototoxic drugs or drugs that cause neuromuscular blockade, or if the patient has significant renal dysfunction.

Vancomycin should not be administered for routine empiric therapy because of the increased risks of selecting for VRE and of nephrotoxicity. A recent meta-analysis revealed that the addition of a glycopeptide as part of empiric therapy did not shorten the febrile episode or reduce mortality in neutropenic patients. But a gly-

Table 16.3. Anti-infective Therapy for Neutropenic Patients

Agent	Dosing (see text for duration)
Parenteral antibiotics, monotherapy	
Cefepime, or	2 g q8h
imipenem, or	500 mg q6h
meropenem, or	1 g q8h
piperacillin–tazobactam	4.5 g q6h
Parenteral antibiotics, dual therapy	
Aminoglycoside, plus	Tobramycin: 5–6 mg/kg first dose; gentamicin: 5–6 mg/kg first dose;
anti-pseudomonal β-lactam, or	amikacin: 15 mg/kg first dose; then dose daily based on levels (for β-lactam dosing, see the above monotherapy section
cefepime, or carbapenem	
Parenteral vancomycin (see text for indications)	
Add vancomycin to monotherapy or dual therapy only if criteria are met	1 g q12h
Oral therapy (low-risk adults only)	
Ciprofloxacin, plus	500 mg q12h
amoxicillin–clavulanate	875 mg q12h
Fungal coverage (see text for indications)	
Caspofungin	70 mg on day 1, then 50 mg daily
Liposomal amphotericin B	5 mg/kg IV daily
Amphotericin B deoxycholate	0.6–1.2 mg/kg IV daily
Voriconazole	400 mg PO q12h, or 6 mg/kg IV q12h on day 1, then 4 mg/kg q12h
Posaconazole	200 mg PO q8h

copeptide antibiotic should be added if an intravascular device infection is suspected, if colonization with methicillin-resistant *S. aureus* is known to exist, if blood cultures are positive for gram-positive cocci before final identification and sensitivity testing, or if the patient is hypotensive or has other evidence of cardiovascular compromise. Linezolid has been shown to be therapeutically equivalent to vancomycin in the neutropenic patient. However, in combination with selective serotonin-reuptake inhibitors, linezolid has been associated with severe myelosuppression in bone marrow transplant patients.

In approximately 30% of cases, blood cultures will be positive, and in the patient with positive blood cultures who becomes afebrile in 3 to 5 days, antibiotic coverage should be adjusted to the least toxic regimen. However, broad-spectrum coverage should be maintained to prevent breakthrough bacteremia. Anti-infective therapy should be continued for a minimum of 7 days. Duration also depends on clinical response and the ability to sterilize the bloodstream. The Infectious Diseases Society of America recommends that antibiotics usually be continued until the neutrophil count rises above 500/mm³.

If the neutropenic patient with a low risk profile becomes afebrile in 3 to 5 days, and if cultures are negative, intravenous antibiotics can be switched to oral ciprofloxacin and amoxicillin–clavulanate. For the high-risk patient, intravenous antibiotics should be continued for a minimum of 7 days and until the neutrophil count rises above 500/mm^3.

If the patient remains febrile after 3 to 5 days, all clinical findings must be re-evaluated. Cultures should be thoroughly reviewed, and a complete physical exam repeated, paying careful attention to skin, mucosal surfaces, and intravenous catheter sites. Additional imaging studies should be considered, depending on the physical findings and the patient's complaints. Antibiotic serum levels (particularly aminoglycosides) should be checked, and cultures should be repeated.

If fever persists for more than 5 days, the patient does not appear septic, no new findings have been uncovered, and the neutrophil count is expected to recover quickly, continue the same antibiotics. However, if clinical worsening or persistent sepsis is noted, the antibiotic regimen should be changed. Switch from monotherapy to dual therapy and consider adding vancomycin if the criteria are appropriate as described earlier. Add antifungal therapy if the neutropenia is expected to persist for more than 5 to 7 days. Several antifungal agents are available: caspofungin or liposomal amphotericin B (amphotericin B deoxycholate is a less expensive, but more toxic alternative) are currently recommended by most experts. Depending on the incidence of aspergillosis and mucormycosis in the specific institution, other agents that can be used are voriconazole and posaconazole (see Table 16.3).

The duration of antibiotic therapy is an important consideration given the fragile nature of bone marrow transplant patient. This decision must be applied in two major instances:

1. **The Afebrile Patient**. If the patient is afebrile after 3 to 5 days of therapy, and if the neutrophil count has been above 500/mm^3 for 2 days, antibiotics can be discontinued after the patient has been afebrile for 48 hours. If the neutrophil count remains below 500/mm^3, and if the patient was initially low-risk and is not currently septic, then antibiotics can be discontinued when the patient has been afebrile for 5 to 7 days. If the patient was initially high-risk, and if the neutrophil count is below 100/mm^3, or if the patient has mucositis or unstable vital signs or other unstable findings, antibiotics should be continued.

2. **The persistently febrile patient**. If the patient continues to have fever despite empiric antibiotic therapy and if the neutrophil count is above 500/mm^3, antibiotics can be discontinued after the neutrophil count has remained at that level for 4 to 5 days. The patient should then be reassessed. Otherwise, if the neutrophil count is below 500/mm^3, the antibiotic therapy should be continued for 2 weeks, with reassessment at that time. Then, if no infection is evident and the patient is

> ### KEY POINTS
> #### About Management of the Neutropenic Patient[1]
>
> 1. Conduct a careful physical examination, especially lungs, perirectal area, and skin. Biopsy new skin lesions.
> 2. Culture all sites, including blood.
> 3. Obtain a chest x-ray. If infiltrate is seen, consider bronchoscopy with lavage.
> 4. Empiric antibiotics can include
>   a) monotherapy with cefepime, imipenem, piperacillin–tazobactam; and
>   b) dual therapy with β-lactam plus an aminoglycoside or a fluoroquinolone.
>   c) Add vancomycin for catheter-related infection or colonization with methicillin-resistant *Staphylococcus aureus*.
> 5. Reassess at 96 hours. If fever persists, add antifungal therapy.
> 6. Outpatient management of fever is increasing in popularity.
> 7. Routine antibiotic prophylaxis in the afebrile non-septic neutropenic patient is not recommended.

clinically stable, antibiotics can be discontinued. Antiviral therapy is not indicated in neutropenic patients unless a specific viral infection is documented.

Antibiotic prophylaxis has been studied in the neutropenic patient, and such therapy was found to reduce the incidence of febrile episodes and to modestly reduce *E. coli* bacteremia in one trial. However, prophylaxis has not been shown to affect mortality. Furthermore, prophylaxis with levofloxacin was associated with significantly higher rates of antimicrobial resistance. Given the modest benefit, and high risk of selecting for antibiotic-resistant pathogens, antibiotic prophylaxis is not recommended.

THE FEBRILE NON-NEUTROPENIC PATIENT

The organisms that can cause infection in the febrile non-neutropenic patient population is so large in number that empiric therapy is *not* recommended unless a specific site of infection is identified or unless, after evaluation, a specific pathogen is thought to be the most likely cause. Even cellulitis may have a nonbacterial origin. However, empiric therapy may be given for central catheter or urinary tract infections, because the usual organisms continue to cause these infections.

Community-acquired infections, both bacterial and viral, are also a problem for susceptible patients, and evaluation of an infectious illness should consider the community context. A thorough history—including details about the onset of the fever, family illnesses, the underlying reason for immunosuppression, and the dose and length of time on immunosuppressive therapy—is therefore important. Patients who have lived in certain geographic areas may experience reactivation of latent infections or succumb to specific infections, such as histoplasmosis in the Ohio River valley or coccidioidomycosis in the Southwest, but none of the specific infections in this patient population requires immediate empiric therapy. Emergent anti-infective therapy is usually not life-saving in this patient population.

Certain sites of infection do require urgent diagnostic action, however:

1. Patients with a headache or other central nervous system complaint should undergo a lumbar puncture if that procedure can be safely performed. Cryptococcal or *Listeria* meningitis are the most urgent diagnoses, and these illnesses require immediate treatment.

2. Blood, urine, and any suspicious sites should be cultured. A urinalysis is helpful because these patients are not neutropenic.

3. An inflamed central line may be treated presumptively for gram-positive infection.

4. If a chest radiograph is abnormal, and if the patient is producing sputum, a sample should be obtained for culture and for Gram, acid-fast, and silver staining. If no sputum is being produced, urgent pulmonary and infectious diseases consultations for a diagnostic evaluation should be requested. Because the number of possible causes of pulmonary infection is so large in this population, empiric therapy is not recommended (unless respiratory failure has begun).

5. If the patient is febrile, but none of the foregoing tests has yielded a diagnosis, an infectious diseases consultation should be sought. The possible entities causing fever in the setting of a negative initial evaluation are so diverse that much time and many resources can easily be wasted.

Although the approach outlined above is most applicable to the transplant population, clinicians must not forget that people receiving corticosteroids represent the greatest number of immunosuppressed patients. Much debate has occurred concerning the lowest dosage of corticosteroid that will predispose to infection. A useful general rule is to assume that any dose above physiologic maintenance may be immunosuppressive. Doses as low as 10 mg daily of prednisone have led to invasive pulmonary aspergillosis. Therefore, when faced with a febrile non-transplant patient on corticosteroids for an inflammatory disorder, the diagnostic points discussed in this subsection should be kept in mind. Also, because immunosuppressive agents may blunt an inflammatory response, clinicians should consider that even low-grade fever may indicate the presence of a serious infection.

Prevention

Given the long-term nature of immunosuppression in graft recipients, preventive measures play a critical role in preventing morbidity and mortality. The recommended preventive measures can be categorized by pathogen type:

- **Bacteria**. In the patient with a documented reduction in IgG level to below 400 mg/dL, intravenous IgG may be given to prevent sinus and pulmonary infections resulting from *S. pneumoniae* infection.

- **Viruses.** CMV remains one of the most significant concerns, and CMV IgG serum titers should be obtained for all transplant patients and donors. If recipient and donor are both negative, prophylaxis is not required. However, all platelet and blood transfusions should be CMV-negative or cleansed of all leukocytes. If the recipient or donor, or both, are CMV–positive. then the patient should receive prophylaxis for the first 100 days with oral valganciclovir (900 mg daily). Because of a lower incidence of disease, preemptive therapy is preferred by many experts for the CMV-positive recipient with a CMV-negative donor. If this strategy is chosen, the patient must undergo periodic screening or quantitative PCR for CMV. If these tests are positive, the patient should be treated with intravenous ganciclovir 5 mg/kg twice daily for 14 to 21 days or oral valganciclovir 900 mg twice during the first 24 hours for induction, and then 900 mg daily.

Another major concern is herpes simplex virus. Anti–herpes simplex IgG titers should be measured in all potential recipients before transplantation. Bone marrow transplant patients with a positive titer should receive prophylaxis during the induction phase and during the first 30 days after transplant (phase I) with either oral valacyclovir (1000 mg twice or three times daily) or oral valganciclovir (900 mg twice daily) if the patient also requires CMV prophylaxis.

Other transplant patients undergoing high-level immunosuppression should also be considered for prophylaxis. Reactivation of varicella virus can lead to serious morbidity and also requires preventive measures. The recipient and all family members should be vaccinated with the live attenuated

KEY POINTS

About the Management of Patients with Depressed Cell-Mediated Immunity

1. Empiric antibiotics are generally *not* recommended.
2. The number of possible organisms is very large.
   a) Samples for biopsy and culture are strongly recommended.
   b) A thorough epidemiologic history is often helpful.
3. Emergent management is required for
   a) central nervous system symptoms such as headache and confusion—consider Cryptococcus and Listeria.
   b) infected central lines—institute empiric antibiotics.
   c) infiltrate on chest radiographs: seek a pulmonary consultation (bronchoscopy is often required).
4. Even low-grade fever in the patient on corticosteroids is a matter of concern.

vaccine at least 4 weeks before the transplant procedure.

- **Fungi.** Allogeneic bone marrow transplant patients have a high incidence of *Candida albicans* infection during phase I and should receive oral fluconazole 400 mg daily or posaconazole (200 mg three times daily) for prophylaxis.

- **Pneumocystis jiroveci.** Throughout the period of immunosuppression, transplant patients are at risk of infection with this organism, and oral trimethoprim–sulfamethoxazole (1 double-strength tablet 3 times weekly, or 1 single-strength tablet daily) is recommended.

PREVENTIVE MEASURES IN SOLID-ORGAN AND BONE MARROW TRANSPLANT PATIENTS

1. *Immunoglobulin G (IgG) should be administered if IgG levels fall below 400 mg/dL.*
2. *Recipients or donors positive for cytomegalovirus should receive valganciclovir.*

3. *Bone marrow recipients with positive IgG titer for herpes simplex virus should receive valacyclovir.*
4. *Vaccine for varicella virus should be given to patients and household contacts before a transplantation procedure,*
5. *Allogeneic transplant patients should receive fluconazole or posaconazole to prevent fungal infections.*
6. *All transplant recipients should receive trimethoprim–sulfamethoxazole to prevent Pneumocystis infection.*

CONCLUSIONS

Continuing advances in the treatment of malignancies and transplantation will maintain a large population of medically compromised hosts. These patients fit into two general categories that predispose them to infections that are usually controlled either by neutrophils or by T cells. Bone marrow or stem-cell transplant patients fit into both categories depending on how much time has passed since transplantation. The febrile neutropenic patient can be considered to be a near medical emergency requiring empiric antibacterial therapy with one or two broad-spectrum antibiotics. Conversely, the patient with suppression of cell-mediated immunity requires a thorough evaluation and empiric antibiotic therapy should be avoided unless the cause of the fever is known on presentation. It is advisable that these patients receive care from infectious disease specialists. Outpatient management of these patients can be expected to become increasingly common.

FURTHER READING

Centers for Disease Control and Prevention (CDC). Chagas disease after organ transplantation—Los Angeles, California, 2006. *MMWR Morb Mortal Wkly Rep.* 2006;55:798–800.

Bliziotis IA, Michalopoulos A, Kasiakou SK, et al. Ciprofloxacin vs an aminoglycoside in combination with a beta-lactam for the treatment of febrile neutropenia: a meta-analysis of randomized controlled trials. *Mayo Clin Proc.* 2005;80:1146–1156.

Bow EJ, Rotstein C, Noskin GA, et al. A randomized, open-label, multicenter comparative study of the efficacy and safety of piperacillin–tazobactam and cefepime for the empirical treatment of febrile neutropenic episodes in patients with hematologic malignancies. *Clin Infect Dis.* 2006;43:447–459.

Bucaneve G, Micozzi A, Menichetti F, et al. Levofloxacin to prevent bacterial infection in patients with cancer and neutropenia. *N Engl J Med.* 2005;353:977–987.

Cornely OA, Maertens J, Winston DJ, et al. Posaconazole vs. fluconazole or itraconazole prophylaxis in patients with neutropenia. *N Engl J Med.* 2007;356:348–359.

Cullen M, Steven N, Billingham L, et al. Antibacterial prophylaxis after chemotherapy for solid tumors and lymphomas. *N Engl J Med.* 2005;353:988–998.

Denning DW, Kibbler CC, Barnes RA. British Society for Medical Mycology proposed standards of care for patients with invasive fungal infections. *Lancet Infect Dis.* 2003;3:230–240.

Fischer SA, Graham MB, Kuehnert MJ, et al. Transmission of lymphocytic choriomeningitis virus by organ transplantation. *N Engl J Med.* 2006;354:2235–2249.

Fishman JA, Rubin RH. Infection in organ-transplant recipients. *N Engl J Med.* 1998;338:1741–1751.

Fukuda T, Boeckh M, Carter RA, et al. Risks and outcomes of invasive fungal infections in recipients of allogeneic hematopoietic stem cell transplants after nonmyeloablative conditioning. *Blood.* 2003;102:827–833.

Hachem RY, Hicks K, Huen A, Raad I. Myelosuppression and serotonin syndrome associated with concurrent use of linezolid and selective serotonin reuptake inhibitors in bone marrow transplant recipients. *Clin Infect Dis.* 2003;37:e8–e11.

Hamour IM, Mittal TK, Bell AD, Banner NR. Reversible sirolimus-associated pneumonitis after heart transplantation. *J Heart Lung Transplant.* 2006;25:241–244.

Hughes WT, Armstrong D, Bodey GP, et al. 2002 Guidelines for the Use of Antimicrobial Agents in Neutropenic Patients with Cancer. *Clin Infect Dis.* 2002;34:730–751.

Jaksic B, Martinelli G, Perez-Oteyza J, Hartman CS, Leonard LB, Tack KJ. Efficacy and safety of linezolid compared with vancomycin in a randomized, double-blind study of febrile neutropenic patients with cancer. *Clin Infect Dis.* 2006; 42:597–607.

Kalil AC, Levitsky J, Lyden E, Stoner J, Freifeld AG. Meta-analysis: the efficacy of strategies to prevent organ disease by cytomegalovirus in solid organ transplant recipients. *Ann Intern Med.* 2005;143:870–880.

Marty FM, Lee SJ, Fahey MM, et al. Infliximab use in patients with severe graft-versus-host disease and other emerging risk factors of non-*Candida* invasive fungal infections in allogeneic hematopoietic stem cell transplant recipients: a cohort study. *Blood.* 2003;102:2768–2776.

Patterson TF, Boucher HW, Herbrecht R, et al. Strategy of following voriconazole versus amphotericin B therapy with other licensed antifungal therapy for primary treatment of invasive aspergillosis: impact of other therapies on outcome. *Clin Infect Dis.* 2005;41:1448–1452.

Raad, II, Escalante C, Hachem RY, et al. Treatment of febrile neutropenic patients with cancer who require hospitalization: a prospective randomized study comparing imipenem and cefepime. *Cancer.* 2003;98:1039–1047.

Rolston KV, Manzullo EF, Elting LS, et al. Once daily, oral, outpatient quinolone monotherapy for low-risk cancer patients with fever and neutropenia: a pilot study of 40 patients based on validated risk-prediction rules. *Cancer.* 2006;106:2489–2494.

Sipsas NV, Bodey GP, Kontoyiannis DP. Perspectives for the management of febrile neutropenic patients with cancer in the 21st century. *Cancer.* 2005;103:1103–1113.

Vardakas KZ, Samonis G, Chrysanthopoulou SA, Bliziotis IA, Falagas ME. Role of glycopeptides as part of initial empirical treatment of febrile neutropenic patients: a meta-analysis of randomised controlled trials. *Lancet Infect Dis.* 2005;5:431–439.

Viscoli C, Varnier O, Machetti M. Infections in patients with febrile neutropenia: epidemiology, microbiology, and risk stratification. *Clin Infect Dis.* 2005;40(Suppl 4):S240–S245.

Walsh TJ, Pappas P, Winston DJ, et al. Voriconazole compared with liposomal amphotericin B for empirical antifungal therapy in patients with neutropenia and persistent fever. *N Engl J Med.* 2002;346:225–234.

Wisplinghoff H, Seifert H, Wenzel RP, Edmond MB. Current trends in the epidemiology of nosocomial bloodstream infections in patients with hematological malignancies and solid neoplasms in hospitals in the United States. *Clin Infect Dis.* 2003;36:1103–1110.

HIV Infection

Time Recommended to Complete: 3 days

Bernard Herschel, M.D.

GUIDING QUESTIONS

1. How is HIV primarily transmitted, and how do genital ulcers increase the risk of HIV transmission?

2. Which cells does the HIV virus primarily infect?

3. What are the symptoms and signs of primary HIV infection?

4. What is the preferred test for diagnosis of HIV, and how is AIDS defined?

5. What is meant by the term "the window period"?

6. How is HIV activity monitored?

7. What is the CD4 count below which the host begins to experience opportunistic infections?

8. What are the indications for initiating antiretroviral therapy?

9. What are the goals for therapy, and what are the factors that increase the risk of developing resistance?

POTENTIAL SEVERITY

Management of HIV is challenging and complex. The associated opportunistic infections are often difficult to diagnose and frequently life-threatening.

EPIDEMIOLOGY

Having originated in Eastern Africa between 1910 and 1950, by transmission of a precursor virus from a chimpanzee, HIV infection has now spread across the world. Sub-Saharan Africa remains the epicenter of the epidemic: 3 to 4 million new infections occur annually, 30 million Africans are living with HIV, and more than 10 million have already died. Uganda alone has lost 2.5 million people to AIDS: 300 to 400 deaths daily, every day from 1985 to 2006, in a country with a population of 20 million. In the sub-Saharan countries, transmission occurs predominantly by heterosexual intercourse, with as many women as men being infected. On average, infected women are younger than infected men, but overall, the most productive age strata is where the infection predominates, contributing to the disastrous socioeconomic impact of the AIDS epidemic.

The problems of North America and Western Europe pale in comparison with those of Africa. Nonetheless, the number of HIV-infected people living in the United States has reached almost 1 million. Incidence figures are difficult to determine, because most newly acquired infections are not diagnosed. Judging from the number of first positive tests (which may be the result of an infection acquired years earlier), infection rates declined during the 1990s, reaching a plateau around 1998. Some reports claim that infections have increased slightly since 1998, perhaps because of an increase in sexual-risk taking linked to a false sense of security created by the existence of highly active antiretroviral therapy (HAART). However, by decreasing viremia, HAART may also be having a positive effect on transmission of HIV.

The probability of acquiring an HIV infection varies depending on the type of exposure. Transfusion with a unit of HIV-infected blood is almost certain to infect the recipient. In the absence of treatment, the child of an HIV-positive mother has about a 30% chance of

---

KEY POINTS

About the Epidemiology of HIV Infection

1. Highest incidence is found in Africa where the virus originated:
   a) New infections occur at a rate of 3 to 4 million annually.
   b) About 30 million are living with AIDS.
   c) Transmission is mainly heterosexual, with the incidence in men and women being about equal.
2. North America and Europe have lower incidences and prevalences:
   a) Prevalence in the United States approaches 1 million.
   b) Incidence has increased slightly since 1998 because of a change in attitude caused by highly active antiretroviral therapy.
3. Risk of HIV infection is
   a) very high with a contaminated blood transfusion.
   b) about 1 in 300 for a needle stick.
   c) about 30% for a child of an untreated infected mother.
   d) about 0.01% to 1% for vaginal or anal intercourse. Genital ulcers increase risk by a factor of 10; condoms prevent transmission. Circumcision reduces risk by 50%.
4. Preventive measures are far more cost-effective than treatment.

---

infection. The chance of acquiring an infection after a needle-stick injury involving infected bodily fluids is about 1 in 300. Most infections occur with sexual exposure, the primary determinant of infectivity being the level of viremia, which is particularly elevated during primary HIV infection. Local genital factors modulate that risk. Inflammation such as may be caused by sexually transmitted diseases attracts lymphocytes. In an infected person, these may harbor HIV, and in the recipient, they may provide a reservoir of cells vulnerable to HIV infection. Recently, circumcision was found to reduce a man's risk of contracting HIV by approximately 50%.

Depending on the level of viremia, the risk of HIV infection varies from roughly 1% to 0.01% for each act of vaginal or anal intercourse. Compared with infection rates for other sexually transmitted diseases, this risk is quite low, although in the presence of genital ulcers, infection rates as high as 10% have been reported. These rates

compare with rates of infection of 20% to 40% after exposure to syphilis or gonorrhea. Nonetheless, repeated sexual exposure—as occurs in a serodiscordant couple—entails substantial risk, typically reaching 1% per month. The risk is likely higher during the first months of a sexual partnership than later. Indeed, some studies show an HIV-specific, potentially protective cellular immune response in seronegative sexual partners of seropositive individuals. However, absence of infection in the past is no guarantee for the future: increasing immune deficiency and viremia are part of the natural history of untreated HIV infection, and they carry with them an increased risk of transmission.

Anal and vaginal intercourse are approximately equally effective in transmitting HIV. Some (but not all) studies have found that the risk of transmission from an HIV-infected man to a woman is higher than the reverse. Compared with vaginal or anal intercourse, oral sex is certainly much less risky—specifically, it is too low to be quantified. However, any sizable HIV center encounters examples of transmission by oral sex. Condoms are effective in preventing transmission. Transmission has never been observed in a large series of couples who declared "always" to have used condoms. However, perfect compliance with condom use, and avoidance of slippage and breakage is difficult to achieve in practice.

Preventive efforts have had varying success:

- Transmission of HIV infection through infected blood products has almost been eliminated. Rare cases may still occur (less than 1 transmission in 500,000 blood transfusions) if blood is donated during the "window period."
- Use of antiretroviral therapy in the mother has the potential to decrease mother-to-child transmission from more than 30% to less than 1%. Such transmission has now become very rare in Western Europe and the United States, and is almost always the result of some procedural failure.
- Needle exchange programs and methadone or even heroin substitutions have reduced the incidence of HIV infection in intravenous drug users by more than 90%.
- As noted earlier, condoms are effective in decreasing HIV transmission, particularly in stable couples. Incidence rates of HIV have declined in homosexual communities that practice safer sex. The decrease in the prevalence of HIV may also have contributed to a reduced rate of infection among younger homosexual men, even without necessarily perfect adherence to safer-sex guidelines. Among both homosexual and heterosexual communities, some subgroups continue high-risk practices, with a concomitant high incidence of sexually transmitted diseases and HIV. From 1999 to 2004, several instances of small epidemics of syphilis were reported in Dublin, Bristol, Baltimore,

Paris, and California. Interestingly, these epidemics were nowhere accompanied by a rise in HIV infections. As noted earlier, the explanation for this seeming paradox may lie in the protective effect of HAART.

When contemplating the use of scarce resources to fight HIV infection, it is important to realize that prevention is much more cost-effective than cure. Even with unrealistically favorable assumptions regarding the efficacy and costs of HAART, costs per life–year saved are 20 to 100 times lower for condoms than for anti-retroviral treatment. But it is the sick who are crying for help, not the healthy who are crying for condoms . . . .

PATHOGENESIS

The primary targets of the human immunodeficiency virus are probably the dendritic cells in the mucosa of the genital tract. The virus uses a specific receptor called DC-SIGN to attach to those cells. The dendritic cells then transport HIV into lymph nodes, where the virus infects lymphocytes.

The receptors for HIV are mainly the CD4 molecules on the surface of a sub-population of T lymphocytes. A co-receptor is also necessary for infection. Viruses that preferentially interact with the co-receptor CCR5 are called "R5 viruses" (or "monocytotropic," or "nonsyn-cytium–inducing"), and they predominate in early infection. Later on, HIV often acquires the capacity to interact with the CXCR4 receptor; such viruses are called "X4" ("syncytium-inducing," or "lymphocy-totropic"). The CD4 lymphocytes whose T-cell receptor is specific for HIV proteins proliferate and are preferentially infected. This preferential infection (followed by destruction) may explain the specific deficiency of immunity to HIV as described next.

More than 98% of lymphocytes are localized in the lymph nodes and spleen. Nonetheless, the viruses produced by the newly HIV-infected lymphocytes flood the blood and are transported into all tissues within a matter of days. Viremia reaches high levels—up to millions of HIV genomes per cubic millimeter. During this time, many patients become symptomatic with fever, skin lesions, pharyngitis, and swollen lymph nodes. This self-limiting disease (Figure 17.1), lasting usually a few days to a few weeks, is called "primary HIV infection," "acute retroviral syndrome," or "seroconversion syndrome." Then, the immune response kicks in; antibodies directed against HIV appear in the blood, and cytotoxic T cells specific for HIV-infected cells proliferate. This HIV immune response rapidly achieves partial control of the HIV infection. Viremia levels decrease by several orders of magnitude, stabilizing at a lower level, called "plateau level." This level can vary from fewer than 50 to several hundred thousand copies of HIV RNA per cubic millimeter, and it correlates closely with further evolution toward immune deficiency: the higher the level, the faster the development of AIDS.

A progressive reduction in the level of CD4 T cells is the hallmark of HIV-induced immune deficiency. A fall from the normal level of approximately 1000 CD4 cells per cubic millimeter occurs during acute HIV infection. After seroconversion, the level of CD4 lymphocytes again rises, but rarely returns to normal. Later, during the chronic phase of HIV infection, a progressive annual loss of about 70 cells per cubic millimeter occurs. However, the speed at which immune deficiency progresses is extremely variable. In rare individuals, AIDS may appear as early as 1 or 2 years after infection. An incubation period of 10 years is more typical, but occasionally other

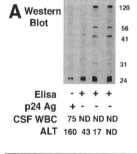

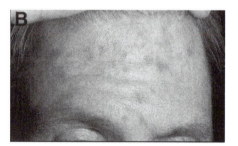

Figure 17–1. Acute retroviral syndrome with seroconversion (from www.aids-images.ch;). **A.** Appearance of bands on successive Western blots. Note the negative enzyme-linked immunoabsorbent assay (ELISA) and early positive *p24* antigen (Ag), plus the pleocytosis in the cerebrospinal fluid (CSF) and elevated serum transaminase level. **B.** Acneiform lesions can develop. **C.** Macules on the chest. **D.** Ulceration in the oral cavity (arrow). *See color image on color plate 3*

A Western Blot			120
			56
			41
			31
			24
Elisa	−	+	+ +
p24 Ag	+	−	− −
CSF WBC	75	ND	ND ND
ALT	160	43	17 ND

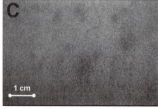

1 cm

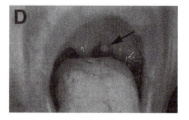

patients, called "long-term nonprogressors" or "elite controllers," show no evidence of damage to the immune system at all. These nonprogressors survive many years with low viremia and a normal number of CD4 cells.

An enormous amount of research has been conducted to find factors that influence the rate of progression. A number of genetic traits are thought to correlate with faster or slower development of immune deficiency. Age at the time of infection also plays a role: the older the individual, the more likely it is that progression will be rapid. (The late fetal and perinatal period is an exception; HIV acquired neonatally may progress very rapidly.) Unfortunately, neither age nor genetic inheritance is easily changed, and no easily influenced factors for progression ("Drink carrot juice, and you'll never get AIDS") has been found so far.

The CD4 cells are the conductors of the immunologic orchestra; they are critical for some of its most important functions, including development of specific CD8 T cell cytotoxic responses, and production of neutralizing antibodies. When the number of CD4 cells declines below a critical level of about $200/\mu m^3$, the "AIDS defining diseases" start to appear. The list

of these diseases (see Table 17.1) is relatively short: *Pneumocystis jiroveci* pneumonia (PCP) rather than aspergillosis, Kaposi's sarcoma and lymphoma rather than tumors of other types. Some of these infections—for example, PCP—are highly suggestive of HIV infection; others—pneumococcal pneumonia, *Candida* stomatitis, and tuberculosis—also occur in patients with normal immune systems or with immune deficiencies caused by conditions other than AIDS. Most of the opportunistic diseases are caused by reactivation of latent herpes viruses [for example, cerebral lymphoma resulting from Epstein–Barr virus, or retinitis from cytomegalovirus (CMV)], by fungi (PCP), or by bacteria (tuberculosis). Other infections—such as salmonellosis or cryptococcosis—may be newly acquired.

As described earlier, the nascent HIV immune response controls the runaway viral proliferation observed during acute HIV infection. How can the eventual failure of this immune response be explained?

Despite thousands of papers written on the subject, a clear answer is not currently available. The long-term nonprogressors tend to have a vigorous HIV-specific cytotoxic immune response, but overlap with populations showing progression is considerable. The role of antibodies to HIV is also unclear; individual cases show no clear correlation between the existence of neutralizing antibodies and progression. Attention has recently shifted to the nonspecific components of the immune system such as natural killer cells and toll-like receptors. The extreme mutability of HIV leads to the emergence of HIV quasispecies that are no longer recognized by the immune response (the "immune escape phenomenon"). In addition, HIV preferentially infects proliferating lymphocytes, but the lymphocytes that proliferate in response to HIV infection are precisely those whose receptors recognize HIV-derived peptides. Infection of these lymphocytes eventually leads to their destruction.

Effective therapy reverses most of the immune deficiency. Given enough time, recovery of the CD4 cell count occurs even in patients who have practically no cells left when treatment starts. Cell counts continue to increase for several years, finally reaching a plateau of 500 to $1000/\mu m^3$. The immune response to the most important pathogens recovers, as can be seen by the disappearance of opportunistic diseases. But one exception remains: the immune response to HIV itself stays deficient even after successful treatment.

In North America and Western Europe, most patients come to medical attention during the latent or plateau period of chronic HIV infection, when clinical signs and symptoms are rare or absent. Nonetheless, the infection remains active, with the production of 10^9 to 10^{11} viral particles daily. At the

Table 17.1. Indicator Conditions in the Case Definition of AIDS in Adults[a]

Condition	n (%)
Candidiasis of esophagus, trachea, bronchi, or lungs	3846 (16)
Cervical cancer, invasive	144 (0.6)
Coccidioidomycosis, extrapulmonary	74 (0.3)
Cryptococcosis, extrapulmonary	1168 (5)
Cryptosporidiosis with diarrhea for more than 1 month	314 (1.3)
Cytomegalovirus of any organ other than liver, spleen, or lymph nodes; or of eye	1638 (7)
Herpes simplex with mucocutaneous ulcer for more than 1 month, or bronchitis, pneumonitis, or esophagitis	1250 (5)
Histoplasmosis, extrapulmonary	208 (0.9)
HIV-associated dementia (disabling cognitive or other dysfunction interfering with occupation or activities of daily living)	1196 (5)
HIV-associated wasting [involuntary loss of more than 10% of baseline weight, plus chronic diarrhea (2 or more loose stools daily for 30 days or more), or chronic weakness and documented enigmatic fever for 30 days or more]	4212 (18)
Isospora belli infection with diarrhea for more than 1 month	22 (0.1)
Kaposi's sarcoma	1500 (7)
Lymphoma:	
Burkitt's	162 (0.7)
Immunoblastic	518 (2.3)
Primary central nervous system	170 (0.7)
Mycobacterium avium, disseminated	1124 (5)
Mycobacterium tuberculosis	
Pulmonary	1621 (7)
Extrapulmonary	491 (2)
Nocardiosis	– (<1)
Pneumocystis jiroveci pneumonia	9145 (38)
Pneumonia, recurrent bacterial (2 or more episodes in 12 months)	1347 (5)
Progressive multifocal leukoencephalopathy	213 (1)
Salmonella septicemia (non-typhoid), recurrent	68 (0.3)
Strongyloidiasis, extraintestinal	None
Toxoplasmosis of internal organ	1073 (4)
Wasting syndrome because of HIV	1980 (18)

[a] The listed numbers and percentages indicate the frequencies of occurrence in the database of the Swiss HIV cohort study, an ongoing registry of more than 11,000 patients.

same time, several billion CD4 cells are destroyed and replaced each day. Production of 10^{11} viral particles daily provides the potential for a mutation at every single nucleotide position. Unsurprisingly, under the selective pressure of a partially effective immune response or partially effective therapy, resistant mutations rapidly emerge. To obtain a durable antiviral effect, several drugs must be combined to completely abolish viral production. Once this goal is achieved, emergence of resistance becomes much less likely, and in those circumstances, patients may be treated for many years without viral breakthrough. Nonetheless, the virus persists in reservoirs that are not accessible to current treatment. These reservoirs may include nonproductive infection in pools of long-lived lymphocytes. Sensitive molecular techniques suggest that the half-life of this type of reservoir may reach several years, making eradication by continuous treatment unrealistic.

CLINICAL MANIFESTATIONS OF PRIMARY HIV INFECTION

The incubation period for symptomatic infection is 2 to 4 weeks, but can be as prolonged as 10 weeks. Onset of fever can be abrupt and is associated with diffuse lymphadenopathy and pharyngitis. The throat is usually erythematous, without exudates or enlarged tonsils. Painful ulcers can develop in the oral and genital mucosa (Figure 17.1). Gastrointestinal complaints are common, with many patients experiencing nausea, anorexia, and diarrhea. A skin rash often begins 2 to 3 days after the onset of fever and usually involves the face, neck, and upper torso. The lesions are small pink-to-red macules or maculopapules (Figure 17.1). Headache is another prominent symptom, and aseptic meningitis is noted in about one quarter of patients. Headache is often retro-orbital and worsened by eye movement. Findings in the cerebrospinal fluid (CSF) are consistent with viral meningitis: lymphocytes, normal glucose, and mildly elevated protein. Guillain–Barré syndrome and palsy of the VIIth cranial nerve have been reported. Peripheral leukocyte count may be normal or slightly below normal, with a decrease in CD4 lymphocytes and an increase in CD8 lymphocytes (the CD4:CD8 ratio is commonly below 1.0). Liver transaminase values may be moderately elevated. The illness is self-limiting, with severe symptoms usually resolving over 2 weeks. Lethargy and fatigue may persist for several months.

KEY POINTS

About the Clinical Manifestation of Primary HIV Infection

1. Abrupt onset of fever 2 to 4 weeks after exposure.
2. Accompanied by
   a) non-exudative pharyngitis and lymphadenitis.
   b) maculopapular skin rash on the head, neck, and upper torso.
   c) headache and aseptic meningitis.
   d) anorexia, nausea, diarrhea.
3. The acute illness lasts 2 to 6 weeks. Lethargy and fatigue can persist for several months.

■ LABORATORY EVALUATION OF HIV INFECTION

DIAGNOSIS

Infection with HIV is diagnosed by the detection of HIV-specific antibodies in plasma or serum. These antibodies appear a few weeks after infection, shortly before or after the symptoms of the acute retroviral syndrome. From studies in which the date of infection is precisely known (for instance, in individuals infected by a blood transfusion), the delay to the appearance of antibodies can be determined: about 5% of patients seroconvert within 7 days, 50% within 20 days, and more than 95% within 90 days. Therefore, a period exists (called the "window period") during which, although the patient is infected, antibodies cannot be detected in the plasma. For a few days, the HIV-specific p24 antigen is detectable alone, without antibodies [Figure 17.1(A)]. Therefore, screening tests now combine the detection of antigen and antibody. Gene amplification tests [polymerase chain reaction (PCR), as well as other hybridization techniques] for the detection of viral genomes should not be used for early diagnosis. They are much more expensive than the antibody tests. Antibody tests remain positive for the lifetime of HIV-infected people, except possibly in very rare cases when treatment was started before seroconversion.

Antibody tests for HIV are among the most reliable of all medical tests, with specificity and sensitivity largely exceeding 99%. Nonetheless, in view of the importance of the diagnosis and the possibility of clerical errors (mislabeled tubes and such), confirmation of the diagnosis by a second blood sample is recommended. Confirmation is especially important when the pre-test probability is low, raising the proportion of false positive results.

True false-positives are much rare than "Indeterminate" test results. An indeterminate result arises when substances in the patient's plasma interact with impurities in the HIV antigen preparations. Usually, the color reaction of the enzyme-linked immunoabsorbent assay is above the threshold for positivity, but much below the results of a routine positive test. To diminish these indeterminate reactions, manufacturers are using recombinant technology to purify the HIV protein. In the presence of an indeterminate test, and particularly in the absence of risk factors for HIV infection, the patient should be reassured that the result is negative, with the negativity confirmed by a second test using a different method. Such a method might involve use of the Western blot. In a Western blot test, the HIV proteins are first separated by electrophoresis and then blotted onto a nitrocellulose membrane (Figure 17.1). This membrane is incubated with a dilution of the patient's serum. Specific antibodies fix to the respective HIV proteins, producing a colored band after a coloring reaction. The position of the band permits a deduction concerning whether the reaction is nonspecific or the result of an HIV-specific protein.

CLASSIFICATION

The stages of HIV infection are defined by clinical events and by CD4 lymphocyte count (Table 17.2). This classi-fi-cation, established in 1992, indicates clearly the immuno-suppression and symptomatic status of the patient.

The meaning of the word "AIDS" is not the same on both sides of the Atlantic. In the United States, every person with a CD4 count below $200/\mu m^3$ is considered to have AIDS (shaded area in Table 17.2); alternatively, patients may be considered to have AIDS if they have an AIDS defining opportunistic infection (Table 17.1). In Europe, the CD4 count does not enter into the definition of AIDS, which remains synonymous with the occurrence of an opportunistic disease as those defined in Table 17.1. The stage of HIV infection is defined by the CD4 lymphocyte count (biologic stage 1, 2, or 3) and clinical events (A, B, or C). Occurrence of a type C disease defines AIDS. In addition, in the United States, AIDS is also defined by a CD4 count below $200/\mu m^3$ (categories C1, C2, C3, A3, or B3).

Table 17.2. Stages of HIV Infection

CD4 cell category	Patients (%)	Clinical category		
		A^a	B^b	C^c
		Asymptomatic, or PGL, or acute HIV infection	Symptomatic (not A or C)	AIDS indicator conditions (1987)
1) $>500/\mu m^3$	($\geq$29)	A1	B1	C1
2) $200–499/\mu m^3$	(14–28)	A2	B2	C2
3) $<200/\mu m^3$	(<14)	A3	B3	C3

[a] Clinical signs associated with stage A are primary HIV infection, persistent generalized lymphadenopathy (PGL), or lack of symptoms (asymptomatic patients).

[b] Clinical signs and symptoms associated with stage B are oral candidiasis, relapsing vaginal candidiasis, herpes zoster, localized neoplasia of the cervix, any other clinical manifestations not defined by categories A and C.

[c] Corresponds to the occurrence of an "AIDS-defining opportunistic disease" as listed in Table 17.1.

[d] Dark shaded areas designate the stages of illness that are defined as AIDS in the United States.

TREATMENT AND PROGNOSIS

Monitoring Tests

Infection with HIV has been likened to a train speeding towards a wreck: the speed corresponds to the level of viremia, and the distance to the site of the wreck corresponds to the CD4 count.

To determine viral load, genomic tests are now almost universally used. These tests measure HIV genomes per cubic millimeter of plasma. Because the genomes consist of RNA, the RNA first has to be transcribed into DNA, which is then amplified, most often by PCR. Patients with untreated HIV infection typically have 500 to 1 million copies of HIV RNA per cubic millimeter; with treatment, this number declines to undetectability. Depending on the test being used, "undetectability" means fewer than 5 to 50 copies of HIV RNA. Ideally, after 2 to 6 months of treatment, all patients on modern antiretroviral therapy should have fewer than 50 copies of HIV RNA per cubic millimeter.

Many studies have shown that the long-term prognosis for untreated HIV infection depends on the viremia. However, within this broad correlation, large inter-individual variations occur, with patients remaining in good health for many years despite viremia exceeding 100,000 copies per cubic millimeter.

For short-term prognosis, the CD4 count is more useful. The occurrence of opportunistic infections and tumors is unusual with CD4 counts above $200/\mu m^3$. Below this value, the incidence of such infections rises exponentially. It is very unusual for patients to die of AIDS with CD4 counts above $50/\mu m^3$.

Antiretroviral Resistance Tests

Although antiretroviral combination therapy is effective in most patients, resistance may occur, and treatment may need to be adjusted. To guide the choice of therapy, tests measuring antiretroviral resistance have been developed.

KEY POINTS

About Tests for HIV Drug Resistance

1. Genotype testing detects specific mutations and is used to predict resistance.
2. Phenotype testing inserts viral genes into a standardized viral strain and measures sensitivities. It is time consuming and expensive.
3. Testing may allow ineffective drugs to be discontinued.

Two types of tests are currently in use:

1. **Genotypic tests.** Determine the sequence of the relevant viral genes: the reverse transcriptase, protease, gp-41, and integrase genes. The sequence shows the presence or absence of mutations that are associated with antiretroviral resistance. However, with rare exceptions, the occurrence of a specific mutation does not predict a specific resistance phenotype. Rather, the combination of many mutations must be considered. A prediction of resistance from such a combination of mutations has been marketed as a "virtual phenotype."
2. **Phenotypic tests.** Excise the relevant gene from amplified patient virus and insert the excised portion into a standard virus of known growth properties. This recombinant virus is then exposed to various drugs and its resistance is ascertained. Phenotypic tests are more expensive than genotypic tests, and they take 1 to 3 weeks to complete.

The value and use of resistance tests are subjects of continuing controversy. It has been difficult to show that they improve the outcome of treatment, but they may allow ineffective drugs to be discontinued, thus sparing side effects and costs. The use of resistance testing is further discussed in the subsection on HIV therapy later in this chapter.

Caveats Regarding Laboratory Tests

Modern antiretroviral treatment would be impossible without the use of laboratory tests. However, physicians

---

KEY POINTS

About Tests for Monitoring Treatment and Prognosis

1. Level of viremia correlates with speed of progression; copies of HIV RNA per cubic millimeter is usually measured by polymerase chain reaction.
2. The number of copies of HIV RNA per cubic millimeter varies from 500 to 1 million; treatment should reduce that number to below 50 within 6 months.
3. "Undetectable" levels of HIV RNA vary depending on the sensitivity of the test used; individual tests vary by a factor of 2.
4. A CD4 count below $200/\mu m^3$ puts the patient at risk of opportunistic infections and tumors.
5. The CD4 count varies by 10% to 30% between counts.

---

and patients need to be aware of the limits of the tests and, in particular, of the need to avoid over-interpretation of small changes. The precision of measurements of viral load is only about 0.3 log (a factor of 2). This means that values of 200 and 400 copies per cubic millimeter may actually be the same. Another problem with the interpretation of HIV viremia is the expression "undetectable" viremia. Detectability depends on the assay used. Experimental assays with sensitivities as low as 1 or 3 copies per cubic millimeter actually show viremia in almost all patients who have started their treatment during chronic HIV infection. Whether viremia that is very low (for example, fewer than 10 copies per cubic millimeter) is better for the patient than viremia that is detectable but between 10 and 50 copies per cubic millimeter is unknown.

In patients with viremia that is low on treatment, some values may nonetheless exceed 50 or 100 copies from time to time. These "blips" of viremia are of no great prognostic significance, and they should not prompt a change in treatment. On the other hand, values that rise above 500 copies per cubic millimeter are clearly predictive of subsequent resistance and escape.

Similarly, the CD4 count is not a precise measure. It results from the multiplication of two percentages (the percentage of lymphocytes among leukocytes and the percentage of CD4-positive lymphocytes among all lymphocytes). The number of lymphocytes varies during the day, depending on food intake, physical activity, and steroid levels, among other factors. In addition, laboratories and lab technicians vary in their interpretation of the morphology of leukocytes. Therefore, CD4 counts may vary as much as 10% to 30% when counts are repeated at frequent intervals within the same individual.

■ MODERN ANTI-HIV THERAPY

INTRODUCTION

The Ten Principles
of Antiretroviral Treatment

Since 1996, treatment with HAART, consisting usually of two nucleoside reverse-transcriptase inhibitors (NRTIs) plus an HIV protease inhibitor (PI), has been widely used. These regimens produced durable suppression of viral replication, with undetectable plasma levels of HIV RNA, in more than half of treated patients. Immunity recovered, and morbidity and mortality fell by more than 80%. Treatment was thought to be particularly effective when started early; HAART was therefore recommended for essentially all HIV-infected people willing to commit themselves to lifelong therapy.

But besides these successes, HAART also produced problems. Present-day drugs do not eradicate HIV, and often, patients cannot comply with long-term combination treatment. Moreover, HAART causes unexpected and ill-understood side effects. The dogma of earliest possible treatment has therefore come under attack.

Table 17.3 summarizes the Ten Principles governing antiretroviral treatment. Starting and maintaining HAART is complex. Within the last few years, the numbers of antiretroviral agents, of their known and potential interactions with each other and with non-HIV drugs, and of their side effects have all increased exponentially. Usually, a physician specializing in HIV care should be consulted whenever HAART is started or changed. It is this specialist's job to guarantee that the treatment chosen is optimal for the particular patient. Mismanagement of antiretroviral therapy can lead to untoward toxicities and the development of resistant viruses that can no longer be treated.

CAVEATS ABOUT HAART

A physician specializing HIV should be consulted whenever highly active antiretroviral therapy (HAART) is started or changed.
   Mismanagement of antiretroviral therapy can lead to untoward toxicities and resistant viruses.

Indications for Starting Treatment

The patient's CD4 count indicates the degree of immune deficiency and predicts short-term risk of opportunistic disease. Without treatment, that risk is less than 1% per year when the CD4 count is above $500/mm^3$, but rises to 30% when the CD4 count falls below $100/\mu m^3$. In the long term, prognosis is also determined by the viral load—that is, the number of HIV RNA copies per cubic millimeter of plasma. An elevated viral load predicts a more rapid progression toward AIDS in population-based studies, although inter-individual variations are enormous. The destruction by HIV of CD4 cells and lymph node architecture causes progressive immunodeficiency. Antiretroviral treatment suppresses viral replication, prevents further destruction of the immune system, and even allows for considerable repair in patients who start treatment while already immunosuppressed.

Treatment must be adapted to the patient, taking into account the speed of progression, acceptance of treatment by the patient, the likelihood of compliance, and possible side effects. The recommendations presented in Table 17.4

Table 17.3. Ten Principles for Highly Active Antiretroviral Therapy

1. Indication	The presence of HIV infection establishes theoretically the indication for treatment, but treatment does not usually start until subclinical immune deficiency is apparent.
2. Combination	Antiretroviral treatment consists of at least three drugs.
3. First chance = best chance	The choice of drugs during a first treatment course determines which possibilities remain when a second and different treatment becomes necessary later on. Chances for success are best first. Later on, alternatives are limited by selection of resistant mutants.
4. Complexity	Antiretroviral treatment is complex, in particular because of drug interactions and side effects.
5. Resistance	Selection of resistant quasispecies occurs frequently. Within substance classes, cross-resistance is complete among available non-nucleoside reverse transcriptase inhibitors, and partial among protease inhibitors, and nucleoside reverse transcriptase inhibitors.
6. Information	Starting and maintaining effective antiretroviral treatment is time-consuming, because the information needs of physician and patients are considerable.
7. Motivation and compliance	The patient's willingness to take the drugs regularly at prescribed times and dosages will largely determine the success of treatment. Patients must understand the relationship between insufficient compliance and drug resistance.
8. Monitoring	Efficacy of antiretroviral treatment is established by regular measures of viral RNA and of CD4 counts.
9. Goals of treatment	The goal of treatment is durable suppression of viral RNA below 50 copies per cubic millimeter of plasma. Such suppression minimizes selection of resistant mutants and assists in immune reconstitution and avoidance of morbidity and mortality.
10. Studies	Antiretroviral treatment continues to evolve toward greater simplicity and efficacy. Patients should be encouraged to participate in clinical studies that aim to optimize therapy.

Table 17.4. Indications for Starting Antiretroviral Treatment

Clinical stage Acute HIV infection	Laboratory values Irrelevant	Recommendations Consider HAART, obtain specialized consultation	
	CD4 count	**Viral load**	
		<50,000	**>50,000**
Chronic asymptomatic	>500	Wait	Wait
HIV infection	350–500	Wait	Consider HAART
(stage A)	<350	Treat	Treat
Symptomatic chronic	Irrelevant	Treat	
HIV infection			
(stage B or C)			

HAART = highly active antiretroviral therapy.

Table 17.5. Potential Advantages and Disadvantages of Early Antiretroviral Treatment

Possible advantages	Possible disadvantages
Maximal suppression of viral replication; as a consequence, lesser risk of selection of resistant mutants	Risk of resistance as a consequence of suboptimal compliance
Prevention of immune deficiency and more complete immune reconstitution	Duration of efficacy of treatment may be limited
Less risk of side effects in patients whose general state of health is excellent	Loss of quality of life through short-term side effects, and possible long-term toxicity
	Cost
Healthy carriers are less contagious when treated (Lesser number of new infections?)	Transmission of new infections with drug-resistant viruses

are therefore only approximations, because individual factors, although often decisive, do not lend themselves to abstractions in a table. Table 17.5 outlines the advantages and disadvantages of an early start to treatment.

TIMING OF ANTIRETROVIRAL THERAPY

The course of HIV infection has been compared to a train speeding toward a wreck. The patient's CD4 count represents the distance to the site of the wreck, and the viral load represents the train's speed. In the absence of symptoms, those two factors are used to determine the timing of antiretroviral therapy so as to prevent AIDS.

Four different classes of drugs are currently available:

1. The Nucleoside reverse transcriptase inhibitors (NRTIs), such as abacavir (ABC), didanosine (ddI), emtricitabine (FTC), lamivudine (3TC), stavudine (d4T), tenofovir (TDF), and zidovudine (AZT)
2. The non-nucleoside reverse-transcriptase inhibitors (NNRTIs), such as efavirenz (EFV) and nevirapine (NVP)
3. The PIs, such as amprenavir (APV), darunavir (DRV), indinavir (IDV), lopinavir/ritonavir (LPV/r), nelfinavir (NFV), ritonavir (RTV), and saquinavir (SQV) and tipranavir (TPV)
4. The fusion inhibitor enfurvitide.

Two further classes of drugs are in advanced stages of development and may become available during 2007-08:

the inhibitors of the CCR5 receptor (maraviroc a promising candidate) and the integrase inhibitors (MK-0518).

Optimal suppression of viral replication requires a regimen to whcih HIV can only become resistant with multiple mutatons. At the present time, no single drug (with the possible exception of the ritonavir-boosted protease inhibitors) fulfills this requirement. Combination therapy with at least three drugs: one or two NRTIs with one or two PIs or with an NNRTI is necessary. Choice of drugs is determined by several factors, including drug interactions, dosage intervals (that is, the need to accommodate professional activity), future therapeutic options, or possible pregnancy.

Currently, no clear criteria are available to assist in making the choice between PIs and NNRTIs in initial treatment. Treatment experience with PIs is greater. Table 17.7 describes some advantages and disadvantages of the two classes of drugs.

The following treatment options are not recommended:

- Therapy with only one or two drugs
- Combinations of zidovudine plus d4T (antagonism), or TDF plus ddI (dosage adjustment necessary because of an increase in the area-under-the-curve for ddI), d4T plus ddI (overlapping toxicity), ABC plus TDF (rapid emergence of mutants with the resistance mutation K65R)
- Use of protease inhibitors without concomitant ritonavir (insufficient drug levels). Atazanavir is an exception to this rule, and can be used without ritonavir at a dose of 400 mg/day.

Monitoring Treatment

TOLERANCE AND SIDE EFFECTS

Nucleoside reverse-transcriptase inhibitors can be toxic to mitochondria, producing liver damage, lactic acidosis,

Table 17.6. Anti-HIV drugs available in 2007

Generic name (Abbreviation)	Trade name	Usual Dosage in the absence of renal failure	Class
Abacavir (ABC)	Ziagen	300 mg bid, or 600 mg qd	NRTI
Didanosine (ddI)	Videx	300-400 mg qd*	NRTI
Emtricitabine (FTC)	Emtriva	200 mg qd	NRTI
Lamivudine (3-TC)	3-TC	150 mg bid or 300 mg qd	NRTI
Stavudine (d4T)	Zerit	30 mg bid**	NRTI
Tenofovir (TFV)	Viread	245 mg qd	NRTI
Zidovudine (AZT)	Retrovir	250 mg bid	NRTI
AZT + 3-TC	Combivir	1tab bid	NRTI
AZT + 3-TC + ABC	Trizivir	1tab bid	NRTI
ABC + 3-TC	Epzicom (US), Kivexa (Europe)	1 tab qd	NRTI
TDF + FTC	Truvada	1 tab qd	NRTI
TDF + FTC + EFV	Atripla	1 tab qd	NRTI
Efavirenz (EFV)	Sustiva or Stocrin	600 mg qd	NNRTI
Nevirapine (NVP)	Viramune	200 mg bid	NNRTI
Etravirine (ETV)	Undetermined as of 8/07	400 mg bid	NNRTI
Atazanavir (ATZ)	Reyataz	300 mg qd***, or 400 mg qd	PI
Darunavir (DRV)	Prezista	600 mg bid***, or 800 mg qd***	PI
Fosamprenavir (FPV)	Lexiva (US), Telzir (Europe)	700 mg bid***, or 1400 mg qd***	PI
Indinavir (IDV)	Crixivan	800 mg bid***	PI
Lopinavir/ritonavir (LPV/r)	Kaletra	400/100 mg bid***	PI
Nelfinavir (NFV)	Viracept	1250 mg bid	PI
Ritonavir (RTV)	Norvir	100 mg ****	PI
Saquinavir hard gel (SQVh)	Invirase	1000 mg bid***	PI
Maraviroc (MVC)	Selzentry	300 mg bid	CCR5 inhibitor
Raltegravir (RTG)	Isentress	400 mg bid	Integrase inhibitor
Enfuvirtide (T-20)	Fuzeon	90 mg bid	Fusion inhibitor

NRTI = nucleoside reverse-transcriptase inhibitors; NNRTI = non-nucleoside reverse-transcriptase inhibitors; PI = protease inhibitors

* 250-300 mg qd if weight < 60 kg; adjust dose in case of renal failure

** 30 mg bid if weight < 60 kg; adjust dose in case of renal failure

*** when co-administered with 100 mg of RTV

**** 100 mg when used to boost serum concentration of other protease inhibitors

lipoatrophy, and polyneuropathy. Protease inhibitors cause nausea, vomiting, and diarrhea; elevate plasma cholesterol and triglycerides; induce insulin resistance and glucose intolerance; and contribute, together with NRTIs, to the redistribution of fatty tissue (atrophy in the face and extremities, contrasting with fat accumulation in breasts and abdomen). Treatment of dyslipidemia with statins is problematic because of the potential for drug interactions.

All drugs produce various specific side effects; Table 17.8 presents an overview. In the table, gray shading means that the corresponding side effect has been reported in 5% or more of patients; black shading designates a

Table 17.7. PIs compared to NNRTIs in initial treatment, when combined with NRTIs

	Advantages	Disadvantages
Protease inhibitors	• well documented clinical efficacy • relatively slow selection for resistance when treatment is suboptimal • partial cross-resistance only; possible efficacy of a second PI in case of failure	• heavy pill burden, no combination pills available • GI side effects • elevation of serum cholesterol and triglycerides • glucose intolerance • lipodystrophy • osteopenia?
Non-nucleosides	• only a few pills to swallow • better compliance • possibly less lipodystrophy	• rapid development of resistance when treatment is suboptimal • cross resistance among currently used NNRTIs • cutaneous side effects, including rare cases of Stevens-Johnson syndrome

Table 17.8. Frequent Side Effects of Anti-HIV Drugs

| | Reverse-Transcriptase Inhibitors | | | | | | | | Protease Inhibitors | | | | | | | |
| | NRTIs | | | | | | NNRTIs | | | | | | | | | |
Clinical symptom	ABC	AZT	DdC	ddI	d4T	3TC	EFV	NVP	APV	DRV**	IDV	LPV	NFV	RTV	SQV	TPV*
Abdominal pain											■				■	
Alterations of taste								■						■		
Bleeding																■
CNS symptoms							■									
Diarrhea	■		■					■	■		■	■	■			■
Drug rash	■						■	■								
Fat accumulation							?	?	■		■	■	■	■	■	■
Fat loss	■	■	■	■	■	■	?	?								
Fatigue				■												
Fever	■							■								
Headaches					■	■		■			■		■			
Hypersensitivity syndrome	■							■								
Kidney stones											■					
Myalgia		■														
Nausea		■	■			■		■	■					■		■
Pancreatitis				■												
Paresthesias									■					■		
Polyneuropathy			■	■	■											
Sleep disturbances	■				■	■										
Stomatitis				■												
Vertigo		■					■									
Vomiting								■							■	

(Continued)

Table 17.8. Frequent Side Effects of Anti-HIV Drugs (*Contd...*)

Clinical symptom	Reverse-Transcriptase Inhibitors								Protease Inhibitors							
	NRTIs						NNRTIs									
	ABC	AZT	DdC	ddI	d4T	3TC	EFV	NVP	APV	DRV**	IDV	LPV	NFV	RTV	SQV	TPV*
Laboratory tests																
Amylase↑				gray												
Bilirubin↑											black					
Cholesterol↑							gray			?		black	gray	black	gray	gray
Creatinine↑											gray					
Cytopenias		black														
Glucose↑										?	gray	gray	gray	gray		?
GOT/GPT↑								gray				gray	gray	black	gray	gray
Lactate↑	gray		gray	gray	black											
Macrocytosis		gray			gray											
Triglycerides								gray	gray	?	gray	gray	gray	gray	gray	gray

Key: Black = principle side effect, gray = side effect in > 5% of patients
* Tipranavir dramatically lowers the plasma concentration of many other drugs, including other protease inhibitors'
** At the time of writing, darunavir has been on the market for less than 6 months. Other, rare side effects may yet appear.

principal side effect of the associated drug. Because drugs have usually been tested in combination, assignment of a particular side effect to a particular drug is often uncertain; this situation is particularly true of the various aspects of the lipodystrophy syndrome. Lipoatrophy and lactic acidosis are more strongly associated with d4T than with other NRTIs, and fat accumulation may be particularly frequent with the combination of saquinavir and ritonavir.

These potential side effects necessitate regular patient visits. One usual schedule requires a telephone consultation after three days and visits after 1, 2, and 4 weeks of treatment; if all goes well, interval between visits may then lengthen to every 2 to 6 months. For surveillance of toxicity, a complete blood count, liver enzymes, lactates, and serum cholesterol and triglycerides are useful.

DRUG INTERACTIONS

Protease inhibitors and NNRTIs are preferentially metabolized by cytochrome P3A. The potential for drug interactions is therefore large. Drugs such as rifamycin or *Hypericum* (St. John's Wort) may lower PI and NNRTI concentrations by inducing cytochrome P3A. Other drugs may accumulate because they compete with NNRTIs and PIs for cytochrome P3A. Examples include ergot alkaloids (dramatic cases of ergotism with amputation have been published) and many benzodiazepines. Hardly a week goes by without new interactions being reported; consultation of Web resources for up-to-date information is recommended. Among the best of the available sites are those produced by the Liverpool HIV Pharmacology Group of the University of Liverpool (www.hiv drugin-teractions.org) and the electronic journal Medscape (http://medscape.com/hiv).

Ritonavir deserves special mention. It is the most powerful inhibitor of cytochrome P3A known in medical

---

KEY POINTS

About Monitoring Drug Toxicity

1. Follow-up visit should be scheduled at 1, 2, and 4 weeks after initiation of a new treatment.
2. If all goes well, the interval between visits may then lengthen to every 2 to 3 months.
3. Tests for surveillance of toxicity should include a complete blood count, liver enzymes, lactates, and serum cholesterol and triglycerides.

therapeutics. Its capacity to inhibit metabolism of other PIs can be put to good use: increasingly, other PIs such as indinavir, lopinavir, saquinavir, ripranavir, darunavir and amprenavir, are being combined with small doses of ritonavir (100 mg twice daily) to boost plasma drug levels and to lengthen intervals between dosages.

UTILITY OF RITONAVIR

Ritonavir is the most powerful inhibitor of cytochrome P3A known in medical therapeutics. It can be used to boost plasma levels of other protease inhibitors.

COMPLIANCE

Patients must acquire an adequate understanding of HIV pathogenesis, of the goals of HIV treatment, and of pharmacokinetics. They should be able to recognize the most frequent side effects and know how to manage them.

Aids to improve compliance abound, although few have been tested rigorously. Pill boxes are popular; these contain all the drugs taken during one week in separate compartments. The establishment of a detailed written schedule, showing how and when to take prescribed drugs in relation to meals and drinks, is recommended. More elaborate and expensive procedures involve use of electronic pill boxes, involving a device that records each time a bottle cap is unscrewed; the information can be downloaded into a computer and discussed with the patient. Directly observed therapy is becoming a possibility with once-daily regimens; this approach may be particularly appropriate in combination with methadone maintenance.

EFFICACY

Viral suppression as measured by decline in the viral load, a rise in the CD4 count, and clinical efficacy are all closely related. Above approximately 50 copies per cubic millimeter, the nadir of viral load reached through treatment predicts duration of viral suppression. Time to optimal viral suppression depends on the initial viral load and on the sensitivity of the viral load test. Combination treatment must produce a rapid fall in viral load, which should drop to fewer than 400 copies per cubic millimeter after 12 weeks and to fewer than 50 copies after 24 weeks. Measurements of viral load and CD4 count are recommended every 3 months.

TREATMENT RESULTS MUST MEET EXPECTATIONS

Viral load should drop to 400 or fewer copies per cubic millimeter after 12 wks, and 50 or fewer copies after 24 weeks.

RESISTANCE TESTS

Suboptimal treatment, lack of compliance, insufficient bioavailability, or drug interactions can result in prolonged periods of low blood and tissue drug concentrations with continued viral replication and selection of resistant mutants. The presence of resistance genotypes and phenotypes can be detected using commercially available methods. Studies show that these tests are useful mainly for excluding drugs to which the virus is resistant; they are less helpful for finding drugs to which the virus is sensitive. Resistance tests are recommended in patients who are yet untreated, but who have likely been infected since 1997, because they may harbor a primarily resistant HIV variant. Resistance tests are also recommended after early treatment failure.

MEASUREMENT OF PLASMA DRUG CONCENTRATIONS

In prospective studies, trough concentrations of PIs correlated well with degree and duration of viral suppression. However, the utility of these measures in clinical practice is not established. They are recommended in cases of unexpected toxicity, of suspected problems with compliance that cannot be otherwise investigated, or when multiple medications may produce unforeseeable pharmacokinetic interactions.

KEY POINTS

About Resistance Testing

1. Resistance tests are useful mainly for excluding ineffective drugs.
2. Resistance tests should be ordered before treatment commences in patients who are likely to have been infected in 1997 or later.

Treatment Modification and Simplification

Once a complicated drug regimen has suppresse viremia, patients and physicians would like to simplify treatment. When the PI is replaced by an NNRTI, viral suppression persists for at least 2 years. It is also possible to replace a PI+2NRTI combination with the three NRTIs ABC/ AZT/3TC, provided that patients had received no antiretroviral drugs before starting triple therapy. Scheduled treatment interruptions have been evaluated in clinical trials, the largest of which (the SMART trial) showed a 1.6% per year increase in AIDS and death among those who interrupted treatment, compared to those who continued therapy. These AIDS/death events were more frequent in those with lower CD4 counts. When treatment is interrupted, it would seem prudent to limit the length of interruption to less than four months, and to start treatment again before the CD4 count falls below 350 per cubic millimeter.

Procedures in Case of Failure

Treatment must often be changed because of intolerance, drug interactions, or side effects. If viremia is below 50 copies per cubic millimeter, a single offending drug can be replaced. In cases of lipodystrophy replacement of stavudine, ddI or AZT with tenofovir or abacavir may be helpful: however, patience is necessary, as an increase in limb fat usually takes over 6 months. In cases of virologic failure—that is, viremia that does not decline to fewer than 50 copies per cubic millimeter after 6 months (9 months if the initial viremia exceeded 1 million copies per cubic millimeter) or that rises to more than 200 copies requires a different approach. In this situation, a new combination should be chosen, containing (if possible) a drug from a class that had not already been used. At least one additional drug should also be replaced by another to which the patient is unlikely to be resistant, given personal medication history and resistance tests.

KEY POINTS

About Failing Regimens

1. A new combination should be chosen, containing (if possible) a drug from a class that has not already been used.
2. At least one additional drug should also be replaced by another to which the patient is unlikely to be resistant.
3. In the absence of alternatives, a virologically failing regimen should be maintained. Such a regimen often preserves the CD4 count.

However, changes to new therapy are not automatic, especially in patients who have experienced long-standing failure, with exposure to many drugs. Such patients often maintain CD4 counts at relatively high levels and are thus protected against clinical complications. On the other hand, salvage regimens may be ineffective or toxic, and drug holidays may produce falling CD4 counts. Maintenance of a virologically failing regimen is therefore often the best option.

Start and End of Prophylaxis for Opportunistic Infections

Efficacious antiretroviral treatment—provided that it is started in time—prevents immune deficiency and obviates the need for prophylaxis of opportunistic infections. Even if started late, effective HAART is followed by immune reconstitution. Prophylaxis of opportunistic infections can be discontinued after the patient's CD4 count has risen above a given level for at least 3 months. This level is $100/\mu m^3$ for stopping prophylaxis of CMV and non-tuberculous mycobacteria, and $200/\mu m^3$ for stopping prophylaxis of PJP and *Toxoplasma* encephalitis.

CONCLUSIONS AND OUTLOOK

Antiretroviral treatment has profoundly changed the prognosis of HIV infection, but such treatment is complex. Chances for success are best in the previously untreated; therefore, every effort must be made to optimize the first treatment given. A specialist should be consulted when starting or changing antiretroviral treatment. Compliance remains essential for treatment success; all drugs must be taken as prescribed. In asymptomatic patients with CD4 counts above $350/\mu m^3$, it is better to abstain than to risk failure through insufficient treatment. Talking reluctant patients into accepting drugs makes no sense; refusal of HAART must be respected.

Treatments continue to evolve. In 2006, a once-a-day combination pill combining efavirez, FTC and tenofovir (Atripla) has become available. Drugs for new targets will follow. Within 5 years, judicious use of strategic treatment interruption and of immune stimulation may permit survival in good health, without drugs, at least for some patients.

RESPECTING PATIENT CHOICE

It makes no sense to talk reluctant patients into accepting drugs; refusal of HAART must be respected.

OPPORTUNISTIC DISEASES

CASE 17.1

A 28–year-old black man was admitted to the hospital with a 3-week history of progressive shortness of breath accompanied by a nonproductive cough. Two weeks earlier, he had been seen by his local doctor for the same complaints and had been given an oral antibiotic at that time. He noted no improvement in his symptoms.

An epidemiologic history noted that the patient reported multiple episodes of unprotected homosexual intercourse 3 years earlier, but several months' abstinence recently. The patient denied intravenous drug use and said that he had never smoked cigarettes. This was an anxious-appearing man who was short of breath.

On physical examination a temperature of 38.2°C, a pulse of 120 per minute, a blood pressure of 110/60 mm Hg, and a respiratory rate of 34 per minute were recorded. No lymphadenopathy was evident, but white plaques consistent with thrush were seen on the posterior pharynx. Breath sounds were clear, with no rales or rhonchi. A II/VI systolic ejection murmur was noted, but no rubs or gallops. No organomegaly was evident on abdominal exam, and the genitalia was within normal limits. Skin was clear, and no edema of the extremities was noted.

On laboratory workup, arterial blood gasses measured pH 7.44, $PaCO_2$ 32 mm Hg, PaO_2 62 mm Hg, HCO_3 20 mEq/L on room air. Chest x-ray revealed bilateral, interstitial, diffuse, fluffy infiltrates forming a butterfly pattern. Bronchial lavage with Giemsa stain revealed P. jiroveci (Figure 17.2).

The patient was started on intravenous methylprednisolone and trimethoprim–sulfamethoxazole. His shortness of breath gradually improved over the next 3 days, and he was discharged on oral trimethoprim-sulfamethoxazole. An antibody test for HIV was positive, subsequently confirmed by Western blot. The patient's CD4 count was $150/\mu m^3$.

Case 17.1 represents a typical example of a primary episode of symptomatic AIDS. Opportunistic infections typically represent reactivation of latent infection or acquisition of a new infection, often caused by microorganisms of intrinsically low virulence. *Toxoplasma gondii*, CMV, viruses of the herpes group, PCP papovavirus JC (the agent of progressive multifocal leukoencephalopathy), and *Mycobacterium tuberculosis* have usually been acquired years before, but lie dormant as long as the immune response is intact. Once immune deficiency is profound, these microorganisms may start to proliferate. Some of these agents can be isolated long before clinical signs appear. Progressively, however, organ damage and symptoms occur—for example, stomatitis and symptomatic esophagitis from *Candida albicans*.

In advanced stages of immune suppression, agents that are usually nonpathogenic can have devastating consequences. Examples include destruction of the retina by CMV, or cachexia caused by *Mycobacterium avium*, present in the blood of 25% of patients with CD4 counts below $10/\mu m^3$. Several infections can be present at the same time, greatly complicating diagnosis and treatment.

Even before HAART, the prevention of opportunistic infections by antibiotics and antiretrovirals prolonged survival and improved quality of life. Since 1996, HAART has made an enormous difference. Advanced stages of AIDS with chronic diarrhea, cachexia, and central nervous system (CNS) and pulmonary manifestations have become rare in the United States and Western Europe.

PRIMARY AND SECONDARY PROPHYLAXIS

Primary prophylaxis prevents the first occurrence of a disease; secondary prophylaxis prevents relapses after a first episode. In AIDS, many opportunistic infections can be prevented. Patients who should receive prophylaxis are identified by their CD4 lymphocyte count and by serologic tests with evidence of previous exposure to the infectious agent. For instance, the presence of immunoglobulin G (IgG) against *Toxoplasma gondii* in a patient whose CD4 count is below $100/\mu m^3$, identifies a high risk of cerebral toxoplasmosis. Regular measures of the CD4 count, combined with serologic

---

KEY POINTS

About Prophylaxis

1. Latent infections often reactivate as cell-mediated immunity wanes.
2. Use serologic and skin testing to detect latent infections on initial evaluation.
3. Prophylaxis is recommended for a CD4 count below $200/\mu m^3$.
4. After treatment of active infections, secondary prophylaxis is often necessary to prevent relapse.
5. Prophylaxis can be discontinued after highly active antiretroviral therapy has been instituted, when the CD4 count is durably above $200/\mu m^3$.

Table 17.9. Prophylaxis of Opportunistic Infections

Disease	Indications	Drugs and dosage	Comments
Pneumocystis jiroveci pneumonia (PCP)	Primary prophylaxis if CD4 count is below 200/μm^3 or after an episode of PCP	Trimethoprim–sulfamethoxazole 1 double-strength tablet 3 times weekly, or 1 single-strength tablet q24h	Most effective; also protects against cerebral toxoplasmosis
		Pentamidine aerosols 300 mg once monthly	Doesn't protect against cerebral toxoplasmosis
		Dapsone 50 mg q24h, plus pyrimethamine 50 mg q24h	Add folinic acid 15 mg twice weekly
Cerebral toxoplasmosis	Primary prophylaxis if CD4 count is below 100/μm^3	Trimethoprim–sulfamethoxazole 1 double-strength tablet 3 times weekly, or 1 single-strength tablet q24h	Also protects against pneumocystosis
	Secondary prophylaxis	Sulfadiazine 2 g q24h, or clindamycin 600 mg q8h, plus pyrimethamine 25 mg q24h	
Mycobacterium (other than tuberculosis)	Primary prophylaxis if CD4 count is below 50/μm^3	Azithromycin 1200 mg weekly, or rifabutin 300 mg q24h	Rifabutin has many drug interactions, in particular with protease inhibitors
Tuberculosis	Primary prophylaxis if skin induration exceeds 5 mm with a 5-U tuberculin test	Isoniazid 5 mg/kg q24h (maximum 300 mg q24h) for 6 months with vitamin B$_6$ 40 mg PO q24h	Skin reaction is difficult to interpret with moderate-to-advanced immune deficiency
Cryptococcosis	Primary prophylaxis if CD4 count is below 50/μm^3	Fluconazole 400 mg weekly, or 200 mg 3 times weekly	Only in regions with a high incidence
	Secondary prophylaxis after an episode of cryptococcosis	Fluconazole 200 mg q24h	
Cytomegalovirus retinitis	Primary prophylaxis if CD4 count is below 50/μm^3	Valganciclovir 450 mg PO q24h	
	Secondary prophylaxis after an episode of retinitis		

tests on initial evaluation are necessary for a timely start to prophylaxis.

Opportunistic infections have a tendency to relapse. Therefore, as long as the underlying immune deficiency is not corrected, secondary prevention is necessary. Of course, preventive therapy has risks and side effects such as allergies, drug interactions, and development of resistance, but the risk–benefit ratio has been proven favorable, especially for prevention of PCP and cerebral toxoplasmosis by trimethoprim–sulfamethoxazole. On the other hand, once antiretroviral therapy is efficacious and the patient's CD4 count has risen durably above 200/μm^3, these preventive measures can be discontinued. Table 17.9 summarizes the common preventive regimens.

PULMONARY INFECTIONS

The differential diagnosis of pulmonary disease in HIV-infected patients depends on the patient's epidemiologic history (presence of intravenous drug abuse, previous episodes of bacterial pneumonia, exposure to tuberculosis), CD4 lymphocyte count, and use of preventive therapy. (see Table 17.9)

During the early years of the AIDS epidemic, PCP was the initial opportunistic infection in one third of cases. The infection remains frequent, but its incidence has greatly decreased because of the use of trimethoprim–sulfamethoxazole and HAART. Bacterial pneumonia, in particular that caused by *Streptococcus pneumoniae*, is 10 to 100 times more frequent in HIV-positive than in HIV-negative patients. Tuberculosis can occur at any degree of immune deficiency, but it is particularly frequent in patients who grew up in developing countries.

With a lobar infiltrate in a patient with a CD4 count above 200/μm^3, the presumptive diagnosis is bacterial pneumonia. Empiric treatment should start with amoxicillin–clavulanate, a cephalosporin, or one of the quinolones with activity against gram-positive bacteria. If immune deficiency is more profound (CD4 count is below 200/μm^3), PCP is most likely, except if the patient has faithfully taken trimethoprim–sulfamethoxazole prophylaxis. The chest x-ray pattern is helpful in narrowing the diagnostic possibilities (see Table 17.10). However, in all patients, whatever their degree of immune suppression, a definitive diagnosis usually requires bronchoalveolar lavage.

Pneumocystis Jiroveci Pneumonia

DIAGNOSIS AND TREATMENT

As illustrated in case 17.1, PCP is a subacute disease. With rare exceptions, its occurrence is limited to immunosuppressed patients with a CD4 count below 200/μm^3. Symptoms originate in the respiratory tract (dry cough, dyspnea) and are accompanied by fever (always), weight loss, and fatigue. A prominent symptom is dyspnea on exertion. Initially, patients experience shortness of breath with exercise, but do not complain of shortness of breath at rest. Alveolar fluid accumulation associated with *Pneumocystis* infection interferes with oxygen exchange, and patients quickly outstrip the ability of their lungs to supply arterial oxygen.

Lung auscultation is usually normal. Chest radiographs, which can be normal, typically show a reticulonodular bilateral infiltrate that can be asymmetrical (see Table 17.11 and Figure 17-2). Classically, the infiltrates form a butterfly pattern, mimicking pulmonary edema associated with left-sided congestive heart failure. Occasionally, a standard chest x-ray shows cystic lesions or a pneumothorax. When PCP prophylaxis is delivered by pentamidine inhalation, the chest x-ray is often atypical, with asymmetrical infiltrates limited to the lung apex.

Table 17.10. Lung Diseases Linked to HIV

Diagnosis	Signs and symptoms	Laboratory results	Radiology	Initial treatment
Bacterial pneumonia (*Streptococcus pneumoniae*)	Rapid onset of fever, dyspnea, cough, and sputum production	Leukocytosis with neutrophilia; blood cultures often positive	Lobar or diffuse infiltrate	Amoxicillin–clavulanate or cephalosporin
Pneumocystis jiroveci pneumonia	Fever, dyspnea, cough for several weeks; auscultation is usually normal	Hypoxemia, elevated lactate dehydrogenase; diagnosis through bronchoalveolar lavage	Diffuse reticulonodular interstitial infiltrate	Trimethoprim–sulfamethoxazole
Tuberculosis	Weight loss, fever, cough, night sweats, lymphadenopathy	Positive sputum smear by Ziehl stain; positive sputum and blood cultures; typical histopathology of lymph nodes	Mediastinal adenopathy; variable pulmonary infiltrate; cavitary upper lobe lesions are rare	Isoniazid, plus rifampin, plus pyrazinamide, plus ethambutol
Kaposi's sarcoma	Usually associated with skin or mucosal lesions	Typical lesions seen on bronchoscopy	Nodular infiltrates with perihilar location	Treatment for HIV; rarely requires radiotherapy or chemotherapy
Interstitial lymphoid pneumonia	Transitory fever and dyspnea	No specific findings	Reticulonodular infiltrates	Possibly steroids; diagnosis by exclusion!

Table 17.11. Chest Radiograph Results and Possible Causes

Chest radiograph[1]	Cause
Normal	Bronchitis *Pneumocystis jiroveci* pneumonia (PCP),
Lobar or other focal infiltrates	Bacterial pneumonia including Rhodococcus equi Tuberculosis (TB) PCP Cryptococcosis
Diffuse interstitial infiltrates	PCP TB Bacterial pneumonia Atypical pneumonia Interstitial lymphocytic pneumonia
Pleural effusion	Bacterial pneumonia TB Kaposi's sarcoma PCP rare
Mediastinal adenopathy	TB Atypical mycobacteria Lymphoma Kaposi's sarcoma
Cavities	Lung abscess *Mycobacterium kansasii* *Rhodococcus equi* TB *Staphylococcus aureus*
Cysts or bullae	PCP

[1] Note that all types of pneumonia can be associated with hilar lymphadenopathy

KEY POINTS

About the Clinical Manifestations, Diagnosis, and Treatment of *Pneumocystis jiroveci* Pneumonia

1. *Pneumocystis jiroveci* pneumonia (PCP) is a subacute disease that develops in HIV-infected patients with a CD4 count below $200/\mu m^3$.
2. Primary symptoms are fever, dyspnea on exertion, dry cough, weight loss, and fatigue.
3. Pulmonary exam is usually normal.
4. Chest x-ray may be normal, but usually demonstrates an interstitial butterfly pattern.
5. Lactate dehydrogenase is usually elevated, and PaO_2 depressed.
6. Trimethoprim–sulfamethoxazole is the drug of choice for treatment.
7. If PaO_2 is below 70 mm Hg, give prednisone before anti-PCP therapy.

Tests of the peripheral blood are usually nonspecific, but lactate dehydrogenase (LDH) is found to be elevated in more than 90% of patients with *Pneumocystis* infection. Higher values and a persistent elevation despite appropriate therapy are associated with a poorer prognosis. The ^{67}Ga citrate scan is very sensitive and demonstrates increased uptake in infected areas of the lung. However,

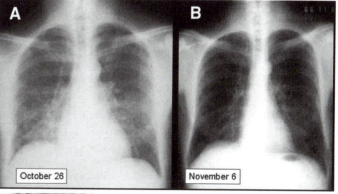

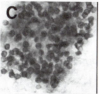

Figure 17-2. *Pneumocystis jiroveci* pneumonia (from www.aids-images.ch;). **A.** Chest radiograph shows symmetric infiltrates of the lower lobes similar in appearance to pulmonary edema. **B.** Repeated chest radiograph after 11 days of treatment. **C.** Sample of bronchoalveolar lavage stained with toluene blue, showing multiple organisms.

this test is expensive, time-consuming (usually taking 2 days to complete), and nonspecific. Gallium scan is most useful in patients with suspected PCP who have a normal chest x-ray.

The diagnosis of PCP is established by special stains of bronchoalveolar lavage fluid or of sputum induced by a 30-minute inhalation of 3% NaCl. If clinical suspicion of PCP is high, starting treatment before confirmation of the diagnosis is recommended, because PCP can still be found in lavage fluid 1 to 3 days later. In rare cases, the diagnosis may necessitate a transbronchial biopsy—particularly if pentamidine inhalations have been used.

Treatment modality will depend on the gravity of PCP. Patients who are very short of breath, with a PaO_2 of less than 70 mm Hg, particularly if accompanied by nausea or vomiting, will usually be admitted to hospital and treated intravenously. If signs of grave disease are absent, and if the patient is not nauseated, outpatient treatment is possible. The drug of choice is high-dose trimethoprim–sulfamethoxazole, 2 double-strength tablets (sulfamethoxazole 1600 mg and trimethoprim 320 mg every 8 hours for 21 days), followed by secondary prophylaxis with sulfamethoxazole 400 mg and trimethoprim 80 mg daily until the patient's CD4 count durably exceeds $200/\mu m^3$.

Trimethoprim–sulfamethoxazole has numerous side effects, of which drug rash is the most frequent. If the skin lesions are extensive (and, in particular, if mucosal involvement is evident), if leukopenia and thrombocytopenia are severe, or if renal or hepatic toxicity or serious vomiting occurs, alternative treatment is necessary. In an attempt to reduce the incidence of bone marrow

suppression, folinic acid has been added to the treatment regimen; however, it diminishes the efficacy of treatment and is not recommended. Many alternatives to trimethoprim–sulfamethoxazole are available, but their efficacy is in general inferior, and many have other serious side effects. Table 17.12 summarizes the alternatives.

At the start of the AIDS era, patients with *Pneumocystis*, even if correctly treated, often experienced increased respiratory distress and worsening lung infiltrates during the first few days. In many cases, this initial deterioration necessitated intubation or caused death. Severe respiratory compromise that necessitates intubation can be prevented by giving steroids (prednisone 1 mg/kg daily for 5 days, then 40 mg daily for 5 days, followed by 20 mg daily for 11 days) in cases of severe pneumocystosis with a PaO2 below 70 mmHg. Prednisone should be given before or simultaneously with initiation of anti-*Pneumocystis* therapy.

PREVENTION

In HIV patients with CD4 counts below $200/\mu m^3$, the annual risk of PCP is roughly 20%. The risk of relapse after a first episode is even higher: 40% after 6 months.

KEY POINTS

About Prophylaxis of *Pneumocystis jiroveci* Pneumonia

1. In HIV patients with a CD4 count below $200/\mu m^3$ not on prophylaxis, the annual incidence of *Pneumocystis jirovecii* pneumonia (PCP) is 20%.
2. Trimethoprim–sulfamethoxazole is the drug of choice: efficacious, inexpensive, and equally active in preventing toxoplasmosis.
3. Alternatives are not as effective:
   a) Dapsone does not cover toxoplasmosis; pyrimethamine must be added.
   b) Pentamidine is associated with cough and asthma.
   c) Atovaquone is expensive.

Table 17.12. Treatment of *Pneumocystis jiroveci* pneumonia: trimethoprim–sulfamethoxazole and alternatives

Agent	Dosage	Side effects
Trimethoprim–sulfamethoxazole	Two double-strength tablets PO q8h, or 15 mg/kg IV daily divided q8h	Skin rash, nausea and vomiting, anemia, leukopenia
Dapsone, plus trimethoprim	100 mg PO q24h 5 mg/kg PO q8H	Rash, nausea, and vomiting; hemolytic anemia in patients with G6PD deficiency
Clindamycin, plus primaquine	600 mg PO or IV Q8H 30 mg PO q24h	Rash, nausea, and vomiting; hemolytic anemia in patients with G6PD deficiency
Atovaquone	750 mg PO q12h	Skin lesions, nausea, vomiting, and diarrhea; less efficacious but better tolerated than sulfonamides

Primary prophylaxis diminishes the risk of pneumocystis, but if severe immunosuppression persists without HAART, the risk is still 19% after 3 years of prophylaxis with trimethoprim–sulfamethoxazole, and 33% after 3 years of pentamidine aerosols. Primary and secondary prophylaxis strategies use the same treatment options:

- Trimethoprim–sulfamethoxazole 1 double-strength tablet three times weekly, or 1 single–strength tablet daily. Trimethoprim–sulfamethoxazole has the advantages of great efficacy, protection against cerebral toxoplasmosis, and low price. However, almost 50% of patients will develop signs of cutaneous intolerance. Desensitization permits re-administration in most cases, but desensitization has been used mostly in cases of treatment, when alternatives to agents are clearly less satisfactory. The mechanisms of trimethoprim–sulfamethoxazole intolerance are not well understood. Dose dependency is one of the features that argues against "allergy." Another is the observation that up to 60% of patients who have shown cutaneous intolerance do not relapse when re-exposed.

- Dapsone, 100 mg daily, does not protect against cerebral toxoplasmosis. If anti-*Toxoplasma* IgG antibodies are present, add pyrimethamine to dapsone. Daily (dapsone 50 mg, plus pyrimethamine 50 mg) and weekly schedules (dapsone 200 mg, plus pyrimethamine 75 mg) are equivalent.

- Pentamidine by inhalation (Respirgard nebulizer), 300 mg every 4 weeks. Some patients, particularly smokers, cannot tolerate inhaled pentamidine because of cough and asthma. Preventive use of a bronchodilator may be helpful.

- Atovaquone 750 mg divided into two daily doses. Well tolerated, but expensive.

Bacterial Pneumonia

As a complication of HIV infection, bacterial pneumonia produces the same symptoms and signs as pneumonias in HIV-negative patients: sudden onset of fever, chills, cough, and dyspnea. By far the most frequent cause is *S. pneumoniae*, but *Haemophilus influenzae* (particularly in smokers), *Staphylococcus aureus*, *Pseudomonas aeruginosa*, and *Rhodococcus equi* may also be implicated. Bacteremia and relapses are frequent. Empiric treatment consists of amoxicillin–clavulanate, or a second-or third-generation cephalosporin; treatment duration is 10 to 14 days (see Chapter 4).

Tuberculosis

Tuberculosis usually presents as a subacute disease with weight loss, cough, fever, night sweats, and lung lesions. However, if immune suppression is very advanced, the

---

KEY POINTS

About Mycobacterium tuberculosis in AIDS

1. Tuberculosis (TB) is usually a subacute disease with weight loss, cough, fever, night sweats, and lung lesions.
2. With severe immunosuppression, TB can present as miliary disease:
   a) Interstitial involvement
   b) Meningitis
   c) Negative sputum smears for acid-fast bacilli, but positive blood cultures
3. Susceptibility testing is critical: multiresistant TB is associated with >50% and extensively resistant TB with a near 100% mortality in AIDS.
4. Four-drug therapy: isoniazid, rifampin, pyrazinamide, and ethambutol. Delay HAART therapy when possible.

---

chest x-ray may be atypical for the disease. Interstitial infiltrates may predominate, without cavitary lesions; CNS tuberculosis becomes more frequent; mediastinal adenopathy is evident on the chest x-ray, and blood cultures are often positive. Diagnosis relies on acid-fast stain of the sputum; however, this test is frequently negative in disseminated (miliary) tuberculosis. For culture, liquid media are recommended because results are more rapid: growth is usually evident by 10 to 14 days, and presumptive identification of *Mycobacterium* can be made by nucleic acid probes.

Susceptibility testing should always be done, because multiresistant tuberculosis (MDR-TB) is a serious threat to an HIV-positive individual, with mortality exceeding 50%, and extensively resistant tuberculosis (XDR-TB) is associated with a near 100% mortality in HIV patients. Initial treatment should include four drugs: oral isoniazid 300 mg daily (plus vitamin B_6), rifampicin 600 mg daily, pyrazinamide 20 to 30 mg/kg daily, and ethambutol 15 mg/kg daily. This quadruple therapy should be continued during the first 2 months, followed by isoniazid and rifampicin for a further 7 months. Patients respond well to classic antituberculous treatment, but without HAART and reversal of the underlying immune deficiency, a high risk remains of persistent disease and death as a consequence of other complications of AIDS. In cases of isoniazid or rifampicin resistance (or both), consultation with a specialist is advised.

The co-administration of HAART and treatment for TB is a particular problem: on the one hand, PIs and rifampicin mutually modify one another's plasma levels;

on the other hand, concomitant administration of seven or more drugs may be toxic to the liver and gut. In addition, immune reconstitution disease caused by HAART is difficult to distinguish from paradoxical inflammatory reactions that are sometimes observed at the start of anti-TB treatment. If immune suppression is not very advanced, it is often more reasonable to postpone HAART for a few months while anti-TB drugs take effect.

Mycobacterium Kansasii

In HIV-positive patients, *M. kansasii* causes a disease resembling classical TB with fever, cough, weight loss, and pulmonary infiltrates predominating at the apex. Very occasionally, apical cavities are observed. Classical antituberculous drugs such as isoniazid, rifampicin, and ethambutol are efficacious.

Mycobacteria Other Than Tuberculosis

Mycobacterium avium intracellulare (and similar mycobacteria) do not usually cause pulmonary disease, but rather a systemic illness with fever, weight loss, night sweats, and liver involvement. However, mycobacteria other than tuberculosis (MOTT) are frequently found in sputum, where their pathogenic significance remains uncertain.

Pulmonary Kaposi's Sarcoma

In patients with obvious cutaneous Kaposi's sarcoma, involvement of the mucosal surfaces is frequent (30% to 50% of cases) and, in general, asymptomatic. When lung is involved, the chest x-ray shows reticulonodular infiltrates with a perihilar distribution, hilar lymphadenopathy, and occasionally, pleural effusions [Figure 17.3(D)]. Treatment with radiotherapy or chemotherapy is indicated for relief of cough or dyspnea. In general, lung lesions, like other manifestations of Kaposi's sarcoma, improve on antiretroviral combination therapy.

Other Rare Pulmonary Diseases

INTERSTITIAL LYMPHOID PNEUMONIA

Interstitial lymphoid pneumonia is usually diagnosed by exclusion. It is particularly frequent in children and presents with fever and dyspnea. The chest x-ray shows reticulonodular infiltrates that may vary and disappear spontaneously. Pathogenesis is not clear; HIV itself may perhaps be implicated. Treatment relies on corticosteroids.

HISTOPLASMOSIS

In contrast to the localized pulmonary disease observed in immunocompetent populations (see Chapter 4), histoplasmosis in AIDS is often disseminated and accompanied by anemia, enlargement of liver and

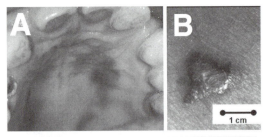
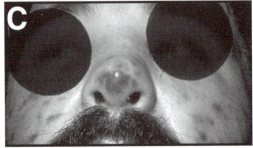
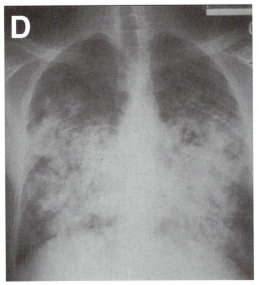

Figure 17-3. Kaposi's sarcoma (from www.aids-images.ch;). **A.** Macular lesions on the palate. **B.** Tumor-like skin lesion. **C.** Facial lesions including on tip of the nose (picture courtesy of J. Sampson) **D.** Typical chest radiograph; note the central nodular densities, with peripheral extension. *See color image on color plate 4*

spleen, and positive blood cultures. Gastrointestinal involvement with ulcers, skin lesions, and lymphadenopathies are also frequent. The diagnosis is established by blood or bone marrow culture. Treatment relies on amphotericin B or fluconazole.

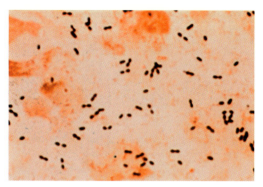

Figure 4–2B. Pneumococcal pneumonia: sputum Gram stain shows *Streptococcus pneumoniae*. Note that the cocci come to a slight point, explaining the term "lancet-shaped."

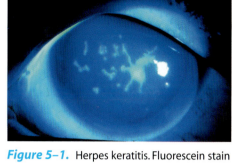

Figure 5–1. Herpes keratitis. Fluorescein stain shows the typical dendritic corneal lesions of herpes simplex.

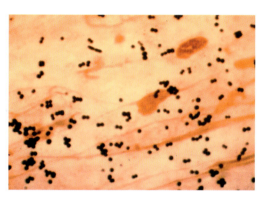

Figure 4–3B. *Staphylococcus aureus* pneumonia: sputum Gram stain shows gram-positive cocci in clusters and tetrads.

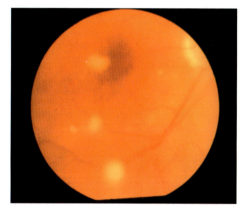

Figure 5–3. *Candida* retinitis. The typical rounded white exudates are caused by seeding from the bloodstream.

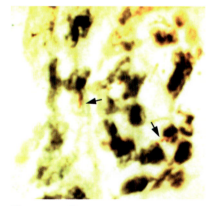

Figure 4–5B. Cavitary pulmonary tuberculosis: sputum smear for acid-fast bacilli confirms the presence of those organisms.

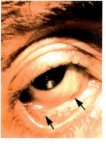 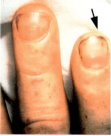

A. **B.**

Figure 7–1. Embolic phenomena in infective endocarditis. **A.** Conjunctival petechiae **B.** Nail-bed splinter hemorrhage: Multiple petechiae are seen on both fingers.

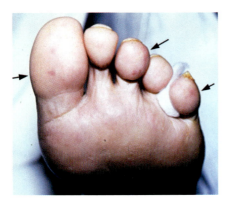

Figure 7–1C. Embolic phenomena in infective endocarditis. Osler nodes

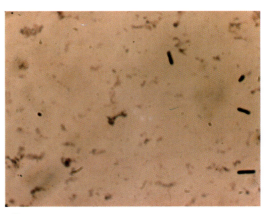

Figure 10–2B. Clostridia myonecrosis. Gram stain of brown fluid obtained from the large blister on the patient's arm. Note the large gram-positive rods and the absence of inflammatory cells.

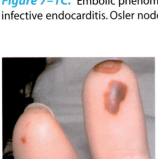

Figure 7–1D. Embolic phenomena in infective endo-carditis.

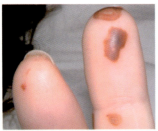

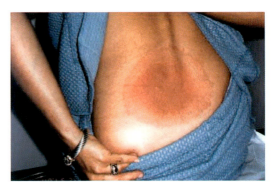

Figure 13–1. Erythema migrans. Note the dark erythematous center.

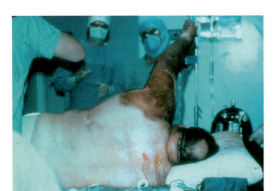

Figure 10–2A. Clostridia myonecrosis. Patient from case 10.3 undergoing surgical debridement. The skin over the left arm and shoulder had a brownish-red appearance.

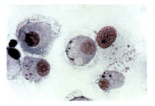

Figure 13–2. Morulae found in human granulocy-totropic ehrlichiosis caused by *Anaplasma phagocy-tophilum*.

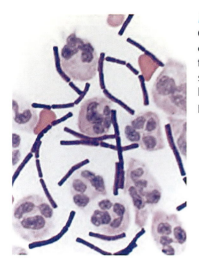

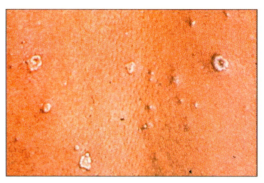

Figure 14–1B. Gram stain of the cerebrospinal fluid demonstrates boxcarlike grampositive rods.

Figure 14–3B. Smallpox. View of individual raised skin lesions.

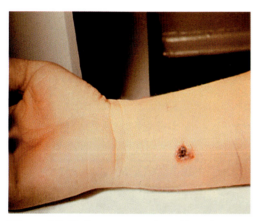

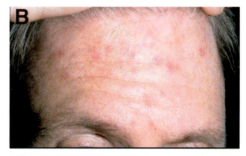

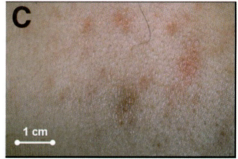

Figure 14–2. Cutaneous anthrax. Note the black eschar and edematous margins of this 7-day-old lesion.

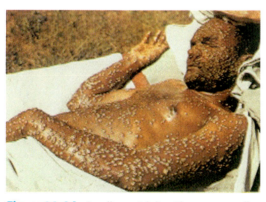

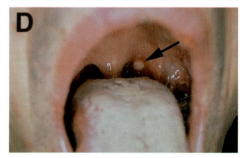

Figure 14–3A. Smallpox. Adult with severe smallpox skin lesions.

Figure 17–1. Acute retroviral syndrome with seroconversion. **B.** Acneiform lesions can develop. **C.** Macules on the chest. **D.** Ulceration in the oral cavity.

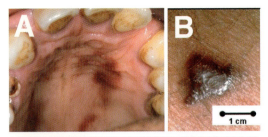

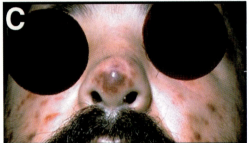

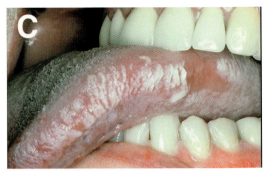

Figure 17-4C. Lesions of the oral cavity in AIDS. Oral leukoplakia.

Figure 17-3. Kaposi's sarcoma. **A.** Macular lesions on the palate. **B.** Tumor-like skin lesion. **C.** Facial lesions including on tip of the nose.

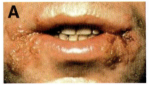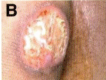

Figure 17.5. Herpesvirus group infections **A.** Herpes simplex virus 1. Chronic perioral lesions. **B.** Ulcer on the buttocks due to herpes simplex virus 2. **C.** Cytomegalovirus retinitis. Left: Initial lesions, showing perivascular sheathing. Right: Later lesions, showing necrosis and hemorrhage.

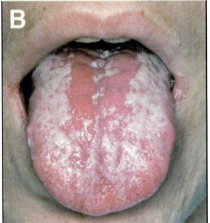

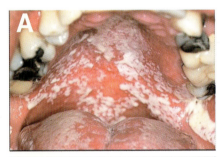

Figure 17-4. Lesions of the oral cavity in AIDS. **A.** Oral thrush involving the soft and hard palate. **B.** Candidiasis of the tongue.

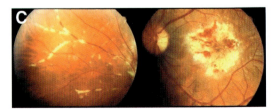

Figure 17.6C. Bottom panel: Progressive multi-focal leukoencephalopathy. Left: MRI T2 weighted image. Right: T1 image without contrast. Note the hypodensities, reflecting loss of myelin.

COCCIDIOMYCOSIS

Coccidiomycosis is restricted to the southwestern United States and to Central America. Symptoms are fever, cough, and reticulonodular infiltrates. Diagnosis relies on culture of sputum or bronchoalveolar lavage fluid. Treatment is by amphotericin B (0.5 to 1 mg/kg daily) or fluconazole (400 to 800 mg daily).

DISSEMINATED TOXOPLASMOSIS

Rarely, and only in the presence of extreme immuno-suppression (CD4 count below 20), *Toxoplasma gondii* can cause a devastating disseminated disease, with prominent lung involvement. Typically, the lactate dehydrogenase (LDH) is extremely elevated. Toxoplasma organisms can be seen in the bronchoalveolar lavage. This form of toxoplasmosis is treated like cerebral toxoplasmosis.

NOCARDIA ASTEROIDES

N. asteroides is a cause of chronic pneumonia and nodular pulmonary lesions. Other organs than the lung, such as the kidney and the brain, can be involved. The disease is diagnosed by direct stain of the sputum, where delicate, gram-labile, branched filaments are detected. Treatment relies on prolonged administration of high doses of trimethoprim-sulfamethoxazole; alternatives are imipenem and the newer fluoroquinolones.

INVASIVE ASPERGILLOSIS

Aspergillosis is often a terminal complication with a disastrous prognosis in hospitalized patients who have received steroids and are experiencing neutropenia. Cardiac and CNS lesions may be associated with pneumonia.

RHODOCOCCUS EQUI

Rhodococcus causes cavitary acute pneumonias that carry a very somber prognosis. Contact with horses is found in about half of patients. Treatment relies on vancomycin, which can be combined with ciprofloxacin. Other regimens include imipenem, amikacin, or rifampin.

GASTROINTESTINAL SYSTEM

Also see Chapter 8 for a discussion of infections that can affect both immunocompetent and immunocompromised individuals.

Oral Cavity and Esophagus

CANDIDIASIS

Candidiasis is the most frequent of the opportunistic infections, occurring in virtually all HIV-positive patients with severe immunosuppression. Usually, oral candidiasis presents with yellowish-white plaques on the oral mucosa ("oral thrush"; see Figure 17.4). These

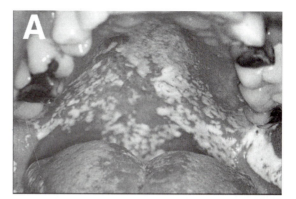
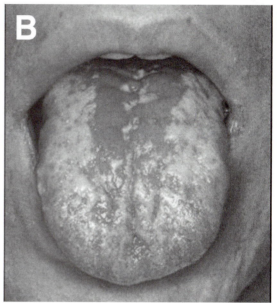
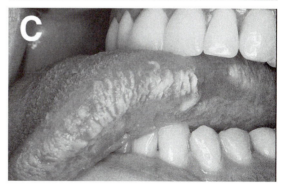

Figure 17-4. Lesions of the oral cavity in AIDS (from www.aids-images.ch;). **A.** Oral thrush involving the soft and hard palate. **B.** Candidiasis of the tongue (Pictures A and B courtesy of J. Sampson). **C.** Oral leukoplakia. *See color image on color plate 4*

Table 17.13. Gastrointestinal Diseases Associated with HIV Infection

Location	Disease	Cause	Signs and symptoms	Diagnosis
Oral cavity	Thrush	Candida stomatitis (*Candida albicans*)	Whitish plaques	Inspection
	Leukoplakia	Epstein–Barr virus	Whitish spots with irregular surface on margin of tongue	Inspection and biopsy
	Aphthous ulcers	Herpes simplex Cytomegalovirus (CMV), idiopathic or unknown	Painful erosions of about 5 mm	Culture or biopsy
Esophagus	Candida esophagitis	*Candida albicans*	Dysphagia, retrosternal pain with coexisting *Candida* stomatitis	Clinical signs and symptoms, endoscopy
	Ulcers and erosions	Cytomegalovirus, or herpes simplex	Dysphagia and retrosternal pain	Endoscopy (longitudinal ulcers) and histology
Stomach	Gastritis	*Candida*, CMV, herpes, *Helicobacter pylori?*	Various signs and symptoms, frequently pH is elevated; malabsorption	Endoscopy and biopsy
Small intestine	Diarrhea	*Cryptosporidium Isospora belli Enterocytozoon bieneusi*	Chronic watery diarrhea; loss of weight; malabsorption	Examination of feces
		Salmonella, Shigella, Campylobacter	Acute or subacute diarrhea and fever	Culture of feces and blood
	Malignant lymphoma		Loss of weight; intestinal obstruction; perforation	Computed tomography scan and biopsy
Biliary system	Cholangitis	CMV? *Cryptosporidium?* HIV? Microsporidium?	Epigastric pain, nausea, anorexia, weight loss	Endoscopy or x-ray examination showing segmental stenosis without gallstones
Liver	Hepatitis	*Mycobacterium avium intracellulare*	Fever; weight loss; abdominal pain	Biopsy or blood culture
Colon	Colitis	CMV or herpes simplex	Diarrhea; abdominal ; pain tenesmus	Biopsy

plaques detach easily, revealing reddish mucosa beneath. The erythematous form of candidiasis consists of brilliant red spots on the tongue or palate. Candidiasis can also present as angular cheilitis or perlèche. The clinical diagnosis is usually evident; cultures are difficult to interpret, because *Candida* is found in the mouth of many people without stomatitis.

Often, *Candida* stomatitis is associated with esophagitis, which may cause dysphagia and retrosternal

pain. *Candida* esophagitis is one of the designated AIDS-defining opportunistic infection; patients with this complication are stratified into class C. Patients with stomatitis only are stratified into class B.

Oral imidazoles, especially fluconazole, have become the treatment of choice. In previously untreated patients, single doses of 150 to 400 mg are effective. Options for subsequent management vary. Relapses can be prevented by HAART's reversal of immune suppression. If achieving

---

KEY POINTS

About Oral Candidiasis

1. Develops in all HIV-infected patients with serious immunocompromise.
2. Typically seen as white plaques that detach when scraped, or as red spots on the tongue and palate.
3. Often accompanied by esophagitis, an AIDS-defining illness.
4. Fluconazole is the treatment of choice.
5. Recurrent pharyngitis is common; suppression often results in resistance.

KEY POINTS

About Esophagitis in HIV

1. *Candida albicans* is the most common cause.
2. Cytomegalovirus is less common, causing longitudinal ulcers and viral inclusions on biopsy.
3. Herpes simplex virus type 1 is moderately frequent; type 2 and herpes zoster are less common. Diagnosis is made by culture or immunofluorescence.
4. Thalidomide may help idiopathic esophageal ulcers.

---

reversal is not possible, some physicians prefer to wait for a relapse, which they then re-treat; others favor preventive therapy—for instance, fluconazole 50 mg daily or 150 mg weekly.

After years of intermittent treatment or prevention, relapses become more frequent and resistance of *Candida* is common. Such cases may present difficult problems of management. Other imidazoles—such as itraconazole solution, voriconazole, or ketoconazole—may remain effective. In other cases, intravenous therapy with amphotericin B at doses of 20 to 30 mg daily, are necessary. Newer agents such as the echinocandins (See Chapter 1) are easier to administer.

MOUTH ULCERS AND APHTHOUS STOMATITIS

Superficial lesions of the oral and esophageal mucosa can cause pain and dysphagia. Differential diagnoses includes herpes simplex, CMV, medication side effects (f), and idiopathic ulcers. If the lesion persists, a biopsy with viral culture or immunofluorescence is often necessary for diagnosis.

ORAL HAIRY LEUKOPLAKIA

Oral hairy leukoplakia, a whitish lesion with an irregular border located along the lateral part of the tongue, is caused by Epstein–Barr virus. Often, the lesion is bilateral. Histology shows epithelial hyperplasia. Usually, treatment is not necessary, but in resistant cases, topical application of podophyllotoxin can be effective. Acyclovir can also be administered, but usually it causes only temporary regression of the lesions (see Chapter 15).

TUMORS

Kaposi's sarcoma frequently involves the oral cavity. It produces painless macules or nodules with characteristic purple coloration on the palate, gingivae, or tongue.

SALIVARY GLANDS

Benign lymphoepithelial lesions and cystic hyperplasia involve mostly the parotid gland. They can be associated with xerostomia. The clinical picture is similar to that in Sjögren's syndrome. The parotid lesions are particularly frequent in children; they are attributed to HIV itself.

DIFFERENTIAL DIAGNOSIS OF ESOPHAGITIS

As noted earlier, the most frequent cause of esophagitis is infection by *Candida albicans*. However, when esophageal symptoms occur in a patient who does not have clear evidence of *Candida* stomatitis, other causes must be sought.

- Cytomegalovirus causes longitudinal ulcers. The lesion can be diagnosed only by biopsy: characteristic viral inclusions are seen in endothelial, epithelial, or smooth-muscle cells.

- Involvement of the esophagus by herpes is most often caused by herpes simplex type 1 and less commonly by herpes type 2 or by herpes zoster. Lesions are typically small. Diagnosis is made by biopsy plus immunofluorescence, or culture, or both.

- Idiopathic ulcer is a diagnosis by exclusion. Treatment with thalidomide may bring relief.

Small and Large Intestine

DIARRHEA

Diarrhea associated with weight loss is one of the hallmarks of AIDS, particularly in Africa, where AIDS, diarrhea, and weight loss are practically synonymous ("slim disease"). Infection with HIV itself, plus many opportunistic pathogens and tumors, can involve the small and large intestine and cause diarrhea. The differential diagnosis is vast. This subsection briefly comments on the most frequent causes (also see Chapter 8).

Drugs. Many of the antiretroviral drugs can cause diarrhea—in particular all protease inhibitors, and didanosine. Because patients with HIV often receive antibiotics, the possibility of colitis associated with *Clostridium difficile* must often be considered, and the *C. difficile* toxin must be sought in feces.

Salmonella, Campylobacter, Shigella. These organisms are frequent causes of acute gastroenteritis both in non-HIV and HIV-infected populations. In HIV infection, bacteremia is extremely frequent, particularly as a result of infection with *S. typhimurium* or *S. enteritidis*.

Abdominal Tuberculosis. Abdominal tuberculosis presents with fever, pain, weight loss, or obstruction. These symptoms are difficult to distinguish from those of abdominal lymphoma. Often, the diagnosis is made only at laparoscopy.

MOTT. Infections with "mycobacteria other than tuberculosis" are often caused by *M. avium*, but other mycobacterial species cause similar clinical signs and symptoms, and may be more difficult to diagnose, because they grow poorly in culture (for instance, *M. genavense*). The MOTT organisms cause a systemic illness with fever, weight loss, and positive blood cultures. In biopsies of the gastrointestinal tract, the submucosa may be filled with characteristic acid-fast microorganisms. Diarrhea and abdominal pain dominate the clinical picture.

Cytomegalovirus Colitis. Diseases caused by CMV are typically the result of reactivation of latent CMV infection—that is, IgG antibodies against CMV were present before symptoms started—in immunosuppressed patients, usually those with a CD4 count below $50/\mu m^3$.

Symptoms may be severe, with diarrhea, abdominal pain, tenesmus, and fever. Colonoscopy shows multiple erosions, and biopsies reveal the characteristic intranuclear inclusions. Cytomegalovirus is also implicated in some cases of cholangitis and pancreatitis.

Cryptosporidium. In immunocompetent individuals, *C. parvum* causes asymptomatic infections and acute diarrhea. In immunosuppressed patients, diarrhea becomes chronic, causing malabsorption. Oocysts can be found in the feces. No treatment has so far proven effective, although oral paromomycin (500 to 750 mg every 8 hours), macrolides such oral azithromycin (1250 mg daily), oral clarithromycin (500 mg twice daily), and oral albendazole (400 mg daily) can be tried, in addition to symptomatic treatment of diarrhea (loperamide, narcotics).

Microsporidia. Three types of *Microsporidia* are found in cases of diarrhea:

- *Enterocytozoon bieneusi* (most frequent)
- *Encephalitozoon intestinalis* (which can also involve the biliary tract)
- *Encephalitozoon cuniculi*

Some patients do not exhibit symptoms; however, more often, patients experience profuse diarrhea, abdominal pain, and weight loss. Up to 30% of cases of chronic diarrhea in immunosuppressed HIV-positive patients may be a result of *Enterocytozoon bieneusi*. A special stain (modified trichrome stain) reveals the parasite in feces. Past treatments were not very effective, and eradication of the organism was usually impossible. Fumagillin (20 mg three times daily for 2 weeks) clears the spores and prevents relapse in most patients (see Chapter 8). Albendazole (400 mg twice daily) is useful in cases of *Encephalitozoon intestinalis* infection.

Isospora belli. Diarrheas caused by *I. belli* are frequent in developing countries (in African countries and Haiti, for instance). The treatment of choice is trimethoprim–sulfamethoxazole, which is also effective in primary and secondary prophylaxis.

Rectum and Anus

Many HIV-infected patients are at risk for other sexually transmitted infections such as gonococcal proctitis, syphilis, and venereal warts. Herpes simplex can cause rectitis with tenesmus and bleeding; in addition, in severely immunosuppressed patients, herpes simplex may cause persistent and debilitating ulcerations (see Figure 17.5). Such lesions may necessitate admission to hospital and parenteral therapy with high-dose acyclovir. Resistance to acyclovir may develop; the alternative treatment is foscarnet. Less commonly, such ulcerations can be caused by CMV.

KEY POINTS

About HIV-Associated Diarrhea

1. Diarrhea can be caused by HIV infection alone.
2. Antiretroviral drugs and antibiotics can cause diarrhea (with *Clostridium difficile*, for example).
3. Salmonella gastroenteritis is more commonly associated with bacteremia in HIV patients.
4. *Mycobacterium tuberculosis* and atypical mycobacteria can result in diarrhea.
5. Cytomegalovirus colitis in patients with a CD4 count below $50/\mu m^3$ can be diagnosed by biopsy.
6. Infecting protozoa include *Cryptosporidium*, *Microsporidia*, and *Isospora belli*. Search for oocysts, and use trichrome stain for *Microsporidia*.

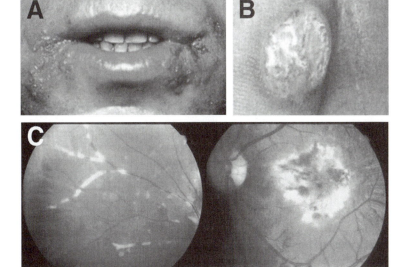

Figure 17-5. Herpesvirus group infections (from www.aidsmages.ch;) **A.** Herpes simplex virus 1. These chronic perioral lesions have become resistant to acyclovir. **B.** Ulcer on the buttocks resulting from infection with herpes simplex virus 2 (diameter: 5 cm). **C.** Cytomegalovirus retinitis. Left: Initial lesions, showing perivascular sheathing. Right: Later lesions, showing necrosis and hemorrhage.

(picture courtesy of E. Baolivo).

See color image on color plate 4

Anal and rectal carcinoma are particularly frequent in homosexual patients. The development of that tumor is related to the human papilloma virus. Screening programs in homosexual patients for this virus have been considered, analogous to those that screen for cervical cancer, as well as vaccination of adolescents have been considered, but are not yet part of routine clinical practice.

Tumors of the Digestive System

KAPOSI'S SARCOMA

When patients with cutaneous Kaposi's sarcoma undergo endoscopy, gastric or intestinal involvement is found in about one half of cases. However, such involvement is usually asymptomatic, and involvement of the gastrointestinal tract without involvement of skin is rare. Occasional complications include bleeding, obstruction, invagination, and perforations.

LYMPHOMA

The AIDS-associated lymphomas preferentially involve the gastrointestinal tract (and the brain), causing diarrhea, abdominal pain, fever, and weight loss. Symptoms of lymphoma are therefore difficult to distinguish from those of opportunistic infections. Chemotherapy is theoretically effective, but often very difficult to administer to these severely immunosuppressed patients.

Liver

VIRAL HEPATITIS

Transmission of both HCV and HIV occurs parenterally; which is why HIV–HCV co-infection is particularly frequent in intravenous drug abusers and patients with hemophilia. Transmission of HBV occurs sexually, and its incidence is increased in men who have sex with men.

In HIV–HCV co-infection, the two viruses influence one another. Co-infected patients tend to have unfavorable prognostic indices for hepatitis C: higher incidence of infection with HCV type 1, cirrhosis, and high levels of HCV viremia. Conversely, HCV influences HIV infection: notably, the CD4 response to HAART is less vigorous in co-infected patients than in those infected with HIV alone. Experience with interferon treatment of

---

KEY POINTS

About Coinfection with HIV and Hepatitis C Virus

1. Co-infection is frequent in intravenous drug abusers and people with hemophilia.
2. Patients infected with HIV tend to have more severe hepatitis C (HCV): they have a higher incidence of HCV type 1 cirrhosis, and higher levels of HCV viremia.
3. Patients infected with HCV have a reduced response to highly active antiretroviral therapy (HAART).
4. The combination of HAART with pegylated interferon and ribavirin is demonstrating increased responsiveness.

HIV–HCV co-infection was previously disappointing. However, as a consequence of HAART for HIV and combination therapy with pegylated interferon and ribavirin for HCV response to therapy has improved.

Nevertheless, treatment of HCV in co-infected patients remains a challenge. Interactions between liver disease and HAART are frequent and unfavorable, and contraindications to the use of interferon (for instance, a history of depression) and of ribavirin (anemia) are frequent.

Lamivudine (3TC) Lamivudine (3-TC), emtricitabine (FTC), and tenofovir (TDF) are active against both HIV and HBV. In HBV–HIV co-infected patients, HAART that includes lamivudine diminishes HBV viremia. After years of therapy, however, the risk of development of lamivudine resistance is high. Lamivudine-resistant HBV is also resistant to emtricitabine. However, tenofovir remains effective.

LIVER DAMAGE INDUCED BY ANTIRETROVIRAL DRUGS

Almost all antiretroviral agents may cause liver damage. However, the nature of that damage varies with the drug:

- The NRTIs occasionally cause severe steatosis associated with elevated plasma lactate levels. This side effect is more frequent with stavudine than with other NRTIs.
- The PIs indinavir and atazanavir cause asymptomatic hyperbilirubinemia (pseudo–Gilbert's syndrome). Ritonavir and nelfinavir can occasionally cause cholestasis and hepatitis.
- The NNRTIs are also associated with toxic hepatitis. Severe cases, with death and liver transplantation, have been reported after use of nevirapine. Risk factors include female sex, pregnancy, obesity, and CD4 counts above 400. Such severe cases have not been reported with efavirenz.

CENTRAL NERVOUS SYSTEM

Table 17.14 summarizes the CNS diseases most often seen in HIV infection. See also Chapter 6 for a discussion of infections that can affect both immunocompetent and immunocompromised individuals.

Primary HIV Infection

About half of patients with the acute retroviral syndrome complain of headaches, and in 5% to 20%, clinical signs of meningitis such as neck stiffness or photophobia are evident. Encephalitis, with symptoms ranging from confusion to coma, is rare. In the CSF, lymphocytes predominate, with a cell count of 5 to 200/μm^3. Cranial nerve involvement may occur. Symptoms usually disappear spontaneously.

HIV Encephalopathy

The disease called HIV encephalopathy is synonymous with HIV dementia or AIDS-related dementia. This syndrome includes cognitive, behavioral, and motor symptoms and signs. The diagnosis is often one of exclusion, after neuroradiologic and CSF examinations have failed to show an opportunistic disease.

The first signs are usually memory problems, mental slowness, and lack of precision. Apathy and withdrawal may be interpreted as a depression. Clinical examination shows difficulties in comprehension and coordination, abnormal gait, nystagmus, and archaic reflexes. Without treatment, dementia progresses within a few months. Convulsions may appear. Neuroradiologic investigation usually shows cerebral atrophy. O magnetic resonance imaging (MRI) scan, the T2 signal is increased in the subcortical white matter, preferentially in the parasagittal regions. The CSF shows a variable increase in protein and mononuclear cells.

Since the introduction of HAART, the incidence of HIV dementia has greatly decreased. In established dementia, the effect of HAART is variable, but spectacular improvements are noted in some patients. Despite HAART, many patients continue to complain of subtle symptoms, such as forgetfulness and difficulties with concentration. This may represent a milder form of HIV-related dementia, perhaps related to the lack of penetration of HARRT into the CNS.

Focal CNS Lesions

Cerebral toxoplasmosis, primary cerebral lymphoma, and progressive multifocal leukoencephalopathy (Figure 17-6) cause 90% of focal lesions of the CNS in HIV infection. Differential diagnosis relies upon computed tomography (CT) scan, MRI, and PCR amplification of the DNA from the putative infectious agents in the CSF. Cerebral biopsy remains an option in exceptional cases.

KEY POINTS

About HIV Encephalopathy

1. The diagnosis is made by exclusion.
2. Dementia symptoms are accompanied by apathy and withdrawal that can be mistaken for depression.
3. Magnetic resonance imaging shows an increased T2 signal in the subcortical white matter preferentially in parasagittal regions.
4. Highly active antiretroviral therapy has dramatically decreased the incidence of HIV dementia.

Table 17.14. Central Nervous System Involvement in HIV Infection

Diagnosis	Symptoms and signs	Laboratory and CSF findings	CT/MRI/ PET–SPECT findings	Treatment of choice	Evolution
Cerebral toxoplasmosis	Focal deficit, headache, fever, seizures	CD4 count <200/μm^3; presence of IgG antitoxoplasmosis antibodies; PCR positive if untreated	Multiple corticomedullary lesions with contrast enhancement; edema; PET scan shows hypodense lesions	Sulfadiazine, plus pyrimethamine, plus folinic acid	Better than 80% response to treatment Prophylaxis until immune reconstitution
Primary cerebral lymphoma	Slow onset of reduced consciousness, headache, or focal deficits	CD4 count <100/μm^3; CSF PCR always positive for EBV; cytology is seldom positive	Variable number of lesions; periventricular contrast enhancement; lesions are positive in PET scan	Radiotherapy with or without chemotherapy	Very serious prognosis
Progressive multifocal leukoencephalopathy	Progressive decline in superior cerebral functions, focal lesions	CD4 count <100/μm^3; CSF usually positive for papovavirus JC	Reduced density of white substance on CT, no contrast enhancement or edema; increased T2 signal in MRI without gadolinium enhancement	No specific treatment; cidofovir (?); intensify anti-HIV treatment	Has improved since HAART
Cryptococcal meningitis	Fever, headache; meningeal signs can be present or absent	CD4 count <100/μm^3; blood and LCR positive for cryptococcal antigen; direct stain of CSF	No useful information	Amphotericin B with or without flucytosine, or fluconazole	Better than 80% response; prophylaxis with fluconazole until immune reconstitution
HIV encephalopathy and dementia	Cognitive and motor impairment	CD4 <200/μm^3; rise in HIV in the CSF; moderate rise in CSF cells and proteins	Cortical or subcortical atrophy; MRI shows enhanced T2 signal	Intensify antiretroviral treatment	Progressive dementia within a few months
Aseptic meningitis	Headache, neck stiffness, photophobia, nausea during primary HIV infection	Moderate or no immunosuppression; moderate rise in CSF cell count	Normal	No specific treatment	Spontaneous resolution
CMV encephalitis	Confusion, lethargy, cranial nerve palsies, nystagmus	CD4 <50/μm^3; PCR in the LCR is positive	Periventricular contrast enhancement	Foscarnet and ganciclovir	Bad prognosis

CSF = cerebrospinal fluid; CT = computed tomography; MRI = magnetic resonance imaging; PET–SPECT = positron emission tomography–single-photon emission computed tomography; IgG = immunoglobulin G; PCR = polymerase chain reaction; EBV = Epstein–Barr virus; LCR.

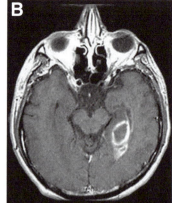

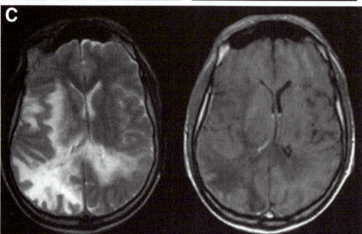

Figure 17-6. Neurologic complication of AIDS (from www.aids-images.ch;). Upper left panel: Toxoplasmosis encephalitis. Magnetic resonance imaging (MRI) scan with contrast shows typical ring-enhancing lesions. Insert: Toxoplasma gondii tissue cyst contains thousands of bradyzoites (100 to 300 mm). Upper right panel: Central nervous system lymphoma. This MRI scan with contrast shows a typical ring-enhancing lesion (picture from Sakaie KE, Gonzalez RG. Imaging of neuroAIDS. NeuroAIDS. 1999;2:online;). Bottom panel: Progressive multifocal leukoencephalopathy. Left: MRI T2 weighted image. Right: T1 image without contrast. Note the hypodensities, reflecting loss of myelin.

(picture courtesy of R. Dupasquier).

TOXOPLASMA ENCEPHALITIS

Toxoplasma encephalitis (Figure 17.6) follows from reactivation of latent *Toxoplasma* infection. Such latent infection is present in 10% (in the United States) to more than 90% (in developing countries) of HIV-infected people.

Toxoplasma encephalitis usually starts with a focal deficit (hemiplegia, for instance), convulsions, headaches, fever, or confusion. In a preponderance of cases, the CD4 count is below $200/\mu m^3$, and if performed, testing for *Toxoplasma* IgG antibody will be positive. If antibody is absent, or if the patient has taken trimethoprim–sulfamethoxazole prophylaxis, another diagnosis should be considered first. The CT or MRI scan shows abscesses that are usually multiple and preferentially located at the corticomedullary junction and in the basal ganglia. Annular contrast or gadolinium enhancement is typical, as is marked edema.

If the IgG antibody are positive and the images are typical, empiric treatment is warranted. If the diagnosis is

---

KEY POINTS

About Central Nervous System Toxoplasmosis

1. Usually presents with focal findings, in the presence of a CD4 count below $200/\mu m^3$ and a positive test for *Toxoplasma* immunoglobulin G antibody.

2. Computed tomography (CT) or magnetic resonance imaging (MRI) scan demonstrates multiple contrast-enhancing ring-like lesions.

3. Empiric treatment is indicated if symptoms and MRI findings are typical. Polymerase chain reaction testing of the cerebrospinal fluid is confirmatory.

4. Treat using a combination of sulfadiazine and pyrimethamine, with added folinic acid.

5. Follow-up CT or MRI scan at 2 weeks should demonstrate improvement.

6. After treatment, secondary prophylaxis is required.

in doubt, *Toxoplasma gondii* DNA can be amplified from the CSF. The rate of DNA positivity decreases when PCR is attempted after treatment has already started. The treatment of choice is a combination of oral sulfadiazine (1 to 1.5 g every 6 hours) and oral pyrimethamine (200 mg the first day, then 50 mg every 6 hours) combined with folinic acid (10 mg daily) to prevent bone marrow toxicity. Steroids (intravenous dexamethasone 4 mg every 6 hours) may be administered to diminish the cerebral edema. This treatment should be continued for 4 to 6 weeks; after that, secondary prevention using oral sulfadiazine 2 g daily and oral pyrimethamine 25 mg daily is indicated. The foregoing regimen will also prevent PCP. After 2 weeks, improvement on repeat brain CT or MRI scan is expected.

Often, treatment of toxoplasmosis is not well tolerated because of cutaneous, renal, or hepatic toxicity from sulfadiazine and bone marrow toxicity from both sulfadiazine and pyrimethamine. As an alternative, clindamycin (600 mg every 6 hours, and then 600 mg every 12 hours) can be combined with pyrimethamine; tolerance of that regimen is usually better, but efficacy is reduced. Another alternative is atovaquone suspension (750 mg every 12 or 8 hours) combined with pyrimethamine.

PRIMARY BRAIN LYMPHOMA

HIV infected patients can develop highly malignant B cell brain lymphoma consisting of large immunoblastic lymphocytes. The tumor always contains the genome of Epstein–Barr virus. Clinical signs usually progress rapidly over a few weeks, with confusion, focal signs, and headache. A CT or MRI scan shows one or several lesions with irregular contrast enhancement and preferential periventricular localization (Figure 17.6). Occasionally, lymphomatous cells can be seen in the CSF, where PCR for Epstein–Barr virus is almost always positive. Newer techniques such as single-photon emission computed tomography and positron emission tomography show hyperactivity in the lesions and are useful to differentiate lymphoma from cerebral toxoplasmosis and from progressive multifocal leukoencephalopathy. Although these tumors are sensitive to radiation and to chemotherapy, the prognosis is poor. Long-term survivors are predominantly those with CD4 counts above $200/\mu m^3$ at diagnosis.

PROGRESSIVE MULTIFOCAL LEUKOENCEPHALOPATHY

Progressive multifocal leukoencephalopathy follows reactivation of papovavirus JC, to which 75% of the population is seropositive. The virus infects oligodendrocytes, which are localized in the white matter. Their destruction causes demyelination.

The disease starts insidiously with loss of memory or dysphasia, visual disturbances, aphasia, or motor signs—or, more rarely, with convulsions. A CT or MRI scan shows one or several subcortical lesions without contrast enhancement or edema (Figure 17.6). These lesions are MRI hyperintense in T2 scans. Usually, a PCR test of the CSF is positive for papovavirus JC. No specific treatment is available (cidofovir and cytosine arabinoside have been tried, with inconsistent results). HAART is a double-edged sword; after starting HAART symptoms may worsen; however over time stabilization and even clinical improvement may ensue.

KEY POINTS

About Central Nervous System Lymphoma in HIV

1. A B cell lymphoma caused by Epstein–Barr virus (EBV).
2. Headache, focal signs, and confusion progress rapidly.
3. Magnetic resonance imaging or computed tomography scan shows 1 or 2 irregular enhancing lesions
4. Polymerase chain reaction of the cerebrospinal fluid is usually positive for EBV.
5. Positron emission tomography and single-photon emission computed tomography scans are helpful in differentiating lymphoma from toxoplasmosis and progressive multifocal leukoencephalopathy.
6. Sensitive to radiation and chemotherapy, but prognosis poor if the patient's CD4 count is below $200/\mu m^3$.

KEY POINTS

About Progressive Multifocal Leukoencephalopathy

1. Caused by reactivated papovavirus JC, infects oligodendrocytes and causes demyelinization.
2. Produces dementia, aphasia, and motor deficits.
3. On MRI, shows as hyperintense T2 images in subcortical regions.
4. Polymerase chain reaction testing of the cerebrospinal fluid is positive for papovavirus JC.
5. Treat with highly active antiretroviral therapy.

Meningitis

CRYPTOCOCCAL MENINGITIS

Cryptococcus neoformans, a yeast, is the most frequent cause of meningitis in HIV infected patients. Cryptococcosis occurs in profoundly immunosuppressed patients and is particularly frequent in Africa and in the United States.

The disease usually starts with headaches and fever; curiously, meningeal signs can be absent. The diagnosis can be made by direct examination of CSF stained with India ink, by finding of cryptococcal antigen in the CSF or in the blood, or by culture of CSF or blood. The CSF shows moderate pleocytosis and an increase in protein; however, in some cases, the CSF formula is only minimally abnormal. A CT or MRI scan is noncontributory (see Chapter 6 for a complete discussion).

Treatment in severe cases consists of intravenous amphotericin B (0.7 mg/kg) for at least 2 weeks. Some authorities recommend the addition of flucytosine (25 mg/kg every 6 hours), but that drug has substantial gastrointestinal and bone marrow toxicity. After 2 weeks, the amphotericin B is replaced with fluconazole 400 mg daily for 6 to 10 weeks, and then 200 mg daily until immune function recovers. In less severe cases (without intracranial hypertension, with normal mental status, and with cryptococcal antigen in the CSF at less than 1:1000 dilution), fluconazole can be used from the start. Itraconazole is not a good choice because it does not penetrate well into the CSF.

CNS Infection by Cytomegalovirus

Cytomegalovirus can cause various nervous system diseases in HIV infection: polyradicular myelitis,

peripheral neuropathy, and encephalitis. Patients with encephalitis are usually profoundly immunosuppressed with a CD4 cell count below $50/\mu m^3$.

Diagnosis is difficult and is usually made after exclusion of other more frequent causes in patients who are confused and lethargic, and who are showing cranial nerve palsies and nystagmus. The typical finding in an MRI or CT scan is periventricular contrast enhancement. A PCR test of the CSF is more than 80% sensitive, and specific. Although foscarnet and ganciclovir should theoretically be effective, the prognosis is unfavorable.

Cerebrovascular Diseases

Cerebrovascular accidents are much more frequent in the HIV-infected populations than in comparable populations of the same age. The pathogenesis is uncertain, but direct involvement of HIV in vasculitis is suspected. Transient ischemic attacks have also been described.

Other Rare Cerebral Disorders

Rare focal diseases in the HIV-infected population include cryptococcoma (in these cases, the cryptococcal antigen test in CSF and blood can be negative), tuberculoma, varicella virus encephalitis, and secondary or tertiary syphilis. In intravenous drug abusers, septic emboli may be associated with cerebral abscesses and mycotic aneurisms.

Peripheral Neuropathy

DISTAL SYMMETRIC POLYNEUROPATHY

Distal symmetric polyneuropathy may cause painful paresthesia and dysesthesia in hands and feet, associated with diminished reflexes and motor weakness in the legs, and autonomic dysfunction.

These polyneuropathies can be very difficult to manage. Amitriptyline or carbamazepine may be useful. Aggravating circumstances include concomitant vitamin deficiencies, diabetes, alcohol abuse, and use of medications such as dapsone, vincristine, and isoniazid. Among antiretroviral drugs, and stavudine cause neuropathy, as do didanosine and lamivudine on occasion. The foregoing drugs can usually be replaced by other nucleosides if necessary.

INFLAMMATORY DEMYELINATING POLYNEUROPATHY

Inflammatory demyelinating polyneuropathy usually occurs during the early stages of HIV infection. Presentation is similar to that of Guillain–Barré syndrome. With steroids, plasmapheresis, or intravenous immunoglobulins, evolution is usually favorable. In some cases, CMV infection is involved.

KEY POINTS

About Cryptococcal Meningitis in HIV

1. *Cryptococcus neoformans* is the most common cause of meningitis in HIV-infected patients.
2. Headache and fever are the most common complaints; neck stiffness is absent.
3. Lymphocytosis of the cerebrospinal fluid (CSF) is usual, but the CSF formula may be only minimally abnormal.
   a) India ink test positive.
   b) Antigen testing of the CSF or blood is positive.
   b) Culture of CSF or blood is frequently positive.
3. Treat with amphotericin B with or without flucytosine for 2 weeks; followed with fluconazole.

Mononeuritis Multiplex

Sudden palsies of one or several nerves, including cranial and laryngeal nerves, can occur at any stage of HIV infection. Varicella virus can be the cause in cases of advanced immunodeficiency.

Myelopathy

Myelopathy presents with gait disturbance, ataxia, spastic paraparesis, and urinary or fecal incontinence. An MRI scan is usually normal, but edema or even enhancing lesions may be seen. Autopsy findings show vacuolization of myelin and an accumulation of macrophages. No specific treatment is available, but potentially reversible causes of myelopathy such as epidural abscess, toxoplasmosis, infection with human T lymphotropic virus type 1, herpes simplex or zoster, CMV, or a vitamin B_{12} deficit should be excluded.

OPHTHALMOLOGY

Also see Chapter 5 for a discussion of infections that can affect both immunocompetent and immunocompromised individuals.

HIV Retinopathy

HIV retinopathy is frequent and benign; it does not require treatment. "Cotton wool" exudates are characteristically observed; these correspond to focal lesions of ischemia. Besides exudates, intraretinal hemorrhages, telangiectasias, and microaneurysms may occur; these conditions must be distinguished from retinal lesions caused by diabetes or hypertension. HIV retinopathy does not interfere with vision.

KEY POINTS

About Peripheral Neuropathies in HIV

1. In distal symmetrical polyneuropathy associated with paresthesias and weakness, drugs that cause neuropathy should be discontinued. Treat with amitriptyline or carbamazepine.
2. Treat inflammatory demyelinating polyneuropathy with plasmapheresis or a cytomegalovirus regimen.
3. Mononeuritis multiplex can be caused by varicella virus.
4. Myelopathy can lead to spastic paraparesis; look for reversible causes.

Cytomegalovirus Retinitis

Chorioretinitis from CMV occurs in patients with profound immunosuppression (CD4 count below $50/\mu m^3$); CMV IgG antibodies are invariably present. Before HAART became available, 25% to 30% of patients with AIDS developed retinitis before death. All patients with HIV should be repeated questioned about changes in vision—blurring of vision, loss of central vision or other blind spots, floaters, or flashing lights.

Cytomegalovirus retinitis is a subacute disease in which visual deficits progress within a few weeks. The diagnosis is easily made by examining the retina, which shows a characteristic mix of exudates, hemorrhages, and atrophy. Exudates often sheath the vessels. Without treatment, lesions invariably progress to retinal detachment with progressive loss of vision. Often, both eyes are involved, as are other organs such as the colon, esophagus, or brain.

Treatment starts with high doses of medication, followed by secondary prophylaxis using the same drugs at lower doses. Three drugs are available: ganciclovir, foscarnet, and cidofovir.

KEY POINTS

About Cytomegalovirus Retinitis

1. Before the advent of highly active antiretroviral therapy, 35% to 30% of AIDS patients developed this infection.
2. Visual symptoms—blurred vision, scotomas, floaters, or flashing lights—are subacute in onset.
3. Retinal findings are characteristic: mix of exudates, hemorrhages, and atrophy; vascular sheathing.
4. Treatment is required to prevent progression to retinal detachment and blindness.
   a) Ganciclovir is the drug of choice; causes bone marrow toxicity, and dosing must be corrected for renal dysfunction.
   b) Foscarnet is associated with renal failure; intravenous NaCl is protective.
   c) Cidofovir, a once-weekly therapy, is associated with renal failure 25% of patients; probenecid and intravenous NaCl are helpful protective measures.
5. Maintenance therapy is required in patients with a CD4 count below $100/\mu m^3$; primary prophylaxis reduces the incidence, but is expensive and associated with side effects.

- Ganciclovir 5 mg/kg is administered intravenously every 12 hours. Its main side effects are leukopenia and thrombocytopenia. Ganciclovir accumulates in patients with renal failure, and doses have to be adapted. Oral valganciclovir (450 mg BID) has good bioavailability and is as efficacious as iv ganciclovir for treatment as well as for maintenance therapy.
- Foscarnet 60 mg/kg is administered every 8 hours. It is nephrotoxic (hydration with 1 L 0.9% NaCl is necessary) and causes numerous electrolyte disturbances (hypocalcemia, hypokalemia, hypophosphatemia, and hypomagnesemia), convulsions, and genital ulcers.
- Cidofovir has the advantage of infrequent administration (5 mg/kg once weekly for 2 weeks, then 5 mg/kg every 2 weeks), but it is also nephrotoxic in 25% of patients and may cause neutropenia. Nephrotoxicity can be diminished, but not eliminated, by administering oral probenecid 2 g before the cidofovir and 1 g at 1 and 8 hours after, in conjunction with intravenous NaCl. Particular care is needed when cidofovir is co-administered with tenofovir.

After an initial treatment course lasting at least 2 weeks, doses can be lowered: valganciclovir 450 mg daily, foscarnet 100 mg/kg daily 5 days per week, cidofovir 5 mg/kg every 2 weeks. Treatment with intravenous ganciclovir or foscarnet (or both) necessitates use of a permanent catheter.

Secondary prophylaxis of CMV retinitis is onerous. In patients with a good response to HAART and a durable rise in CD4 count above $100/\mu m^3$, treatment can be discontinued without risk of relapse.

Patients with persistently low CD4 counts should be regularly examined so as to detect CMV retinitis and institute early treatment to prevent loss of vision. Preventive administration of oral valganciclovir diminishes the incidence of CMV retinitis by at least 50%. However, because of expense, inconvenience, and side effects, such prevention has not commonly been used. Of course, the best prevention of all is correction of the underlying immunodeficiency by effective HAART.

Retinal Necroses

Retinal necrosis is a medical emergency necessitating treatment within hours. This disease is caused by varicella virus. Two clinical presentations can be distinguished:

- **Acute Retinal Necrosis**. Acute retinal necrosis (ARN) causes orbital pain and inflammation visible in the anterior ocular segment with hypopyon. At the same time, peripheral retinal necrosis with vasculitis occurs. Without treatment, progression to retinal detachment and blindness is rapid.

- **Progressive Outer Retinal Necrosis**. In contrast to ARN, progressive outer retinal necrosis (PORN) causes no pain. However, the patient notices a marked loss of visual acuity. Often, these patients have recently had herpes zoster. The anterior segment does not show evidence of inflammation; however, peripheral lesions of retinal necrosis occur. Again, there is a major risk of rapid vision loss. For both ARN and PORN, treatment involves high doses of intravenous acyclovir, and ganciclovir if a possibility of CMV retinitis exists.

Other Infectious Eye Diseases

P. jiroveci may occasionally involve the retina. Cryptococcal meningitis may be complicated by papillary edema. Particularly in intravenous drug abusers, *Candida albicans* and other bacteremia may cause retinitis. Uveitis can complicate the administration of rifabutin, particularly when rifabutin levels are boosted by co-administration of macrolides or PIs.

SKIN DISEASES

It is important to recognize skin diseases during HIV infection. The development of a new skin rash often warrants immediate action (see Table 17.15). For instance, new acneiform lesions accompanied by fever suggest primary HIV infection. New onset of a maculopapular total body rash is indicative of a drug reaction. New crops of macular, papular, pustular, or vesicular lesions may represent the first manifestation of an opportunistic infection. Even benign skin diseases may have a major psychological impact when they reveal the patient's HIV status to the outside world.

Table 17.15. Skin Diseases in HIV

Disease	Signs and symptoms	Diagnosis	Treatment	Comments
Acute HIV infection	Reddish macules on trunk, face, palms of hands, and soles of feet	Rise in viremia and P24 antigenemia	HAART	Standard screening test for HIV can still be negative
Oral leukoplakia	Whitish plaques on the lateral aspect of the tongue	Clinical aspect	No treatment	Associated with advancing immunodeficiency
Kaposi's sarcoma (result of HHV8)	Macules, papules, or nodules of purple to dark blue color; edema and ulcers are possible	Inspection and histology	HAART; local treatment; cryotherapy, radiotherapy, and systemic chemotherapy	
Bacillary angiomatosis (*Bartonella henselae*)	Red-to-violet papule or nodule	Histology (culture is difficult)	Antibiotics (macrolides, quinolones, and tetracyclines)	Rare; associated with advanced immunodeficiency
Herpes zoster	Vesicles on a red surface, necrosis, dermatomal distribution	Thorough inspection, possibly confirmed by culture and immunofluorescence	Oral valacyclovir, or famciclovir, or acyclovir; in serious cases, IV acyclovir	Chronic and disseminated forms are possible in advanced immunodeficiency
Seborrheic dermatitis (mold, *Malassezia?*)	Red and squamous plaques on face and trunk	Inspection	Topical ketoconazole	Prevalence > 30%
Acute condylomata	Wart-like papules resembling a rooster's comb	Inspection, or histology and typing of HPV	Curettage, podophyllin, electrocoagulation, or laser	Treat sexual partner at the same time
Molluscum contagiosum (virus pox)	Umbilicated papules	Inspection and histology	Curettage or electrocoagulation	
Herpes simplex	Painful vesicles or ulcers that can become very large	Inspection, culture, and immunofluorescence	Valacyclovir, or famciclovir; possibly IV acyclovir	Lesions are primarily perianal, vulvar, or peribuccal
Prurigo nodularis	Isolated, very itchy squamous papules	Histology	Symptomatic treatment	Possibly with UV irradiation

HHV8 = human herpesvirus 8; HPV = human papilloma virus; UV = ultraviolet.

Primary HIV Infection

Primary HIV infection causes erythematous macules or papules with ill-defined borders and symmetrical distribution on the front and back of the trunk, the face, and sometimes on the palms and soles. The skin lesions neither itch nor hurt. They resemble Gilbert's pityriasis or the lesions of secondary syphilis, which are the principal differential diagnoses. Other differentials include viral exanthema as a result of Epstein–Barr virus, CMV, rubella, or a toxic or allergic reaction to medication. The lesions persist for a median of 2 weeks, and then fade spontaneously. Less commonly, painful mucosal ulcers occur (Figure 17-1).

Opportunistic Infections with Skin or Mucosal Involvement

CHRONIC HERPES SIMPLEX

In severely immunosuppressed patients, herpes simplex type I or II may cause persistent genital, perianal or perioral ulcerations. Although herpes simplex is by far the most likely causative agent, the differential diagnosis is large, including infections by fungi, mycobacteria, CMV, and varicella virus, and malignant skin tumors. Confirmation is obtained by biopsy and immunofluorescence or by culture of a virus. The preferred treatment is valacyclovir 500 mg or famciclovir 125 mg twice daily. Herpes simplex virus may become resistant to acyclovir and its derivatives, necessitating alternative treatment with foscarnet.

HERPES ZOSTER

Herpes zoster caused by reactivation of varicella virus occurs almost 20 times more frequently in HIV-positive individuals than in HIV-negative individuals of the same age, and the condition can present at any stage of immunosuppression. In the severely immunosuppressed patient, herpes zoster may extend beyond one or two dermatomes, causing atypical, ulcerated, and painful lesions that are difficult to treat. In cases in which the skin lesions are atypical, biopsy with direct immunofluorescence establishes the diagnosis. Particularly in cases in which immune suppression is severe, treatment is indicated: use valacyclovir 1 g every 8 hours or famciclovir 500 mg twice daily. In patients with severe immune suppression, intravenous acyclovir may be preferred.

KAPOSI'S SARCOMA

Kaposi's sarcoma is a very unusual "tumor." Infection by a virus—human herpesvirus 8 (HHV8)—is a necessary but not sufficient condition. Kaposi's sarcoma appears in patients who are HHV8 seropositive and who have a variable degree of immunosuppression. Very often, Kaposi's sarcoma is multifocal from the start. Karyotypic anomalies have not been described. Lesions resemble reactive hypoplasia rather than typical malignancies. In the United States and in Europe, Kaposi's sarcoma is essentially a disease of patients who acquired their HIV infection by homosexual contact. Although cases can occur in patients with a nearly normal CD4 count, immune suppression greatly increases the risk.

The lesions of Kaposi's sarcoma are macules, papules, or nodules of characteristic purple color. Preferred locations are the extremities, the tip of the nose, and the palate. Often, the lesions are only slowly progressive and do not cause pain. In rare cases, Kaposi's sarcoma may run an aggressive course with nodular, ulcerated lesions; limb edema; and gastrointestinal and pulmonary involvement. Kaposi's sarcoma is easy to recognize; when in doubt, a

---

> ### KEY POINTS
>
> ### About Kaposi's Sarcoma
>
> 1. Associated with human herpesvirus 8; in the United States and Europe, is found mainly in HIV-infected homosexual men.
> 2. Manifests as macules, papules, or nodules of distinctive purple color, usually on the extremities, the tip of the nose, and the palate.
> 3. Disease is occasionally aggressive, with limb edema and gastrointestinal and pulmonary involvement.
> 4. Histopathologic examination shows vascular proliferation and fusiform cells.
> 5. May be refractory to therapy.
>   a) HAART usually induces remissions.
>   b) For local disease, cryotherapy or radiotherapy can be used.
>   c) In severe disease, liposomal doxorubicin or vincristine plus bleomycin, or α-interferon are favored.

---

skin biopsy showing vascular proliferation and fusiform cells will yield the diagnosis.

The incidence and severity of Kaposi's sarcoma is favorably influenced by HAART, which has become the mainstay of treatment. If the lesions persist or enlarge, local treatment by cryotherapy or radiotherapy is recommended. Systemic treatment is necessary in cases with edema of extremities, genitalia, or the face, or in cases of massive visceral involvement. Many chemotherapeutic agents produce remissions, but these are rarely of long duration. For reasons of relative lack of side effects and good efficacy, liposomal preparations of doxorubicin, used at a dose of 40 mg/m^2 every 2 to 3 weeks are currently popular. The combination of bleomycin 10 mg/m^2 and vincristine 2 mg is also effective, as is high-dose intravenous α-interferon (up to 50×10^6 U 5 days per week) in patients with a CD4 count above $200/\mu m^3$.

BACILLARY ANGIOMATOSIS

Bacillary angiomatosis is caused by *Bartonella henselae*, the agent that is responsible for cat scratch disease (see Chapter 13). In HIV infection, *B. henselae* causes papules and nodules of a red-to-violet color. These are present in variable numbers, are not painful, and may be ulcerated. Patients are usually febrile and extremely immunosuppressed. Liver ("peliosis hepatitis") and bone may be involved.

A biopsy with silver impregnation stain can show the *Bartonella* and differentiate the disease from Kaposi's sarcoma. A serologic test is also available. Prolonged treatment with clarithromycin 500 mg twice daily, azithromycin 250 mg daily, or ciprofloxacin 500 mg twice daily is necessary.

SEBORRHEIC DERMATITIS

Seborrheic dermatitis is frequent in the general population. However, in HIV-infected patients, the disease may be particularly severe. Reddish plaques covered by small scales appear on the face (nose, between the eyebrows), the scalp, and the sternum. Ketoconazole creams and shampoos are efficacious.

MOLLUSCUM CONTAGIOSUM

The lesions of molluscum contagiosum are caused by poxvirus. The multiple, umbilicated, painless flesh-colored papules or nodules appear particularly on the face and the genitalia. In immunosuppressed patients, they can persist for months and become extremely numerous. The lesions can be destroyed by curettage, electrocoagulation, or cryotherapy. Cidofovir may be effective in extreme cases.

Drug Reactions

Drug rashes are frequent during HIV infection and can constitute an emergency. Conjunctivitis or lesions of the buccal mucosa, generalized erythroderma, and detachment of the skin are alarming; these signs necessitate hospitalization and specialized consultation. However, drug rashes are more often mild and will disappear even if the drug is continued—particularly in the case of early reactions to efavirenz and nevirapine. Because alternative treatments often have disadvantages of their own, an effort should be made to "treat through" drug eruptions that are not severe.

Skin Diseases Aggravated by HIV

Many common skin diseases—for instance, dryness of the skin, psoriasis, reactions to insect stings, and dermatomycosis—seem to be more severe in patients who also have HIV infection.

KEY POINTS

About Drug Rashes in HIV-Infected Patients

- -

1. Conjunctivitis, buccal mucosa lesions, erythroderma, and skin detachment are danger signs.
2. "Treat through" milder drug eruptions.

SEXUALLY TRANSMITTED DISEASES

The occurrence of sexually transmitted diseases (also see Chapter 9) in an HIV-positive patient is a reminder of unsafe sexual practices and an occasion to reinforce educational messages about the need to prevent transmission of HIV.

Syphilis

Treatment of syphilis in the HIV-infected individual has elicited a great deal of controversy. Contrary to widespread belief, serologic tests for syphilis are as valid in HIV-infected people as in an uninfected population. The recommended treatment regimens are benzathine penicillin 2.4×10^6 U intramuscularly at weeks 0, 1, and 2 in cases of secondary or latent tertiary syphilis, and a prolonged course of high-dose intravenous penicillin or ceftriaxone in cases of suspected neurosyphilis.

FURTHER READING

Some of the best (and certainly the most up-to-date) resources can be accessed via the Internet.

General

University of California–San Francisco. HIV InSite [Web page]. San Francisco, Calif.: UCSF; 2007. [Available online at: http://hivinsite.ucsf.edu/InSite; cited]

Medscape. HIV/AIDS [Web page]. New York, NY 2007: Medscape; n.d. [Available online at: http://medscape.com/hiv; cited]

Drug Interactions

University of Liverpool. Liverpool HIV Pharmacology Group www.hiv-druginteractions.org home page [Web site]. Liverpool, U.K.: University of Liverpool; 2007. [Available online at: http://www.hiv-druginteractions.org; cited]

Epidemiology

United Nations, Joint UN Programme on HIV/AIDS. Home page [Web page]. Geneva, Switzerland: UNAIDS; 2007. [Available online at: http://www.unaids.org; cited]

Up-to-Date Treatment Guidelines

United States, Department of Health and Human Services. AIDSinfo, clinical guidelines. Rockville, MD: DHHS; 2007. [Available online at: http://aidsinfo.nih.gov/Guidelines/Default.aspx? MenuItem?Guidelines; cited]

Index

Page numbers in *italics* denote figures; those followed by "t" denote tables

A

Abacavir, 407, 408*t*
Abdominal tuberculosis, 423
Abscess
  brain, 157–163
  hepatic, 214–215
  intracranial, 163
  orbital, 135
  pancreatic, 215–216
  perivalvular, 181
  skin, 260*t*, 268–269
  spinal epidural, 164–165
Acid-base disturbances, in sepsis syndrome, 61
Actinomyces israelii, 99
Actinomycosis, 99
Acute diarrhea, 196
Acute retinal necrosis (ARN), 431
Acyclovir, 49–53, 51*t*, 368, 381
Adenoviruses, 121*t*, 185, 205
Adult respiratory distress syndrome (ARDS), 61–62
Afebrile patients, 392
African tick-bite fever, 334
Agammaglobulinemia, 152
Alanine aminotransferase (ALT), 219
Albendazole, 298–299*t*
Alkaline phosphatase, 215, 219
Alphavirus, 155*t*
ALT (alanine aminotransferase), 219
Amantadine, 52*t*, 56, 378
Amblyomma americanum, 337
American Academy of Pediatrics, 130
Amikacin, 24*t*, 111*t*, 391*t*
Amikin, 24*t*, 111*t*
Aminoglycosides, 23–27
  chemistry and mechanisms of action, 23
  dosing, 24*t*
  nephrotoxicity of, 23
  for neutropenic patients, 391*t*
  organisms susceptible to, 24*t*
  ototoxicity of, 23
  pharmacokinetics of, 23–26
  spectrum of activity, 26–27
  treatment recommendations, 26–27
Aminopenicillins, 15
Aminotransferases, 219
Amoebiasis, 205–207
  clinical features of, 206
  diagnosis of, 206–207
  epidemiology of, 205–206
  life cycle of, 205–206
  treatment of, 207

Amoebic liver abscess, 214
Amoxicillin, 15
  antimicrobial spectrum of, 15
  dosing, 14*t*
  treatment recommendations, 15
    for chronic arthritis, 327*t*
    for leptospirosis, 327*t*
    for Lyme diseases, 326, 327*t*
    for otitis media, 128*t*, 131
    for sinusitis, 128*t*, 137
Amoxicillin-clavulanate, 14*t*, 128*t*, 137, 238*t*, 261*t*, 391*t*
Amoxil, 14*t*
Amphotericin B, 298*t*
Amphotericin B, 42–45
Amphotericin B deoxycholate, 391*t*
Ampicillin, 15
  antimicrobial spectrum of, 15
  dosing, 14*t*
  treatment recommendations, 15
    for bacterial meningitis, 147*t*
    for infective endocarditis, 178*t*
    for pyelonephritis, 238*t*
Ampicillin-sulbactam, 14t, 261*t*
Amprenavir, 408*t*
Anal carcinoma, 424
Anaplasma, 327*t*
       Anaplasma phagocytophilum, 331, 336–337, 338*f*
Ancef, 17*t*
Ancylostoma duodenale, 309–310
Aneurysms, 177
Anidulafungin, 47–48
Animal bites, 270–271
Anopheles funestus, 289
Anopheles gambiae, 289
Anthrax, 350–356
  case study of, 351–352
  clinical features of, 351–354
  cutaneous, 352–353
  diagnosis of, 354–355
  epidemiology of, 351
  gastrointestinal, 354
  inhalation, 353–354
  microbiology of, 351
  pathogenesis of, 351
  prophylaxis for, 355–356
  treatment of, 355, 356*t*
Antibiotic-associated diarrhea, 200–204
  clinical features of, 201–202
  diagnosis of, 202–203
  epidemiology of, 201

  microbiology of, 201
  pathogenesis of, 201
  potential severity of, 200
  prevention of, 203
  treatment of, 203
Antibiotic lock therapy, 184
Antibiotics, 11–41. *See also* specific drugs
    and classes
  aminoglycosides, 23–27
  antibiogram of, 9*f*
  in anti-infective therapy, 6–10
  carbapenems, 22
  cephalosporins, 18–21
  chloramphenicol, 34–35
  clindamycin, 31–32
  daptomycin, 39–40
  degradation or modification of, 3
  dosing, 4–5
  enzyme modification of, 3
  glycopeptide, 27–29
  ketolides, 29–31
  ß-lactam antibiotics, 11–13
  macrolides, 29–31
  metronidazole, 40
  micafungin, 47–48
  microbial resistance to, 2–4
  monobactams, 21–22
  oxazolidones, 37–38
  penicillins, 13–18
  quinolones, 35–37
  for specific infections
    bacterial diarrhea, 198–200
    bacterial meningitis, 146–148
    brain abscess, 161–162
    infective endocarditis, 177–180
    intravascular catheter-related infections, 184–185
    necrotizing fasciitis, 262–263
    sepsis syndrome, 62–63
    sexually transmitted diseases (STDs), 242–244*t*
    sinusitis, 137
    urinary tract infections (UTIs), 237–239
    zoonotic, 327–328*t*
  spectrum of activity, 8*t*
  streptogramins, 38–39
  sulfonamides, 40–42
  tetracyclines, 32–34
Antibiotics (*con't*)
  toxicities of, 25*t*
  trimethoprim, 40–42

Antifungal agents, 42–49
  amphotericin B, 42–45
  anidulafungin, 47–48
  azoles, 45–47
  caspofungin, 47–48
  dosing, 43*t*
  flucytosine, 48–49
  toxicities of, 43*t*
Anti-infective therapy, 1–56
  antibiotics for, 11–41
  antifungal agents for, 42–49
  antiviral drugs for, 49–56
  basic strategies for, 6–10
  case study of, 10
  colonization *vs.* infection in, 10
  dosing, 4–5
  microbial resistance to, 1–4
Anti-influenza viral agents, 56
Antimicrobial resistance, 1–4
  biomechanical mechanisms for, 3–4
  genetic modifications leading to, 2–3
  odification of antibiotic target, 4
    alterations in cell wall precursors, 4
    alterations in ribosomal binding site, 4
    changes in target enzymes, 4
    reduction of antibiotic concentration, 3–4
    interference with antibiotic entry, 3–4
    production of efflux pumps, 4
Antipseudomonal ß-lactam, 391*t*
Antiretroviral resistance, 404
Antiretroviral therapy, 405–412
  advantages and disadvantages of early treatment, 407*t*
  compliance in, 410
  and diarrhea, 422
  drug interactions in, 410
  drugs for, 407, 408*t*
  efficacy of, 410–411
  failure of, 411–412
  indications for starting, 405–406
  liver damaged from, 425
  measurement of plasma drug concentrations in, 411
  modification and simplification of, 411
  principles for, 405, 406*t*
  prophylaxis for opportunistic infections, 412
  resistance tests, 411
  side effects of, 407–410
  timing of, 407
  tolerance for, 407–410
Antiviral drugs, 49–56
  acyclovir, 49–53
  amantadine, 56
  cidofovir, 53–54
  dosing, 51*t*
  famciclovir, 49–53
  foscarnet, 54–55
  ganciclovir, 53
  interferons, 55–56
  neuramidase inhibitors, 56
  ribavirin, 55
  rimantadine, 56
  toxicities of, 50*t*

  valacyclovir, 49–53
  valganciclovir, 53
Aphthous stomatitis, 421
Aplastic anemia, 301
Arachnoid, 139
Arboviruses, 155*t*
ARDS (adult respiratory distress syndrome), 61–62
Argyll Robertson pupils, 251
ARN (acute retinal necrosis), 431
Artemisin, 294
Arteritis, 251
Arthralgias, 172
Ascaris, 298*t,* 306
Aseptic meningitis, 151, 426*t*
Aspartate aminotransferase (AST), 219
Aspergillosis, 419
Aspergillus, 137, 387
Aspiration pneumonia, 97–99
  from anaerobic and aerobic mouth flora, 98
  bronchial obstruction, 98
  case study of, 97–98
  chemical burn pneumonitis, 98
  diagnosis of, 98–99
  treatment of, 99
AST (aspartate aminotransferase), 219
Astroviruses, 205
Asymptomatic filariasis, 318
Atovaquone, 298*t*
Atovaquone-proguanil, 294
Atrial myxoma, 70
Atypical pneumonia, 96–97, 113–114
Augmentin, 14*t,* 137
Autoimmune diseases, 71–72
Azactam, 17*t*
Azithromycin, 29–31
  antimicrobial spectrum of, 31
  chemistry and mechanism of action, 29–30
  dosing, 28*t*
  pharmacokinetics of, 30–31
  toxicity of, 30
  treatment recommendations, 31
    for babesiosis, 298*t*
    for bacterial diarrhea, 199*t*
    for *Bartonella* lymphatic disease, 327*t*
    for *Mycobacterium* infections, 414*t*
    for sinusitis, 137
Azoles, 45–47
Aztreonam, 17*t,* 21–22, 147*t,* 238*t*

B
Babesia, 296–297
Babesiosis, 296–299
  case study of, 296–297
  clinical features of, 296–297
  diagnosis of, 297–299
  epidemiology of, 296
  life cycle of, 296
  prevalence of, 296
  treatment of, 297–299
Bacillary angiomatosis, 343, 433–434
Bacillus anthracis, 351
Bacillus cereus, 125
Bacitracin, 122

Back pain, 172
Bacteremia, 58, 169–170
Bacterial diarrhea, 190–200
  case study of, 191
  clinical features of, 196–198
  diagnosis of, 198
  pathogenesis of, 191–196
    Campylobacter, 193–194
    Escherichia coli, 193–194
    Salmonella, 191–193
    Shigella, 193
    Vibrio cholera, 195–196
    Vibrio parahaemolyticus, 196
    Yersinia, 196
  potential severity of, 190
  prevention of, 200
  treatment of, 198–200
Bacterial infections, 336–339. *See also*
    specific infections
  anthrax, 350–356
  antibiotics for, 11–41
  Bartonella infections, 341–344
  bite wounds, 270–271
  brain abscess, 157–163
  brucellosis, 344–347
  burn wounds, 265–266
  cellulitis, 257–259
  conjunctivitis, 121
  corneal, 121
  diarrhea, 190–200
  endophthalmitis, 125–126
  epiglottitis, 129
  fever of undetermined origin (FUO) in, 69–70
  folliculitis, 266–267
  furunculosis, 267–268
  Helicobacter pylori-associated peptic ulcer, 217–218
  hepatic abscess, 214–215
  immunocompromised host, 386
  impetigo, 266
  infective endocarditis, 167–181
  intravascular catheter-related, 181–185
  leptospirosis, 328–331
  Lyme disease, 322–328
  mastoiditis, 131–132
  meningitis, 140–150
  myonecrosis, 263–265
  necrotizing fasciitis, 259–263
  neutropenia, 385
  osteomyelitis, 273–283
  otitis externa, 130
  otitis media, 130–131
  pericarditis, 186–188
  peritonitis, 210–214
  pharyngitis, 127–129
  plague, 357–358
  prostatitis, 239–240
  prosthetic joints, 283–284
  Q fever, 339–341
  rickettsial diseases, 331–334
    Rocky Mountain spotted fever, 331–334
    spotted fevers, 334–335
    typhus, 335–336

septic arthritis, 284–286
sexually transmitted diseases (STDs), 240–245
sinusitis, 132–137
skin abscesses, 268–269
syphilis, 248–254
tularemia, 258–260
urinary tract, 232
urinary tract infections (UTIs), 231–239
Bacterial meningitis, 140–150
case study of, 143
chemoprophylaxis for, 150
clinical features of, 143–145
complications of, 148–149
diagnosis of, 145–146
epidemiology of, 140–141
initial management of, 145*f*
major pathogens of, 140–141
mortality rate, 148–149
pathogenesis of, 142
prevention of, 149–150
treatment of, 146–148
vaccines for, 149–150
Bacterial pneumonia, 418
Bacterial sinusitis, 136–137
Bacterial vaginosis, treatment of, 244*t*
Bannworth's syndrome, 324
Barium enema, 169*t*
Bartonella henselae, 341–343
Bartonella infections, 341–344
bacillary angiomatosis, 343
bacteremia in, 343
cat scratch disease, 342–343
clinical features of, 342
diagnosis of, 343–344
epidemiology of, 341
pathogenesis of, 341–342
treatment of, 344
Bartonella lymphatic disease, treatment of, 327*t*
Bartonella quintana, 343–344
Batson's plexus, 274
B cells, 185
Behcet's syndrome, 247*t*
Benzathine penicillin, 14t, 128*t*, 253
Benznidazole, 298*t*, 304
β-Lactam antibiotics, 3, 11–13
chemistry and mechanisms of action, 11–12
toxicities of, 12–13, 12*t*
Biaxin, 28*t*
Biologic weapons, 349
Bioterrorism, 349–363
anthrax, 350–356
approach to management of, 350
definition of, 349
ideal biologic agents for, 349
plague, 357–358
potential severity of, 349
small pox, 360–363
tularemia, 358–360
BioThrax, 355
Black fever, 301
Blackwater fever, 293
Blood-brain barrier, 18–19, 158

Blood cultures, 74, 174–175
Blood transfusions, 397–398
Body temperature, 66
Bone marrow transplantation, 388–389
Borrelia burgdorferi, 285, 297, 322–323
Borrelia lonestari, 322
Boutonneuse fever, 334
Bradycardia, in sepsis syndrome, 61
Brain abscess, 157–163
case study of, 157
clinical features of, 159–160
diagnosis of, 160
computed tomography scan, 160
lumbar puncture, 161
magnetic resonance imaging (MRI), 160–161
microbiology of, 158–159
in immigrants, 158–159
in immunocompromised host, 158–159
neurologic deficits in, 160*t*
pathogenesis of, 157–158
direct spread, 157–158
hematogenous spread, 158
potential severity of, 157
prevalence of, 157
treatment of, 161–163
antibiotics, 161–162
glucocorticoids, 162–163
surgery, 162
Brill-Zinsser disease, 335
Bronchopneumonia, 85
Bronchoscopy, 169*t*
Brucella, 344–347
Brucellosis, 344–347
case study of, 345
clinical features of, 345–346
diagnosis of, 346
pathogenesis of, 344–345
potential severity of, 344
treatment of, 327–328*t*, 346–347
Brudzinski's nape-of-the-neck sign, 143
Brugia malayi, 299*t*, 317–319
Brugia timori, 317
Bubo, 357
Bullae, 262
Bunyavirus, 155*t*
Burn infections, 265–266
clinical features of, 265–266
pathology of, 265
treatment of, 266

C
Calabar swellings, 319
California group encephalitis, 155*t*
Campylobacter, 192*t*, 193–194, 422
Candida, 387, 421
Candida albicans, 125, 169, 183, 422
Candida krusei, 169
Candidiasis, 401*t*, 420–421
Capastat, 111*t*
Capreomycin, 111*t*
Carbapenems, 22
chemistry and pharmacokinetics of, 22
dosing, 21*t*

for neutropenic patients, 391*t*
spectrum of activity, 22
treatment recommendations, 22
Carboxypenicillins, 16–18
Carbuncles, 268
Cardiovascular infections, 167–188
infective endocarditis, 167–181
intravascular catheter-related, 181–185
myocarditis, 185–186
pericarditis, 186–188
Cardiovascular syphilis, 251
Case studies
acute pneumonia, 82–83
anthrax, 351–352
anti-infective therapy, 10
aspiration pneumonia, 97–98
babesiosis, 296–297
bacterial diarrhea, 191
bacterial meningitis, 143
brain abscess, 157
brucellosis, 345
cellulitis, 258
chicken pox, 367–368
corneal infections, 122
echinococcosis, 312
ehrlichiosis, 337–338
Epstein-Barr virus (EBV), 369
fever of undetermined origin (FUO), 68–69, 70–71
hantavirus pulmonary syndrome (HPS), 373
hematogenous osteomyelitis, 274–275
immunocompromised hosts, 385
infective endocarditis, 171
intravascular catheter-related infections, 181–182
leptospirosis, 329
Lyme disease, 323
malaria, 292
mastoiditis, 131
myonecrosis, 264
necrotizing fasciitis, 261–262
opportunistic HIV infections, 412–413
prosthetic joint infections, 283
Rocky Mountain spotted fever, 332–333
schistosomiasis, 315
sepsis syndrome, 60–61
septic arthritis, 285
sinusitis, 133–134
Still's disease, 70–71
Strongyloides infection, 307–308
tuberculosis, 103–104
urinary tract infections (UTIs), 234
viral diarrhea, 205
viral encephalitis, 154
viral meningitis, 150
Caspofungin, 47–48, 391*t*
Cat bites, 270–271
Catheters, 182
Cat scratch disease, 342–343
Cavernous sinus thrombosis, 135
CD4 cells, 399–401
CD14 receptor, 59
Ceclor, 17*t*
Cefaclor, 17*t*, 19

Cefadroxil, 260*t*
Cefazolin, 17*t*, 18–19, 178*t*, 260*t*
Cefepime, 20–21
  dosing, 17*t*
  for malignant otitis externa, 128*t*
  for neutropenic patients, 391*t*
  for pyelonephritis, 238*t*
  for sepsis syndrome, 63*t*
Cefixime, 17*t*, 20
Cefizox, 17*t*
Cefotan, 17*t*
Cefotaxime, 17*t*, 19–20, 128*t*, 147*t*
Cefotetan, 17*t*, 19
Cefoxitin, 17*t*, 19
Cefpirome, 17*t*, 21
Cefpodoxime, 128*t*
Cefpodoxime proxetil, 17*t*, 238*t*
Cefprozil, 128*t*
Ceftazidime, 17*t*, 128*t*, 147*t*
Ceftin, 17*t*
Ceftizoxime, 17*t*
Ceftriaxone, 19–20
  antimicrobial spectrum of, 19
  dosing, 17*t*
  treatment recommendations, 19–20
    for bacterial diarrhea, 199*t*
    for bacterial meningitis, 147*t*
    for epiglottitis, 128*t*
    for heart block or meningitis, 327*t*
    for infective endocarditis, 178*t*
    for leptospirosis, 327*t*
    for Lyme diseases, 327*t*
    for mastoiditis, 128*t*
    for pyelonephritis, 238*t*
    for sepsis syndrome, 63*t*
    for sinusitis, 128*t*
Cefuroxime, 17*t*, 128*t*, 327*t*
Cefuroxime-axetil, 17*t*, 326
Cellulitis, 257–259
  case study of, 258
  clostridial, 259
  diagnosis of, 259
  erysipelas, 258–259
  non-clostridial anaerobic, 259
  orbital, 135
  periorbital, 135
  predisposing factors for, 258
  treatment of, 259
Cell walls, 58
Centers for Disease Control and Prevention
  (CDC), 246, 350
Centor clinical criteria, 127
Central nervous system (CNS) infections,
  139–165
  bacterial meningitis, 140–150
  brain abscess, 157–163
  cerebrospinal fluid (CSF) profiles in, 146*t*
  cryptococcal meningoencephalitis, 153–154
  encephalitis, 152–157
  in HIV infection, 425–430
    cerebrovascular diseases, 429
    cryptococcal meningitis, 429
    cytomegalovirus infection, 429
    focal CNS lesions, 425–428

    primary brain lymphoma, 428
    progressive multifocal
      leukoencephalopathy, 428
      Toxoplasma encephalitis, 425–428
    HIV encephalopathy, 425
    peripheral neuropathy, 429–430
      distal symmetric polyneuropathy, 429
      inflammatory demyelinating
        polyneuropathy, 429
      mononeuritis multiplex, 429
      myelopathy, 429–430
    in primary HIV infection, 425
  intracranial epidural and subdural
    abscess, 163
  potential severity of, 139
  spiral epidural abscess, 164–165
  tuberculosis meningitis, 152
  viral encephalitis, 154–157
  viral meningitis, 150–152
Cephalexin, 17*t*, 260*t*
Cephalosporins, 18–21
  allergy to, 147
  for clostridia, 265
  dosing, 17*t*
  for ear, nose, and throat infections, 128*t*, 137
  for endocarditis, 177
  first-generation, 18–19
  fourth-generation, 20–21
  organisms susceptible to, 18*t*
  for osteomyelitis, 279*t*
  second-generation, 19
  for sinusitis, 137
  third-generation, 19–20
Cephradine, 17*t*
Cerebral lymphoma, primary, 426*t*
Cerebral toxoplasmosis, 414*t*, 426*t*
Cerebritis, 158, 160
Cerebrospinal fluid (CSF), 139, 142, 146*f*
Cerebrovascular diseases, 429
Cervical cancer, 401*t*
Cervical necrotizing fasciitis, 261
Chagas' disease, 302–304
  clinical features of, 303
  diagnosis of, 303–304
  epidemiology of, 303
  life cycle of, 303
  potential severity of, 302
  prevalence of, 303
  treatment of, 298*t*, 304
Chagoma, 303
Chancroid
  clinical features of, 247*t*
  treatment of, 244*t*
Chemical burn pneumonitis, 98
Chemosis, 135
Chemotherapy, 281
Chest pain, 83–84
CHF (congestive heart failure), 180–181
Chickenpox, 365–369
  case study of, 367–368
  clinical features of, 366
  complications of, 367–368
  diagnosis of, 366–367
  epidemiology of, 365

  pathogenesis of, 366
  vs. smallpox, 361–362
Chlamydia pneumoniae, 96–97
Chlamydia psittaci, 69–70
Chlamydia trachomatis, 121, 240–241
Chlamydophila pneumoniae, 31
Chloramphenicol, 34–35
  antimicrobial spectrum of, 34–35
  chemistry and mechanisms of action, 34
  dosing, 28*t*
  pharmacokinetics of, 34
  toxicity of, 34
  treatment recommendations, 34–35
    for bacterial meningitis, 147*t*
    for plague, 356*t*
    for spotted fever, 327*t*
Chloromycetin, 28*t*
Chloroquine, 294–295
Cholangitis, 216–217
  clinical features of, 216
  diagnosis of, 216–217
  pathogenesis of, 216
  treatment of, 217
Cholecystitis, 216–217
  clinical features of, 216
  diagnosis of, 216–217
  pathogenesis of, 216
  treatment of, 217
Chronic arthritis, treatment of, 327*t*
Chronic diarrhea, 205–209
  immunocompromised hosts, 208–209
  parasitic, 205–208
Chronic fatigue syndrome, 372
Chronic hepatitis B, 226–227
Chronic herpes simplex, 433
Chronic pneumonias, 103–118
  atypical mycobacteria, 113–114
  coccidiomycosis, 116–118
  histoplasmosis, 114–116
  tuberculosis, 103–113
Cidofovir, 51*t*, 53–54, 362–363, 431
Cipro, 111*t*
Ciprofloxacin, 35–37
  antimicrobial spectrum of, 35–37
  pharmacokinetics of, 35
  treatment recommendations, 35–37
    for bacterial diarrhea, 199*t*
    for *Bartonella* lymphatic disease, 327*t*
    for bioterror bacterial agents, 356*t*
    for bite infections, 261*t*
    for infective endocarditis, 179*t*
    for malignant otitis externa, 128*t*
    for neutropenic patients, 391*t*
    for sepsis syndrome, 63*t*
    for tuberculosis, 111*t*
    for urinary tract infections (UTIs),
      238*t*
Claforin, 17*t*
Clarithromycin, 28*t*, 29–31, 327*t*, 356*t*
Cleocin, 28*t*
Clindamycin, 31–32
  antimicrobial spectrum of, 32
  chemistry and mechanisms of action,
    31–32

dosing, 28*t*
pharmacokinetics of, 32
toxicity of, 32
treatment recommendations, 32
    for anthrax, 356*t*
    for babesiosis, 298*t*
    for cerebral toxoplasmosis, 414*t*
    for osteomyelitis, 279*t*
    for skin and soft tissue infections,
        260–261*t*
Clonorchis sinensis, 299*t,* 317
Clostridial cellulitis, 259
Clostridium difficile, 192*t,* 201–204
Clostridium septicum, 263–264
Clostridium sordellii, 263–264
Cloxacillin, 14t
Coccidioides immitis, 388
Coccidiomycosis, 116–118, 401*t,* 419
Colchicine, 188
Colonoscopy, 169*t*
Computed tomography (CT) scan, 160
    echinococcosis, 312–313
    fever of undetermined origin (FUO) in, 75
    osteomyelitis, 276–278
    sinusitis, 134–136
    vs. magnetic resonance imaging (MRI), 161
Condoms, use of, 398
Congestive heart failure (CHF), 180–181
Conjugation, 2
Conjunctival petechiae, 173*f*
Conjunctivitis, 120–122
    allergic, 121
    bacterial, 121
    chlamydial, 121
    clinical features of, 120–121
    diagnosis of, 121–122
    fungal, 121
    parasitic, 121
    potential severity of, 120
    predisposing factors for, 120
    toxic, 121
    treatment of, 121–122
    viral, 121
Copegus, 51*t*
Corneal infections, 122–125
    bacterial, 123
    case study of, 122
    clinical features of, 122
    diagnosis of, 123–124
    fungal, 123
    in herpes simplex, 380
    potential severity of, 122
    predisposing factors for, 122
    protozoal, 123
    treatment of, 124–125
    viral, 123
Corticosteroids, 64–65, 371–372
Corynebacterium, 386
Corynebacterium diphtheriae, 127
Cough, 83
Cowpox virus, 363
Coxiella burnetii infection, 339–341
C-reactive protein (CRP), 275
Creatine kinase antibodies, 185–186

Creatine phosphokinase (CPK), 330
Cryptococcal meningitis, 426*t,* 428–429
Cryptococcal meningoencephalitis, 153–154
    clinical features of, 153
    diagnosis of, 153
    mortality from, 154
    treatment of, 153–154
Cryptococcosis, 70, 401*t,* 414*t*
Cryptococcus neoformans, 153, 388, 428–429
Cryptosporidium, 208–209, 423
CSF (cerebrospinal fluid), 139, 142, 146*f*
Cultures, 74
Cutaneous anthrax, 352–353
Cutaneous leishmaniasis, 301
Cycloserine, 111*t*
Cysticercosis, 313–314
    clinical features of, 313
    diagnosis of, 313–314
    epidemiology of, 313
    life cycle of, 313
    potential severity of, 313
    prevalence of, 313
    treatment of, 299*t,* 313–314
Cystic fibrosis, 133
Cystitis, 235
    symptoms of, 234*t*
    treatment of, 238*t*
Cystoscopy, 169*t*
Cytochrome P450, 46
Cytokines, 59
Cytomegalovirus (CMV) infections, 381–382
    clinical features of, 381
    diagnosis of, 381–382
    in HIV infection, 401*t,* 414*t,* 429
    pathophysiology of, 381
    in suppression of T cell functions, 388
    treatment of, 53, 382
Cytomegalovirus colitis, 422–423
Cytomegalovirus retinitis, 414*t,* 430–431
Cytovene, 51*t*

D
Dalfopristin, 38
Dapsone, 414*t*
Daptomycin, 39–40
    antimicrobial spectrum of, 39–40
    chemistry and mechanisms of action, 39
    pharmacokinetics of, 39
    toxicity of, 39
    treatment recommendations, 39–40
        for infective endocarditis, 179*t*
        for severe cellulitis, 260*t*
DC-SIGN receptor, 399
Debridement, 282
Delta agent, 227
Dementia, HIV-associated, 401*t,* 426*t*
Dental procedures, and endocarditis,
        169–170
Dermacentor andersoni, 332
Dermacentor variabilis, 332
Dermatitis, 287
Dexamethasone, 148
Diabetic patients
    necrotizing fasciitis in, 261

osteomyelitis in, 274
urinary tract infections (UTIs) in, 232
Diarrhea, 190–209
    antibiotic-associated, 200–204
    bacterial, 190–200
        Campylobacter, 193–194
        case study of, 191
        clinical features of, 196–198
        diagnosis of, 198
        Escherichia coli, 193–194
        pathogenesis of, 191–196
        potential severity of, 190
        prevention of, 200
        Salmonella, 191–193
        Shigella, 193
        treatment of, 198–200
        Vibrio cholera, 195–196
        Vibrio parahaemolyticus, 196
        Yersinia, 196
    chronic, 205–209
    in HIV infection, 422–423
    immunocompromised hosts, 208–209
    parasitic, 205–208
    potential severity of, 190
    viral, 204–205
        astrovirus, 205
        case study of, 205
        clinical features of, 205
        diagnosis of, 205
        enteric adenoviruses, 205
        epidemiology of, 204–205
        norovirus, 204
        pathogenesis of, 204–205
        potential severity of, 204
        rotavirus, 204–205
        treatment of, 205
Dicloxacillin, 14t, 260*t*
Didanosine, 408
Diethylcarbamazine, 299*t*
Dilantin, 72
Diphtheria-pertussis-tetanus (DPT)
        vaccine, 270
Direct spread, 157–158
Dirofilariasis, 319
Disseminated gonococcal disease, 286–287
    clinical features of, 286–287
    diagnosis of, 287
    pathogenesis of, 286
    predisposing factors for, 286
    treatment of, 242*t,* 287
Distal symmetric polyneuropathy, 429
Dog bites, 270–271
Dog heartworm, 319
Dog tick, 332
Donovanosis
    clinical features of, 247*t*
    treatment of, 244*t*
Dosing, 4–5
Doxy, 28*t*
Doxycycline, 33
    antimicrobial spectrum of, 33
    dosing, 28*t*
    pharmacokinetics of, 33
    treatment recommendations, 33

Doxycycline (*con't*)
for bacterial diarrhea, 199*t*
for bioterror bacterial agents, 356*t*
for Lyme diseases, 326
for Rocky Mountain spotted fever, 334
for zoonotic infections, 327–328*t*
DPT (diphtheria-pertussis-tetanus) vaccine, 270
Drotrecogin alpha, 65
Drug abuse, and risk for hepatitis C, 228
Drug fever, 72–73
Duncan syndrome, 370
Dura mater, 139
Duricef, 17*t*
Dynapen, 14t
Dysuria, 234

E
Ear infections, 130–132
mastoiditis, 131–132
otitis externa, 130
otitis media, 130–131
Eastern equine encephalitis, 155*t*
EBV. *See* Epstein-Barr virus (EBV) infection
Echinocandins, 47–48
Echinococcosis, 311–313
case study of, 312
clinical features of, 312
diagnosis of, 312–313
epidemiology of, 311–312
life cycle of, 311–312
potential severity of, 311
prevalence of, 311–312
treatment of, 299*t*, 312–313
Echinococcus granulosus, 299*t*, 311–313
Echinococcus multilocularis, 299*t*, 311–313
Echocardiography, 175
Eczema, 380
Efavirenz, 408*t*
Efflux pumps, 4
Ehrlichia, 331
Ehrlichia chaffeensis, 336–337
Ehrlichiosis, 336–339
case study of, 337–338
clinical features of, 337–338
diagnosis of, 338–339
epidemiology of, 336–337
pathogenesis of, 337
potential severity of, 336
treatment of, 327*t*, 338–339
Eikenella corrodens, 271
ELISA (enzyme-linked immunosorbent
assay), 202, 325–326
Elite controllers, 400
Empyema, 101–103
causes of, 101–102
clinical features of, 102
pathophysiology of, 102
treatment of, 102–103
Encephalitis, 152–157
cryptococcal meningoencephalitis, 153–154
in herpes simplex, 380
in HIV infection, 426*t*
potential severity of, 152
viral, 154–157

Encephalitozoon cuniculi, 423
Encephalitozoon intestinalis, 423
Endocarditis, 346
Endophthalmitis, 125–126
acute post-operative, 125
clinical features of, 126
diagnosis of, 126
hematogenous, 125
posttraumatic, 125
potential severity of, 125
predisposing factors for, 125
treatment of, 126
with uncontrolled keratitis, 125
Endotoxemia, 58
Endotoxin, 58–59
Enema, 169*t*
Entamoeba dispar, 207
Entamoeba histolytica, 205–207
Entamoeba moshkovskii, 207
Enteric adenoviruses, 205
Enteric fever, 197
Enteroaggregative *E. coli,* 194
Enterobius, 298*t*, 306–307
Enterocolitis, 196–197
Enterocytozoon bieneusi, 423
Enterohemorrhagic *E. coli,* 194–195
Enteroinvasive *E. coli,* 194–195
Enteropathogenic *E. coli,* 194
Enterotoxigenic *E. coli,* 194
Enteroviruses, 121*t*, 185
Enzyme-linked immunosorbent assay
(ELISA), 202, 325–326
Epidemic typhus, 336
Epidural abscess, 163
Epiglottitis, 129
antibiotic therapy for, 128*t*
potential severity of, 129
Epstein-Barr viral nuclear antigens
(EBNAs), 370
Epstein-Barr virus (EBV) infection, 369–372
case study of, 369
clinical features of, 369–370
complications of, 370
diagnosis of, 370–371
epidemiology of, 369
pathophysiology of, 369–370
serologic testing for, 371*t*
treatment of, 371–373
chronic fatigue syndrome, 372
infectious mononucleosis, 371–372
oral hairy leukoplakia, 372
Ergosterols, 42
Ertapenem, 22, 260*t*
Erysipelas, 258–259
Erysipelothrix infection, 269
Erythema migrans, 323–324
Erythromycin, 28*t*, 29–31, 122, 128*t*, 260*t*
Escherichia coli infection, 194–195
bacterial diarrhea, 194–195
enteroaggregative, 194
enterohemorrhagic, 194–195
enteroinvasive, 195
enteropathogenic, 194
enterotoxigenic, 194

epidemiology of, 192*t*
sepsis, 58
urinary tract, 232
Esophagitis, 422
Ethambutol, 111*t*
Ethionamide, 111*t*
Exotoxins, 351
Extended-spectrum ß-lactamases (ESBLs), 3
Eye diseases, 120–126
conjunctivitis, 120–122
corneal infections, 122–125
endophthalmitis, 125–126
in HIV infection, 430–431
cytomegalovirus retinitis, 430–431
HIV retinopathy, 430
other eye infections, 431
retinal necroses, 431

F
Factitious fever, 73
Famciclovir, 49–53, 51*t*, 381
Famvir, 51*t*
Fasciola hepatica, 299*t*, 317
Febrile neutropenic patients, 389–392
Febrile non-neutropenic patients, 392–393
Febrile paroxysms, 292
Fever, 66–78
in bacterial meningitis, 143
benefits of, 66
in febrile neutropenic patients, 389–392
in febrile non-neutropenic patients, 392–393
harmful effects of, 66–67
in infective endocarditis, 172–173
in intensive care patients, 77–78
in malaria, 292–293
quintan, 343
in sepsis syndrome, 60–61
and temperature regulation, 66
treatment of, 67
underlying mechanisms of, 66
Fever of undetermined origin (FUO), 67–77
case study of, 68–69, 70–71
causes of, 68–73
autoimmune disease, 71–72
drug-related, 72–73
infection, 69–70
neoplasm, 70–71
definition of, 67–68
diagnostic tests for, 74–76
cultures, 74
imaging studies, 75
invasive procedures, 75–76
peripheral blood tests, 74–75
skin tests, 74
smears, 74
history for, 73
in HIV-infected patients, 76–77
physical examination in, 73
potential severity of, 67
prognosis for, 76
treatment of, 76
Filariasis, 317–319
asymptomatic, 318
clinical features of, 318

diagnosis of, 318
epidemiology of, 317–318
inflammatory, 318
life cycle of, 317–318
obstructive, 318
prevalence of, 317
treatment of, 318–319
Fimbriae, 232
Flavivirus, 155*t*
Flea-borne typhus, 335
Flucloxacillin, 279*t*
Fluconazole, 46–47, 414*t*
Flucytosine, 48–49
Flukes, 317
Flumadine, 52*t*
5-Fluorocytosine (5-FC), 48–49
Fluorodeoxyglucose, 75
Fluoroquinolones
    for microbial infections, 122
    for sinus infections, 137
5-Fluorouracil (5-FU), 48
Folliculitis, 266–267
Fortaz, 17*t*
Foscarnet, 51*t*, 54–55, 423, 430–431
Foscavir, 51*t*
Fournier's gangrene, 261
Francisella tularensis, 358–360
Frontal sinusitis, 136
Fungal infections. *See also* specific infections
    candidiasis, 420–421
    coccidiomycosis, 419
    conjunctivitis, 121
    corneal, 123
    cryptococcal meningoencephalitis, 153–154
    drug therapy for, 42–49
    endophthalmitis, 125–126
    folliculitis, 266–267
    histoplasmosis, 419
    in immunocompromised host, 385–386
    intravascular catheter-related, 183
    invasive aspergillosis, 419
    sinusitis, 137
Fungal pneumonia, 114–118
    coccidiomycosis, 116–118
    histoplasmosis, 114–116
Fungal sinusitis, 137
Fungi, 385–386
Furunculosis, 267–268

G

Gallium scan, 415
Ganciclovir, 51*t*, 53, 430
GAS (group A streptococci), 127, 256
Gastroenteritis, 196–198
Gastrointestinal anthrax, 354
Gastrointestinal diseases, in HIV infection, 420–425
    liver, 423–425
        damage from antiretroviral drugs, 423–425
        viral hepatitis, 423–425
    oral cavity and esophagus, 420–423
        candidiasis, 420–421
        esophagitis, 422

Kaposi's sarcoma, 422
    mouth ulcers and aphthous stomatitis, 421
    oral hairy leukoplakia, 422
    salivary gland lesions, 422
rectum and anus, 423
small and large intestine, 422–423
    diarrhea, 422–423
    tumors of digestive system, 423
    Kaposi's sarcoma, 423
    lymphoma, 423
Gatifloxacin, 35–37, 128*t*
Gemifloxacin, 37
General paresis, 251
Genital ulcers, 246–248
    causes of, 246–247
    clinical features of, 247–248
    diagnosis of, 248
    treatment of, 243–244*t*, 248
Genitourinary tract infections, 231–240
    potential severity of, 231
    prostatitis, 239–240
    urinary tract infections (UTIs), 231–239
Genotypic tests, 404
Gentamicin, 24*t*, 178*t*, 199*t*, 238*t*, 279*t*, 356*t*
Giardia lamblia, 207–208
Giardiasis, 207–208
    clinical features of, 208
    diagnosis of, 208
    epidemiology of, 207–208
    life cycle of, 207–208
    treatment of, 208
Giemsa stain, 74
Gingivostomatitis, 379
Glasgow coma score, 144*t*
Glomerulonephritis, 177
Glucocorticoids, 162–163
Glucose-6-phosphate dehydrogenase (G6PD) deficiency, 41
Glycopeptide antibiotics, 27–29
    antimicrobial spectrum of, 29
    chemistry and mechanisms of action, 27
    dosing, 28*t*
    pharmacokinetics of, 27
    toxicity of, 27
    treatment recommendations, 29
Gonococcal urethritis, treatment of, 242*t*
Gram-negative bacteria, 58
Gram-positive bacteria, 58–59
Granulocytes, 337
Granulomatous diseases, 72
Gray hepatization, 81
Group A streptococci (GAS), 127, 256
Guarnieri bodies, 361
Guillain-Barré syndrome, 368, 370, 381, 402
Gum chewing, 169*t*
Gummas, 251–252
Gynecomastia, 45

H

HAART (highly active anti-retroviral therapy). *See* Antiretroviral therapy
Haemophilus influenzae B (HiB) vaccine, 140
Haemophilus influenzae infection, 94
    conjunctivitis, 121*t*

epiglottitis, 129
    meningitis, 141
    pneumonia, 94
Hantavirus pulmonary syndrome (HPS), 373–374
    case study of, 373
    clinical features of, 373
    diagnosis of, 373–374
    epidemiology of, 373
    pathophysiology of, 373
    prevention of, 374
    treatment of, 374
H antigens, 194
Heart block, treatment of, 327*t*
Helicobacter pylori-associated peptic ulcer, 217–218
    clinical features of, 217–218
    diagnosis of, 217–218
    microbiology of, 217
    pathogenesis of, 217
    potential severity of, 217
    treatment of, 31, 218
Hemagglutinin, 376
Hematogenous osteomyelitis, 274–278
    case study of, 274–275
    clinical features of, 275
    diagnosis of, 275–278
    microbiology of, 274
    pathogenesis of, 274
    treatment of, 278
Hematogenous spread, 158
Hematuria, 177
Hemodynamic changes, in sepsis syndrome, 61
Hemoglobinuria, 293
Heparin, 136
Hepatic abscess, 214–215
    clinical features of, 215
    diagnosis of, 215
    microbiology of, 214
    pathogenesis of, 214
    potential severity of, 215
    treatment of, 215
Hepatitis, viral, 218–220
    clinical features of, 218–220
    potential severity of, 218
    stages of, 218
Hepatitis A, 220–222
    clinical features of, 219*t*, 221–222
    diagnosis of, 221–222
    epidemiology of, 220–221
    pathogenesis of, 220–221
    prevention of, 222
    treatment of, 222
Hepatitis B, 223–227
    chronic, 226–227
    clinical features of, 219*t*, 224–225
    diagnosis of, 224–225
    epidemiology of, 223–224
    in HIV infection, 423–425
    pathogenesis of, 223
    prevention of, 225–226
    treatment of, 225–226
    virology of, 223

Hepatitis C, 228–229
    clinical features of, 219*t*, 228–229
Hepatitis C (*con't*)
    diagnosis of, 228–229
    epidemiology of, 228
    in HIV infection, 228, 423–425
    pathogenesis of, 228
    prognosis for, 229
    treatment of, 229
    virology of, 228
Hepatitis D, 227
Hepatitis D + B, 219*t*
Hepatitis E, 219*t*, 222–223
Herpes gladiatorum, 380
Herpes simplex virus (HSV) infection,
        379–381
    clinical features of, 379–380
    complications of, 380
    in conjunctivitis, 121*t*
    diagnosis of, 380–381
    epidemiology of, 379
    in HIV infection, 401*t*, 433
    pathophysiology of, 379–380
    treatment of, 243–244*t*, 381
    ulcers in, 247*t*
Herpes zoster, 433
Histoplasma capsulatum, 114–116, 388
Histoplasmosis, 114–116
    clinical features of, 114–115
    diagnosis of, 115–116
    epidemiology of, 114
    fever in, 70
    in HIV infection, 401*t*, 419
    pathogenesis of, 114
    treatment of, 116
HIV. *See* Human immunodeficiency virus
        (HIV) infection
HIV encephalopathy, 425, 426*t*
HIV retinopathy, 430
Hodgkin lymphoma, 70
Hookworm, 298*t*
    clinical features of, 310
    diagnosis of, 310
    epidemiology of, 309–310
    life cycle of, 309–310
    prevalence of, 309–310
    treatment of, 310
HPS. *See* Hantavirus pulmonary
        syndrome (HPS)
HPV (human papillomavirus), 254
HSV (herpes simplex virus), 247
Human bites, 271
Human herpesvirus (HHV8), 433
Human immunodeficiency virus (HIV)
infection, 397–434
    antiretroviral therapy for, 405–412
    classification of, 403
    clinical features of primary infection, 402
    diagnosis of, 402–403
    epidemiology of, 397–399
    fever of undetermined origin (FUO) in,
        76–77
    and hepatitis C, 228
    indicator conditions, 401*t*

infection rates, 397–398
    laboratory testing of, 404–405
        for antiretroviral resistance, 404
        caveats for, 404–405
        for monitoring treatment and
            prognosis, 404
    mortality from, 397
    opportunistic diseases in, 412–434
        case study of, 412–413
        central nervous system diseases, 425–430
            cerebrovascular diseases, 429
            cryptococcal meningitis, 428–429
            cytomegalovirus infection, 429
            distal symmetric polyneuropathy, 429
            HIV encephalopathy, 425
            inflammatory demyelinating-
                polyneuropathy, 429
            mononeuritis multiplex, 429
            myelopathy, 429–430
            primary brain lymphoma, 428
            in primary HIV infection, 425
            progressive multifocal leukoen-
                cephalopathy, 428
            Toxoplasma encephalitis, 425–428
        eye diseases, 430–431
            cytomegalovirus retinitis, 430–431
            HIV retinopathy, 430
            other eye infections, 431
            retinal necroses, 431
        gastrointestinal diseases, 420–425
            diarrhea, 422–423
            esophagitis, 422
            Kaposi's sarcoma, 422, 424
            lymphoma, 423
            mouth ulcers and aphthous
                stomatitis, 421
            oral and esophageal candidiasis,
                420–421
            oral hairy leukoplakia, 422
            rectal and anal, 423
            salivary gland lesions, 422
            viral hepatitis, 423–425
        prophylaxis for, 413, 414*t*
        pulmonary infections, 413–419
            aspergillosis, 419
            bacterial pneumonia, 418
            coccidiomycosis, 419
            histoplasmosis, 419
            interstitial lymphoid pneumonia, 419
            Kaposi's sarcoma, 419
            mycobacteria other than
                tuberculosis, 418
            Mycobacterium kansasii infection, 418
            nocardiosis, 419
            Pneumocystis jirovecii pneumonia,
                414–417
            Rhodococcus equi infection, 419
            tuberculosis, 418
        skin diseases, 431–434
            bacillary angiomatosis, 433–434
            chronic herpes simplex, 433
            drug reactions, 434
            herpes zoster, 433
            Kaposi's sarcoma, 433

            molluscum contagiosum, 434
            in primary HIV infection, 431–433
            seborrheic dermatitis, 434
            syphilis, 434
    pathogenesis of, 399–402
    primary, 399
    stages of, 403*t*
    and syphilis, 254
Human papillomavirus (HMV), 254
Hydrocephalus, 313
Hydroxychloroquine, 327*t*
Hyperbilirubinemia, 39
Hypercarbia, 148
Hypernephroma, 70
Hypnozoites, 289
Hypoglycorrachia, 145
Hyponatremia, 156, 333
Hypotension, in sepsis syndrome, 61

I
Icterus, 219
IL-1 (interleukin 1), in sepsis syndrome, 59
Imipenem, 22, 260*t*, 279*t*, 356*t*, 391*t*
Imipenem-cilastatin, 238*t*
Immigrants, 159
Immunocompromised hosts, 384–394. *See
        also* Human immunodeficiency virus
        (HIV) infection
    anti-infective therapy for, 391*t*
    in bone marrow transplantation, 388–389
    in brain abscess, 158–159
    case study of, 388
    chronic diarrheal diseases in, 208–209
    classification of, 385
    cytomegalovirus infection in, 381–382
    definition of, 384–385
    diagnosis of, 389–393
    microbiology of, 386–387
        bacteria, 386
        fungi, 386–387
    neutropenia, 385–394
    pathogenesis of, 385–386
    pathogens in patients with suppression of
            T cell functions, 387–388
        bacteria, 388
        fungi, 388
        viruses, 388
    potential severity of, 384
    prevention of, 393–394
    treatment of, 389–393
        febrile neutropenic patient, 389–392
        febrile non-neutropenic patient, 392–393
Impetigo, 266
Indinavir, 408*t*
Infection, 58, 59–60, 69–70
Infectious mononucleosis, 371–372
Infective endocarditis, 167–181
    case study of, 171
    clinical features of, 171–174
        history, 172
        laboratory findings, 174
        physical findings, 172–173
    complications of, 175–177
        cardiac, 175–176

mycotic aneurysms, 177
neurologic, 177
renal, 177
systemic emboli, 176–177
diagnosis of, 174–175
blood cultures, 174–175
echocardiography, 175
modified Duke criteria, 175
embolic phenomena in, 173*f*
epidemiology of, 167–168
microbiology of, 170–171
pathogenesis of, 168–170
bacteremia, 169–170
bacterial factors, 168–169
host factors, 168
potential severity of, 167
prevention of, 181
prognosis for, 181
treatment of
antibiotics, 177–180
surgery, 180–188
Inflammatory demyelinating
polyneuropathy, 429
Inflammatory filariasis, 318
Inflammatory mediators, in sepsis syndrome, 59
Influenza, 376–379
clinical features of, 377
complications of, 377–378
diagnosis of, 378
epidemiology of, 376–377
pathophysiology of, 377
prevention of, 378–379
risk groups, 378–379
treatment of, 378
vaccination against, 378–379
virology of, 376–377
Inguinal adenopathy, 247–248
Inhalation anthrax, 353–354
Intensive care patients, fever in, 77–78
Interferons, 55–56
Interleukin 1 (IL-1), in sepsis syndrome, 59
Interstitial lymphoid pneumonia, 419
Interstitial pneumonia, 85
Intra-abdominal infections, 209–229
cholangitis, 216–217
cholecystitis, 216–217
Helicobacter pylori-associated peptic ulcer,
217–218
hepatic abscess, 214–215
pancreatic abscess, 215–216
peritonitis, 210–214
viral hepatitis, 218–229
Intracranial epidural and subdural abscess, 163
Intravascular catheter-related infections,
181–185
case study of, 181–182
clinical features of, 183–184
diagnosis of, 183–184
epidemiology of, 182
pathogenesis of, 182–183
potential severity of, 181
treatment of, 184–185
Intubation, 169*t*
Invasive aspergillosis, 419

Isoniazid, 111*t*, 414*t*
Isospora belli, 208–209, 401*t*, 423
Itraconazole, 47
Ivermectin, 298*t*, 299*t*
Ixodes scapularis, 296–297, 323, 337

J
Janeway lesions, 173*f*
Japanese encephalitis, 155*t*
Jaundice, 293

K
Kala-azar, 301
Kaposi's sarcoma, 401*t*, 418–419,
422–424, 433
Kaposi's varicelliform eruption, 366
Kartagener's syndrome, 133
Katayama fever, 313–314, 316
Keflex, 17*t*
Keratitis. *See* Corneal infections
Kernig's sign, 143
Ketek, 28*t*
Ketoconazole, 45
Ketolides, 29–31
antimicrobial spectrum of, 31
chemistry and mechanisms of action, 29–31
organisms susceptible to, 30*t*
pharmacokinetics of, 30–31
toxicity of, 30
treatment recommendations, 31
Kupffer cells, 330

L
Lactic acid, 61
Lamivudine, 408*t*
Latent syphilis, 250, 253
treatment of, 244*t*
Late syphilis, 250–251
Legionella, 387
Legionella pneumophilia, 31, 95–96
Leishmania, 300–301
Leishmaniasis, 300–302
clinical features of, 300–301
cutaneous, 301
epidemiology of, 300
life cycle of, 300
mucosal, 301
potential severity of, 300
prevalence of, 300
treatment of, 298*t*, 302
visceral, 301
Leptomeninges, 139
Leptospira interrogans, 329
Leptospirosis, 328–331
case study of, 329
clinical features of, 329–330
diagnosis of, 330–331
epidemiology of, 328–329
fever of undetermined origin (FUO) in, 69
pathogenesis of, 329
potential severity of, 328
treatment of, 327*t*, 331
Lethal factor, 351
Leukocytosis, 174

Leukoencephalopathy, 401*t*
Leukopenia, 34, 338
Levofloxacin, 37, 128*t*, 199*t*, 238*t*, 356*t*
Linezolid, 37–38, 260*t*
Lipid A, 58
Lipopolysaccharide (LPS), 58–59
Liposomal amphotericin B, 391*t*
Lipoteichoic acid, 58
Listeria, 388
Listeria monocytogenes, 15, 141
Live attenuated influenza vaccine (LAIV), 379
Liver biopsy, 169*t*
Loa loa, 299*t*, 319
Loa loa filariasis, 121*t*
Lobar pneumonia, 85
Lock jaw, 269
Loeffler's syndrome, 309
Loiasis, 319
Lomefloxacin, 238*t*
Lone Star tick, 337
Long-term nonprogressors, 400
Lopinavir, 408*t*
Louse-borne typhus, 336
Low back pain, 172
LPS (lipopolysaccharide), 58–59
Lumbar puncture, 152, 161
Lung abscess, 85
Lyme arthritis, 285
Lyme disease, 322–328
case study of, 323
clinical features of, 323–325
cardiovascular, 324
musculoskeletal, 324–325
nervous system, 324
neurologic, 325
diagnosis of, 325–326
epidemiology of, 322
pathogenesis of, 322–323
potential severity of, 322
prevention of, 326–328
stages of, 323–325
treatment of, 326
Lymphocytes, 399
Lymphocytic choriomeningitis, 151
Lymphogranuloma venerium
clinical features of, 247*t*
treatment of, 244*t*
Lymphoma, 401*t*, 423

M
Macrogametocytes, 290
Macrolides, 29–31
antimicrobial spectrum of, 31
chemistry and mechanisms of action, 29–31
dosing, 28*t*
organisms susceptible to, 30*t*
pharmacokinetics of, 30–31
toxicity of, 30
treatment recommendations, 31
Magnetic resonance imaging (MRI), 160–161
Malaria, 288–295
blood smear findings, 290*f*
case study of, 292
chloroquine-resistant, 294–295

clinical features of, 292–293
diagnosis of, 293
Malaria (con't)
    epidemiology of, 289–290
    life cycle of *Plasmodium* species in, 290–291
    prevalence of, 289
    prophylaxis for, 293–295
    susceptibility to, 291–292
    treatment of, 293–295
Malignant otitis externa, antibiotic therapy
        for, 128*t*
Mannitol, 153
Mannose, 232
MAP (mitogen-activated protein), 351
Mastoiditis, 131–132
    antibiotic therapy for, 128*t*
    case study of, 131
    computed tomography scan of, 132
    potential severity of, 131
Maxipime, 17*t*
Mean bacterial concentration (MBC), 4–5
Measles, 121*t*
Mebendazole, 298*t*
*Medical Management of Biological
        Casualties,* 350
Mediterranean fever, 72
Mediterranean spotted fever, 334
Mefoxin, 17*t*
Meninges, 139
Meningismus, 159
Meningitis, 140–152
    aseptic, 426*t*
    bacterial, 140–150
        case study of, 143
        chemoprophylaxis for, 150
        clinical features of, 143–145
        complications of, 148–149
        diagnosis of, 145–146
        epidemiology of, 140–141
        initial management of, 145*f*
        major pathogens of, 140–141
        mortality rate, 148–149
        pathogenesis of, 153–154
        prevention of, 149–150
        treatment of, 146–148
        vaccines for, 149–150
    in brucellosis, 346
        treatment of, 327*t*
    in tuberculosis, 152
    viral, 150–152
Meningococcemia, 58
Meningoencephalitis, 152
Meropenem, 22, 63*t*, 260*t*, 391*t*
Merozoites, 289–290
Metabolic acidosis, 61
Methicillin-resistant *Staphylococcus aureus*
        (MRSA), 179*t*
Metronidazole, 40
    antimicrobial spectrum of, 40
    chemistry and mechanisms of action, 40
    pharmacokinetics of, 40
    toxicity of, 40
    treatment recommendations, 40
        for bacterial diarrhea, 199*t*

for brain abscess, 161–162
for sinusitis, 128*t*
Micafungin, 47–48
MIC (minimum inhibitory
        concentration), 4–5
Miconazole, 45
Microgametocytes, 290
Microsporidium, 209, 423
Miliary tuberculosis, 69, 107–108
Miltefosine, 302
Minimum inhibitory concentration
        (MIC), 4–5
Minocycline, 28*t*, 33
Mitogen-activated protein (MAP), 351
Modified Duke criteria, 175
Mollaret's aseptic meningitis, 151
Molluscum contagiosum, 254, 434
Monobactams, 21–22
Monocytotropic viruses, 399
Mononeuritis multiplex, 429
Mononucleosis, 421
Moraxella catarrhalis, 121*t*
Mouth ulcers, 421
Moxifloxacin, 37, 128*t*
MRI (magnetic resonance imaging), 160–161
MRSA (methicillin-resistant *Staphylococcus
        aureus*), 179*t*
Mucosal leishmaniasis, 301
Mucositis, 385–387
Mupirocin, 260*t*
Myalgias, 172
Myambutol, 111*t*
Mycobacterium, 414*t*
Mycobacterium avium, 113–114, 401*t*,
        413, 422
Mycobacterium avium intracellulare, 418
Mycobacterium kansasii, 418
Mycobacterium marinum, 269
Mycobacterium tuberculosis, 164–165,
        388, 401*t*
Mycoplasma pneumoniae, 31, 96–97
Mycotic aneurysms, 177
Myelopathy, 429–430
Myocardial abscess, 181
Myocarditis, 185–186
    clinical features of, 185–186
    diagnosis of, 185–186
    pathogenesis of, 185
    potential severity of, 185
    treatment of, 186
Myonecrosis, 263–265
    case study of, 264
    clinical features of, 264
    diagnosis of, 264
    necrotizing infections in, 263
    pathophysiology of clostridial infections
        in, 263–264
    predisposing factors for, 263
    pyomyositis in, 263
    treatment of, 265

N
Nafcillin, 15–16
    antimicrobial spectrum of, 16

dosing, 14*t*
    pharmacokinetics of, 15–16
    treatment recommendations, 16
        for bacterial meningitis, 147*t*
        for cellulitis, 260*t*
        for infective endocarditis, 178–179*t*
        for osteomyelitis, 279*t*
        for sinusitis, 128*t*
Nail-bed splinter hemorrhage, 173*f*
Nasotracheal suction, 169*t*
Natural killer (NK) cells, 369–370
Natural penicillins, 13–15
NBTE (nonbacterial thrombotic
        endocarditis), 168
Necator americanus, 309–310
Necrotizing fasciitis, 259–263
    case study of, 261–262
    cervical, 261
    clinical features of, 261–262
    in diabetic patients, 261
    diagnosis of, 261–262
    Fournier's gangrene in, 261
    predisposing factors for, 259–261
    treatment of, 262–263
    types of, 261
Necrotizing myositis. *See* Myonecrosis
Neisseria gonorrhoeae infection
    conjunctivitis, 121*t*
    disseminated gonococcal, 286–287
    pelvic inflammatory disease, 214–216
    pharyngitis, 127
    septic arthritis, 286–287
    urethritis, 240–241
Neisseria meningitidis, 121*t*, 140–141
Nelfinavir, 408*t*
Nematodes, intestinal, 305–310
    acquired by ingestion, 305–307
        Ascaris, 306
        Enterobius, 306–307
        Trichuris trichiura, 305–306
    acquired by skin penetration, 307–310
        hookworm, 309–310
        Strongyloides, 307–309
    life cycles of, 306*f*
Neomycin, 122
Neonatal tetanus, 270
Neoplastic disorders, 70–71
Nephrotoxicity, 23, 42
Netilmicin, 24*t*
Neuramidase inhibitors, 56, 376
Neurocysticercosis, 313–314
Neutropenia, 385–394
    in ehrlichiosis, 338
    microbiology of, 386–387
    pathogenesis of, 385–386
    pathogens in patients with suppression of
        T cell functions, 387–388
        bacteria, 388
        fungi, 388
        viruses, 388
    prevention of, 393–394
    as side effect of anti-infective
        therapy, 53
    treatment of, 389–393

febrile neutropenic patient, 389–392
febrile non-neutropenic patient, 392–393
Neutrophils, 337, 386
Nevirapine, 408*t*
New World hookworm, 309–310
Nifurtimox, 298*t*, 304
Nitazoxanide, 203, 298*t*
Nitrofurantoin, 238*t*
Nocardia, 99–100, 388
Nocardia asteroides, 41, 158, 419
Nocardiosis, 99–100, 401*t*, 419
Nodular lesions, 85
Nonbacterial thrombotic endocarditis
(NBTE), 168
Non-clostridial anaerobic cellulitis, 259
Non-gonococcal urethritis (NGU), 241, 242*t*
Non-nucleoside reverse-transcriptase
inhibitors (NNRTIs), 408*t*, 425
Non-syncytium-inducing viruses, 399
Non-treponemal tests, 252
Norfloxacin, 238*t*
Norovirus, 204
Nosocomial pneumonia, 100–101
Nydrazid, 111*t*

O
O antigens, 194
Obstructive filariasis, 318
Ocular syphilis, 253
Ofloxacin, 238*t*
Old World hookworm, 309–310
Oliguria, in sepsis syndrome, 61
Omnipen, 14*t*
Onchocerca volvulus, 121*t*, 299*t*, 319
Onchocerciasis, 319
Ophthalmology. *See* Eye diseases
Opisthotonus, 269
Opsonins, 149
Oral hairy leukoplakia, 372, 422
Oral irrigation device, 169*t*
Orbital access, 135
Orbital cellulitis, 135
Oseltamivir, 51*t*, 378
Osler nodes, 173*f*
Osteomyelitis, 273–283
acute *vs.* chronic, 273
classification of, 273–274
hematogenous, 274–278
case study of, 274–275
clinical features of, 275
diagnosis of, 275–278
microbiology of, 274
pathogenesis of, 274
treatment of, 278
microbiology of, 275*t*
potential severity of, 273
principles for management of, 281–283
antimicrobial therapy, 281–282
clinical response assessment, 282–283
surgical management, 282
tissue sampling, 281
secondary to contiguous infection, 278–280
causes of, 279–280
clinical features of, 278–279

primary infections associated with,
278–279
secondary to vascular inefficiency in
diabetic patients, 280–281
clinical features of, 280
diagnosis of, 280–281
treatment of, 281
treatment of, 279*t*
Otitis externa, 130
diagnosis of, 130
malignant, 130
potential severity of, 130
Otitis media, 130–131
antibiotic therapy for, 128*t*
diagnosis of, 130–131
potential severity of, 130
treatment of, 131
Ototoxicity, 23
Outer membrane proteins, 332
Outer surface proteins, 322
Oxacillin, 15–16
antimicrobial spectrum of, 16
dosing, 14*t*
treatment recommendations, 16
for bacterial meningitis, 147*t*
for cellulitis, 260*t*
for infective endocarditis, 178–179*t*
for sepsis syndrome, 63*t*
for sinusitis, 128*t*
Oxamniquine, 299*t*
Oxazolidones, 37–38
antimicrobial spectrum of, 38
chemistry and mechanisms of action, 37–38
pharmacokinetics of, 38
toxicity of, 38
treatment recommendations, 38

P
Pachymeninges, 139
Pancreatic abscess, 215–216
Papular genitourinary lesions, 254–255
Para-aminosalicylic acid, 111*t*
Paragonimus westermani, 299*t*
Parasites, 159
Parasitic diarrhea, 205–208
amoebiasis, 205–207
giardiasis, 207–208
Parasitic infections, 288–319
blood protozoa, 288–299
babesiosis, 296–299
malaria, 288–295
intestinal helminths, 304–310
acquired by ingestion, 305–307
acquired by skin penetration, 307–310
tissue and blood helminths, 310–319
cysticercosis, 313–314
dirofilariasis, 319
echinococcosis, 311–313
filariasis, 317–319
loiasis, 319
onchocerciasis, 319
schistosomiasis, 314–317
trichinosis, 310–311
tissue protozoa, 300–304

Chagas' disease, 302–304
leishmaniasis, 300–302
Trypanosoma brucei complex, 304
Parinaud's oculoglandular syndrome, 343
Pasteurella, 270–271
Patient management, 63–64
PBPs (penicillin-binding proteins), 4
PCR (polymerase chain reaction), 151
Pegasys, 51*t*
PEG-Intron, 51*t*
Pel-Ebstein fever, 70
Pelvic inflammatory disease, 241–246
clinical features of, 245
diagnosis of, 245–246
pathogenesis of, 241–245
treatment of, 242–243*t*
Penicillin, 147*t*
Penicillinase-resistant penicillins, 15–16
Penicillin-binding proteins (PBPs), 4
Penicillin G, 14, 178*t*, 260*t*, 279*t*, 327*t*, 356*t*
Penicillins, 13–18
allergic reactions to, 13
aminopenicillins, 15
carboxypenicillins, 16–18
dosing, 14*t*
natural, 13–15
organisms susceptible to, 15*t*
penicillinase-resistant, 15–16
ureidopenicillins, 16–18
Penicillin VK, 128*t*
Pentamidine, 414*t*
Peptidoglycan, 58
Pericarditis, 186–188
clinical features of, 187
diagnosis of, 188
pathogenesis of, 186–187
potential severity of, 186
treatment of, 188
tuberculous, 187–188
Periodontal surgery, 169*t*
Periorbital cellulitis, 135
Peripheral blood tests, 74–75
Peritoneal dialysis, 213–214
Peritonitis, 210–214
primary or spontaneous, 210–211
clinical features of, 210
diagnosis of, 210–211
microbiology of, 210
mortality rate, 211
pathogenesis of, 210
potential severity of, 210
treatment of, 211
secondary, 211–214
associated with peritoneal dialysis,
213–214
clinical features of, 212
diagnosis of, 212–213
microbiology of, 211–212
pathogenesis of, 211–212
potential severity of, 211
treatment of, 212–213
Perivalvular abscess, 181
Pet animal bites, 270–271
Pharyngitis, 127–129

antibiotic therapy for, 128*t*
clinical features of, 127–129
diagnosis of, 127
potential severity of, 127
treatment of, 127
Phenotypic tests, 404
Photophobia, 151
Pia mater, 139
Pin worm, 298*t*, 306–307
Piperacillin, 279*t*
Piperacillin-tazobactam, 14t, 63*t*, 128*t*, 238*t*, 260*t*, 391*t*
Plague, 357–358
clinical features of, 357–358
diagnosis of, 358
pathogenesis of, 357
prophylaxis for, 358
treatment of, 356*t*, 358
Plasmodium falciparum, 289–295
Plasmodium ovale, 291*t*
Plasmodium vivax, 289–291
Plateau level, 399
PMNs. *See* Polymorphonuclear leukocytes (PMNs)
Pneumocystis carinii, 42
Pneumocystis jirovecii pneumonia, 414–417
chest radiographs of, 416*f*
diagnosis of, 414–417
in HIV infection, 401*t*
in immunocompromised host, 394
treatment of, 414–417, 414*t*
Pneumonia, 79–118
actinomycosis, 99
acute, 79–103
aspiration, 97–99
atypical, 96–97, 113–114
case study of, 82–83
causes of, 79–80
chronic, 103–118
clinical features of, 82–85
chest discomfort, 83–84
cough, 83
epidemiology, 84–85
rigor, 84
community-acquired, 90–103
empiric treatment of, 88, 89–90*t*
empyema, 101–103
fungal, 114–118
coccidiomycosis, 114–116
histoplasmosis, 114–116
in HIV infection, 401*t*
influenza, 378
laboratory tests in, 85–88
mortality from, 90
nocardiosis, 99–100
nosocomial, 100–101
pathogenesis of, 80–81
pathology of, 80–81
potential severity of, 79
predisposing factors for, 81–82
prevalence of, 79
tuberculosis, 103–113
Podofilox, 254
Polyarthritis syndrome, 287

Polymerase chain reaction (PCR), 151
Polymorphonuclear leukocytes (PMNs)
in bacterial meningitis, 142
in central nervous system infections, 145–146
in conjunctivitis, 122
function of, 81
urinary tract infections (UTIs), 233
Polymyxin B, 122
PORN (progressive outer retinal necrosis), 431
Posaconazole, 47, 391*t*
Pott's puffy tumor, 136
PPI (proton pump inhibitor), 218
Praziquantel, 299*t*
Pregnancy, urinary tract infections (UTIs) in, 232
Pre-shock, 61
Primary brain lymphoma, 428
Primary HIV infection, 399, 425
Primary syphilis, 249, 253
Primary tuberculosis, 107
Pristinamycin, 38
Probenecid, 13
Procaine PCN G, 14*t*
Progressive multifocal leukoencephalopathy, 426*t*, 428
Progressive outer retinal necrosis (PORN), 431
Prostaphlin, 14*t*
Prostatitis, 239–240
clinical features of, 239–240
diagnosis of, 240
pathogenesis of, 239
potential severity of, 239
treatment of, 240
Prosthetic joint infections, 283–284
case study of, 283
clinical features of, 283
diagnosis of, 283
microbiology of, 283
pathogenesis of, 283
treatment of, 283–284
Protease inhibitors (PIs), 408*t*, 425
Protective antigen, 351
Protein C, 65
Proteinuria, 177
Proteus mirabilis, 15, 232
Proteus vulgaris, 334
Proton pump inhibitor (PPI), 218
Pseudomonas aeruginosa, 16, 63*t*, 121*t*, 130, 418
Pulmonary emboli, 73
Pulmonary infections, 79–118
acute pneumonias, 79–103
aspergillosis, 419
bacterial pneumonia, 418
chronic pneumonia, 103–118
atypical mycobacteria, 113–114
coccidiomycosis, 116–118
histoplasmosis, 114–116
tuberculosis, 103–113
coccidiomycosis, 419
community-acquired pneumonia
actinomycosis, 99
aspiration pneumonia, 97–99

atypical pneumonia, 96–97
Haemophilus influenzae, 94
Legionella pneumophilia, 95–96
nocardiosis, 99–100
nosocomial pneumonia, 100–101
Staphylococcus aureus, 94–95
Streptococcus pneumoniae, 90–94
empyema, 101–103
hantavirus pulmonary syndrome (HPS), 373–374
histoplasmosis, 419
in HIV infection, 413–419
aspergillosis, 419
bacterial pneumonia, 418
coccidiomycosis, 419
histoplasmosis, 419
interstitial lymphoid pneumonia, 419
Kaposi's sarcoma, 418–419
mycobacteria other than tuberculosis, 418
Mycobacterium kansasii infection, 418
nocardiosis, 419
Pneumocystis jirovecii pneumonia, 414–417
Rhodococcus equi infection, 419
tuberculosis, 418
Punch tenderness, 219
Purified protein derivative (PPD) test, 112–113
Purulent arthritis, 287
Pyelonephritis, 232, 234*t*, 238*t*
Pyomyositis, 263
Pyrantel pamoate, 298*t*
Pyrimethamine, 414*t*

Q
Q fever, 339–341
clinical features of, 340
diagnosis of, 340–341
pathogenesis of, 339–340
potential severity of, 339
treatment of, 327*t*, 341
Quasi-species, 228
Quinidine, 294–295
Quinine, 294, 298*t*
Quinolones, 35–37
antimicrobial spectrum of, 35–37
chemistry and mechanisms of action, 35
dosing, 36*t*
for osteomyelitis, 279*t*
pharmacokinetics of, 35
toxicity of, 35
treatment recommendations, 35–37
Quintan fever, 343
Quinupristin, 38

R
Rabies encephalitis, 155–156
Rapid plasma reagin (RPR) test, 248, 252
Rash, 381
Rebetol, 51*t*
Rectal carcinoma, 423
Rectitis, 423
Red hepatization, 81
Red man syndrome, 27
Relenza, 51*t*

Renal dysfunction, 177
Research Institute of Viral Preparations, 360
Respiratory alkalosis, 61
Respiratory changes, in sepsis syndrome, 61
Retinal necroses, 431
Retinopathy, 430
Reye's syndrome, 378
Rhipicephalus sanguineus, 332
Rhodococcus equi, 419
Ribavirin, 51*t,* 55
Ribosomes, 4
Rickettsia, 331
Rickettsia africae, 334
Rickettsia akari, 334
Rickettsial infections, 331–341
    ehrlichiosis, 336–339
    fever of undetermined origin (FUO) in, 69
    Rocky Mountain spotted fever, 332–334
    spotted fevers, 334–335
    typhus, 335–336
Rickettsialpox, 334–335
Rickettsia prowazekii, 335
Rickettsia tsutsugamushi, 336
Rifabutin, 414*t*
Rifadin, 111*t*
Rifampin, 111*t,* 147*t,* 178–179*t,*
    327–328*t,* 356*t*
Rigor, 84
Rimactane, 111*t*
Rimantadine, 52*t,* 56, 378
Ritonavir, 408*t*
River blindness, 319
Rocephin, 17*t*
Rocky Mountain spotted fever, 332–334
    case study of, 332–333
    clinical features of, 332–333
    diagnosis of, 333–334
    epidemiology of, 332
    pathogenesis of, 332
    treatment of, 327*t,* 334
Rosetting, 290
Rotavirus, 204–205
RPR (rapid plasma reagin) test, 248, 252
Rugose, 195
R5 viruses, 399

S
Sacroiliitis, 345
Salivary gland lesions, 422
Salmonella, 15, 191–193, 401*t,* 422
Saquinavir, 408*t*
SBE (subacute bacterial endocarditis), 69
Schistosoma haematobium, 121*t,* 314–317
Schistosoma japonicum, 314–317
Schistosoma mansoni, 314–317
Schistosomiasis, 314–317
    case study of, 315
    clinical features of, 315–316
    diagnosis of, 316
    epidemiology of, 314–315
    life cycle of, 314–315
    prevalence of, 314–315
    treatment of, 299*t,* 316–317
Scrub typhus, 336

Seborrheic dermatitis, 434
Secondary syphilis, 249–250, 253
Secondary tuberculosis, 108–109
Secreted factors, 58–59
Sepsis syndrome, 57–65
    case study of, 60–61
    clinical features of, 60–62
        acid-base disturbances, 61
        fever, 60–61
        hemodynamic changes, 61
        respiratory changes, 61–62
    definition of, 58
    diagnosis of, 62
    pathogenesis of, 58–60
        cell wall factors, 58
        cytokines and inflammatory
            mediators, 59
        host cell receptors for bacterial products,
            59–60
        infection, 59–60
        secreted factors, 58–59
    pathophysiology of, 60*f*
    prevalence of, 57–58
    treatment of, 62–65
        adjunctive therapies, 64
        antibiotics, 62–63
        corticosteroids, 64–65
        drotrecogin alpha, 65
        patient management, 63–64
Septic arthritis, 284–286
    in brucellosis, 345
    case study of, 285
    clinical features of, 284
    diagnosis of, 284–285
    microbiology of, 284–285
    pathogenesis of, 284–285
    potential severity of, 284
    predisposing factors for, 284–285
    treatment of, 285
Septic shock, 58, 59–60
Seroconversion syndrome, 399
Serogroups, 149
Seromycin, 111*t*
Serratia marcescens, 121*t*
Severe acute respiratory syndrome (SARS),
    374–376
    clinical features of, 374–375
    diagnosis of, 375
    epidemiology of, 374
    pathogenesis of, 374
    prevention of, 375–376
    probable, 375*t*
    suspected, 375*t*
    treatment of, 375
Sexually transmitted diseases (STDs),
    240–255
    genital ulcers, 246–248
    papular genitourinary lesions, 254–255
    pelvic inflammatory disease, 241–246
    potential severity of, 240
    syphilis, 248–254
    treatment of, 242–244*t*
    urethritis, 240–241
Shigella, 193, 422

Shigella flexneri, 15
Sigmoidoscopy, 169*t*
Sinusitis, 132–137
    antibiotic therapy for, 128*t,* 137
    case study of, 133–134
    clinical features of, 133–134
    complications of, 135–136
        cavernous sinus thrombosis and
            meningitis, 135
        orbital abscess, 135
        orbital cellulitis, 135
        periorbital cellulitis, 135
    diagnosis of, 134–135
    frontal, 136
    fungal, 137
    microbiology of, 136–137
    potential severity of, 132
    predisposing factors for, 132–133
    sphenoid, 136
    treatment of, 137
SIRS (systemic inflammatory response
    syndrome), 58, 62
Sjögren's syndrome, 422
Skin abscesses, 268–269
Skin and soft tissue infections, 256–271
    anatomic sites of, 257*f*
    animal bites, 270–271
    burns, 265–266
    carbuncles, 268
    cellulitis, 257–259
    classification of, 256–257
    folliculitis, 266–267
    furunculosis, 266–267
    in HIV infection, 431–434
        bacillary angiomatosis, 433–434
        chronic herpes simplex, 433
        drug reactions, 433
        herpes zoster, 433
        Kaposi's sarcoma, 433
        molluscum contagiosum, 434
        in primary HIV infection, 431–433
        seborrheic dermatitis, 434
    human bites, 271
    impetigo, 266
    indolent, 269
    myonecrosis, 263–265
    necrotizing fasciitis, 259–263
    skin abscesses, 267–269
    tetanus, 269–270
    treatment of, 260–261*t*
Skin tests, 74
Slim disease, 422
Small pox, 360–363
    as biologic weapon, 361
    clinical features of, 361–362
    epidemiology of, 360–361
    pathogenesis of, 360–361
    prevention of, 363
    treatment of, 362–363
    virology of, 360–361
    vs. chickenpox, 361–362
Smears, 74
Sodium stibogluconate, 298*t*
Sonication method, 184

Southern tick-associated rash illness (STARI), 322
SPEA (streptococcal pyrogenic exotoxin A), 59
Sphenoid sinusitis, 136
Spinal epidural abscess, 164–165
Splenectomized patients, 385
Splenic rupture, 372
Splenomegaly, 343
Sporotrichosis, 269
Sporozoites, 289
Spotted fever, 327*t*, 334–335
Sputum, 86–88
St. Louis encephalitis, 155*t*
Staphylococcus aureus infection, 94–95
  bacterial pneumonia, 418
  conjunctivitis, 121*t*
  infective endocarditis, 169, 172–173, 179–180
  intravascular catheter-related infections, 184
  neutropenia, 386
  sepsis syndrome, 59
  septic arthritis, 285
  skin abscesses, 268–269
  skin and soft tissues, 256
Staphylococcus epidermis, 164
STARI (Southern tick-associated rash illness), 322
Statins, 39
Stavudine, 408*t*
Still's disease, 70–72
Stomatitis, 421
Streptococcal gangrene. *See* Necrotizing fasciitis
Streptococcal pyrogenic exotoxin A (SPEA), 59
Streptococcal toxic shock syndrome. *See* Necrotizing fasciitis
Streptococcus bovis, 169
Streptococcus pneumoniae infection, 90–94
  in bacterial meningitis, 140
  clinical features of, 92
  in conjunctivitis, 121*t*
  diagnosis of, 92
  in HIV infection, 413, 418
  pathogenesis of, 90–91
  predisposing factors for, 91–92
  prevalence of, 91–92
  prevention of, 93–94
  treatment of, 31, 92–93
Streptococcus pyogenes, 31, 59, 127, 129
Streptococcus viridans infection, 169, 179–180, 386
Streptogramins, 38–39
  antimicrobial spectrum of, 39
  chemistry and mechanisms of action, 38
  pharmacokinetics of, 39
  toxicity of, 38–39
Streptomyces, 23
Streptomycin, 24*t,* 111*t,* 356*t*
Strongyloides infection, 307–309
  case study of, 307–308
  clinical features of, 307–309
  diagnosis of, 309

  epidemiology of, 307
  in HIV infection, 401*t*
  life cycle of, 307
  prevalence of, 307
  treatment of, 309
Subacute bacterial endocarditis (SBE), 69
Sulfadiazine, 41*t,* 414*t*
Sulfamethoxazole, 41*t*
Sulfonamides, 40–42
  antimicrobial spectrum of, 41–42
  chemistry and mechanisms of action, 40
  effects on bacterial folate pathway, 40*f*
  organisms susceptible to, 41*t*
  pharmacokinetics of, 41
  toxicity of, 41
  treatment recommendations, 41
Summer flu, 297
Superantigens, 59
Superinfections, 387
Super spreaders, 374
Suprax, 17*t*
Surgical drainage, 162
Sutton's law, 74, 76
Swimmer's ear. *See* Otitis externa
Symadine, 52*t*
Symmetrel, 52*t*
Synercid, 38–39
Syphilis, 248–254
  cardiovascular, 251
  clinical features of, 247*t,* 249–252
  diagnosis of, 252–253
    non-treponemal tests, 252
    specific treponemal tests, 252–253
  epidemiology of, 249
  in HIV infection, 434
  late benign gummas, 251–252
  latent, 250, 253
  neurosyphilis, 253
  ocular, 253
  pathogenesis of, 249–252
  potential severity of, 248
  primary, 249, 253
  secondary, 249–250, 253
  tertiary or late, 250–251
  treatment of, 244*t*
Systemic emboli, 176–177
Systemic inflammatory response syndrome (SIRS), 58, 62

T
Tache noire, 334
Tachycardia, in sepsis syndrome, 61
Tachypnea, in sepsis syndrome, 61
Taenia solium, 121*t,* 299*t,* 313–314
Talithromycin, 28*t,* 29–31
Tamiflu, 51*t*
Targocid, 28*t*
T cells, 185, 369–370, 387–388
TEE (transesophageal echocardiography), 175
Teicoplanin, 27–29, 28*t,* 279*t*
Tenofovir, 408*t*
Tenosynovitis, 287
Tertiary syphilis, 250–251
Tetanospasmin, 269

Tetanus toxoid, 270
Tetracyclines, 32–34
  antimicrobial spectrum of, 33–34
  chemistry and mechanisms of action, 32–33
  dosing, 28*t*
  organisms susceptible to, 33*t*
  pharmacokinetics of, 33
  toxicity of, 33
  treatment recommendations, 33–34
Thermotherapy, 302
Three-day rule, 7–10
Throat infections, 126–129
Thrombocytopenia, 34, 53, 177, 333, 338
Ticarcillin, 15
Ticarcillin-clavulanate, 14*t,* 63*t,* 128*t,* 238*t,* 260*t,* 269–270
Tigecycline, 28*t,* 33–34
Timentin, 14*t*
Tissue helminth infections, 310–319
  cysticercosis, 313–314
  dirofilariasis, 319
  echinococcosis, 311–313
  filariasis, 317–319
  flukes, 317
  loiasis, 319
  onchocerciasis, 319
  schistosomiasis, 314–317
  trichinosis, 310–311
TLR (toll-like receptor), 59
TMX-sulfa, 199*t*
TNF-alpha (tumor necrosis factor alpha), 59
Tobramycin, 24*t,* 122, 391*t*
Tolevamer, 203–204
Toll-like receptor (TLR), 59
Tooth brushing, 169*t*
Toxic shock syndrome, 59
Toxic shock syndrome toxin 1 (TSST), 59
Toxoplasma encephalitis, 425–428
Toxoplasma gondii, 158–159, 413
Toxoplasmosis, 401*t*
Transduction, 2
Transesophageal echocardiography (TEE), 175
Transformation, 2
Transthoracic echocardiography (TTE), 175
Transurethral prostatectomy, 169*t*
Trecator, 111*t*
Treponema pallidum, 127, 249
Triazoles, 45
Trichinella, 298*t,* 310–311
Trichinella spiralis, 121*t*
Trichinosis, 310–311
  clinical features of, 311
  diagnosis of, 311
  epidemiology of, 311
  life cycle of, 311
  potential severity of, 310
  prevalence of, 311
  treatment of, 311
Trichomoniasis, treatment of, 244*t*
Trichuris, 298*t*
Trichuris trichiura, 305–306
Triclabendazole, 299*t*

Trimethoprim, 40–42
  antimicrobial spectrum of, 41–42
  chemistry and mechanisms of action, 40
  effects on bacterial folate pathway, 40*f*
  organisms susceptible to, 41*t*
  pharmacokinetics of, 41
  toxicity of, 41
  treatment recommendations, 41
    for conjunctivitis, 122
    for urinary tract infections (UTIs),
238*t*
Trimethoprim-sulfadiazine, 260*t*
Trimethoprim-sulfamethoxazole, 147*t*, 238*t*,
  260*t*, 414*t*
Tropical myositis, 263
Trypanosoma brucei complex, 304
Trypanosoma cruzi, 185, 302–304
Trypomastigotes, 303
TSST-1 (toxic shock syndrome toxin 1), 59
TTE (transthoracic echocardiography), 175
Tuberculosis, 103–113
  abdominal, 422
  case study of, 103–104
  clinical features of, 107–109
  diagnosis of, 109
  direct observed therapy for, 111*t*
  drugs for, 111*t*
  epidemiology of, 105–107
  in HIV infection, 418
  miliary, 107–108
  pathogenesis of, 104–105
  potential severity of, 103
  prevention of, 112–113
  primary, 107
  prophylaxis for, 414*t*
  secondary, 108–109
  toxicities of drugs, 110*t*
  treatment of, 109–112
Tuberculosis meningitis, 152
Tuberculous pericarditis, 187–188
Tubzid, 111*t*
Tularemia, 358–360
  clinical features of, 359–360
  diagnosis of, 360
  mortality from, 360
  pathogenesis of, 359
  prevention of, 360
  treatment of, 356*t*, 360
Tumor necrosis factor alpha (TNF-alpha), in
  sepsis syndrome, 59
Tygecil, 28*t*
Typhoid fever, 197
Typhus, 335–336
  clinical features of, 335–336
  diagnosis of, 336
  epidemiology of, 335–336
  pathogenesis of, 335–336
  potential severity of, 335
  treatment of, 327*t*, 336
Tzanck test, 381

U
Unasyn, 14*t*
Unipen, 14*t*

Upper gastrointestinal endoscopy, 169*t*
Ureaplasma urealyticum, 241
Ureidopenicillins, 16–18
Urethra, 232
Urethral catheter, 169*t*
Urethral dilatation, 169*t*
Urethritis, 240–241
  causes of, 240–241
  clinical features of, 241
  diagnosis of, 241
  non-gonococcal, 240–241
  symptoms of, 241
  treatment of, 241
  vs. cystitis, 235
Urinary tract infections (UTIs), 231–239
  case study of, 234
  causes of, 233
  clinical features of, 234–235
  diagnosis of, 235–237
  empiric therapy for, 238*t*
  management of, 236*f*
  pathogenesis of, 232–233
    bacterial factors, 232–233
    host factors, 232–233
  treatment of, 237–239
    lower tract disease, 237
    upper tract disease, 237–239
U.S. Army Medical Research Institute for
  Infectious Diseases
  (USAMRIID), 350
Uveitis, 431

V
Vaccination, 378–379
Vaccines, 149–150
Vaccinia immune globulin (VIG), 363
Vaccinia virus, 363
Vaginosis, treatment of, 244*t*
Valacyclovir, 49–53, 51*t*, 381
Valcyte, 51*t*
Valganciclovir, 51*t*, 53, 414*t*
Valtrex, 51*t*
Vancomycin, 27–29
  antimicrobial spectrum of, 29
  chemistry and mechanism of action, 27
  dosing, 28*t*
  pharmacokinetics of, 27
  toxicity of, 27
  treatment recommendations, 29
    for anthrax, 356*t*
    for bacterial diarrhea, 199*t*
    for bacterial meningitis, 147*t*
    for cellulitis, 260*t*
    for infective endocarditis, 178–179*t*
    for neutropenic patients, 391*t*
    for osteomyelitis, 279*t*
    for sepsis syndrome, 63*t*
Vancomycin-resistant enterococci (VRE),
  38, 387
Vantin, 17*t*
Varicella, 121*t*, 151
Varicella-zoster virus (VZV) infection,
  365–369
  case study of, 367–368

  clinical features of, 366
  complications of, 367–368
  diagnosis of, 366–367
  epidemiology of, 365
  pathogenesis of, 366
  prevention of, 368–369
  treatment of, 368
Variola virus, 360–361
Velocef, 17*t*
Venereal Disease Research Laboratory
  (VDRL) test, 252
Venereal warts, 254
Venezuelan equine encephalitis, 155*t*
Venturi effect, 168
Vibramycin, 28*t*
Vibrio cholera, 192*t*, 195–196
Vibrio parahaemolyticus, 192*t*, 196
Vibrio vulnificus, 263
Viral diarrhea, 204–205
  astrovirus, 205
  case study of, 205
  clinical features of, 205
  diagnosis of, 205
  enteric adenoviruses, 205
  epidemiology of, 204–205
  norovirus, 204
  pathogenesis of, 204–205
  potential severity of, 204
  rotavirus, 204–205
  treatment of, 205
Viral encephalitis, 154–157
  case study of, 154
  clinical features of, 155–156
  diagnosis of, 156
  epidemiology of, 154–155
  treatment of, 156–157
Viral infections, 360–363. *See also* specific
  infections
  conjunctivitis, 121
  corneal, 123
  cytomegalovirus, 381–382
  diarrhea, 204–205
  encephalitis, 154–157
  Epstein-Barr virus (EBV), 369–372
  hantavirus, 373–374
  hantavirus pulmonary syndrome (HPS),
    373–374
  hepatitis, 218–229
  herpes simplex virus (HSV), 379–381
  human immunodeficiency virus (HIV),
    397–434
  in immunocompromised host, 388
  influenza, 376–379
  meningitis, 150–152
  molluscum contagiosum, 434
  myocarditis, 185–186
  pericarditis, 186–188
  pharyngitis, 127–129
  pneumonia, 378
  severe acute respiratory syndrome (SARS),
    374–376
  sinusitis, 132–137
  small pox, 360–363
  varicella, 365–369

varicella-zoster virus (VZV), 365–369
Viral meningitis, 150–152
    case study of, 150
    epidemiology of, 150–151
Viremia, 397–398
Virions, 361
Virtual phenotype, 404
Virus-like particles (VLPs), 254
Visceral leishmaniasis, 301
Vistide, 51*t*
Vitamin B6 414*t*
Voriconazole, 45–47, 391*t*
VRE (vancomycin-resistant enterococci),
    38, 387

W
Walking pneumonia, 96
Wasting, HIV-associated, 401*t*
Weil's disease, 330
Western equine encephalitis, 155*t*
West Nile encephalitis, 155*t*
Whip worm, 305–306
White blood counts (WBCs), 145, 174, 325

Whitlow, 380
Wood tick, 332
Woolsorters' disease, 353–354
Wright stain, 74
Wuchereria bancrofti, 299*t*, 317–319

X
Xerostomia, 422
X-linked lymphoproliferative syndrome, 370
X4 viruses, 399

Y
Yersinia, 192*t*, 196
Yersinia enterocolitica, 196
Yersinia pestis, 357–358

Z
Zalcitabine, 408*t*
Zanamivir, 51*t*, 378
Zidovudine, 408*t*
Zinacef, 17*t*
Zithromax, 28*t*

Zoonotic infections, 322–347
    Bartonella infections, 341–344
        bacillary angiomatosis, 343
        cat scratch disease, 342–343
    brucellosis, 344–347
    ehrlichiosis, 336–339
    leptospirosis, 328–331
    Lyme disease, 322–328
    Q fever, 339–341
    Rocky Mountain spotted fever, 332–334
    spotted fevers, 334–335
    typhus, 335–336
Zoster, 365–369
    case study of, 367–368
    clinical features of, 366
    complications of, 367–368
    diagnosis of, 366–367
    epidemiology of, 365
    pathogenesis of, 366
Zosyn, 14t
Zovirax, 51*t*